Book of Abstracts of the 54th Annual Meeting of the European Association for Animal Production

The EAAP Book of Abstracts is published under the direction of Ynze van der Honing

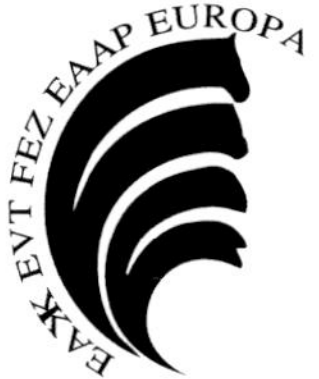

EAAP - European Association for Animal Production

The European Association for Animal Production wishes to express its appreciation to the
Ministero delle Politiche Agricole e Forestali (Italy) and the
Associazione Italiana Allevatori (Italy)
for their valuable support of its activities.

Book of Abstracts of the 54th Annual Meeting of the European Association for Animal Production

Rome, Italy, 31 August -3 September 2003

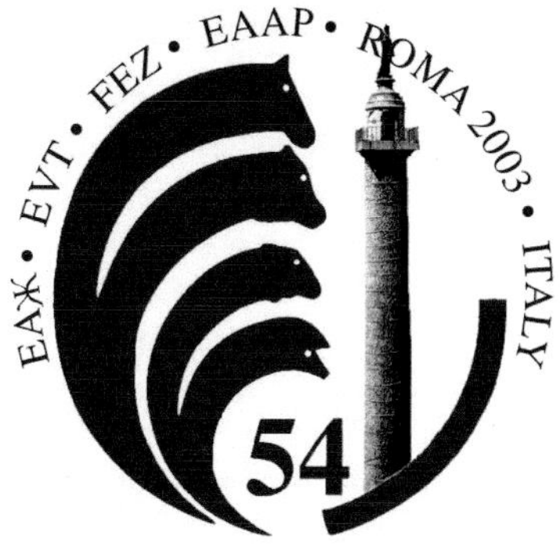

Ynze van der Honing, Editor-in-chief

A. Hofer, G. Zervas, E. von Borell, C. Knight, C. Lazzaroni, M. Sneeberger, C. Wenk, W. Martin-Rosset

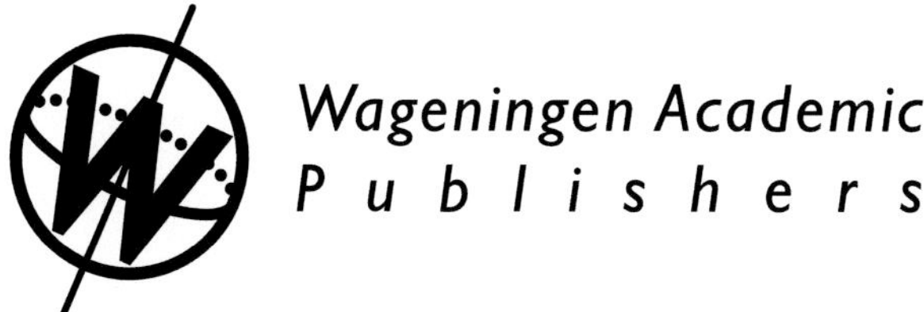

CIP-data Koninklijke Bibliotheek
Den Haag

ISSN 1382-6077
ISBN 9076998205
NUGI 835

The individual contributions in this publication and any liabilities arising from them remain the responsibility of the authors.

Subject headings:
animal production,
book of abstracts

The designation employed and the presentation of material in this publication do not imply the expression of any option whatsoever on the part of the European Association for Animal Production concerning the legal status of any country, territory, city or area or of its authorities, or concerning the delimitation of its frontiers or boundaries.

Wageningen Academic Publishers
The Netherlands, 2003

Printed in The Netherlands

Preface

The 54th annual meeting of the European Association for Animal Production (EAAP) was held in Rome, Italy, 31 August to 3 September 2003. The annual EAAP meeting gives the opportunity to present new scientific results and discuss their potential applicability in animal production practices. This year's meeting is of particular interest for participants from a wide range of animal production organisations and institutions. Discussions stimulate developments in animal production and encourage research on relevant topics. In Rome the main theme is "Product quality from livestock systems". Of the 37 sessions in total, 11 joint sessions of two or more Study Commissions are planned on:

- *Product quality from livestock systems -Animal health and welfare aspects;*
- *Product quality from livestock systems -Human health and consumer aspects;*
- *Long term effects of pre- and post-natal conditions, including nutrition, on growth and development;*
- *Functional genomics applied to growth, tissue development and meat quality in farm animals;*
- *Tissue development and meat quality: The role of lipids and antioxidants;*
- *Large-scale cattle units - health, welfare and economics;*
- *Use of small ruminants and horses for landscape conservation and non agricultural use;*
- *Feeding and meat quality in heavy pigs;*
- *Metabolic disorders in high yielding dairy cows in the transitional period;*
- *Nutrition and feeding of dairy sheep and goats;*
- *Impact of feed processing in horse nutrition.*

The book of abstracts is the main publication of the scientific contributions to this meeting; it covers a wide range of disciplines and livestock species. It contains the full programme and abstracts of the invited as well as the contributing speakers, including posters, of all 37 sessions. The number of abstracts submitted for presentation at this meeting (842) is a true challenge for the different study commissions and chairpersons to put together a scientific programme. In addition to the theatre presentations, there will be a large number of poster presentations during the conference.

Several persons have been involved in the development of the book of abstracts. Mike Jacobs has been responsible for organising the administrative and editing work and the production of the book. The contact persons of the study commissions have been responsible for organising the scientific programme and communicating with the chairpersons and invited speakers.

The programme is very interesting and I trust we will have a good meeting in Rome. I hope that you will find this book a useful reference source as well as a reminder of a good meeting during which a large number of people actively involved in livestock science and production have met and exchanged ideas.

Ynze van der Honing
Editor-in Chief

EAAP Program Foundation

Aim

EAAP aims to bring to our annual meetings, speakers who can present the latest findings and views on developments in the various fields of science relevant to animal production and its allied industries. In order to sustain the quality of the scientific program that will continue to entice the broad interest in EAAP meetings we have created the "EAAP Program Foundation". This Foundation aims to support

- Invited speakers by funding part or all of registration and travel costs.
- Delegates from less favoured areas by offering scholarships to attend EAAP meetings
- Young scientists by providing prizes for best presentations

The "EAAP Program Foundation" is an initiative of the Scientific Advisory committee (SAC) of EAAP. The Foundation is aimed at stimulating the quality of the scientific program of the EAAP meetings and to ensure that the science meets societal needs . In its first year (2003), the "EAAP Program Foundation" concentrates on the program of the Genetics commission. For the coming years the activities will be broadened to entire meeting. The Foundation Board of Trustees oversees theses aims and seeks to recruit sponsors to support its activities.

Sponsorships

We distinguish three categories of sponsorship: Student award sponsor, Gold sponsor, and Sponsor. The sponsors will be acknowledged during the scientific sessions commission. of the Genetics commission. The names of Student Award sponsors will be linked to the awards given to young scientists with the best presentation. Gold Sponsors and Student Award sponsors will have opportunity to advertise their activities during the meeting and their support for EAAP.

Contact and further information

If you are interested in becoming a sponsor of the "EAAP Program Foundation" or want to have further information, please contact the secretary of the Foundation, Dr Andreas Rosati (e-mail: rosati@eaap.org).

Sponsors of 2003 meeting

The board of Trustees wants to thank the following organisations for their support:

Student award sponsor:
CR-Delta, Arnhem, The Netherlands
www.cr-delta.nl
CR-Delta is a reliable source for breeding dairy cows world wide.

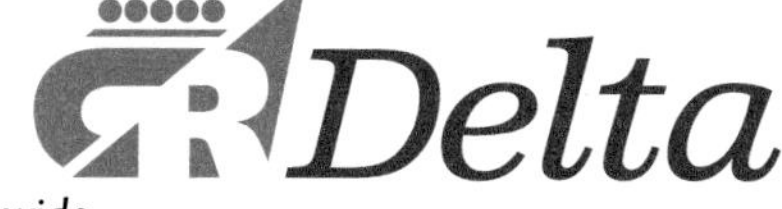

Gold Sponsor:
Animal Sciences Group of Wageningen UR
The Netherlands, www.asg.wur.nl
Wageningen UR: for quality of life.

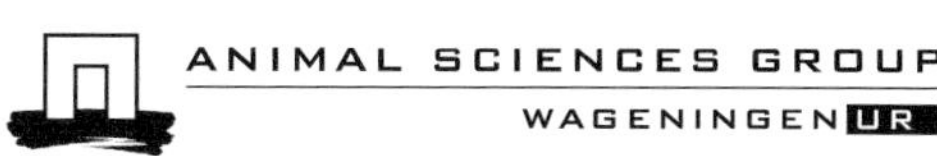

European Association for Animal Production (EAAP)

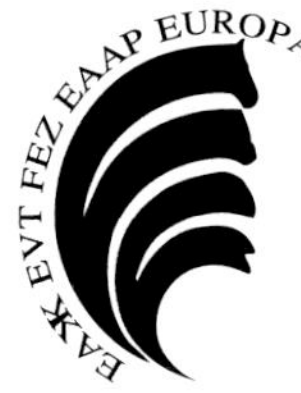

President	Mr A.L. Aumaitre
Executive Vice-President	Dr. Andrea Rosati
Address	Villa del Ragno, Via Nomentana 134, I-00161 Rome, Italy
Phone	+39 06 86329141
Telefax	+39 06 86329263
E-Mail	eaap@eaap.org

In cooperation with

Ministero delle Politiche Agricole e Forestale (MiPAF)
Istituto Sperimentale per la Zootecnia (ISZ)
Università degli Studi della Tuscia (Viterbo)
Consiglio Nazionale delle Ricerche (CNR)
Associazione Italiana Allevatori (AIA)

Organizing Committee

Giancarlo Rossi	Scientific Association for Animal Production (ASPA)
Sergio Gigli	Animal Production Research Institute (ISZ)
Giuseppe Ambrosio	Ministry of Agriculture (MiPAF)
Nino Andena	Italian Breeders Association (AIA)
Giuseppe Enne	Lazzaro Spallanzani National Research Institute
Lino Ferrara	National Research Council (CNR)
Juani Maki-Hokkonen	FAO
Romano Marabelli	Ministry of Health
Donato Matassino	ConSDABI
Carlo Perone-Pacifico	University of Tuscia - Viterbo
Giacomo Pirlo	Animal Production Research Institute (ISZ)
Vincenzo Russo	Scientific Association for Animal Production (ASPA)

Scientific advisory Committee

Alessandro Nardone	University of Tuscia - Viterbo
Bianca Moioli	Animal Production Research Institute (ISZ)
Giuseppe Bertoni	University of Piacenza (UCSC)
Giovanni Bittante	University of Padova
Paolo Brandano	University of Sassari
Tullio Di Lella+	University of Napoli
Alessandreo Giorgetti	University of Firenze
Alfio Lanza	University of Catania
Archimede Mordenti	University of Bologna
Francesco Panella	University of Perugia
Pierlorenzo Secchiari	University of Pisa
Franco Valfrè	University of Milano

Organizing Committee

Istituto Sperimentale per la Zootecnia (ISZ)
Via Salaria, 31 0016 Monterotondo, Roma, Italy
Tel. 39-06-9066689 - Fax 39-06-90558616
e-mail: eaap.roma2003@isz.it

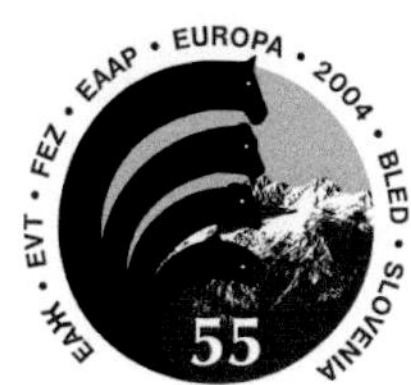

55th Annual Meeting of the European Association for Animal Production

The 54th Annual Meeting will take place in Bled, Slovenia, September 5 - 9, 2004

Organizing Committee
University of Ljubljana
Biotechnical Faculty
Zootechnical Department
Groblje 3, 1230 Domzale, Slovenia
Phone: +386 1 7217 855
Fax: +386 1 7241 005
E-mail: EAAP2004@bfro.uni-lj.si
Web: www.bfro.uni-lj.si/eaap2004

Abstract submission
Please find the abstract form on the internet:
www.WageningenAcademic.com/eaap
Submission of the completed abstract form exclusively in digital format as an attachment before March 1, 2004 to:
EAAP2004@WageningenAcademic.com

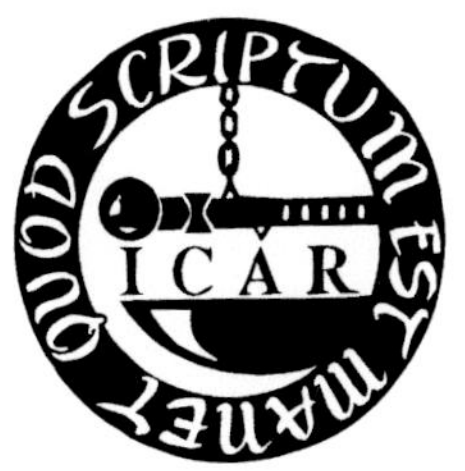

34th ICAR Session and INTERBULL Meeting

May 29 - June 3, 2004, Sousse, Tunisia

Organizing Committee

Tunisian ICAR member:
Office de l'Elevage et des Pâturages
30, Rue Alain Savary – 1002 Tunis – TUNISIA
Tel : 00 216 71 790 795 – 71 782 960
Fax : 00216 71 793 603
Email : dg.oep@email.ati.tn

Timetable

Thursday, August 28th (National Research Council)

15.30-17.30	Interbull Bussiness Meeting

Friday, August 29th (Conference Centre)

08.00-17.30	Registration of partecipants
13.30-15.30	EAAP Scientific Advisory Commitee Meeting
16.00-18.00	Livestock Production Science Board Meeting
08.30-18.00	Interbull Open meeting
08.30-17.30	Workshop: Writing and Presenting Scientific Papers (restricted participation)
13.45-19.45	Workshop: Rare Breeds International

Saturday, August 30th (Conference Centre)

08.00-17.30	Registration of partecipants
09.30-12.30	Joint Session of Council with Presidents and Secretaries of Study Commissions, Presidents of Working groups and Representatives of International Organizations
17.30-20.00	An G R W.G.
13.00-18.30	IGA board
14.30-17.30	Council Meeting (102nd)
08.30-15.00	Interbull Open Meeting
15.30-17.30	Interbull Business Meeting
09.30-16.30	Symposium: Effects of the robotic milking system on milk quality with reference to typical products
09.30-16.30	Symposium: Recent progress in buffalo reproduction
09.30-17.30	AFAnet/EAAP Workshop: Teaching for Learning Animal Breeding (restricted participation)
08.00-18.00	Workshop: National Coordinators

Sunday, August 31st (Conference Centre)

08.00-17.30	Registration of partecipants
08.30-09.00	"Animal Production after BSE" Report of an EAAP Working group. Prof P.Cunningham
09.15-13.15	Session I of Study Commission
09.30-13.30	Cattle network working group meeting
15.00-16.30	Round Table " Changing consumers...changing Animal production?"
16.00-18.30	Opening Ceremony (Awards Ceremony, General Assembly, part I)
18:45	Welcome Cocktail

Monday, September 1st (Conference Centre)

08.00-17.30 Registration of partecipants
08.30-12.30 Session II of Study Commssions
13.30-17.30 Sessione III of Study Commissions
20:30 Conference dinner

Tuesday, September 2nd (Conference centre)

08.00-17.30 Registration of partecipants
8:30 Council Meeting (103rd)
08.30-12.30 Session IV of Study Commissions
08.30-9.30 Business Meeting
10.00-12.30 Free Communications
13.30-17.30 Session V of Study Commissions
17.30-19.30 Poster Session
17.45-19.30 General Assembly (part II)

Wednesday, September 3rd (Conference Centre)

08.00-12.00 Registration of participants
08.30-12.30 Session Vi of Study Commission
11.30-12.30 Council Meeting (104th)
12.30-13.00 SAC Meeting
13.00-21.00 Conference Tours
21.00-24.00 Farewell dinner

Thursday, September 4th

(Hotel Palatino)
09.00-17.00 Symposium: Sustainable breeding for European farm animals
Tuscia University
09.00-18.30 Symposium: Interactions between climate and animal production

Departure for post Conference tour

Scientific programme EAAP-2003

Session I
Sunday 31 August
8:30 - 12:30

Product quality from livestock systems
-Animal health and welfare aspects
Sorensen (DK)
(M* + N + C + S +L with FAO)

Incorporating molecular information in breeding schemes
Bovenhuuis (NL)
(G)

Importance of milk bioactive components for the adaptation and survival of the new-born and its subsequent growth
Baldi (I)
(Ph)

Genetic factors regulating feed intake in growing pigs
Knap (D)
(P)

Welfare and behaviour of horses
Kennedy (UK)
(H)

Session II
Monday 1 September
8:30 - 12:30

Product quality from livestock systems-Human health and consumer aspects
Jacobsen (DK)
(N* + C + S +L with FAO)

Genetics of behaviour
Rydhmer (SE)
(G)

Electronic identification in farm animals and traceability
Geers (B)
(M with OIE and ICAR)

Role of IGFs and related hormones on tissue differentiation and development
Vestegaard (DK)
(Ph)

Genetic strategies to improve sow fertility
Kovac (SI)
(P)

Locomotion and execise in Horses
Barrey (F)
(H)

Session III
Monday 1 September
13:30 - 17:30

Long term effects of pre- and post-natal conditions, including nutrition, on growth and development
Knight (UK)
(Ph* + P + N)

Use of small ruminants and horses for landscape conservation and non agricultural use
Schneeberger (CH)
(S* + H)

Metabolic disorders in high yielding dairy cows in the transitional period
Bertoni (It)
(C* + M)

Air quality in animal housing
Hartung (De)
(M)

Free Communications in Genetics
Le Roy (F)
(G)

Key to Commissions (subject areas): (G – Genetics; N – Animal Nutrition; M- Animal Management and Health; Ph – Animal Physiology; C – Cattle Production; S – Sheep and Goat Production; P – Pig Production; H – Horse Production; L – Livestock Farming Systems)
* = Organising Commission

Scientific programme EAAP-2003

Session IV Tuesday 2 September 8:30 - 12:30	Session V Tuesday 2 September 13:30 - 17:30	Session VI Wednesday 3 September 8:30 - 12:30
Functional genomics applied to growth, tissue development and meat quality in farm animals *Williams (UK)* (Ph* +G)	Tissue development and meat quality: The role of lipids and antioxidants *Torrallardona (E)* (P* and Ph)	Large-scale cattle units - health, welfare and economics *Brascamp (NL)* (C* + M)
Free Communications Animal Genetics *Le Roy (F)*	Impact of feed processing in horse nutrition *Miraglia (I)* (H* + N)	Feeding and meat quality in heavy Pigs *Piva (I)* (N* + P)
Free Communications Animal Nutrition *Oldham (UK)*	Locomotor disorders in Cattle, Pigs and Poultry *Metz (NL)* (M)	Nutrition and feeding of dairy sheep and goats *Bocquier (F)* (S* + N)
Free Communications Animal Management and Health *Fourichon (F)*	Changes in cattle husbandry-knowledge transfer and farmer attitudes *Kuipers (NL)* (C)	Tissue development and meat quality: muscle fibres and collagen *Maltin (UK)* (Ph)
Free Communications Animal Physiology *Sejrsen (DK)*	New developments in sheep breeding *Bodin (F)* (S)	Genetics and quality of animal products *Carnier (I)* (G)
Free Communications Cattle Production *Gigli/ Lazzaroni (I)*	Advances in computing strategies for animal breeding *Emmerling (D)* (G)	Horse production in Italy *Silvestrelli (I)* (H)
Free Communications Sheep and Goat Production *Teixeria (E)*		
Free Communications Pig Production *Wenk (CH)*		
Free Communications Horse Production *Ellis (NL)*		

Key to Commissions (subject areas): (G – Genetics; N – Animal Nutrition; M- Animal Management and Health; Ph – Animal Physiology; C – Cattle Production; S – Sheep and Goat Production; P – Pig Production; H – Horse Production; L – Livestock Farming Systems)

* = Organising Commission

Agendas of Study Commissions

Commission on Animal Genetics (G)

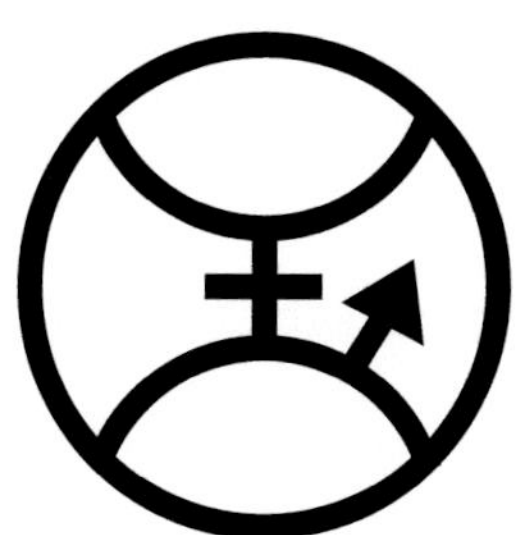

President
Prof.Dr.ir. J.A.M. van Arendonk
Wageningen UR
Zodiac
Postbus 338
6700 AH Wageningen
NEDERLAND
0317 482 335
0317 483 929
Johan.vanArendonk@Alg.VF.WAU.nl

Secretary 1
Dr A. Hofer
SUISAG
AG für Dienstleistungen in der Schweineproduktion
Allmend
6204 Sempach
SWITZERLAND
0041 41 462 65 56
0041 41 462 65 49
hofer@inw.agrl.ethz.ch

Secretary 2
Dr E. Martyniuk
Warsaw Agricultural University
ul. Przejazd 4
05840 Brwinów
POLAND
+48 22 729 62 14
+48 22 729 59 15
eshz@perytnet.pl

INCORPORATING MOLECULAR INFORMATION IN BREEDING SCHEMES

Session 1

Date	31-aug-03
	8:30 - 12:30 hours
Chairperson	Bovenhuis (NL)

Genetics

Theatre

Poster

Poster

Poster

FREE COMMUNICATIONS / GENETICS OF BEHAVIOUR

Session 2

Date	01-sep-03 8:30 - 12:30 hours
Chairperson	Rydhmer (SE)

Theatre (Free communications)

Theatre (Genetics of behaviour)

Poster

FREE COMMUNICATIONS

Session 3

Date	01-sep-03 13:30 - 17:30 hours
Chairperson	Le Roy (F)

Genetics

Theatre

Poster

Poster

Genetics

Poster

Poster

Genetics

Poster

Poster

Genetics

Poster

Poster

G3 no. Page

FREE COMMUNICATIONS: SECONDARY TRAITS / OPTIMISATION OF SELECTION

Session 4

Date	02-sep-03
	8:30 - 12:30 hours
Chairperson	Bagnato (I)

Theatre

G4 no. Page

Theatre

FUNCTIONAL GENOMICS APPLIED TO GROWTH, TISSUE DEVELOPMENT AND MEAT QUALITY IN FARM ANIMALS

Session 4

Joint session with the commission on Animal Physiology

Date	02-sep-03 8:30 - 12:30 hours
Chairperson	Williams (UK)

ADVANCES IN COMPUTING STRATEGIES FOR ANIMAL BREEDING

Session 5

Date 02-sep-03
13:30 - 17:30 hours
Chairperson Emmerling (D)

Theatre

Poster

GENETICS AND QUALITY OF ANIMAL PRODUCTS

Session 6

Date 03-sep-03
8:30 - 12:30 hours
Chairperson Carnier (I)

Theatre

Poster

Poster

Commission on Animal Nutrition (N)

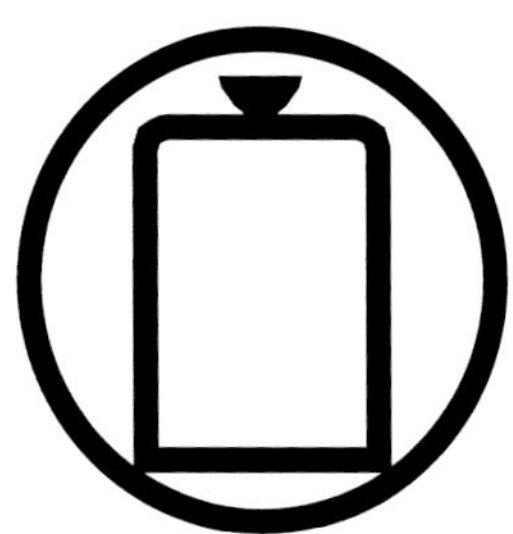

President
Prof. J.D. Oldham
Scottish Agricultural College - SAC
Pentland Building
Sir Stephen Watson Building, Bush Estate
EH26 0PH Penicuik Midlothian
UNITED KINGDOM
0044 131 535 32 01
0044 131 535 31 21
j.oldham@ed.sac.ac.uk

Secretary 1
Dr. G. Zervas
Agricultural University of Athens
Iera Odos 75
11855 Votanikos, Athens
GREECE
+301-529441 1-12
+301-5294413
gzervas@aua.gr

Secretary 2
Dr G.M. Crovetto
University of Milan
Faculty of Agriculture
Via Celoria 2
20133 Milano
ITALY
0039 02 7064 94 37
0039 02 7063 80 83

PRODUCT QUALITY FROM LIVESTOCK SYSTEMS: ANIMAL HEALTH AND WELFARE ASPECTS

Session 1

Joint session with the commissions on Animal Management and Health, Cattle Production, Sheep and Goat Production, Livestock Farming Systems and the FAO

Date	31-aug-03
	8:30 - 12:30 hours
Chairperson	Sorensen (DK)

PRODUCT QUALITY FROM LIVESTOCK SYSTEMS: HUMAN HEALTH AND CONSUMER ASPECTS

Session 2

Joint session with the commissions on Cattle Production, Sheep and Goat Production, Livestock Farming Systems and the FAO

Date	01-sep-03
	8:30 - 12:30 hours
Chairperson	Jacobsen (DK)

Theatre

Nutrition

Poster

Poster

Poster

LONGTERM EFFECTS OF PRE- AND POST-NATAL CONDITIONS, INCLUDING NUTRITION, ON GROWTH AND DEVELOPMENT

Session 3

Joint session with the commissions on Animal Physiology and Pig Production

Date	01-sep-03 13:30 - 17:30 hours
Chairperson	Knight (UK)

	PhPN3	Page	Page
Papers	**1-8**	**228-232**	**LXV-LXVI**
Posters	**9-24**	**232-240**	**LXVI-LXVII**

PRODUCT QUALITY / FREE COMMUNICATIONS

Session 4

Date	02-sep-03 8:30 - 12:30 hours
Chairperson	Oldham (UK)

Theatre (Product quality) **N4 no. Page**

Nutrition

Theatre (Product quality)

Poster (Free communications)

Poster (Free communications)

Nutrition

Poster (Free communications)

Poster (Free communications)

Poster (Free communications)

IMPACT OF FEED PROCESSING ON HORSE NUTRITION

Session 5

Joint session with the commission on Horse Production

Date 02-sep-03
13:30 - 17:30 hours
Chairperson Miraglia (I)

NUTRITION AND FEEDING OF DAIRY SHEEP AND GOATS

Session 6

Joint session with the commission on Sheep and Goat Production

Date 03-sep-03
8:30 - 12:30 hours
Chairperson Bocquier (F)

	SN6	Page	Page
Papers	1-12	341-346	XCI-XCII
Posters	13-25	347-353	XCII-XCIII

FEEDING AND MEAT QUALITY IN HEAVY PIGS

Session 6

Joint session with the commission on Pig Production

Date	03-sep-03
	8:30 - 12:30 hours
Chairperson	Piva (I)

Theatre

NP6 no. Page

Nutrition

Poster

Commission on Animal Management and Health (M)

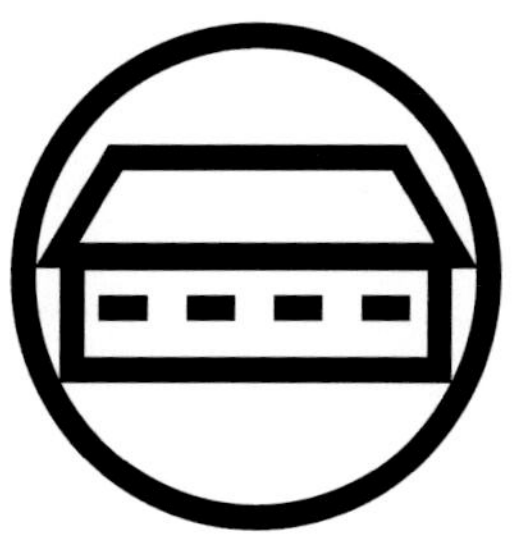

President
Prof.Dr E.H. von Borell
Martin Luther University of Halle
Adam-Kuckhoff-Str. 35
06108 Halle (Saale)
GERMANY
+49 345 55 22 332
+49 345 55 27 105
borell@Landw.uni-halle.de

Secretary 1
Prof.Dr O. Szenci
Szent István University
Faculty of Veterinary Sciences
P.O. Box 2
100 Budapest
HUNGARY
0036 1 478 42 05
0039 1 478 42 07
oszenci@univet.hu

Secretary 2
A. Formigoni
University of Bologna
Veterinary faculty
Via Tolara di Sopra 50
40064 Ozzana Emilia (BO)
ITALY

PRODUCT QUALITY FROM LIVESTOCK SYSTEMS: ANIMAL HEALTH AND WELFARE ASPECTS

Session 1

Joint session with the commissions on Animal Nutrition, Cattle Production, Sheep and Goat Production, Livestock Farming Systems and the FAO

Date	31-aug-03
	8:30 - 12:30 hours
Chairperson	Sorensen (DK)

Management and Health

Theatre

Poster

Poster

Management and Health

Poster

Poster

ELECTRONIC IDENTIFICATION IN FARM ANIMALS AND TRACEABILITY

Session 2

Joint session with the OIE and ICAR

Date	01-sep-03 8:30 - 12:30 hours
Chairperson	Geers (B)

Theatre

Management and Health

Theatre

Poster

METABOLIC DISORDERS IN HIGHYIELDING DAIRY COWS IN THE TRANSITIONAL PERIOD

Session 3

Joint session with the commission on Cattle Production

Date	01-sep-03 13:30 - 17:30 hours
Chairperson	Bertoni (It)

	CM3	Page	Page
Papers	1-8	256-260	LXXIII-LXXIV
Posters	9-18	260-265	LXXIV-LXXV

AIR QUALITY IN ANIMAL HOUSING

Session 3

Date	01-sep-03 13:30 - 17:30 hours
Chairperson	Hartung (D)

Theatre

M3 no. Page

Management and Health

Theatre

Poster

FREE COMMUNICATIONS

Session 4

Date 02-sep-03
8:30 - 12:30 hours
Chairperson Fourichon (F)

Theatre

Theatre

Poster

Management and Health

Poster

LOCOMOTOR DISORDERS IN CATTLE, PIGS AND POULTRY

Session 5

Date	02-sep-03 13:30 - 17:30 hours
Chairperson	Metz (NL)

Theatre

Theatre

Poster

LARGE-SCALE CATTLE UNITS - HEALTH, WELFARE AND ECONOMICS

Session 6

Joint session with the commission on Cattle Production

Date	03-sep-03 8:30 - 12:30 hours
Chairperson	Brascamp (NL)

Commission on Animal Physiology (Ph)

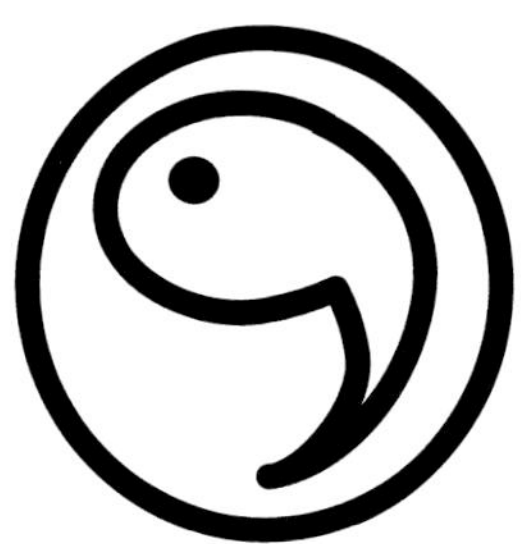

President
Dr. K. Sejrsen
Danish Institute of Agricultural Sciences (DIAS)
Research Centre Foulum
P.O. Box 50
8830 Tjele
DENMARK
0045 89 991 513
0045 89 991 564
kr.sejrsen@agrsci.dk

Secretary 1
Dr B. Kemp
Wageningen UR
Zodiac
Postbus 338
6700 AH Wageningen
NEDERLAND
0317 482 539
0317 485 006
Bas.Kemp@genr.vh.wau.nl

Secretary 2
C.H. Knight
Animal Physiology group
Hannah Research Institute
KA6 5HL Auchincruive, Ayr
UNITED KINGDOM

IMPORTANCE OF MILK BIOACTIVE COMPONENTS FOR THE ADAPTATION AND SURVIVAL OF THE NEW-BORN AND ITS SUBSEQUENT GROWTH

Session 1

Date 31-aug-03
8:30 - 12:30 hours
Chairperson Baldi (I)

Theatre

Theatre

Poster

Physiology

ROLE OF IGFS AND RELATED HORMONES ON TISSUE DIFFERENTIATION AND DEVELOPMENT

Session 2

Date	01-sep-03
	8:30 - 12:30 hours
Chairperson	Vestegaard (DK)

Theatre

Poster

Poster

LONG TERM EFFECTS OF PRE- AND POST-NATAL CONDITIONS, INCLUDING NUTRITION, ON GROWTH AND DEVELOPMENT

Session 3

Joint session with the commissions on Pig Production and Animal Nutrition

Date 01-sep-03
13:30 - 17:30 hours

Chairperson Knight (UK)

Theatre

Physiology

Theatre

Poster

Poster

FREE COMMUNICATIONS

Session 4

Date	02-sep-03 8:30 - 12:30 hours
Chairperson	Sejrsen (UK)

Theatre

Physiology

FUNCTIONAL GENOMICS APPLIED TO GROWTH, TISSUE DEVELOPMENT AND MEAT QUALITY IN FARM ANIMALS

Session 4

Joint session with the commission on Animal Genetics

Date 02-sep-03
8:30 - 12:30 hours
Chairperson Williams (UK)

Theatre

Poster

TISSUE DEVELOPMENT AND MEAT QUALITY: THE ROLE OF LIPIDS AND ANTIOXIDANTS

Session 5

Joint session with the commission on Pig Production

Date 02-sep-03
13:30 - 17:30 hours
Chairperson Torrallardone (E)

TISSUE DEVELOPMENT AND MEAT QUALITY: MUSCLE FIBRES AND COLLAGEN

Session 6

Date 03-sep-03
8:30 - 12:30 hours
Chairperson Maltin (UK)

Theatre

Poster

Commission on Cattle Production (C)

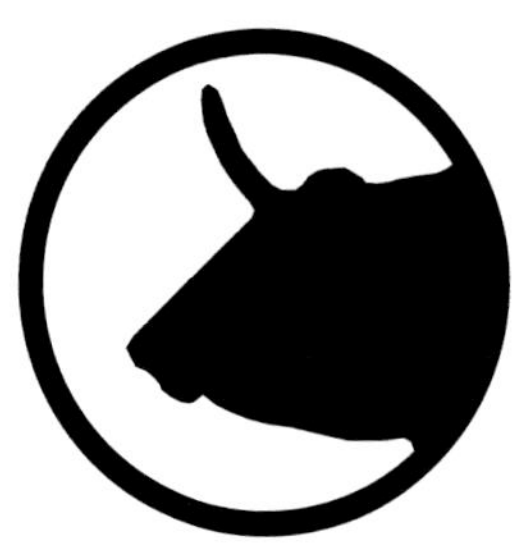

President
Dr S. Gigli
Animal Production Research Institute
Istituto Sperimentale per la Zootecnia
Via Salaria 31
00016 Monterotondo Scalo (Roma)
ITALY
0039 06 900 90 209
0039 06 906 15 41
isz@flashnet.it

Secretary 1
Dr D. Pullar
Meat and Livestock Commission
Winterhill House, Snowdown Drive
P.O. Box 44
MK6 1AX Milton-Keynes
UNITED KINGDOM
+44 1908 677 577
+44 1908 609 221
duncan_pullar@mlc.org.uk

Secretary 2
Dr C. Lazzaroni
University of Torino
Via Leonardo da Vinci 44
10095 Grugliasco (Torino)
ITALY
+39 011 670 85 64
+39 011 670 85 63
carla.lazzaroni@unito.it

PRODUCT QUALITY FROM LIVESTOCK SYSTEMS: ANIMAL HEALTH AND WELFARE ASPECTS

Session 1

Joint session with the commissions on Animal Nutrition, Animal Management and Health, Sheep and Goat Production, Livestock Farming Systems and the FAO

Date	31-aug-03
	8:30 - 12:30 hours
Chairperson	Sorensen (DK)

	MNCS1	Page	Page
Papers	**1-7**	**165-168**	**LI-LII**
Posters	**8-43**	**168-186**	**LII-LV**

PRODUCT QUALITY FROM LIVESTOCK SYSTEMS: HUMAN HEALTH AND CONSUMER ASPECTS

Session 2

Joint session with the commissions on Animal Nutrition, Sheep and Goat Production, Livestock Farming Systems and the FAO

Date	01-sep-03
	8:30 - 12:30 hours
Chairperson	Jacobsen (DK)

	NCS2	Page	Page
Papers	**1-6**	**103-105**	**XXXIX**
Posters	**7-45**	**106-125**	**XL-XLII**

METABOLIC DISORDERS IN HIGHYIELDING DAIRY COWS IN THE TRANSITIONAL PERIOD

Session 3

Joint session with the commission on Animal Management and Health

Date	01-sep-03
	13:30 - 17:30 hours
Chairperson	Bertoni (It)

Cattle

Theatre

Poster

Poster

FREE COMMUNICATIONS

Session 4

Date 02-sep-03
8:30 - 12:30 hours
Chairperson Lazzaroni (I)

Theatre

Cattle

Theatre

Poster

Poster

Cattle

Poster

Poster

Cattle

CHANGES IN CATTLE HUSBANDRY: KNOWLEDGE TRANSFER AND FARMER ATTITUDES

Session 5

Date 02-sep-03
13:30 - 17:30 hours
Chairperson Kuipers (NL)

Theatre

Poster

Poster

LARGE-SCALE CATTLE UNITS - HEALTH, WELFARE AND ECONOMICS

Session 6

Joint session with the commission on Animal Management and Health

Date 03-sep-03
8:30 - 12:30 hours
Chairperson Brascamp (NL)

Theatre

Cattle

Theatre

Poster

Commission on Sheep and Goat Production (S)

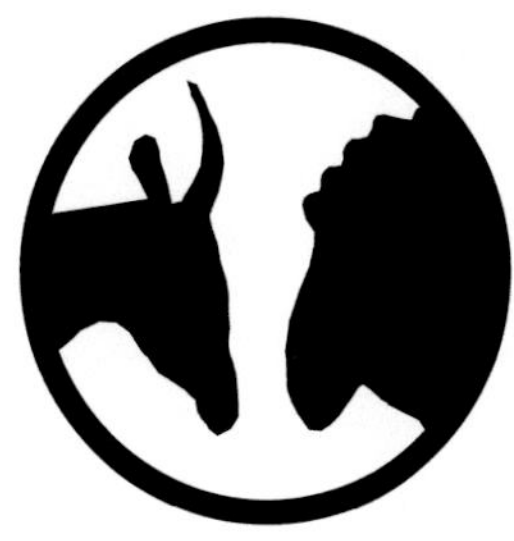

President
Dr D. Gabiña
Mediterranean Agronomic Institute of Zaragoza
IAMZ-CIHEAM
Apdo. 202
50080 Zaragoza
SPAIN
0034 976 716 000
0034 976 716 001
gabina@iamz.ciheam.org

Secretary 1
Dr L. Bodin
INRA
Centre de recherches de Toulouse
P.O. Box 27
31326 Castanet-Tolosan Cedex
FRANCE
0033 5 61 28 52 73
0033 5 61 28 53 53
bodin@toulouse.inra.fr

Secretary 2
Dr M. Schneeberger
Swiss Sheep Breeders Association
P.O. Box 76
3360 Herzogenbuchsee
SWITZERLAND
0041 62 956 68 69
0041 62 956 68 79
schneeberger@pop.agri.ch

PRODUCT QUALITY FROM LIVESTOCK SYSTEMS: ANIMAL HEALTH AND WELFARE ASPECTS

Session 1

Joint session with the commissions on Animal Nutrition, Animal Management and Health, Cattle Production, Livestock Farming Systems and the FAO

Date	31-aug-03 8:30 - 12:30 hours
Chairperson	Sorensen (DK)

Sheep and Goat

	MNCS1	Page	Page
Papers	1-7	165-168	LI-LII
Posters	8-43	168-186	LII-LV

PRODUCT QUALITY FROM LIVESTOCK SYSTEMS: HUMAN HEALTH AND CONSUMER ASPECTS

Session 2

Joint session with the commissions on Animal Nutrition, Cattle Production, Livestock Farming Systems and the FAO

Date	01-sep-03 8:30 - 12:30 hours
Chairperson	Jacobsen (DK)

	NCS2	Page	Page
Papers	1-6	103-105	XXXIX
Posters	7-45	106-125	XL-XLII

USE OF SMALL RUMINANTS AND HORSES FOR LANDSCAPE CONSERVATION AND NON AGRICULTURAL USE

Session 3

Joint session with the commission on Horse Production

Date	01-sep-03 13:30 - 17:30 hours
Chairperson	Schneeberger (CH)

Theatre **SH3 no. Page**

Theatre

Poster

FREE COMMUNICATIONS

Session 4

Date	02-sep-03 8:30 - 12:30 hours
Chairperson	Teixeira (E)

Theatre

Sheep and Goat

Theatre

Poster

Poster

Sheep and Goat

Poster

NEW DEVELOPMENTS IN SHEEP BREEDING

Session 5

Date	02-sep-03 13:30 - 17:30 hours
Chairperson	Bodin (F)

Theatre

Theatre

Poster

Sheep and Goat

Poster

NUTRITION AND FEEDING OF DAIRY SHEEP AND GOATS

Session 6

Joint session with the commission on Animal Nutrition

Date 03-sep-03
8:30 - 12:30 hours
Chairperson Bocquier (F)

Theatre

Sheep and Goat

Theatre

Poster

Poster

Commission on Pig Production (P)

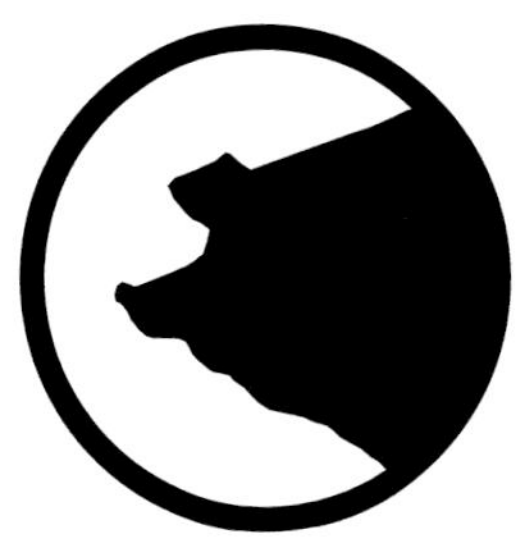

President
Prof.dr. C.Wenk
ETH-Zentrum
Institute of Animal Science
Clausiusstrasse 50 , CLU
8092 Zürich
SWITZERLAND
+41 1 632 32 55
+41 1 632 11 28
caspar.wenk@inw.agrl.ethz.ch

Secretary 1
Dr M. Kovac
University of Ljubljana
Groblje 3
1230 Domzale
SLOVENIA
00386 1 721 78 70
00386 1 7241 005
milena@mrcina.brfo.luni-lj.si

Secretary 2
Dr. D.Torrallardona
IRTA
Center de Mas Bové
Apartat 415
43280 Reus
SPAIN

GENETIC FACTORS REGULATING FEED INTAKE IN GROWING PIGS

Session 1

Date	31-aug-03 8:30 - 12:30 hours
Chairperson	Knap (D)

Theatre

Pig

Theatre

Poster

LONGTERM EFFECTS OF PRE- AND POST-NATAL CONDITIONS, INCLUDING NUTRITION, ON GROWTH AND DEVELOPMENT

Session 3

Joint session with the commissions on Animal Nutrition and Animal Physiology

Date 01-sep-03
13:30 - 17:30 hours
Chairperson Knight (UK)

FREE COMMUNICATIONS

Session 4

Date 02-sep-03
8:30 - 12:30 hours
Chairperson Wenk (CH)

Theatre

P4 no. Page

Pig

Theatre

Poster

Poster

Poster

TISSUE DEVELOPMENT AND MEAT QUALITY: THE ROLE OF LIPIDS AND ANTIOXIDANTS

Session 5

Joint session with the commission on Animal Physiology

Date 02-sep-03
13:30 - 17:30 hours
Chairperson Torrallardone (E)

Theatre

Poster

Poster

FEEDING AND MEAT QUALITY IN HEAVY PIGS

Session 6

Joint session with the commission on Animal Nutrition

Date	03-sep-03
	8:30 - 12:30 hours
Chairperson	Piva (I)

Commission on Horse Production (H)

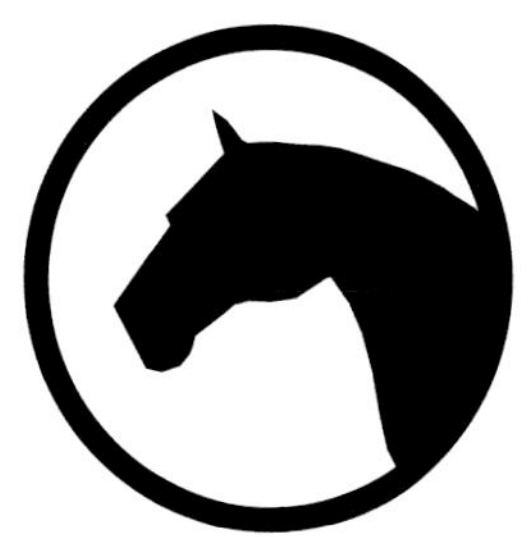

President
Dr W. Martin-Rosset
INRA
Centre of Research Clermont-Ferrand / Theix
63122 Saint Genès Champanelle
FRANCE

Secretary 1
Dr T. Jezierski
Polish Academy of Science
Inst. Animal Genetics & Breeding
Jastrzebiec
05552 Wolka Kosowska
POLAND
0048 22 756 17 11
0048 22 756 16 99
tjezierski@rocketmail.com

Secretary 2
Dr E. Gerber
Swedish University of Agricultural Sciences
P.O. Box 7023
75007 Uppsala
SWEDEN
0046 18 672 789
0046 18 672 648
elisabeth.olsson@hgen.slu.se

WELFARE AND BEHAVIOUR OF HORSES

Session 1

Date	31-aug-03
	8:30 - 12:30 hours
Chairperson	Kennedy (UK)

Theatre

H1 no. Page

Theatre

EQUINE EXERCISE PHYSIOLOGY

Session 2

Date 01-sep-03
8:30 - 12:30 hours
Chairperson Barrey (F)

Theatre

Horse

Theatre

Poster

Poster

USE OF SMALL RUMINANTS AND HORSES FOR LANDSCAPE CONSERVATION AND NON AGRICULTURAL USE

Session 3

Joint session with the commission on Sheep and Goat Production

Date	01-sep-03 13:30 - 17:30 hours
Chairperson	Schneeberger (CH)

Horse

FREE COMMUNICATIONS

Session 4

Date	02-sep-03
	8:30 - 12:30 hours
Chairperson	Ellis (NL)

Theatre

Poster

Poster

Poster

IMPACT OF FEED PROCESSING ON HORSE NUTRITION

Session 5

Joint session with the commission on Animal Nutrition

Date 02-sep-03
13:30 - 17:30 hours
Chairperson Miraglia (I)

Theatre

Theatre

Poster

HORSE PRODUCTION IN ITALY

Session 6

Date	03-sep-03
	8:30 - 12:30 hours
Chairperson	Silvestrelli (I)

Theatre

Horse

Theatre

Poster

ANIMAL GENETICS [G]

Theatre G1.1

Incorporating molecular genetic information in a global approach to genetic improvement for low and medium input systems

J.P. Gibson, International Livestock Research Institute, P.O. Box 30709, Nairobi, Kenya

In the developing world, despite the potential benefits, investment has been low for QTL detection and QTL selection has not been applied. A global approach to use of molecular genetic information might provide greater incentives for investment. Populations that are isolated from each other will often evolve different genetic adaptations to a given selection pressure. If such populations (breeds) can be identified and brought together, synthetic or crossbred populations could be created with substantially better trait expression than original breeds. A global strategy would first use molecular genetic information to determine genetic distance among breeds. The most distantly related breeds with desirable characteristics could then be chosen. Crosses between such breeds would be created and the hypothesis that they carry different genes controlling the desirable traits tested using QTL mapping. An optimised genetic improvement program, which might or might not involve MAS, would then follow from the crossbred population. The global survey of molecular diversity need be completed only once, and the QTL mapping provides information that is essential for the design of the genetic improvement program, even if the optimum design turns out not to use QTL information in selection decisions. This approach assures value of the molecular genetic information whether or not it proves useful in selection, a feature that should prove attractive to funding and executing agencies.

Theatre G1.2

A pedigree-free method for estimating coancestry using markers and population history

J. Hernández-Sánchez, C.S. Haley and J.A. Woolliams Roslin Institute, Roslin (Edinburgh), Midlothian, EH25 9PS, UK*

Coancestry is the probability that any two alleles sampled at random from a population are copies of a single ancestral allele. Thus, coancestry measures genetic relatedness among individuals within populations. Coancestry has been estimated at a locus using linked markers and pedigree information, in order to be used to map quantitative trait loci via variance components estimation. The usual underlying assumption is to consider pedigree founders as unrelated, non-inbred and in linkage equilibrium, i.e. zero coancestry. However, pedigree founders are likely to be related in most livestock species, i.e. > zero coancestry. We have developed a multiple regression model to estimate coancestry among pedigree founders given their marker genotypes, and population parameters, i.e. Ne and the age of the population. Hence, this is a pedigree-free method that makes use of the linkage disequilibrium expected to arise given a specific population history. We have compared our method with a published one and have found very good agreement between the two. However, our model uses the theory of long-term genetic contributions, which can accurately predict linked gene flow patterns under complex scenarios, e.g. including overlapping generations and selection. Therefore, an obvious advantage of our model is the potential to expand an adapt to more realistic population histories.

Theatre G1.3

Simulation of transmission disequilibrium tests for QTL detection in outbred livestock populations

D. Kolbehdari and G.B. Jansen, Centre for Genetic Improvement of Livestock, Univ. of Guelph, Canada, N1G 2W1.*

This study investigated the performance of several transmission disequilibrium tests (TDTs) for detection of QTL in data structures typical of outbred livestock populations. We considered factorial mating designs with 10 sires and either 50 or 200 dams, each family having 2, 5 or 8 full sibs. A single marker and QTL, both biallelic, were simulated using a disequilibrium coefficient based on complete initial disequilibrium and 50 generations of recombination [i.e. $D=D_0(1-c)^{50}$]. The QTL explained either 10% (small QTL) or 30% (large QTL) of the genetic variance for a trait with heritability 0.3. We found that methods Q-TDT, 1-TDT and S-TDT (e.g. Sun *et al.*, 2000) were effective tests for association and linkage between the QTL and a tightly linked marker ($c<0.02$) in these designs. For a large QTL, c=0.01, and 5 full sibs per family, the empirical power for Q-TDT, 1-TDT and S-TDT was 0.965, 0.643 and 0.975, respectively, in the large population, versus 0.686, 0.424 and 0.651, respectively, in the small population. TDTs based on analogous linear models, which incorporated the polygenic covariance structure, provided only small increases in power compared to the simpler tests.

Theatre G1.4

Several QTL affecting calving traits in Danish Holstein Cattle identified using a multiple QTL and multiple trait approach

P. Sorensen, M. Borup, B. Guldbrandtsen and M.S. Lund, Department of Animal Breeding and Genetics, Danish Instititute of Agricultural Sciences, P.O. Box 50, 8830 Tjele, Denmark.*

The objective was to identify QTL affecting calving traits in Danish Holstein Cattle using a multiple QTL and multiple trait approach. Three calving traits, calf size, calving ease, and calf survival were registered in the Danish Holstein Cattle population. The calving characters were assessed as direct and maternal effects in first lactation and later lactations. In total twelve traits were used in the scan for QTL on fifteen chromosomes. Several QTL were identified using the multiple QTL and multiple trait approach. This approach has two important advantages. First the variances attributed by the identified QTL are estimated in a single model that accounts for all QTL simultaneously. Accounting for all QTL in a single model will reduce the problem of overestimating the variances attributed by individual QTL. Second the genetic (co) variances are estimated in a multiple trait model that simultaneously partition the genetic (co) variances into a QTL component and a polygenic component. Partitioning the genetic correlation between traits will be of importance for selection decisions in livestock populations.

Theatre G1.5

Analysis of different selection criteria for selective DNA pooling

M. Dolezal[1], H. Schwarzenbacher[1], J.Soelkner[1], C. Fürst[2], [1]Department of Livestock Sciences, University of Natural Resources and Applied Life Sciences Vienna, Gregor Mendel Straße 33, 1180 Vienna, Austria,[2]ZuchtData EDV-Dienstleistungen GmbH, Universumstrasse 33/8, 1200 Vienna, Austria.*

Selective DNA pooling is an efficient method for QTL mapping applying a daughter design. Former studies used uncorrected estimated breeding values (eBV) for assigning genotypically extreme daughters to the high and low pool. The eBV of a cow is heavily influenced by the eBV of her dam, especially in traits with low heritability. Therefore influence of paternal QTL on the chance of a cow to be selected to the high or low pool could be biased by her dam's eBV. To study the efficiency of selective DNA pooling, records of 18617 daughters (offspring of 5 Simmental sires) were analysed for two traits with medium (h^2 ~0,30) and low (h^2=0,02) heritability, protein yield (kg) and maternal fertility (NRR) respectively. High and low pools were created by means of 5 different selection criteria: yield deviations, yield deviations - corrected by half of the dam eBV, uncorrected eBV, eBV - calculated excluding maternal pedigree information for the cows and eBV - corrected by half of the dam eBV. Those criteria were assessed by their differences in yield deviation and eBV between high and low pools. The averages of dam eBV of the pooled daughters were compared to evaluate the correction for dam eBV.

Theatre G1.6

On the power of the detection of epistatic effects under a bidimensional genomewide threshold value

L. Varona, L. Gomez Raya, W.M. Rauw and J.L. Noguera, Area de Producció Animal, Centre UdL-IRTA, Av. Alc. Rovira Roure 177, 25198 Lleida, Spain.*

The usual model of QTL analysis takes into account the additive and dominance effects, but no epistatic interaction between QTL. Altought there are evidences of epistatic interaction is experimental populations, there are not relevant descriptions of the effect of epistatic interaction between QTL in livestock populations. A simulation study was performed to detect the power on the detection of the epistatic effects. Populations were simulated under a F2 design with 3 different sizes of the population (200, 400 and 800 individuals). Markers and QTL alleles were simulated fixed in the parental populations. Two linkage groups were simulated with two markers and one QTL each one. Two threshold values has been considered: 1) the nominal value of a F test with 4 degrees of freedom in the numerator to detect epistatic effects between to given locations, 2) a threshold value calculated by the simulation of 10,000 replicates with a bidimensional genomic scan thought a simulated genome of 30 Morgans. This threshold can be used to detect epistatic effects between any two locations of the genome. The results suggest that there is enough statistical power to detect epistatic effects between previously detected QTL, but there is not enough power to detect QTL between two arbitrary points of the genome.

Theatre G1.7

Commercial application of marker- and gene-assisted selection in livestock: strategies and lessons

Jack C.M. Dekkers, Animal Breeding & Genetics, Department of Animal Science, 225C Kildee Hall, Iowa State University, Ames, IA, 50011-3150, U.S.A.*

During the past decades, advances in molecular genetics have led to the identification of multiple genes or genetic markers associated with genes that affect traits of interest in livestock, including genes for single gene-traits and genes or genomic regions that affect quantitative traits (quantitative trait loci or QTL).This has provided opportunities to enhance response to selection, in particular for traits that are difficult to improve by conventional selection (low heritability or traits for which measurement of phenotype is difficult, expensive, only possible late in life, or not possible on selection candidates), as has been demonstrated in a number of simulation studies. The objective here is to review strategies for the use of genes or markers in genetic improvement, to assess the extent to which and how marker and gene information has been used in commercial livestock improvement programs, to assess the successes and limitations that have been experienced in such applications, and to discuss strategies to overcome these limitations. Focus will be on the use of QTL information from experimental populations, on detection, verification, and estimation of effects in commercial breeding populations, and on the integration of molecular data in methods for genetic evaluation and in selection strategies. Types of molecular information that will be considered include gene tests for causative mutations and linked markers in population-wide linkage equilibrium or disequilibrium with the QTL.

Theatre G1.8

Targeting QTL in commercial broiler lines using candidate regions

D.J de Koning[1,], D. Windsor[1], P.M. Hocking[1], D.W. Burt[1], C.S. Haley[1], A. Morris[2], J. Vincent[2] and H. Griffin[1], [1]Roslin Institute, Roslin, EH25 9PS, Midlothian, United Kingdom, [2]The Cobb Breeding Company Ltd. Chelmsford, CM3 8BY, Essex, United Kingdom.*

Nine QTL that explained a large proportion of the phenotypic difference between broiler and layer chickens in experimental crosses were evaluated in a commercial broiler line. A three-generation design, consisting of 15 grandsires, 608 half-sib hens, and over 15,000 third generation offspring, was implemented within the existing breeding scheme of a broiler breeding company. Fifty-two markers from candidate regions on chicken chromosome 1, 3, 4, 5, 7, 8, 9, 11, and 13 were selected for their informativeness in the grandsires, and used to genotype the first two generations. Linkage was studied between these markers and 17 growth and carcass traits, using a half-sib approach with unlinked QTL as cofactors. Out of 153 trait x region comparisons, 53 QTL exceeded the threshold for genome-wide significance. QTL for residual feed intake and the dissected weights of bone and muscle in the thigh and drum accounted for most of the detected QTL. This study showed for the first time that QTL that explain differences between broilers and layers were segregating within lines that have been selected for body weight over 50 generations. The results demonstrate the feasibility of QTL detection and the potential for marker-assisted selection within a commercial broiler line, without altering the existing breeding scheme.

Theatre G1.9

Marker assisted selection in German Holstein dairy cattle breeding: Outline of the program and marker assisted breeding value estimation

J. Bennewitz[1], N. Reinsch[1,2], J. Szyda[3], F. Reinhardt[3], C. Kühn[2], M. Schwerin[2], G. Erhardt[4], C. Weimann[4], and E. Kalm[1]. [1]Institut für Tierzucht und Tierhaltung, Christian-Albrechts-Universität, D-24098 Kiel, [2]Forschungsinstitut für die Biologie landwirtschaftlicher Nutztiere, D-18196 Dummerstorf, [3]Vereinigte Informations-systeme Tierhaltung w.V., D-27283 Verden, [4]Institut für Tierzucht und Haustiergenetik der Justus-Liebig-Universität, D-35390 Gießen*

The so-called ADR-project for QTL mapping the German dairy cattle population is a common effort of German AI and breeding companies, several German animal breeding institutes and animal computing centres initiated by the German cattle breeders federation (ADR). The results of this project form the base for the marker assisted selection (MAS) in the German Holstein breeding. The MAS approach is a joint effort of several Holstein breeding companies and follows in principle the Top-Down approach of pre-selection of bulls before entering progeny testing. The MAS program is outlined. Unlike the classical Top-Down approach, the selection criteria for the MAS are marker assisted best linear unbiased prediction (MA-BLUP) estimates of breeding values. This enables the comparison, and hence the MAS, of candidates across families. To keep the number of equations in the model small, a modified sire MA-BLUP model is used, that includes genotyped sires, genotyped bulldams and the genotyped candidates. Further properties of the MAS program (e.g. the organisation structure) and of the MA-BLUP sire model are discussed.

Theatre G1.10

Effect of marker assisted selection for mastitis resistance in a real Danish Holstein pedigree

B. Guldbrandtsen[1], J.R. Thomasen[2], M.S. Lund[1], R. Fernando[3], [1]Dept. of Animal Breeding and Genetics, Danish Institute of Agricultural Sciences, DK-8830 Tjele, Denmark, [2]Borregaardsvej 9, DK-7500 Holstebro, Denmark, [3]Dept. of Animal Breeding, Iowa State University, Ames, IA 50011-3150, USA*

The expected effect of top-down marker assisted selection in a real Danish cattle pedigree was studied. The Swedish-Danish Holstein cattle QTL project has identified a number of heavily used sires heterozygote for QTL affecting mastitis resistance. All bull and heifer calves currently relevant for selection decisions descending from one particular QTL heterozygote sire were identified. All animals from which biological samples were available, were typed for a number of markers linked to the one of the QTL affecting mastitis resistance.

Segregation of the markers was studied to estimate the likely segregation of the mastitis resistance QTL. Segregation was studied using a MCMC descent-graph sampler. Segregation probabilities were used to predict QTL-effects in full and half-sib groups among the calves.

Theatre G1.11

Deterministic evaluation of dairy cattle breeding schemes using QTL information

C. Schrooten[1,2] and H. Bovenhuis[1], [1]Wageningen Institute of Animal Sciences, P. O. Box 338, 6700 AH Wageningen, the Netherlands, [2]Holland Genetics, P. O. Box 5073, 6802 EB Arnhem, The Netherlands.*

In the past decade, molecular techniques have become available that enable the genotypic analysis of animals. In dairy cattle, this has resulted in the localization of a number of Quantitative Trait Loci (QTL), which can be used in the genetic evaluation of selection candidates.
In this paper, a number of closed nucleus breeding schemes in dairy cattle that use information on QTL, have been evaluated. Deterministic simulations were performed using the program SelAction. In the base scheme, the selection index for dams consisted of pedigree information and own performance. The selection index for sires consisted of pedigree information and performance of 100 daughters. In alternative breeding schemes, information on a QTL was accounted for by simulating an additional index trait. The fraction of the variance explained by the QTL determined the correlation between the additional index trait and the breeding goal trait. Information on the QTL became available either at birth or at the embryo level. Other parameters that were varied in the alternative breeding schemes were the number of breeding goal traits (1 or 2), the number of QTL per trait (up to 5, each explaining 10% of the genetic variance) and the number of animals in the breeding program.

Poster G1.12

Effects of complex vertebral malformation on fertility in Swedish Holstein cattle

B. Berglund and A. Persson, Department of Animal Breeding and Genetics, Swedish University of Agricultural Sciences, SE-750 07 Uppsala, Sweden.*

Complex vertebral malformation (CVM) is an autosomal recessive genetic defect in the Holstein breed. It causes embryonic mortality through the entire gestation period thereby leading to economic losses by repeat breeding and involuntary culling of cows. The defect was first reported in Denmark in 1999 and a commercial DNA test for the defect is now available. The aim of this study was to investigate if a reduction in reproductive performance, measured as non-return rate (NR), could be observed in Holstein bulls heterozygous for the CVM gene, compared with non-carrier bulls. All tested Holstein bulls used by the Swedish AI organisations born between 1995 and 1999 were included. Altogether 228 bulls were analysed of which 53 bulls, i.e. 23%, were confirmed CVM carriers and 175 carried the normal genotype. A statistically significant difference between carriers and non-carriers in the relative breeding value for NR was observed for 168 days NR (101.1±0.9 vs. 103.1±0.6, $p<0.05$). There was no difference for 28 days NR whereas the difference approached significance at 56 days NR. No significant effect of CVM genotype/status on the daughter fertility index could be shown. This was probably due to the complexity of traits this index is composed by. In conclusion this study showed that carriers of the CVM defect had an inferior NR compared with non-carriers.

Poster G1.13

The effect of combined defensin genotype on somatic cell count (SCC) in the cow's milk and on dairy production traits

E. Bagnicka, L. Zwierzchowski, Z. Ryniewicz, J. Krzyzewski, N. Strzalkowska, Institute of Genetics and Animal Breeding PAS in Jastrzebiec, 05-552, Poland

Genes coding for defensins seem to be good molecular markers of mammary gland resistance to mastitis and milk performance of dairy cattle. Polymorphism of the defensin genes was studied in the Polish Friesian cows. DNA was isolated from blood samples taken from 217 cows. To determine the polymorphism of defensin genes the RFLP method with enzyme *Taq*I was used. Twenty different polymorphic systems were observed, possibly representing a polymorphism of genes encoding different defensins, but combined defensin genotypes (CDG) which frequency was less then 3% and cows with less than ten records were excluded from statistical analysis. Finally 10 different genotypes of 172 cows were investigated. There were 4074 records about daily milk yield, fat and protein content, and 3468 records about SCC. Combined defensin genotypes had significant effect on all investigated traits. The best CDG for daily milk yield (A1A2/B1/C1) differed significantly from all other CDGs. It had the low frequency (3.49%) in investigated group. This CDG was associated with the lowest fat content, with a very low protein content and low SCC. Animals carrying the most frequent CDG (A1A2/B1B2/C1C2; 38.37%) had a very low daily milk yield but the highest fat and protein content. The lowest SCC was associated with CDG A1/B1/C1C2 of which frequency was 3.49%.

Poster G1.14

Associations between marker gene alleles and Egyptian Suffolk ewes traits

I.F.M. Marai[1], A.A. El-Darawany[1], E. Abu-Fandoud[2] and M.A.M Abdel-Hafez[2], [1]Department of Animal Production, Faculty of Agriculture, Zagazig University, Zagazig, Egypt. [2]Division of Sheep and Goats Research, Department of Animal Production, Institute of Animal Production Research, Ministry of Agriculture, Egypt.

Plasma protein of Egyptian Suffolk (70-90% UK Suffolk 10-30% Ossimi) ewes were examined for biochemical polymorphism of Myosin (M), β-Galactosidase (β -Gal), Phosphorylase β (P), Albumin (Alb), Catalase (Cat) and Aldolase (Ald) by using one-dimensional sodium dodecyl sulfate polyacrylamide gels electrophoresis (SDS-PAGE), with high-range protein molecular weight marker standards as reference bands.

Analysis of the results revealed the existence of associations between productive and reproductive traits of heterozygous ewes and marker gene alleles. The alleles A^{a1}& A^{a2}, A^{b1}& A^{b2} and A^{01}& A^{02} of Alb marker gene were associated with the highest values of age at first lambing and lamb weight at weaning, fertility and lambing interval, respectively. The alleles G^{c1} & G^{c2} and C^{b1}& C^{b2} of β -Gal and Cat marker genes were insignificantly associated with the highest values of lamb weight at birth and kilograms of lambs produced at weaning / ewe / season, respectively.

The positive results may suggest that marker assisted selection could be carried out at a very early age on marker genotypes for improvement of Egyptian Suffolk sheep traits, since such marker genotypes could be scored at early ages.

Poster G1.15

Physiochemical polymorphism in MHC class II peptide binding grove molecule and Somatic Cell Count in Italian Holstein Friesian bulls

M. Longeri[1], I. Taboni[1], M.G. Strillacci[1], A.B. Samorè[2] and M. Zanotti[1], [1]Istituto di Zootecnica, Via Celoria 10, 20134 Milano Italy, [2]Associazione Nazionale Allevatori Frisona Italiana (ANAFI), Via Bergamo 292, 26100 Cremona, Italy.*

A sample of 275 Holstein Friesian bulls, with genetic index for Somatic Cell Count (SCC), has been typed for class II Histocompatibility antigens (MHC-DRB3 exon 2) by PCR-RFLP and the corresponding amino acid (AA) sequence has been considered. Since the T-cell recognition of foreign antigens is not only influenced by the different amino acids in the binding groove of DRB3-MHC molecule, but also by their different charge, we considered the amino acid variability of the three most active residues, corresponding to position 62, 63 and 66 in cattle molecule. Grouping the physiochemical polymorphism by AA residual charge motifs we obtained nine haplotypes, while considering the Isoelectric point (pI) at the three positions we obtained twelve classes.
We estimated the haplotype and the isoelectric point effect on the genetic indexes for somatic cell count by multiple regression analysis. A high isoelectric point and positively charged AA are statistically significant related to a lower SCC, while a neutral pI or lower charged AA are statistically significant with a higher genetic index. Data presented support the hypothesis that a positive charge in the antigen binding groove is favourable for a lower Somatic Cell Count content and therefore for mastitis susceptibility.

Poster G1.16

Population-wide linkage disequilibrium between Precm1 SNP and a milk QTL on BTA6 in Israeli Holsteins

M. Cohen[1], M. Reichenstein[1], J. Heon[2], M Shani[1], H.A. Lewin[2], J.I. Weller[1], M. Ron[1] and E. Serrousi[1], [1]Institute of Animal Sciences, Agricultural Research Organization, The volcani Center, Bet Dagan 50250 Israel, Department of Animal Sciences, [2]University of Ilinois at Urbana-Champaign, Urbana, Illinois 61801, USA.

A cluster of genes coding for proteins of the extra cellular matrix (ECM) that contain sequence motifs essential for integrin-receptor interactions is located on human chromosome 4q21. In cattle this cluster of genes maps to Bos taurus autosome 6 within the critical region of a QTL affecting milk, fat, and protein production. Genes within this ECM cluster were shown to play important role in the formation of bone and lobulo-alveolar structures in mammary gland, as well as kidney function. We cloned a bovine gene related by position to this ECM gene cluster, which we termed *Fam13a1,* as the first member of gene family of unknown function number 13. The 5.1 Kb mRNA capable of encoding 697 amino acids (aa) is similar to mRNAs that are expressed preferentially in normal mammary gland and transcribed from 18-exon orthologous genes in human and mouse, which encode 697 and 693 aa putative nuclear proteins, respectively. Thus, the *FAM13* family of genes may be regulated by adjacent genes via antisense transcription. Genetic analysis of Israeli Holsteins sires revealed population-wide linkage disequilibrium between a SNP in intron 9 of *Fam13a1* and a QTL affecting milk protein production, suggesting that this QTL gene is closely linked to BTA6 ECM cluster.

Poster G1.17

Scrapie genotyping in six ovine italian breeds: preliminary results

M. Blasi[1] A. Lanza[1], M. Motovalian[1], C. Varlotta[1], A. Rosati[1], S. Sangalli[1], N. Nazzarri[2], P. Fraddosio[3], [1]Laboratorio Gruppi Sanguigni, Via dell'edilizia snc, 85100 Potenza, Italy, [2]Assonapa Viale Palmiro Togliatti, 1587 00155 Roma, Italy, [3]A.G.E.A. Roma, Italy

Scrapie is a fatal, infectious, wasting disease affecting the nervous system of adult sheep and belongs to the transmissible spongiform encephalopathy family (TSE). It has been present in Europe for at least 200 years and has been an important disease in the UK since January 1993. For long time has been known that resistance/susceptibility of sheep to scrapie is largely under genetic control. The gene that encodes the normal prion protein (PrP) has polymorphisms at codons 136, 154, and 171. Among all possible combinations of the 3 codons 136 (A/V), 154 (R/H) and 171 (Q/R/H) only five were found: V 136 R 154 Q 171 (VRQ), A 136 R 154 Q 171 (ARQ), A 136 R 154 R 171 (ARR), A 136 H 154 Q 171 (AHQ) e A 136 R 154 H 171 (ARH). Scrapie susceptibility is conferred by the VRQ allele and resistance by ARR and AHQ alleles, with an intermediate situation for ARQ and ARH. In this paper six ovine Italian breeds (Appenninica, Bergamasca, Comisana, Gentile di Puglia, Massese, and Merinizzata) were analyzed to estimate the allelic frequencies relative to PrP gene. Preliminary results showed, for each breed, VRQ allele frequency estimates range from 0,1 for Appenninica to 0,25 for Comisana. ARR and AHQ alleles, determining genetic resistance to the disease, have combined frequencies always larger than 0,50.

Poster G1.18

New nucleotide sequence polymorphisms within 5'-noncoding region of the bovine growth hormone receptor gene

A. Maj, M. Klauzinska, L. Zwierzchowski, Institute of Genetics and Animal Breeding, Polish Academy of Sciences, Jastrzebiec, 05-552 Wólka Kosowska, Poland.*

Growth hormone (GH) plays a central role in the regulation of growth and metabolism in animals. Actions of GH are mediated through its cell-surface receptor - GHR. Genes coding for GH and GHR are obvious candidates for quantitative trait markers in cattle. In this work RFLP polymorphism was studied within 5'-noncoding region of the bovine GHR gene. New RFLP polymorphism was found at a Fnu4HI/TseI site. A C/T transition was determined by sequencing at the position -1104. Two alleles and three genotypes were identified within the analyzed populations of dairy and beef cattle. We showed that the newly found RFLP-Fnu4HI/TseI polymorphic site, as well as previously identified polymorphic sites for restriction enzymes AluI and AccI, are located within the 1.2 kb LINE-1 retrotransposon upstream P1 promoter for exon 1A of bovine GHR gene. Five cows were identified 3 - Polish Red and 2 Bialogrzbietka (Polish native White-Spined) - with the deletion of the LINE-1 element from GHR gene 5' noncoding region; the exact size of the deletion was 1206 bp.

Poster G1.19

Reduction of an immotile short tail sperm defect (ISTS) in the Finnish Yorkshire using a two-marker haplotype

A. Sironen[1], P. Lehtinen[2], J. Vilkki[1], [1]MTT Agrifood Research Finland, Animal Production Research, Animal Breeding, 31600 Jokioinen, Finland, [2]FABA The Finnish Animal Breeding Association PL 40, 01301 Vantaa, Finland

An immotile short tail sperm defect (ISTS) has recently been identified as a hereditary disorder within the Finnish Yorkshire pig population and became a reproductive problem in 1998. The syndrome is inherited as an autosomal recessive disease exclusively expressed in male individuals as shorter sperm tail length and immotile spermatozoa. No adverse effects on reproductive performance of female relatives have been observed. Currently 77 boars are known to have the syndrome. The defect has been mapped on porcine chromosome 16 between microsatellite markers SW1035 and SW419. The two-marker haplotype has been used to reduce the frequency of the disease within the Finnish Yorkshire population. Two haplotypes are linked to the disease and therefore pedigree data are still needed. The test requires a hair sample from an animal under investigation and its parents. All homozygous boars are eliminated based on this test and the carrier information is made available to breeders. The test has an estimated accuracy of 90%. Inaccuracies arise from a recombination with one of the disease associated haplotype, and is therefore also expressed in healthy boars. Since 2002, the test has been implemented and all artificial insemination boars are tested.

Poster G1.20

Attempts for molecular selection of bovine embryos used in milk production improvement

M. Michescu[1],I. Daniela[1], T. Vintila[1], Gh. Ghise[1] and I.Vintila[1], [1]Faculty of Animal Science and Biotechnology, Banat University of Agricultural Sciences and Veterinary Medicine, Calea Aradului No 119, Timisoara 1900, Romania*

At present the bovine embryo transfer is currently used in bovine breeding programs. Specific molecular methods allow the extraction and analyze of DNA from trophoblastic cells. These techniques enable us to develop and implement the bovine selection in embrionary stage by sex determination and genotipization for QTLs or candidate genes.

Two gene located in kappa-casein (k-cn) and beta-lactoglobulin (β-lgb) loci can be used, as molecular markers for obtaining higher milk quality needed to improve the milk manufacturing properties. In order to differentiate the favorable genotype for superior composition and higher cheese yield we used PCR-RFLP analysis. Bovine embryo evaluation also includes their sex determination by PCR amplification of DNA sequences specific to the X and Y-chromosomes.

Therefor, we try to assimilate and developed in our laboratory the specific molecular methods by simple or multiplex PCR reaction. These way we can choose earlier (in embrionary stage) which animal will be promote for reproduction or not, independently of age and sex, and we also can obtain more substantial genetic progress for milk production.

Poster G1.21

Quantification of the sex ratio in sexed bull semen by real time PCR

K. Parati, G. Bongioni and A. Galli, Istituto Sperimentale Italiano Lazzaro Spallanzani, Loc. La Quercia, 26027 Rivolta d'Adda (CR), Italy.

Sexed semen represents an useful tool for the livestock offspring sex preselection which is important for planning matings in management schemes. The cell sorting procedure by flow-cytometry, based on DNA difference, is the only method to produce a significant enrichment of X and/or Y-bearing spermatozoa. In order to verify the purity of the sexed sperm, an accurate assay is required. Nowadays, this kind of evaluation, utilizing microscopy, semi-quantitative PCR or in-situ hybridization, is often approximate or time-consuming.
The aim of this research was to develop a new quantitative real time PCR protocol to establish the sex ratio of sexed bull semen.
Two sets of primers and TaqMan probes were designed on two specific X and Y- chromosome genes. A certificated standard curve, established to calculate the relative percentage of male and female sperms, was built utilizing the fragments obtained from the amplifications of the two genes.
Only two replicates are needed to obtain a repeatability upper of 99% as Ct values. The assay performed on 20 repetitions/sample showed a high accuracy (99.8%) and repeatability (CV=2.8%). The effect of serial diluitions of DNA samples (10^4-10^1 molecules of DNA/reaction) was not significative and not important (P>0.05).
The results showed that this assay is more rapid, reliable and accurate then previous methods.

Poster G1.22

Incorporation of QTL information into routine estimation of breeding values for German Holstein dairy cattle

J. Szyda[1,2], Z. Liu[1], F. Reinhardt[1] and R. Reents[1], [1]United Datasystems for Animal Production (VIT), Heideweg 1, 27-283 Verden, Germany, [2]Department of Animal Genetics, Agricultural University of Wroclaw, Kozuchowska 7, 51-631 Wroclaw, Poland.*

Since 1999 young bulls from German dairy population have undergone routine genotyping. These molecular markers are used both for parentage testing and for marking regions harbouring quantitative trait loci (QTL) influencing traits characterising production performance of dairy cattle. Originally, genotypes of 339 markers have been identified to screen for most likely positions of QTL with largest effects. In the following step a subset of 13 markers has been chosen for routine genotyping. The current dimensions of the genotyped part of the population comprise genotypes of 3867 bulls and their 65 sires.
The national data management and analysis system developed for handling the molecular information and for genetic evaluation under the mixed inheritance model (i.e. separating polygenic and QTL components) is presented. However, the main goal of this contribution is to introduce statistical models used for the incorporation of QTL information into the routine estimation of breeding values. Based on the results from routine genetic evaluation we also show how the estimates of QTL parameters (effect, location) and the polygenic values differ between models with a fixed and a random QTL effect. Finally, the practical use of results by breeding organisations is discussed.

Poster G1.23

Mutation analysis for the identification of melanocyte stimulating hormone receptor (MC1R) locus alleles causing red coat colour in cattle using denaturing high performance liquid chromatography (DHPLC)

L. Pariset, I. Cappuccio, M.C. Savarese and A. Valentini, Dipartimento di Produzioni Animali, Facoltà di Agraria, Università della Tuscia, Viterbo, Italy*

It is often required to exclude from breeding schemes animals carrying alleles resulting in an undesired coat colour. We used the technique of denaturing high performance liquid chromatography (DHPLC) to determine the presence of alleles causing red coat colour in cattle at DNA level.
Genomic DNA was amplified in the polymorphic MC1R region and PCR products were directly used for mutation screening. Some individuals were screened using a PCR-RFLP method previously described to confirm the identified genotypes.
DHPLC analysis proved to be a sensitive and specific method to detect the known mutations, with the advantage of being economic and very fast. The complete analysis after PCR can be performed in just three minutes, the genotypes can be unequivocally determined and potentially new undescribed variant can be detected.

Poster G1.24

Use of AFLP markers to genome mapping in local poultry breeds

C. Targhetta[1], M. De Marchi[1], M. Cassandro[1], G. Barcaccia[2], M. Ramanzin[1] and M. Bonsembiante[1], [1]Department of Animal Science, University of Padova, Agripolis 35020, Legnaro, Padova, Italy, [2]Department of Agronomy, Environment and Crop Production, University of Padova, Agripolis, 35020, Legnaro, Padova, Italy.

AFLP fingerprinting tecnique has been used to enrich existing genetic maps in plants, bacteria and less widely also in animal genomes. Aim of this study was to explore the use of biallelic Amplified Fragment Length Polymorphism (AFLP) markers in a local poultry breed reared in the Veneto region (Italy). Genomic DNA was extracted from whole blood obtained from 12 cocks belonging to Ermellinata di Rovigo breed. AFLP genotyping was carried out using four enzime combinations (*Eco*RI/*Taq*I, *Eco*RI/*Mse*I, *Pst*I/*Taq*I, *Pst*I/*Mse*I), following the protocol described by Barcaccia *et al.*1999 . Results showed that the use of *Mse*I is not appropriate in the breed examined because it doesn't generate polimorphic profiles, while *Taq*I appears more favourable. The highest number of polymorphic bands is obtained using *Taq*I and *Eco*RI, but further experimentation will be necessary to choose the appropriate endonucleases, as only one primer combination for each pair of enzimes has been tested. This study showed the applicability of AFLP markers to the characterisation of the poultry breed examined. Further tests will permit to validate a definitive experimental protocol that might be used also for other poultry breeds.

Poster G1.25

A new protocol for genotyping microsatellites in buffalo

A. Rosati[1], M. Blasi[1], A. Lanza[1], M. Motovalian[1], P. Di Gregorio[2], A. Coletta[3] and L. Gubitosi[3], [1]Laboratorio Gruppi Sanguigni, Via dell'edilizia snc, 85100 Potenza, Italy, [2] Università degli Studi della Basilicata via N. Sauro 85100 Potenza, Italy [3] A.N.A.S.B., Caserta, Italy.*

Knowing the exact genealogy is very important in animal production systems, especially when genealogy information is included in a herd book. Genetic value estimates accuracy is largely dependent of the herd book correctness. Buffalo breeding is on a large scale managed by using natural mating in herds with more than one sire present at the same time. Laboratorio Gruppi Sanguigni defined a working protocol to verify, through DNA microsatellites analysis, the genealogy for each individual. 14 microsatellites in two different multiplex were tested for this purpose (INRA006, CSSM42, CSSM47, CSSM19, D5S2, MAF65, RM4, CYP21 e BM1013 multiplex 1; CSSM70, CSSM60, INRA026, BM0922, BM0922 e BM1706 multiplex 2). The exclusion probability (PE) was estimated by the frequency estimates of alleles for each single microsatellite. The combined PE for the used microsatellites was 0,9999. The method is nowadays largely used to verify the real sire in all buffalo herds whose animals are registered to the Italian national buffalo herd book.

Poster G1.26

Incorporation of high-throughput AFLP[(r)] markers in the RH bovine map

C. Gorni[1], P. Ajmone-Marsan[1], M.J.T. van Eijk[2], H. Heuven[2], M. Zevenbergen[2], R. Negrini[1], D. Waddington[3], J.L. Williams[3], J. Peleman[2], [1]Istituto di Zootecnica, Università Cattolica del S. Cuore, 29100 Piacenza, Italy, [2]Keygene n.v., 6700 AE Wageningen, The Netherlands, [3]Roslin Institute, Midlothian, UK.*

AFLP technology has been adapted to the analysis of Radiation Hybrid panels increasing the number of selective nucleotides present at the 3' end of primers used in the amplification and hence simplifying the electrophoretic profile and reducing overlapping between hamster and bovine bands. Thirty-seven primer pairs have amplified 747 bovine-specific bands in the TM112 3,000 rad RH panel. Among these 650 resulted significantly linked at LOD 4 to 1222 microsatellite markers already located on the 29 autosomes, X and Y bovine chromosomes.
Multipoint mapping of five BTA chromosomes confirms the usefulness of AFLPs for rapidly enriching RH maps with anchor markers.

Poster G1.27

Microarray cytokine expression profiling in Bos Taurus

V. Maran[1-3], P. Parma[1], F. Damin[2], M. Chiari[2], P. Roncada[1-3] and G.F. Greppi[3], [1]LEA Lab. of Applied Epigenomic, Institute L. Spallanzani. Lodi, Italy, [2]Inst. of Chemistry of Molecular Recognition C.N.R. Milan, Italy, [3]Dep. of Veterinary Clinical Science, University of Milan Italy

Microarray technology represent a major advance in postegenomic era. It provides a strategy to monitor gene expression for thousands of genes in parallel. Our task is to create a *Bost taurus* citockine array, that will provide a precious tool to determine citockine profiling expression in different context. Cytokine play a pivotal roles in the regulation of various biological responses, such as immune responses, inflammation, hematopoiesis, oncogenesis. Utilizing the sequences in genebank, for each cytockine we have evaluated the presence and localization of introns, then the probes were designd in the last exon and were evaluated with specific bioinformatics programs for the homogeneity. The probe are oligonucleotide of 80-100 bp obtained via PCR. One of the two primer of the reaction is aminomodified in order to obtain single strand amino modified DNA to be ligated on the matrix of the array slide. The second step lead to the isolation of mRNA and its labelling. Milk was centrifuge, the cellular pellet was washed twice in PBS. mRNA extraction was carried out in specific silica columns and retrotrascribed with specific labelled primer. The cDNA obtained was hybridized on the array.

Poster G1.28

Analysis of chromosome aberrations in transgenic pigs and rabbits

V.A. Bagirov, P.M. Klenovitsky, N.A.Zinoveva, All Russian Research Institute of Animal Science, 142132, Dubrovitcy, Podolsk Distric, Moscow Region, Russia

14 piglets were produced by the method of intertubal insemination using the sperm of mMT1-hGRF transgenic boar kept in the liquid nitrogen during 10 years.

The karyotyping of the produced transgenic and control piglets was performed in comparison to the karyotype of piglets produced by conventional artificial insemination. The karyotype analysis was performed using the digital camera and Image Scope 1 software for the processing and image analysis.

The analysis of the chromosomal pattern indicated the instability of the karyotype in these piglets. The frequency of the cells carrying the aberrations in transgenic piglets was 37.8 percents comparing to 11.2 percents in non-transgenic animals. The cells derived from the control pigs carried about 7.3 percents of aberrant cells.

The cells with the incorrect chromosomal morphology were found in transgenic pigs, whereas in non-transgenic and control pigs such cells were not observed. Probably, the presence of the aberrant chromosomes was appeared due to the transgene integration

Using the same method 38 transgenic rabbits were analyzed. The higher chromosomal instability in transgenic rabbits comparing to non-transgenic animals was proved. The level of chromosomal aberrations was 12.9 and 1,2 percent respectively.

Thus, our results shown, that the integration of the foreign genetic material results in aberrations of the chromosome in transgenic animals.

Poster G1.29

Genetic difference of some sheep breeds in the Republic of Croatia

Martina Bradic, Vesna Pavic and B. Mioc,Department of Animal Production,Faculty of Agriculture, Svetosimunska 25, 10000 Zagreb, Croatia*

About 20 sheep breeds have been raised in the Republic of Croatia, out of which a half belongs to the group of original breeds. During a history, our original breeds were under various influences of foreign breeds, particularly Merino sheep from neighbouring countries. The influence of Merino was particularly strong during the 18th and 19th century. In areas close to the Adriatic coast and on some islands, various sheep population have been grown today, which are defined as separate breeds due to their external appearance, which appeared in a similar way: by improving the autochthonous, local Pramenka with Merino rams. Today, a question of genetic differences of these populations is rightly asked.That is why the aim of this research was to determine differences between Pag, Krk and Dubrovnik sheep, by certain molecular genetic analysis. From 40 blood samples of each breed, the genome DNA was isolated, whose regions were then multiplied by PCR method using specific molecular markers. PCR products were analysed by SSCP method on a polyacrylamide gel, by which difference between individuals of certain breeds were determined. The first results indicate the existence of genetic differences between analysed breeds. The final conclusion of existence of differences between mentioned breeds will be brought after analyses of sequences carried by gene analyser ABI 310.

Poster G1.30

Genome bank of Chianina in Umbria

E. Lasagna[1], F. M. Sarti[1], S. Sorbolini[1], F. Filippini[2], F. Panella[1], [1]Dipartimento di Scienze Zootecniche, Borgo XX Giugno, 74, 06121 Perugia, Italy, [2]A.N.A.B.I.C., S Martino in Colle, 06070 Perugia, Italy.*

The research was carried out in order to obtain a DNA bank for Chianina breed in Umbria. In four years 5100 samples have to be extracted from 4.500 cows and 600 sires. Each sample of DNA must be divided in three parts and stored in three different places, therefore 30-40 μg of DNA are necessary from each animal. In order to optimise the method several solutions have been evaluated. The first tested kit produced a poor quantity of DNA (15-20 μg), so a proof was done using it with only leukocytes instead whole blood. Good quantity of DNA were sometimes obtained but the repeatability was very low, due to the column saturation. To solve this problem a double extraction with two different columns was done, in this way the cost was reduced in comparing with other kits, but to much time was necessary. A special kit able to process large quantity of blood was therefore used. The results were similar to that obtained with the double extractions, the yield was more constant but, unlikely, also in this case the column saturation sometimes occurred. A third kit able to process whole blood samples without using columns was therefore tested; this method allowed to obtain 30-40 μg of DNA from 1.5 ml of blood, with a good repeatability.

Poster G1.31

Genetic variability evaluation of seabream *(Sparus Aurata)* broodstock by microsatellites DNA markers

K. Parati[1], S. Ben Jemaa[1], G. Bongioni[1], A. Cristobal[2], A. Galli[1], [1]Istituto Sperimentale Italiano "Lazzaro Spallanzani", Localita' La Quercia 26027 Rivolta d'Adda, Cremona, Italy, [2]Tinamenor S.A, Marisma de Pesués,39594 Pesués, Spain.

The menagement of a restricted number of reproducers in animal breeding needs a particular care in order to avoid loss in genetic variability across several generations; this is particular true in fish breeding. This work is done in order to study the genetic variability of a gilthead seabream broodstock reared in a hatchery located in north of Spain to evaluate its management approach. For this purpose, 566 individuals, representing the whole broodstock population and divided in 7 ponds, were analysed using six microsatellites. Their Polymorphic Information Content (PIC) was evaluated: four of these microsattelites had PIC>0.80, whereas the two others were less informative (PIC< 0.60). Allele's number found for each microsatellite showed homogenous distribution among ponds and the mean number of alleles didn't show significative difference from one pond to another ($F=2.36$, $P>0.05$). The mean observed heterozygosity in the broodstock, considering the most informative 4 microsatellites, was high ($Ho= 0.91$), reaching that of natural populations.
The Hardy-Weinberg equilibrium (HWE) was verified comparing the observed and expected heterozygosities ($\chi^2= 5.081$, $DF=5$, $P>0.05$).
These results confirm the utility of this methodological approach to support the preservation of the genetic variability of broodstock.

Poster G1.32

Classic breeding methods and molecular genetics in preservation of domestic animals in Hungary

Alice Gy. Molnárné[1], S. Mihók[2], Erzsébet Takács[1], L.Radnóczi[1], I.Bodó[2], [1]National Institut for Agricultural Quality Control H-1024 Budapest, Keleti K-u.24, [2]Debreceni Egyetem Debrecen, Debrecen University H-4032 Debrecen Böszörményi u. 138.*

Immunogenetic and molecular genetic methods are more and more involved in preservation of rare breeds of domestic animals in Hungary.
In Hungarian Grey cattle breed the parentage control was carried out based on blood groups and serum polimorphisms since the sixties of the last century. Recently 2520 blood samples were collected for DNA microsatellite investigation from parents and progeny in order to check the gene frequencies of different subpopulations, genealogical lines and families and for comparison of inbreeding rate measured by different methods and genetic distances among the different groups.
The first results have shown the largest polimorhism on locus TGLA53 and the most balanced one was locus BM1824 with the same frequency of 4 alleles. Interesting was ETH10 locus with 5 allels, 77 % of them produced the same microsatellite length (215 bp).
The aim of investigations is to help the preservation and to reduce the neative impact of genetic drift.
The same research started in traditional Hungarian horse breeds like Nonius, Gidran and Furioso, also in the three colour varieties of Mangalitza pig and in different traditional Hungarian poultry breeds as well.

Theatre G2.1

Predicting the annual effective size of livestock populations

L. Ollivier[1] and J.W. James[2], [1]INRA-SGQA, Domaine de Vilvert, 78350 Jouy-en-Josas, France,[2]Reprogen, University of Sydney, NSW 2006 Australia.*

Effective population size (N_e) is an important parameter determining the genetic structure of small populations. In natural populations, the number of adults (N) is usually known and N_e can be estimated on the basis of an assumed ratio N_e/N, usually found to be close to 0.5. In farm animal populations, apart from using pedigrees or genetic marker information, N_e can be estimated from the number N of breeding animals, and a value of 1 is commonly assumed for the ratio N_e/N. The purpose of this note is to show the relation between effective population size and breeding herd size in livestock species. With overlapping generations, N_e can be predicted knowing the number of individuals entering the population per generation and the variance of family size, the latter being directly related to the replacement policy in the breeding herd. By assuming an ideal replacement policy leading to a geometrical age distribution, the ratio of the annual effective size to the number of breeding animals is shown to be equal to $[1+(a-1)(1-s)]^2/(1-s^2)$, where a is the age at 1st offspring and s the survival rate of the parents between successive births. This expression shows to what extent inbreeding may be determined by demography independently from the actual herd size. Consequences which can be drawn for the management of small populations are discussed.

Theatre G2.2

Inbreeding in the German Holstein cow population

H.H. Swalve[1], F. Rosner[1] and W. Wemheuer[2], [1]Institute of Animal Breeding and Animal Husbandry, University of Halle, D-06099 Halle, Germany, [2]Institute of Veterinary Medicine, University of Göttingen, D-37073 Göttingen, Germany.*

Inbreeding coefficients and additive genetic relationships of important sires with the breed were calculated for a sample of 94,366 cows under milk recording of birth years 1994 to 1997 from Lower Saxony. The sample was drawn extracting all cows of 11 selected counties. Pedigrees on average could be traced for seven generations. 80.3 % of all cows had an inbreeding coefficient > 0. The average coefficient of inbreeding was 1.93 % for all cows and 2.4% for all inbred cows. Sires with the highest average additive genetic relationship with the cow population were R.O.R.A. Elevation, Pawnee Farm Airlinda Chief, SWD Valiant and Hanoverhill Starbuck with coefficients of 11.7%, 9.5%, 8.5%, and 5.4%, respectively. The sire R.O.R.A. Elevation was found in 91% of all pedigrees.

The results indicate that although the German population does not differ much from other Holstein populations with respect to the most influential sires, the average coefficient of inbreeding is substantially lower than found in other populations, and that inbreeding predominantly is caused by bulls born in the Sixties and early Seventies.

Theatre G2.3

Geographic structure of European cattle breeds revealed by AFLP neutral markers

E. Milanesi[1], R. Negrini[1], M. Zanotti[2], R. Bozzi[3], M. Moretti[3], C. Perez Torrecillas[3], A. Bruzzone[4], F. Pilla[4], H. Lenstra[5], I. Nijman[5], E.G. Muro[6], C. Rodellar[6], B. Portolano[7], G. Erhardt[8], I. Olsaker[9], G. Dolf[10], K. Moazami Goudarzi[11], D. Laloë[11], L. E. Holm[12], P. Ajmone Marsan[1], [1]Università Cattolica del Sacro Cuore, Piacenza, Italy, [2]Università degli Studi di Milano, Italy, [3]Università degli Studi di Firenze, Italy, [4]Università degli Studi del Molise, Italy, [5]Utrecht University, The Netherlands, 6Universidad de Zaragoza, Spain, 7Università di Palermo, Italy, 8Justus-Liebig-Universität, Giessen, Germany, 9The Norwegian School of Veterinary Science, Oslo, Norway, 10University of Berne, Switzerland, 11INRA, Jouy en Josas, France, 12Danish Institute of Agricultural Science, Tjele, Denmark.*

Within the EU RESGEN project, we have used the high throughput AFLP technology, to estimate genetic diversity within and between 29 European cattle breeds from Norway, Sweden, Denmark, UK, The Netherlands France, Switzerland, Spain, and Italy. Three highly polymorphic primer pairs revealed 146 AFLP polymorphisms that were binary scored as dominant markers. Multivariate analyses based on Reynolds distance grouped the breeds in three clusters according to their geographic origin: Cluster 1 comprised breeds from Scandinavia, North-East Europe and Channel Islands; cluster 2 comprised all breeds from Central Europe, including Italian breeds from the Alps; cluster 3 comprised all breeds from Central and Southern Italy and Spain. A PCOOA close-up on 16 Italian breeds confirms the strong North-South gradient of genetic distances.

Theatre G2.4

Molecular genetics of behaviour: research strategies and perspectives for animal production

P. Mormède. Laboratoire de Neurogénétique et Stress, INRA, Université Victor Segalen Bordeaux 2, 33077 Bordeaux, France.

Variability of behavioural traits usually results from the influence of numerous genes interacting with each other and with environmental factors. Therefore it would be of interest to know the molecular bases of genetic variation, to improve the efficiency of selection for desirable traits or to eliminate unwanted phenotypes. We can learn from research in laboratory animals the strategies to uncover the genes involved in variation of behavioural traits. The quantitative trait loci (QTL) approach investigates linkage between trait variation and genetic markers in a segregating population (usually an intercross or backcross between two strains contrasting for the trait under study). It allows the detection of genomic regions influencing that trait, and further investigation aims at the identification of the gene(s) located in each of these regions and the molecular polymorphisms involved in phenotypic variation. Available examples show that the mode of inheritance is usually complex, and marker-assisted selection allows the dissection of the trait by its genetic influences.

The examples in farm animal species are still rare, and the success of these approaches will depend on the careful definition of behavioural traits to be studied, and on the efficient mastering of environmental factors. The fast increase in the knowledge of genomic sequences across species will undoubtedly facilitate the application to farm animal species of the knowledge obtained in model organisms.

Theatre G2.5

Mapping of QTL involved in feather pecking behaviour in laying hens

A.J. Buitenhuis[1,], T.B. Rodenburg[2], M. Siwek[1], S.J.B. Cornelissen[1], M.G.B. Nieuwland[3], R.P.M.A. Crooijmans[1], M.A.M. Groenen[1], P. Koene[2], H. Bovenhuis[1] and J.J. van der Poel[1], [1]Animal Breeding and Genetics Group, [2]Ethology Group, [3]Adaptation Physiology Group, Wageningen Institute of Animal Sciences, Wageningen University, Marijkeweg 40, NL-6709 PG Wageningen, The Netherlands.*

Feather pecking (FP) in large group housing systems is a major problem. This behaviour results in denuded areas and wounds of the bird and can ultimately result in cannibalistic behaviour. To date, there is no adequate way to relieve the FP problem, except for beak-trimming. This is, however, not an animal friendly method. It has been shown that a genetic component for FP behaviour exists and that breeding for reduced FP behaviour is feasible. To identify the genes involved in FP behaviour, birds from an F_2 population coming from a cross between two commercial laying lines were characterised for FP behaviour. In addition, these birds were genotyped for 180 micro-satellite markers. Recently, QTL were detected for gentle FP (a mild form of FP) and severe FP (form of FP causing most damage) in adult hens. The QTL identified involved in FP behaviour opens the possibility to relieve the FP problem in practice by breeding techniques. This is of special interest since the EU legislation concerning animal welfare, will prohibit beak-trimming.

Theatre G2.6

Genetic background of maternal behaviour, and its relation to offspring survival

K. Grandinson. Dept. of Animal Breeding and Genetics, Swedish Univ. Agric. Sci., Funbo-Lövsta, 755 97 Uppsala, Sweden.*

Maternal behaviour is becoming increasingly important in animal production. Selection for increased litter size at birth in pigs and sheep put higher demands on the ability of dams to raise large litters. In pig production, the use of loose-housing systems for lactating sows increases the importance of good maternal behaviour. Extensive production systems, e.g. ecological farming and outdoor production, where there is a small degree of supervision of the animals, also leave a greater responsibility with the mother to care for her young. The environment provided by the dam is important for the survival and growth of the offspring in many species. Several behaviour traits of the mother play a role for the offspring's chances of survival and a good start in life. Examples of such behaviour traits are responsiveness towards signals from the offspring (pigs), aggressive behaviour towards the offspring (pigs, sheep), nursing behaviour (pigs, sheep, mice) and fear behaviour (pigs, sheep). Some of these traits are in part genetically controlled, and thus possible to improve by selection. Behaviour traits are, however, often difficult to observe and record on a large scale. By studying behaviour we can gain further understanding about factors affecting survival of the young, and increase our chances to improve maternal behaviour. Improved maternal behaviour would increase the welfare for both mother and young.

Theatre G2.7

Behavioural differences in lactating females in a long-term selection experiment for litter size in mice

W.M. Rauw, L. Gomez Raya, L. Varona and J.L. Noguera, Area de Producció Animal, Centre UdL-IRTA, Av. Alc. Rovira Roure 177, 25198 Lleida, Spain.*

Previous studies showed that non-reproductive adult female mice of a line selected for high litter size at birth (S-line, average of 20 pups per litter) had higher residual food intake (RFI), and higher activity levels in response to a novel environment than female mice of a non-selected control line (C-line, average of 10 pups per litter). Furthermore, during lactation, S-line females had lower RFI than C-line females. The present study investigated activity levels in response to a Runway and an Open-Field in female mice at peak lactation (2 wk in lactation). Lactating females took more time before entering the Runway and ran more slowly than non-lactating females. Lactating S-line females took less time before entering the Runway and ran faster than lactating C-line females. There are no significant differences between the lines in the number of squares crossed in 60 seconds in the Open-Field test. Lactating S-line females crossed a higher number of squares in the middle of the Open-Field than lactating C-line females. The results show that the lower RFI in S-line females during lactation as found in a previous study can not be explained by a lower level of activity in response to a novel environment.

Theatre G2.8

Genetic co-variation in aggression and mothering ability of sows

P. Løvendahl, L.H. Damgaard, B.L. Nielsen, K. Thodberg, K. Skovgaard and G. Su, Danish Institute of Agricultural Sciences, Research Centre Foulum, P.O. Box 50, DK 8830 Tjele, Denmark.

Genetic selection could be used to reduce aggression between sows housed in groups, and to improve mothering ability of sows if the heritabilites of these traits are sufficiently large. This study was designed to estimate genetic variation in aggressive behaviour between sows grouped in pens, and for the same sows their maternal ability recorded as response to vocalisation from their piglets when these were handled by an intruding person. The study included 823 sows observed for number of mild or severe aggressions initiated (AM, AS) for 30 minutes after being penned with seven other sows. Mothering ability was studied in 979 sows as a body-reaction (MBR) and a sound-reaction (MSR) to their piglets being handled on day 3-5 after farrowing. Genetic co-variances were estimated using a multi-trait animal model, assuming traits to be Gaussian. The heritability of aggression traits was intermediate (h^2 AM = 0.21 se 0.11, h^2 AS = 0.27 se 0.10), but heritability of mothering ability traits was lower (h^2 MBR = 0.11 se 0.08; h^2 MSR = 0.09 se 0.07). The genetic correlations between Aggression traits and mothering ability traits were genetically correlated, so that more aggressive sows were also stronger responding mothers. We conclude that aggression in sows is a heritable trait, when aggressive encounters between sows are recorded for the first 30 minutes after being penned together, but selection against aggression may decrease mothering ability as a correlated effect.

Theatre G2.9

Optimising selection in groups with interactions among animals

P. Bijma, Animal Breeding and Genetics Group, Wageningen University, P.O. Box 338, 6700 AH Wageningen, The Netherlands.

When animals are kept in groups, performance of an individual may depend not only on its own merit (called "direct effect"), but also on characteristics of its group mates (so-called "associate effects"). For example, survival of a hen depends on its own genetic merit for survival but also on genetic merit for feather-pecking of its cage mates. Thus, a single phenotype may be affected by multiple breeding values for different traits. Selection experiments in poultry support this expectation.

A bivariate pseudo-BLUP selection index was developed, with the aim to quantify benefits of accounting for associate effects in breeding programs and to study the optimum design of breeding programs in cases where associate effects are important. First results indicate that accounting for associate effects may considerably increase selection response. When ignoring associate effects, it may be difficult to achieve response when direct and associate effects are correlated unfavourably.

Theatre G2.10

Direct and maternal genetic effects on behavior in German Shepherd dogs in Sweden

E. Strandberg[1], J. Jacobsson[1] and P. Saetre[2]. [1]Dept. of Animal Breeding and Genetics, Swedish Univ. Agric. Sci.PO Box 7023, 75007 Uppsala, Sweden, [2]Dept. of Evolutionary Biology, Uppsala Univ., Norbyv. 18 D, 752 36 Uppsala , Sweden.*

Data from 5959 1-2 year-old German Shepherd dogs tested 1989-2001 in the Swedish Dog Mentality Assessment were used to study the genetic (co)variation in behavior. The dogs were exposed to several test situations, in which the intensity of their reactions were scored according to a standardized score sheet. Factor analysis on the 16 subtests revealed 4 main factors, named 1) Curiosity/Fearlessness; 2) Playfulness; 3) Chase-proneness and 4) Aggressiveness. These four traits were analysed using a model containing fixed effects of sex, test protocol (somewhat changed in 1997), month, year, age, and judge, and random effects of litter, dam and animal, the latter two being genetic effects. A multivariate animal model was run to get genetic correlations among traits. The first three traits were moderately highly genetically correlated (around 0.4) with each other, whereas their correlations with aggression were lower (0.14-0.28). Direct heritability estimates were 10-24%, maternal heritability estimates were generally 2-3%, and the direct-maternal correlations were -0.03 to -0.36. Litter variance ratios were 3-10%. A new trait, tentatively named Boldness, consisting of the first three traits, had higher direct heritability (35%) than any of the three component traits, and had a relatively low genetic correlation with aggression (0.22).

Theatre G2.11

The heritability of harmful social behaviour and clinical tail biting in pigs

K. Breuer[1], M.E.M. Sutcliffe[2], J.T. Mercer[3], K.A. Rance[4], N.E. O'Connell[5], I.A. Sneddon[6], S.A. Edwards[1], [1]University of Newcastle, School of Agriculture, Newcastle upon Tyne NE1 7RU, UK., [2]Rattlerow Farms Ltd, [3]Independent Breeding Consultants, [4]University of Aberdeen, [5]Agricultural Research Institute of Northern Ireland, [6]Queens University Belfast.*

Harmful social behaviours in pigs have serious detrimental consequences for both animal welfare and production economics. A 12 month study on a nucleus pig breeding farm, with full pedigree data on each animal, analysed heritabilities of different behavioural traits using DFREML methodology. In a structured experiment, behavioural observations were made on 1011 purebred Landrace (LR) pigs at 7, 14 and 21 weeks of age. Total pig directed behaviour, analysed as a continuous variable, showed a heritability of 0.14 ±0.03, 0.10 ±0.03 and 0.11 ±0.03 respectively. The low frequency data for individual behavioural components were treated as binary data. These heritability estimates were significant but low (0.05-0.20) for most traits, equivalent to 0.1-0.3 when transformed to an underlying continuous distribution. 295 animals (2.8% of Large White and 3.5% of LR, $P<0.10$) in the total farm population were identified as clinical tail biters. For LW, this heritability did not differ from zero. For LR, heritability as a 1-0 trait was estimated as 0.05 ±0.02 ($P<0.05$), equivalent to 0.27 when transformed to an underlying continuous distribution. Tail biting was genetically correlated positively to lean tissue growth rate ($r=0.27$, $P<0.05$) and negatively to backfat thickness at 90 kg ($r=0.28$, $P<0.05$). The low but significant heritability of performance of harmful social behavior offers the possibility of reducing risk of vice outbreaks by selective breeding. This study was funded by the UK Department for Environment, Food and Rural Affairs.

Poster G2.12

Learning behavior - a model and a simulation of a selection experiment

G. Dietl, G. Nürnberg. Forschungsinstitut für die Biologie landwirtschaftlicher Nutztiere, Forschungsbereich Genetik und Biometrie, Wilhelm-Stahl-Allee 2, D-18196 Dummerstorf, Germany*

Farm animal welfare is relevant for an accepted and economic production. Learning behavior can be an important indicator for it. It shows, whether an animal is too burdened or unchallenged by the housing conditions. Learning behavior is genetically determined and it is subject of selective processes. A quantitative genetic model was developed for visual differentiation tasks (choice of the positive stimulus out of 4 offered ones). The model includes the two variables probability of a successful choice (y) and the learning ability (x). Both are connected by a logistic function. The variable x was postulated as the sum of the animals breeding value and the environmental effect. On that basis the marginal distribution of y could be found and the binominal probability for z successful choices of n attempts was given. The simulation was adapted to a population with 36 goats, divergently selected and positive assortativ mated in overlapping generations. The selection responses and the power of their tests were estimated. The results show clear upward and downward selection responses. In ten half-years, y increases from 0.65 to 0.77 as well as decreases to 0.50 in its downward direction. The power of the test of the difference (27 %) against zero was 0.97. Consequently, it is possible to generate subpopulations with different learning abilities in approximately 5 years.

Theatre G3.1

Statistical dissection of quantitative trait variation attributable to bovine chromosome 20

J. Szyda[1,2], *S. Viitala*[3] *and J. Vilkki*[3], [1]*Department of Animal Genetics, Agricultural University of Wroclaw, Kozuchowska 7, 51-631 Wroclaw, Poland,* [2]*United Datasystems for Animal Production (VIT), Heideweg 1, 27-283 Verden, Germany,* [3]*Animal Production Research, MTT, 31600 Jokioinen, Finland.*

The bovine chromosome 20 is already known to host QTL that are responsible for a considerable proportion of quantitative variation of milk production traits. The main goal of our research was to better understand the genetic structure underlying this variation.
For that purpose, following a grand daughter design, a sample of 796 bulls belonging to 23 paternal half sib families were ascertained out of the Finnish Ayrshire population. Each bull and its sire were genotyped for five molecular polymorphisms located within putative candidate genes. The genotypic value of bulls was represented by daughter yield deviations for the 1st and for the later lactations respectively, originated from the 2002 national genetic evaluation.
Several statistical models containing a random polygenic component and a component for modelling the effects of the five polymorphisms were then applied to the data. Comparisons of models differing in terms of statistical description of the non-polygenic component made it possible to test hypotheses on the effects of particular polymorphisms on each of 10 milk production traits studied as well as their interactions.
As a result we observe significant effects of two of the five sites considered. One predominantly affects yields while the other - contents of fat and protein.

Theatre G3.2

Power to discriminate two linked QTL in crossbred populations

H. Gilbert and P. Le Roy, Station de Génétique Quantitative et Appliquée, Institut National de la Recherche Agronomique, 78352 Jouy-en-Josas, France.*

We calculated the power to discriminate two linked QTL from one QTL, based on simulated data. Each QTL determined two traits. The multitrait method was based on a univariate analysis of a linear combination of the traits specific to the couple of tested positions. The linear combination was calculated by a discriminate analysis based on the groups of progeny determined from the couples of haplotypes that they received from their sire at the tested couple of positions.
The designs depended on the distance between the QTL (5, 15, 25, 35 cM) and the density of the genetic map (one marker per 5, 10, 30, 60 cM). The genetic map was 60 cM-long, and the middle of interval between the QTL corresponded to the middle of the map.
When no genetic marker was between the QTL, only the QTL separated by more than 20 cM could be distinguished (in more than 30% of the cases), but this power was not improved until 2 genetic markers were located between the QTL. On the contrary, when the QTL were closer than 20 cM, a great increase of power appeared when at least 1 marker was between the QTL.
It seems that, when the QTL are close enough, the challenge would be to use a genetic marker located between the two locus. When they are distant enough, a good level of power can be reached at the minimum map density generally used.

Theatre G3.3

A method for the analysis of cDNA microarray data

W.W. Kuurman, M.H. Pool, B. Engel, W.G. Buist and L.L.G Janss, Institute for Animal Science and Health, ID-Lelystad, P.O. Box 65, 8200 AB Lelystad, The Netherlands.*

Expression levels for large numbers of genes under different conditions can be measured by using microarrays. In the last few years several statistical methods have been proposed to analyse microarray data, so as to detect genes that are differentially expressed under different conditions. Currently available methods for analysis of microarray data potentially have two drawbacks. First, most methods are devised for oligo-arrays where two samples are measured on different slides, which may not be appropriate for cDNA arrays where two samples are measured on the same slide. Second, in general is the analysis divided in two parts; 1) normalisation and 2) computation and testing of statistics for the expression levels.

In the proposed method, both the normalisation and the computation part are considered integral parts of each other. The proposed method deals with issues such as; variability among gene expression levels, correlation between the difference and the mean of expression levels, correlated observations, multiple testing and the false discovery rate using permutation.

The proposed method was tested with both simulated and real data, and compared to currently available methods, such as the linear mixed model of Wolfinger *et al.* (J. Comput. Biol. 8:625-637, 2001) and the significance analysis of microarrays, a non-parametric method, of Tucher *et al.* (Proc. Natl. Acad. Sci. USA 98:5116-5121, 2001).

Theatre G3.4

SCC, clinical mastitis and milk yield in improving udder health

M. Koivula, E. Negussie, E.A. Mäntysaari, MTT, Agrifood Research Finland, Animal Production Research, FIN-31600 Jokioinen, Finland*

Clinical studies have suggested that breeding for lower somatic cell count (SCC) would be risky when improving mastitis resistance. This paper studies, whether cows with originally lower SCC are more susceptible to clinical mastitis (CM), and how CM and SCC are correlated with milk yield. The data was extracted from the Finnish national milk-recording database and from health recording system. It comprised first and second lactation of 87,861 Ayrshire cows, calving between January 1998 and December 2000. Traits used in the study were conceptual CM (CCM), SCC before and after the CCM, milk sample before and after the CCM. CCM was defined as 1 if cow had been treated for CM and 0 otherwise. Altogether we had ten traits in analysis. Genetic parameters were estimated using multi-trait REML with a sire model. Model included the fixed effect of calving age; the fixed effect of calving season by calving year interaction; the fixed effect of herd; regression of days in milk on trait; random sire additive genetic effect, and the residual effect. Results suggested that cows with genetically low SCC are genetically less susceptible to CM. The genetic correlation between milk and SCC was on average 0.13 in the first lactation but only -0.06 in the second lactation. Thus our result suggest that SCC is a good indicator of mastitis and useful tool in selection of mastitis resistance.

Theatre G3.5

Multivariate threshold model analysis of clinical mastitis in multiparous Norwegian cattle

B. Heringstad[1], Y.M. Chang[2], D. Gianola[1,2] and G. Klemetsdal[1]. [1]Department of Animal Science, Agricultural University of Norway, P.O. Box 5025, N-1432 Ås, Norway; [2]Department of Dairy Science, University of Wisconsin, Madison, USA*

A Bayesian multivariate threshold model was fitted to clinical mastitis (CM) records from 285,947 daughters of 1913 Norwegian Cattle (NRF) sires. All cases of veterinary treated CM from 30 days before first calving to culling or 300 days after third calving were included. Lactations were divided into four intervals: (-30-0), (1,30), (31-120), and (121-300) days after calving. Within each interval, absence or presence of CM was scored as "0" or "1' based on the CM episodes. A 12-variate (3 lactations x 4 periods) threshold model assumed that CM was a different trait in each interval. Residuals were correlated within lactation, but independent between lactations. The model for liability to CM had effects of month-year of calving, age at calving (first lactation) or calving interval (second and third lactation), herd-5-year-period, sire of the cow plus a residual. Posterior mean of heritability of liability to CM was 0.09 and 0.04 in the first and last intervals, respectively, and 0.06-0.07 for other intervals. Posterior means of genetic correlations of liability to CM between intervals ranged from 0.32 to 0.67. Residual correlations ranged from 0.09 to 0.18 for adjacent intervals, and between -0.01 and 0.03 for non-adjacent intervals.

Theatre G3.6

Genotype by environment interaction between automatic and conventional milking systems for production traits and SCS

H.A. Mulder[1], A.F. Groen[1], G. de Jong[2] and P. Bijma[1], [1]Animal Breeding and Genetics Group, Wageningen Institute of Animal Sciences (WIAS), Wageningen University, PO Box 338, 6700 AH Wageningen, The Netherlands, [2]CR Delta, PO Box 454, 6800 AL Arnhem, The Netherlands.*

The objective of this study was to quantify genotype by environment interaction between farms with and without automatic milking systems (AMS), for milk, fat and protein yield and for somatic cell score (SCS). Genetic correlations were estimated in two ways: (1) between farms with and without AMS in the same time period, and (2) within farms between the period before and after introduction of the AMS. Multivariate fixed regression test-day models were used to estimate variance components.
Genetic correlations between farms with and without AMS in the same time period were 0.93, >0.99, 0.98 and 0.79 for respectively milk yield, fat yield, protein yield and SCS. Genetic correlations within farms between the period before and after introduction of the AMS were somewhat different: 0.89, 0.91, 0.87 and >0.99 for respectively milk yield, fat yield, protein yield and SCS. Variances were higher with AMS, especially the residual variance. Therefore, heritability was lower with AMS. It was concluded that genotype by environment interaction was small between automatic and conventional milking systems. A correction for heterogeneity of variance is needed to account for the differences in variances.

Theatre G3.7

Nonparametric analysis of the relationship between performance and inbreeding in Jersey Cows with varying amounts of pedigree information

D. Gulisija[1], D. Gianola[1] and K.A. Weigel[1], [1]Department of Dairy Science, University of Wisconsin-Madison, USA.*

Under dominance, the relationship between a quantitative trait and the inbreeding coefficient (F) should be linear. This is not so if interactions between dominance effects exist. Relationships between yield traits and somatic cell score (SCS) and F were examined via local regression. First lactation records from 139,836, 125,306 and 63,076 Jersey cows having at least 2, 4 or 6 generations of known pedigree, respectively, were used. F ranged between 0 and 33.3% (medians were 4.5, 4.6 and 5.3% for the three groups). LOWESS regressions of BLUP residuals on F were calculated for each trait (BLUP model included herd-year-season, age at calving, days in milk and additive genetic effects). Several spanning parameters and local polynomials were explored. The relationship between BLUP residuals and inbreeding was complex and nonlinear. Yields did not decrease for F up to 7%, and there was no additional depression for F beyond 20%. Curves for cows with at least 6 generations of pedigree and F > 15 suggested a smaller decrease. For SCS, LOWESS curves were flat, suggesting additive action. Effects of inbreeding on performance seem more complex than what is suggested by quantitative genetics theory.

Theatre G3.8

The relationship among ascites related traits, feed efficiency traits and carcass traits in broilers

A. Pakdel,[1] J.A.M. Van Arendonk,[1] A.L.J. Vereijken,[2] and H. Bovenhuis[1], [1]Animal Breeding and Genetics Groups, Wageningen Institute of Animal Sciences, PO Box 338, 6700 AH Wageningen, The Netherlands, [2]Nutreco Breeding Research Center, P.O. Box 220, 5830 AE, Boxmeer, The Netherlands.*

Ascites is a growth-related disorder of broilers that occurs more often in fast growing birds and at low temperature conditions. This study was conducted to determine the relationship among ascites-related traits (AS-traits) measured under cold and normal conditions and performance traits measured under normal conditions. Three different experiments were set up to measure AS-traits (4202 birds), feed efficiency (2166 birds) and carcass traits (2036 birds), respectively. All the birds in different experiments originated from the same group of parents, which enables the estimation of genetic correlations among different traits. The positive genetic correlation between body weight at 7 weeks of age measured under normal conditions and the ratio of right to total ventricular weight (RV:TV) measured under cold conditions (0.30) indicate that birds with higher genetic potential for growth rate are more susceptible to ascites syndrome. In addition the low and non-significant genetic correlation between residual feed intake and ascites indicator traits like RV:TV (-0.16) suggest that more efficient birds are not necessarily more susceptible to ascites syndrome.

Theatre G3.9

Genome scan for QTL to antibody response to SRBC in laying hens

M. Siwek[1], S.J.B. Cornelissen[1], M.G.B. Nieuwland[2], A.J. Buitenhuis[1], H.Bovenhuis[1], J.J.van der Poel[1], H.K.Parmentier[2], R.P.M. Crooijmans[1], M.A.M. Groenen[1], [1]Animal Breeding and Genetics Group, [2]Adaptation Physiology Group, Wageningem Insitute of Animal Sciences, Wageningen University, P.O. Box 338, NL-6700AH Wageningen, The Netherlands.*

The aim of this study is to identify QTL associated with antibody response to SRBC. The experimental F2 population originates from a cross (ISA Warren) between two divergently selected lines for either high (H line) or low (L line) primary antibody response to sheep red blood cells (SRBC) at 5 weeks of age. For the QTL experiment reciprocal crosses have been made to produce 680 F2 animals. Primary antibody response to SRBC, secondary antibody response to SRBC and response to SRBCIgG have been determined. For the genotypic analysis a Genome Scan has been performed using 174 microsatellite markers, equally distributed over the chicken genome, approximately 20 centiMorgan apart. A paternal half-sib and a line-cross analysis model were used to detect QTL involved in antibody response to selection criterion (primary response to SRBC), SRBC secondary and SRBCIgG. QTL detected using half-sib analysis and line-cross analysis model are at different locations. There is only marginal overlap in QTL regions for these antibody responses. These results suggest that different genes are involved in SRBC primary, SRBC secondary and SRBCIgG immune response. Experiments are in progress to improve the (comparative) gene maps in QTL regions.

Theatre G3.10

Assessment of the dynamics and control of microparasite infection in livestock populations by genetic epidemiological modelling

M. Nath, J.A. Woolliams and S.C. Bishop, Roslin Institute (Edinburgh), Roslin, Midlothian EH25 9PS, United Kingdom.*

A stochastic genetic epidemic model was developed and used to assess the relative importance of different genetic control strategies and the effect of genetic structure of the host population in controlling the transmission of microparasitic (viral or bacterial) infection. A genetically homogenous population and a heterogeneous population (comprising three genotypes corresponding to one locus with two alleles), both with 1000 individuals, were considered. A compartmental stochastic epidemic model was used to simulate epidemic dynamics, varying the parameters describing the transmission coefficient, rate of latency, recovery rate, mortality rate and the rate of loss of immunity. The critical parameters influencing the transmission of infection, hence disease incidence, were the transmission coefficient, the latency period and? the recovery rate, whereas the rate of loss of immunity had only trivial effects. Epidemic severities were generally similar in the homogeneous and heterogeneous population, however the heterogeneous population may contain some particularly susceptible animals with little impact on disease risk. By equating the disease transmission parameters with measured traits, the model can be used to identify which disease resistance genes or QTL will be truly effective in helping to develop disease-resistant stocks that suffer fewer epidemics and side effects of infection. It can also help in formulating appropriate genetic control strategies for reducing the incidence of disease in livestock populations.

Poster G3.11

The effect of feeding intensity on telomere length in Holstein heifers -a twin study-

T. Skibbe[1], T. von Zglinicki[2], P. Reinecke[1], U. Müller[1], [1]Humboldt University of Berlin, Institute for Animal Sciences, Philippstr. 13, G-10115 Berlin, [2]General Hospital Newcastle, Institute for the Health of the Elderly, Westgate Road, Newcastle upon Tyne, NE4 6BE, England

Telomeres are some kind of a biological clock in somatic cells and are the repetitive DNA sequences at the end of the chromosomes. These TTAGGG sequence of mammals are important in maintaining the integrity of chromosomes by providing protection against degradation and fusion events as well as anchoring chromosomes to the nuclear matrix. Telomeres shorten with each round of cell division and the length of telomeres decreases in normal human somatic tissues with aging in vivo and with culture in vitro.
In this study we analyze the development of telomeres in lymphocytes of twin heifers. Data from 15 female twin pairs, which were seperated in two differrent feeding groups, were used. The telomeres were collected in a specific period from the first week of life to the 75th week. The detection of the telomeres length were measured by help of the telomere length assay.
The results shown a decrease of 1484 bp in the intensive group and 1649bp in the restriktive group between the first and the 75th week. This decrease was significant in both groups. Furthermore a significant difference was not observed in the telomere length between the both feeding groups.

Poster G3.12

Meiotic stages and incidence of diploid oocytes in Egyptian cattle and buffaloes

Karima Gh.M. Mahmoud, Dept. anim. Reprod. & A.I., National Research Center, Dokki, Cairo, Egypt

The present work describes a cytogenetic study of in vitro matured oocytes from cattle and buffalo to analyze the meiotic stages, to determine the incidence of diploid metaphase II and to evaluate the in vitro maturation progress. Oocytes were collected by aspiration from ovaries of slaughtered buffalo and cattle. A total of 721 cattle and 989 buffalo oocytes were selected for in vitro maturation. The occytes were matured in droplets of maturation medium (TCM-199 medium supplemented with 10% fetal calf serum, 50 ml antibiotic) for two periods 21-24 hrs and 25-28 hrs at 39%C? in 5% CO_2 incubator. Cytogenetic analysis of in vitro matured oocytes revealed that 74.38%, 89.74% in cattle and 75%, 86.93% in buffalo matured at period of 21-24 hrs and 25-28 hrs respectively. The cattle oocytes matured earlier than buffalo oocytes. At period 25-28 hrs there was no any immature oocytes in cattle, but in buffalo, there were 6.53% metaphase I and 2.01% anaphase I satges still immature. The cattle diploid metaphase II increased from 6.15% to 11.7% in the first and second period, while in buffalo the percentage was nearly the same (5.17% and 5.88%). The possible factors that may lead to the formation of diploid M II oocytes observed under in vitro maturation procedure are discussed.

Poster G3.13

Sex ratio and freemartinism in Chios sheep

C. Papachristoforou[1], A.P. Mavrogenis[1], P. Toumazos[2], A. Hadjicostis[2] and M.A. Furguson-Smith[3], [1]Agricultural Research Institute, P.O.Box 22016, Lefkosia, Cyprus, [2]Department of Veterinary Services, Athalassa, 1417, Lefkosia, Cyprus,[3]Department of Clinical Veterinary Medicine, Cambridge University, Madingley Rd, CB3 0ES, Cambridge, UK.*

In the prolific Chios sheep breed, the sex ratio and the incidence of freemartins were investigated using records of 8382 lambs from 4420 parturitions. The number of single lambs was 1396, of twins 4512, of triplets 1857, of quadruplets 512 and of quintuplets 105. The overall sex ratio of 0,494 did not deviate from 0,5, while among singles (0,529) and among twins plus multiples (0,487) differed (P<0,05) from normal. The number of hermaphrodites recorded was 7 and all of them were from multiple litters (5 triplets, one quadruplet, and one quintuplet) with at least one male littermate. The number of such sets was 591 with 1033 F and a sex ratio of 0,46 (P<0,01). The karyotypes of two hermaphrodites born in 2000, showed mosaicism for XX and XY cells confirming the hypothesis that they were freemartins. The possibility of freemartinism is therefore 7/1033 or 0,678% and the incidence is 7/8382 (0,084%). At a young age they looked phenotypically as females but as they grew, they developed male characteristics. They were slaughtered at 11 months of age and examination of the internal genitalia revealed development of testes and male accessory glands and regression of ovaries and of the Mullerian duct system. Circulating testosterone concentrations (nmol/L) were 1,3 to 2,9 in one lamb and 4,1 to 7,3 in the other, while progesterone was less than 2,0 nmol/L.

Poster G3.14

Completion of the hamster-sheep somatic cell hybrids panel characterization by new DNA markers

R. Aït Yahia[1], A. Derrar[1], N. Tabet Aoul[1], N. Boussehaba[1], A. Eggen[2], F. Lantier[3], K. Tabet Aoul[2] and N. Saïdi-Mehtar[1], [1]Laboratoire de Biologie Moléculaire et Génétique Université d'Oran, CRSTRA, Algeria. [2]Laboratoire de Génétique Biochimique et de cytogénétique, Département de génétique Animale, INRA, 78352 Jouy-en-Josas, France. [3]Laboratoire de Pathologie Infectieuse et Immunologie, INRA-Tours, 37380 Nouzilly, France.*

A panel of 24 hamster-sheep somatic cell hybrids, previously obtained by Saïdi-Mehtar and al., 1981, was investiged for sheep gene mapping. A first subchromosomal characterization of this panel showed that ovine chromosomes were fragmented into 130 regions defining segments with variable length (Tabet-Aoul and al., 2000).

Using data available from ruminant maps (sheep, cattle, and goat), we have selected 115 new DNA markers (23 genes and 92 microsatellites) and have analyzed them by PCR using ovine, bovine or caprine primers. The results added 25 markers (8 genes and 17 microsatellites) on 16 different sheep chromosomes. This study provided indications about presence of new break-points on eight ovine autosomes. Consequently, 14 new fragments were defined, increasing the total number of chromosome fragments to 144.

Break-points can be correlated with evolutianary sites; further study will permit to establish relationship between them and regions of chromosome fragility. Identification of these regions will be performed by using sheep radiation hybrid panel.

Poster G3.15

Amplification conditions and multiplex suitability of microsatellite markers from a genome scan in Landrace pigs

S. Schwarz[1], N. Reinsch[1,2], and E. Kalm[1]. [1]Institut für Tierzucht und Tierhaltung,Christian-Albrechts-Universität, D-24098 Kiel,Germany, [2]Forschungsinstitut für die Biologie landwirtschaftlicher Nutztiere, D-18196 Dummerstorf, Germany*

Microsatellites are widely used to perform linkage studies and parentage testing in pigs as well as in other animals. Genotyping work can substantially be reduced by using multiplex PCR, i.e. joint amplification of several microsatellites. However, and in contrast to other species, little has been published on specific multiplex-sets of porcine microsatellites and their PCR conditions.
As a by-product of a whole genome scan in purebred Landrace families we present information on 142 porcine microsatellites, covering all chromosomes with an average marker spacing of 15 cM. In total 96 of these markers were amplified in 45 different multiplex-sets (duplex and triplex reactions) and 46 markers were amplified alone. A Biometra UNO II thermocycler was used for PCR, markers were labelled with fluorescent dyes and marker sets were optimised for separating the amplification products on an ABI 377 sequencer by choosing markers according to fragment length. Details of PCR conditions, observed fragment lengths in Landrace and allele frequencies are given and it is shown in detail, which microsatellites have been combined together. These informations may serve as an aid for the development of more complex multiplex sets, comprising a higher number of simultaneously amplified microsatellites.

Poster G3.16

Phylogenetic relationships among indigenous cattle breeds of Pakistan based on random amplified polymorphic DNA (RAPD) analysis

M.S. Rehman[1], Z. Ahmad[1], M.S. Khan[1] and Y. Zafar[2], [1]Department of Animal Breeding and Genetics, University of Agriculture, Faisalabad, Pakistan, [2]National Institute for Biotechnology and Genetic Engineering, Faisalabad, Pakistan.*

Phylogenetic relationships among ten indigenous cattle breeds of Pakistan viz., Sahiwal, Red Sindhi, Cholistani, Dajal, Dhanni, Rojhan, Lohani, Hissar, Hariana and Tharparkar were assessed using RAPD assay. The genomic DNA bulks were surveyed using 80 arbitrary sequence primers. Of the 80 random decamer primers, screened for their capability of amplifying DNA bulks via the polymerase chain reaction (PCR), 73 generated a total of 604 DNA fragments, with an average of about 8.2 bands per primer. Sixty-eight bands were polymorphic indicating 11.25 % of DNA variation among breeds. The primer OPF-07 could distinguish all breeds without the aid of other primers. The dendrogram obtained using unweighted pair group method of arithmetic means (UPGMA) revealed two main clusters. Hissar, Hariana and Tharparkar breeds were grouped together as cluster A. In the second cluster (B) Cholistani was grouped with Dajal and Rojhan (B_1), Dhanni with Lohani (B_2) and Sahiwal with Red Sindhi (B_3). This indicates that indigenous cattle of Pakistan only recently diverged from each other. However, the results should be interpreted with caution, as the genetic constitutions of these breeds appeared to be highly similar.

Poster G3.17

Evaluation of the genetic diversity in three "*Bos Genus*" populations by microsatellite markers

G. Ceriotti[1] , D. Marletta[2] , S. Conti[3] , C. Barone[4], [1]Dipartimento di Scienze e Tecnologie Veterinarie per la Sicurezza Alimentare, Milano, Italy, [2]DACPA Sezione di Scienze delle Produzioni Animali, Catania, Italy, [3]Dipartimento di Scienze Zootecniche dell'Università, Firenze, Italy, [4]Dipartimento di Scienze zootecniche e Ispezione Alimenti, Portici, Italy*

This study has been carried out within an Italian research project (Cofin 1999) aiming to knowledge, conservation and use of Italian animal germplasm for needs of urban and periurban livestock in hot climate.
The genetic variability of two *Bos indicus* populations reared in Western Africa (Azaouak and Adamawa Gudali) and one *Bos taurus* population reared in Southern Italy (Modicana) was evaluated by 30 microsatellite markers. All microsatellites were polymorphic in each breed. From eight to seventeen alleles were detected per locus. The total allele number among breeds ranged from 274 (Adamawa Gudali) to 234 (Modicana). The examination of allele frequencies revealed different and characteristic distribution in zebuine and taurine breeds. All populations showed high levels of heterozigosity ranging from 0.678 (Azaouak) to 0.750 (Modicana). The gene differentiation coefficient was low, only 7% of the diversity being among breeds and 93% within breeds. A dendrogram, constructed from the genetic distance matrix using Neighbor-Joining algorithm, separated clearly *Bos indicus* and *Bos taurus* populations in two clusters. Principal component analysis confirmed this observation.

Poster G3.18

A study on DNA Fingerprinting of the Native Cattle Breeds in Turkey by RAPD-PCR

Okan Ertugrul[1], Güven Güneren[1], Bilal Akyüz[2], [1]Ankara University, Faculty of Veterinary Medicine, Department of Genetics, Ankara, Turkey, [2]Erciyes University, Faculty of Veterinary Medicine, Department of Genetics, Kayseri, Turkey.*

The preliminary purpose of the study was to investigate the use of RAPD-PCR method in the native cattle breeds in Turkey by estimating the genetic variation within and between breeds. RAPD-PCR method was performed on total 77 animals from four breeds namely Anatolian Black (AB), East Anatolian Red (EAR), South Anatolian Red(SAR) and Turkish Gray(TG). In this method a set of 10 arbitrary 10-mer primers were used to find DNA polymorphism. Primers produced informative patterns of amplified DNA fragments revealing inter and intra-bred differences. Estimation of the distances between the breeds was performed by F_{ST} distant estimation method, and cluster trees were constructed by UPGMA method. Overall average of genetic variances were estimated among the breeds, based on the band sharing method varied from 0,637(in TG) to 0,809 (in SAR); AB and EAR had 0,792 and 0,787 respectively. Estimation of genetic relationships between the breeds revealed two clearly distinct groups of breeds: one was consisted of SAR, EAR and AB; EAR and AB breeds exhibited the closest genetic distance, while SAR was genetically distant from other two. The second group comprised Turkish Gray, which display a clear distinction from the other three breeds.

Poster G3.19

The Saving of Czech Red Cattle

J. Citek[1], V. Rehout[1], L. Panicke[2], [1]Southbohemian University, Dept. of Animal Breeding, Ceské Budejovice, Czech Republic, [2]Res Inst for the Biology of Farm Animals, 18196 Dummerstorf, W. Stahl-Allee 2, Germany*

The Czech Red cattle, an original breed raised in the Czech Republic vanished almost in the 20th century, the program of saving has been started. The goal of the project is to increase the number of pedigree animals. The absorptive crossing of Czech Spotted cows and Czech Red sires should help to enlarge the population. The number of purebred females has increased from 32 in 1992 to 56 in 2001. Involving purebred animals only, the effective population size is Ne=21.7, it is imperative to enlarge it to Ne=50. The average coefficient of inbreeding F in the population owned by the Southbohemian University (crosses and purebred animals) was 1.63, in females 1.32%. It is necessary to breed the population with the aim to rescue its genetic diversity and gene pool. The use of sires of phylogenetic related breeds seems to be of benefit. Furthermore, the genetic diversity was studied in Czech, Polish and German Red cattle, Czech Spotted, Czech Black and White, and German Black and White cattle. The Czech Red breed seems to be genetically somewhat distinct from the other red breeds. The distances at gene reserves were influenced by genetic drift. The genetic diversity of Czech Red cattle was relatively high considering that the breed survives for decades in restricted number.

Poster G3.20

Inbreeding trend and inbreeding depression for birth weight for the Swedish Charolais, Hereford and Simmental populations

A. Stål, S. Eriksson, A. Näsholm and W.F. Fikse, Dept. of Animal Breeding and Genetics, Swedish University of Agricultural Sciences, Box 7023, 75007 Uppsala, Sweden.*

High birth weight is associated with an increased risk at calving, but also with higher growth rate after birth. The few previous studies on inbreeding depression in beef breeds showed a decrease in birth weight with increased inbreeding coefficients. The aim of this study was to estimate the inbreeding trend and inbreeding depression for birth weight in the Swedish purebred Charolais, Hereford and Simmental populations. A coefficient for pedigree completeness (PEC) was calculated for each individual and dam. Birth weight was analysed separately for each breed with an animal model including direct and maternal effects and linear regressions on inbreeding coefficients nested within PEC-groups. Records were available for 62285 Charolais, 31078 Hereford and 18136 Simmental. The size of the populations increased during the studied period, and the inbreeding trends were flat. The average inbreeding coefficient for animals with at least four generations known (PEC >0.8) was lower than 1.4% for all breeds. With 1% increase in inbreeding of the individual, birth weight decreased by 0.06 kg for Charolais and Simmental and 0.04 kg for Hereford. The corresponding effect of inbreeding of dams was 0.04, 0.05 and 0.03 kg for Charolais, Simmental and Hereford, respectively. In the lowest PEC-groups there was a tendency for higher estimates of effect of inbreeding.

Poster G3.21

Introductory results of the survey on genetic separateness of White-back cattle

Z. Litwinczuk, W. Chabuz, P. Stanek and P. Jankowski, Department of Cattle Breeding, Agricultural University of Lublin, Akademicka 13, 20-950 Lublin, Poland

About 100 White-back cattle were localized and described. In 2001, blood was taken from 50 cows to examine genetic differentiation of these cattle. Characteristics of genetic differentiation of White-back cattle carried out in the Institute of Genetics and Animal Breeding in Jastrzebiec on the basis of the number of alleles showed that in the population of 50 cattle, in 26 analyzed loci of DNA micro satellites, 193 alleles were identified. The number of alleles in locus ranged from 2 (locus LSTS005) to 13 (locus TGLA and HEL), which indicates high genetic variability of these cattle. The evaluated White-back cows kept in small individual farms in Eastern Poland represented a similar type to that evaluated by Pajak nearly 50 years ago near Biebrza river. The results of milk protein polymorphism indicate that the frequency of rare genes, such as αs1- Cn C- amounted to 0.15; β- Cn B- 0.15 and κ-Cn B-0.50 and was significantly higher than cows from White-back mass population cows in the Lublin region.

Poster G3.22

Some milk trait characteristics in autochthonous Busha cattle (Bos taurus brachyceros) in Serbia and Montenegro

S. Jovanovic, M. Savic and R .Trailovic, Faculty of Veterinary Medicine, Belgrade, Bulevar JA 18, Serbia and Montenegro*

Busha is a native breed inhabiting mountain region of Balkan as a direct descendant of Bos Taurus brachyceros. Different bio geographic conditions on separate localities allowed development of different types within the breed. Though very adaptable to extremely poor living conditions, Busha population is in decrease for decades due to import of high producing cattle, depopulation trend of the countryside, or due to crossbreeding. A total of 24 animals morphologically identified as Busha, all very small (body weight around 300 kg) bred in satisfactory conditions were submitted to control of milk yield and milk composition.

Average milk yield in sample population was 2 430 l with 5.9 % of milk fat and 3.85% of milk protein. This milk traits, well known disease resistance, especially low frequency of mastitis (upon veterinary data) gives opportunity to use Busha cattle in organic farming in mountain region. Knowing the fact that Busha has never been submitted to planned selection, the data obtained indicates that this breed is having high selective potential for production of high quality milk. Therefore the measures for identification and preservation of remaining individuals on the territory of Serbia and Montenegro have been proposed within the project concerning evaluation and preservation of animal genetic resources.

Poster G3.23

Analysis of melanocortin receptor 1 (*MC1R*) gene polymorphisms in Reggiana bovine breed

V. Russo, L. Fontanesi, S. Dall'Olio, E. Scotti and R. Davoli, DIPROVAL, Sezione di Allevamenti Zootecnici, University of Bologna, Via F.lli Rosselli 107, 42100 Reggio Emilia, Italy.*

Mammalian pigmentation have been indicated to be influenced by several loci. The *extension* (*E*) locus, that has a major role in the regulation of black/brown versus red/yellow pigment synthesis, has been described to be associated to the melanocortin receptor 1 (*MC1R*) gene. In cattle, several mutations in the *MC1R* gene have been recently reported and some have been associated to the three main alleles at this locus with effect on coat colour: E^+, the wild type allele; E^D, that gives black coat colour; *e*, that produces red/yellow coat colour. Reggiana cattle breed has a typical red coat colour (*fromentino*). With the aim to identify DNA markers useful to differentiate the typical Parmigiano Reggiano cheese produced with milk of only Reggiana cows we analysed the *MC1R* gene. The polymorphisms that produce the three mentioned alleles were typed by PCR-RFLP in 135 Reggiana, 26 Italian Friesian and 35 Italian Brown cows. All the Reggiana animals were homozygous for the point deletion that causes allele *e*. Twenty-two Italian Friesian animals resulted E^D/E^D and 4 were E^D/e. All the Italian Brown cows were E^+/E^+. Considering the three bovine breeds studied, these first results may indicate that the *MC1R* polymorphisms could be used to differentiate the cheese produced with milk of only Reggiana cows.

Poster G3.24

Genetic diversity in wild and domestic goats investigated with AFLP markers

P. Ajmone Marsan[1], E. Milanesi[1], R. Negrini[1], P. Crepaldi[2], Y. Zagdsuren[3], O. Ertugrul[4], G. Luikart[5], P. Taberlet[5], [1]Istituto di Zootecnica, Università Cattolica del S. Cuore, 29100 Piacenza, Italy, [2]Istituto di Zootecnia Generale, Università degli Studi, 20100 Milano, Italy, [3]The Agriculture University of Mongolia, Ulambaatar City, Mongolia, [4]Faculty of Veterinary Science, Ankara University, Ankara, Turkey, [5]Laboratoire de Biologie des Populations d'Altitude, CNRS, Grenoble, France.*

A total of 133 AFLP markers have been used to investigate genetic diversity in 222 animals belonging to two wild *Capra* species (*C. ibex* and *C. aegagrus*) and to 9 breeds of domestic goat (*C. hircus*) from Asia (Anatolian Black, Angora, Mongolian Cashmer, Bayendelger Cashmer and Malaysian Native), Africa (West African Dwarf) and Europe (Val Passiria goat, Girgentana, Maltese). In *C. ibex* marker polymorphism and heterozygosity were lower than in *C. aegagrus* and in *C. hircus*. Almost 50% of the total variation at AFLP loci was found between species, while within *C. hircus* the variability at marker loci is mainly maintained within the 9 populations analysed. PCOOA based on Nei's Da distance clearly separates *C. ibex*, *C. aegagrus* and *C. hircus* into three separate groups. The Malaysian native population results half way between *C. aegagrus* and the most geographically distant domestic goat populations analysed. A high correlation ($r=0.75$, $P<0.01$) between genetic and geographic distance was observed within *C. hircus*.

Poster G3.25

Detection of SNPs between Chinese and European sheep breeds by DHPLC analysis

X. Li, L. Pariset, I. Cappuccio, and A. Valentini, Dipartimento di Produzioni Animali, Facoltà di Agraria, Università della Tuscia, Viterbo, Italy*

We applied a new generation markers, single nucleotide polymorphisms (SNPs), to the study of genetic diversity between Chinese and European sheep breeds. We developed an approach of genotyping by denaturing high-performance liquid chromatography (DHPLC), a method that allows a very efficient resolution of identically sized PCR products with a single nucleotide change.
We selected 8 Chinese and 7 Italian sheep breeds. Eight genes with different functions were randomly chosen for polymorphism screening.. Genomic DNA of 3 individuals per breed was therefore amplified in the polymorphic regions and amplification products were therefore subject to DHPLC analysis. Sequencing confirmed the presence of SNPs differentiating breeds from Italy and China. Our results also shows that DHPLC is a sensitive, accurate and cost effective approach to screen sequence variation in sheep genome, allowing a significant reduction of sequencing efforts when searching for novel SNPs.
We report the technical conditions that allowed both the discovery and genotyping of several SNPs among the gene chosen.

Poster G3.26

"Chromosome walking" technique to detect coding DNA regions in proximity of a QTL

F. Napolitano, P. Leone[1], G. Catillo and B. Moioli. ISZ, via Salaria 31, 00016 Monterotondo, Italy [1] IBBA-CNR, via F.lli Cervi 93, 20090, Segrate, Italy*

A linkage disequilibrium in the Chianina breed, between microsatellite IDVGA-46 (chromosome 19q16) and body measurements, was made evident in a Piedmontese x Chianina crossbred population.
It was therefore decided to perform the "chromosome walking" technique starting from both sides of the known DNA fragment (568 bp) containing the microsatellite in order to detect a coding DNA region.
Sequencing was performed on the same clone (about 40 kb) where the microsatellite was identified.
By means of the *Seqaid* software, two single primers were designed, one in the flanking region 5' and the other in 3', allowing to identify two new DNA fragments, each of them on the opposite side of the microsatellite, and consisting of about 450 bp. The new DNA fragments were sequenced on a ABI Prism 310 Analyzer. From the new DNA fragments, new primers were designed in order to move further on the chromosome, from both sides.
As soon as a new flanking sequence was identified, a search in the Gene Bank was performed to: 1. verify similarities between the detected sequences and any existing published sequence, even in other species, in order to find a sequence coding for the searched traits; 2. find the sequence where the new primers should be designed, to proceed with the "walking", while avoiding repeated sequences (SINE in particular) and therefore non-specific primers.

Poster G3.27

Rates of inbreeding in Danish commercial pig populations

P. Berg[*,1] and A. Vernersen[2], [1]Danish Institute of Agricultural Sciences, Dept. Animal Breeding and Genetics, P.O.Box 50, 8830 Tjele Denmark, [2] The National Committee for Pig Production, Danske Slagterier, Axeltorv 3, DK-1609 Copenhagen V, Denmark.*

Use of BLUP methodology in genetic evaluations and short generations interval is expected to result in increased rates of inbreeding. Recently, methods for constraining rates of inbreeding and optimise genetic contributions has been developed. The objective of this study was to evaluate the need for implementing methods to control rates of inbreeding in the Danish pig-breeding program.
Pedigrees on all performance or progeny tested pigs and their ancestors were used for the four breeds Landrace, Yorkshire, Duroc and Hampshire.
Individual inbreeding coefficients, generation intervals, genetic contributions from ancestors, largest genetic contributions to the 2001 year-group and average relationships within and between year-groups were computed.
30 to 67 ancestors in the four breeds contribute 80% of the genes in the 2001 year-group. In all breeds single ancestors contributed more than 14% of the genes in the 2001 year-group.
Annual rates of inbreeding were approximately 0.8% in the Landrace, Duroc and Hampshire breeds, but only 0.4% in the Yorkshire breed. This equals rates of inbreeding close to 1% (L,D,H) and 1/2% (Y) per generation. It is concluded that selection can be improved by controlling rates of inbreeding.

Poster G3.28

Phylogenetic analysis of avian MHC genes

S. Rotundo[1], C. Gorni[1], L. Sironi[1], M. Cassandro[2], M. Baruchello[3], P. Mariani[1], [1]FPTP-CERSA, Via Fratelli Cervi 93, 20090 Segrate, Milan, Italy, [2]University of Padoa, Department of Animal Science, Agripolis, Viale dell'Universita' 16, 35020, Legnaro, Padoa, Italy, [3]Veneto Agricoltura, Regione Veneto, Agripolis, Viale dell'Universita' 16, 35020 Legnaro, Padoa, Italy.*

Although chicken B complex was the second MHC system to be identified, and despite its peculiarity and importance when it comes to resistance to disease, little is known about other avian species MHC system. Nevertheless, from the results of different studies, it becomes apparent that there is high structural variability between avian species.
In the present study we carried out the molecular characterisation of the MHC region in species such as chicken, turkey, duck, guinea fowl and pheasant. With regard to chicken, turkey and duck, the same genomic region was further studied in several local breeds.
We started characterising the MHC region by isolating MHC gene specific sequences. We derived primers specific for classical MHC class I and class II genes, and the *Rfp-Y* region from sequences deposited in GenBank. Conserved regions were determined by aligning the sequences using the program MegAlign. The PCR products were cloned and sequenced and mutations were identified in the regions analysed. Alignments were created by the Clustal W software for each MHC and *Rfp-Y* gene. To evaluate the phylogenetic relationships between the groups implemented in this study, phylogenetic trees were derived using the Phylip software.

Poster G3.29

Phylogenetic relationships of 10 canine Italian breeds (*Canis familiaris*) and wild canids (*Vulpes vulpes, Canis lupus italicus*) by microsatellite and mitochondrial polymorphisms

M. Polli[1], M. Longeri[1], P. Magnetti[2], S.P. Marelli[1], I. Taboni[1], B. Bighignoli[1], M.G. Strillacci[1], M. Zanotti[1] and L. Guidobono Cavalchini[1], [1]Istituto di Zootecnica, Faculty of Veterinary Medicine, [2]Departement of Biology, Faculty of Science, University of Milan, Italy

ENCI (Italian Kennel Club) is committed in better understanding the genetic structure and origin of Italian breeds. The aim of present study is to compare the two main tools of phylogenetic analysis, microsatellite and mitochondrial DNA polymorphism, in evaluating the genetic distances among canids. 10 Italian canine breeds, Italian wolf and red fox have been considered. Genetic variations at 10 canine microsatellite loci and at the 694 bp most polymorphic sequence of the mtDNA D-Loop have been evaluated. All the samples have been collected from animals unrelated in two generations. Microsatellite allele frequencies were examined and evaluated by GENEPOP statistic package. Genetic distances between populations were measured according to Nei's standard genetic distances by DISPAN package. Comparison between the two dendrograms obtained on the some sample with two polymorphism by UPGMA and Neighbor-Joining dendrograms have been performed. Both methods confirm the existence of a lower degree of genetic differentiation among considered dog breeds with the Italian wolf and high genetic distance with other canids. Within canine breeds our data show differences linked to the maternal and the paternal inheritance and the usefulness of integrating genomic and mitochondrial information to genetically characterize breeds.

Poster G3.30

Investigation of blood protein polymorphism and estimation of genetic distances in some dog breeds in Turkey

M. Erdogan[1], C.Uguz[1] and C.Ozbeyaz[2], [1]Departmen of Genetics, Faculty of Veterinary Medicine, University of Afyon Kocatepe, ANS Kampusu 03200, Afyon, Turkey, [2]Departmen of Animal Husbandry, Faculty of Veterinary Medicine, University of Ankara, Diskapi 06110, Ankara, Turkey.

Phylogenetic relationships in some Turkish dog breeds were investigated to determine protein polymorphisms by using electrophoretic analysis. Blood samples were collected from 276 dogs including Kangal, Akbash and German Shepherd as well as Doberman Pinscher, Setter, Pointer and Labrador dog breeds. Enzymes and proteins were separated electrophoretically by using isoelectrofocusing gel, starch gel and polyacrylamide gel. Polymorphism on albumine (Alb), postalbumine-1 (Poa-1), postalbumine-3 (Poa-3), transferrin (Tf), and esterase (ArE) loci was detected, while no polymorphism was observed on the hemoglobin (Hb) locus. These polymorphisms were used to estimate the average heterozygosity value ($\bar{h}_S$), F-statistics and the number of gene flow in each generation (Nm). The genetic distances (d_{ij}) were also compared among these dog breeds. Average heterozygosity values were found to be in the range of 0.3185 (Doberman Pinscher) to 0.4055 (Kangal Shepherd), and significant differences in heterozigosity were found among the dog breeds ($P<0.05$). The estimated values of genetic distance in populations other than Setter breed were between 0.0132 and 0.2442. Cluster analysis (UPGMA) results showed that Pointer and Akbash breeds formed a cluster and then German shepherd joined to this cluster. Finally, Labrador clunched into the cluster. However, Doberman and Kangal shepherd breeds formed a different cluster. Setter breed did not join either and formed its own.

Poster G3.31

The Neapolitan Mastiff: fertility and inbreeding analysis

S.P. Marelli[1], R. Rizzi[2], A. Sommella[1], L. Guidobono Cavalchini[1], [1]Istituto di Zootecnica, Facoltà di Medicina Veterinaria Università degli Studi di Milano, Via Celoria 10, 20133 Milano, [2]Dipartimento VSA, Facoltà di Medicina Veterinaria Università degli Studi di Milano, Via Celoria 10, 20133 Milano.*

The Neapolitan Mastiff is an ancient breed selected over centuries by breeders with very precise objective attempting to fix some particular traits described in the breed standard. The annual entries recorded in the Italian Kennel Club (ENCI) studbooks were analysed from 1974 to 2001 with a total number of 23202dogs. The entire Italian pedigree population of Neapolitan Mastiffs was analysed. Data about demographic, fertility and inbreeding parameters were calculated using SAS® statistic package. More than 60% of the bitches produced only one litter during their whole life. Litter size analysis showed a mean of four puppies per litter. In annual dam/sire ratios the maximum value was 1.59. The distribution of the number of sires divided per year of age shows the highest frequency (26.6%) for two years old dogs. The majority of the stud dogs (>53%) produced only one litter in their life.

Mean F values are clearly high (0.09). Average F per year and maximum F per year were calculated and alternate trends were observed. Typical Italian breeds like Neapolitan Mastiff need a gene pool as wide as possible in order to prevent the loss of genes. Therefore fertility parameters and inbreeding values should be constantly monitored.

Poster G3.32

Costs of gene banks for breed reconstruction

A Stella[1], F. Pizzi[2], P. Boettcher[2], and G. Gandini[3], [1]FPTP-CERSA and [2]IBBA-CNR, 20090 Segrate, Italy, [3]VSA, University of Milan, 20133 Milan, Italy.*

The objective of this study was to calculate the costs of semen or embryos required to establish a gene bank for the future reconstruction of a breed. A breed was considered to be reconstructed when at least 25 females and 25 males (or their semen) of breeding age were simultaneously available and the level of purity of the reconstructed breed was >98% (for schemes using 100% semen). The average level of relationship among members of the reconstructed population was required to be <5.0%. Three different scenarios of reconstruction were considered: 1) using only frozen semen, 2) using exclusively frozen embryos, and 3) using a combination of the two. Costs of the scenarios were calculated for a range of prices and rates of fertility and survival corresponding to a number of common livestock species. None of the three strategies was universally the most cost efficient, as the optimal strategy depended upon values used for the parameters regarding the cost and reproductive efficiency of a given reconstruction scheme. Using current prices for commercially available dairy semen and embryos as an example, costs of establishing a gene bank would be approximately €200,000 for use of only semen; €38,000 for exclusive use of embryos; and €23,000 for a combination of the two using half the maximum number of embryos.

Poster G3.33

Segregation analysis for continuous versus discrete polygenic traits

H. Ilahi and H.N. Kadarmideen, Statistical Animal Genetics Group, Institute of Animal Sciences, ETH Zurich CH-8092 Switzerland*

Segregation analysis was applied to continuous (normal) and discrete (categorical) traits using simulated data to compare bias and accuracy of the estimated parameters. Data were simulated using a mixed inheritance model (polygene + major gene) and according to a hierarchical and balanced family structure: one population consists of 20 sire families with 100 dams per sire, and 3 performances per dam were simulated. The standardized normal data was transformed into categorical data (5 categories) based on the existence of 4 chosen thresholds, corresponding to 4 category incidences (50, 25, 15 and 10%). The analyses were carried out on both normal and categorical data sets with 50 replications.
All the parameters estimated under mixed inheritance (H_1) for continuous trait were similar to the true values of parameters used in the simulation. However, for discrete trait, the genetic parameters were underestimated (e.g. true value of h^2=0.41 and r=0.52 *vs.* estimates of 0.25 and 0.37, respectively) and the estimated genotype frequencies were generally similar to the true frequencies. On the other hand, the estimated parameters under polygenic inheritance (H_0) were generally overestimated. These preliminary results show that the estimated parameters for discrete trait are more biased than continuous trait. More research on statistical methods and software development is needed to detect major genes segregating in binary or categorical traits with good accuracy.

Poster G3.34

Procedure for standardisation and normalisation of cDNA microarrays

M.H. Pool, W.W. Kuurman, B. Hulsegge, L.L.G Janss, J.M.J. Rebel, S. van Hemert. Institute for Animal Science and Health, ID-Lelystad, P.O. Box 65, 8200 AB Lelystad, The Netherlands.*

Expression levels for large numbers of genes under different conditions can be measured by using microarrays. In livestock species often cDNA-arrays are used for this purpose, because the complete genome sequences are not yet available to engineer oligo-arrays, and use of cDNA arrays allows the direct use of available cDNA libraries. However, cDNA-arrays exhibit larger variability than oligo arrays and therefore require more care in order to reduce noise, standardise and normalise the data, and require some different statistical approaches for analysis because two samples are measured on the same slide, unlike in oligo-array technology. This poster describes procedures developed to treat such data consisting of: (1) correction for background using special blank spots; (2) automatic outlier treatment using iteratively reweighted analysis to allow for a robust fit, similar to using medians; (3) a lowess fit to allow for dye-bias on the ratio's with varying intensity; (4) a procedure to identify poor duplicated values (1 duplicate is made within slide) fitting a heterogeneous variance contour to allow for increasing repeatability with increasing intensity; (5) fitting of a heterogeneous variance contour for sample values to allow for decreasing variance with increasing intensity, used to provide weights for a weighted analysis. The procedure is illustrated on a data set showing differences in gene expression levels between malabsorption syndrome infected and control chickens.

Poster G3.35

Simulation of selected sampling in microarray studies

A. Stella[1] and P. Boettcher[2], [1]CERSA-FPTP and [2]IBBA-CNR, via F. Cervi 93, 20090 Segrate, Italy.*

The objective of this research was to use simulation to help design microarray studies. The basis of the proposed microarray study is to detect differentially expressed genes between groups of animals with extreme phenotypes for a quantitative trait. The simulation was used to optimise the number of animals sampled and rate of false positives among genes declared to be differentially expressed. Both gene expression and the quantitative trait were modelled as phenotypes with a given heritability. Differentially expressed genes were simulated to have genetic correlations with the trait ranging from 0.25 to 0.75. Sensitivity to a range of heritabilities was studied, with values ranging from 0.10 to 0.50 for the trait and from 0.30 to 0.50 for gene expression. The simulated array contained 5000 sequences, of which 200 were differentially expressed. The population included 500 animals and pooling of mRNA samples from the *n* highest and lowest animals was simulated, with *n* varying from 1 to 250. The 50 genes with the highest associations with the trait were considered differentially expressed and rates of false positives were calculated and compared. To obtain a 10% rate of false positives, pools of only 3 animals were needed when both the trait and expression had heritabilities of 0.50, but all animals were needed when respective heritabilities were 0.10 and 0.30.

Poster G3.36

Expression analysis of ESTs derived from differential display, subtractive hybridization and cDNA libraries in bovine preimplantation stage embryos

D. Tesfaye, S. Mamo, N. El-Halawany, K. Schellander, K. Wimmers, M. Gilles and S.Ponsuksili, Institute of Animal Breeding Science, Endenicher Allee 15, 53115 Bonn, Germany*

Quantitative expression profiling was performed for three ESTs 4C20, C242 and C112, which are derived from differential display, subtractive hybridization and cDNA libraries respectively, throughout the pre-implantation stages of vitro-produced bovine embryos. For this mRNA isolated from pooled bovine matured oocytes, 2-cell, 4-cell, 8-cell, 16-cell, morula and blastocyst stage were subjected to real time PCR using specific primers and SYBR® Green as DNA binding dye. The sequences of 4C20, C242 and C112 showed significant similarity with bovine NADH dehydrogenase subunit 2 (AF493541), enlongation factor 1a (BTA238405) and human TATA box binding protein-associated factor (NM_016285) respectively, which are reported to play important role in various aspects of embryogenesis. The EST 4C20, derived from 8-cell stage in DD-PCR, was found to be highly expressed in 8- and 16-cell stages compared to the other developmental stages. The EST C242, obtained from a blastocyst enriched subtractive library, was found to be highly expressed in 2-cell, 4-cell and blastocyst stages. The transcript C112, which is obtained from single blastocyst cDNA libraries, detected at higher level in matured oocytes and in 2-cell stages than in other developmental stages. The differential expression of these transcripts in bovine preimplantation stages may suggest their potential role in various developmental transitions occur during bovine embryogenesis.

Poster G3.37

Toward the construction of a B.*bubalus* tissue CDNA microarray

M. Strazzullo[1,2], C. Campanile[3], M. D'Esposito[1] and L. Ferrara[3], [1]Institute of Genetics and Biophysics "A.Buzzati Traverso" CNR, Naples Italy, [2]Biogem-SCARL, Italy, [3]ISPAAM-CNR, Naples, Italy

Livestock farming constitutes between the 30%-40% of agriculture, thus taking an undoubtable importance for the economics of most of the world countries.
Among them, water buffalo represent an important specie for Italian food industry, especially in Southern Italy. In spite of these considerations, it lacks a systematic approach to the understanding of the water buffalo genome, a condition which is indispensable for its genetic improvement. Animal genomics will, however, be cost efficient as a beneficiary of the Human Genome Project, in consideration of the overall similarity of the livestock genomes to human genome.
We are taking advantage of technologies we already set up for the structural and functional analysis of the Human Genome, such as long range sequencing, cDNA libraries construction and arrangement and microarray development. Our interest is to construct tissue specific cDNA libraries from muscle, brain and mammary gland of B.bubalis.
We wish to derive B.bubalis tissue specific microarray and to analyze specific genes and specific biochemical pathways important for cellular functions.
We extracted total RNA from targeted tissues and checked its quality by retrotranscription and subsequent gene specific PCR. We used gene specific primers to amplify myostatin and leptin genes, involved, in mammals, in muscle development and fat metabolism in adypocite, respectively. Progress in gene characterization and library construction will be reported.

Poster G3.38

Weaning performance of the Charolais beef cattle in Hungary

Z. Lengyel[1], Z. Domokos[2], F. Szabó[1], D. Márton[3], I. Erdei[1], Zs. Wagenhoffer[1], P.J., Polgar[1] [1]University of Veszprém, Georgikon Faculty of Agricultural Science, H-8360 Keszthely, Deák F. str. 16. 2Association of Hungarian Charolais Breeders, H-3525 Miskolc, Vologda u. [3]Hungarian Hereford, Angus and Galloway Association, H-7400. Kaposvár, Dénes Major

Weaning performance of 11672 purebred offspring (5059 male and 6613 female) of 155 sire were analised with sire model in thirteen farms. Heritability, repetability, breeding value, genetic and environmental variance of weaning weight (WW), preweaning daily gain (PDG), 205-day weight (CWW), and the genetic, phenotypic and environmental correlation between WW and PDG were calculated. Farm, number of calving, year of birth, season of birth, sex, were treated as fixed, the sire was treated as random effect. The age of the calves at weaning was fitted as a covariant. Data were analyzed with Harvey's (1990) Least Square Maximum Likelihood Computer Program. The overall mean value and standard error of WW, PDG and CWW were 231±8.43 kg, 1130±39.02 g/day and 231±8.02 kg, respectively. The age of the calves at weaning was 205 days. The effect of sire was small 1.5% in the examined traits. Among the fixed effects the largest influence was the sex (75-78%). The heritability of WW and PDG was 0.34±0.05, 0.32±0.04 and CWW was 0.34±0.04, respectively. The genetic, phenotypic and environmental correlations between WW and PDG were strong and positive.

Poster G3.39

Weaning performance and calving difficulty of Hereford beef cattle in Hungary

F. Szabó[1], Z. Lengyel[1], D. Márton[2], I. Márton[2] I. Erdei[1], Zs. Wagenhoffer, [1]University of Veszprém, Georgikon Faculty of Agricultural Science, H-8360 Keszthely, Deák F. str. 16. [2]Hungarian Hereford, Angus and Galloway Association, H-7400. Kaposvár, Dénes Major 2.

Weaning performance of 1468 purebred offspring (731 male and 737 female) of 39 sire and calving difficulty of 1540 purebred offspring (769 male and 771 female) were analised with sire model in two farms. Heritability, repetability, breeding value, genetic and environmental variance of weaning weight (WW), preweaning daily gain (PDG), 205-day weight (CWW), calving difficulty (CD) and the genetic, phenotypic and environmental correlation between WW and PDG were calculated. Farm, year of birth, season of birth, sex, number of calving were treated as fixed, the sire was treated as random effect. The age of the calves at weaning was fitted as a covariant. Data were analyzed with Harvey's (1990) Least Square Maximum Likelihood Computer Program. The overall mean value and standard error of WW, PDG, CWW and CD were 192±13.28 kg, 842±67.72 g/day, 202±13.85 kg and 1.02±0.01 score, respectively. The age of the calves at weaning was 198 days. The sex of calves did not have any effect on calving difficulty because the distribution of assisted calvings was similar in the sexes. The heritability of traits varies between 0.15-0.23. The genetic, phenotypic and environmental correlations between WW and PDG were strong and positive. The repetability of the investigated traits were small.

Poster G3.40

Some population genetic parameters of a Limousine herd in Hungary

Zs. Wagenhoffer, Z. Lengyel and F. Szabó, University of Veszprem, Georgikon Faculty, Keszthely, Hungary*

The aim of our study was to determine the most important population genetic parameters of a Limousine herd kept under extensive condition in Hungary. Data of 1543 calves (901 male and 642 female) for a period of seven years (1992-1998) were computed. Gestation length (G), age at first calving (AC), weaning weight (WW), 205 day weight (CW), preweaning growth (WG), season (S) as well as sire (Si) effect were evaluated. Mean of G for 1400 calving was 289±4.4 day with a maximum of 300 days. AC was 34.6±3.6 months with a maximum of 39 months. WW were 216±4.56 and 202±4.58, while CW were 225±4.33 and 206±4.34 for male and female calves respectively. WG were 1102±20.14 for bull calves and 1033±20.21 for heifers. As the herd is grazed all year long apart from winter, when beef cows are fed with forage and hay, season effect on WW and WG were also evaluated. According to the results, best calving period is March and April. Correction indices were calculated for each season (winter, spring, summer and autumn) as well as for each calving (according to the results, only 1st; 2nd; 9th and 10th calving should be corrected). Sires (n=21) used as mating bull during the examined period were ranked according to their breeding value for G, AC, WW, CW and WG.

Poster G3.41

Analysis of gene action in growth traits of Hereford x Czech Pied catttle

V. Jakubec[1], I. Majzlík[1], D. Kadlecová[1] and J. Říha[2], [1]Czech University of Agriculture, 165 21 Prague, [2]Research Institute of Cattle Production, 788 13 Rapotín, Czech Republic*

Gene action in 210-day and 365-day weights and average daily gains (birth-210 days, birth-365 days and 210-365 days) was analysed by fitting the genetic additive-dominance model according to *Mather and Jinks*. Least squares means and their standard errors of growth traits of Hereford (sire breed) and Czech Pied cattle (dam breed) and their crossbreds F_1, B_1, B_{11} a B_{111} (backcrosses to the Hereford) were used for the estimation of the following genetic parameters: μ-mean, direct and maternal population effect (g a g^M), direct and maternal heterosis (h a h^M). The parameters were estimated by using the weighted least squares method. The adequacy of the additive-dominance model was tested by the goodness of fit (χ^2) and it was found that there was a good agreement between the observed and expected generation means for all growth traits. The maternal population effects were in all traits (with the exception of daily gains from 210 to 365 days) more important than the direct population effects. The direct heterosis was in all traits negative. The maternal heterosis was in the 210-day weight and average daily gains from birth to 210 days positive and in the other traits negative.

Poster G3.42

Multi trait and random regression analysis of dry matter intake and weight gain of station tested Holstein Frisian bulls

E. Tholen[1], W. Muesch[2], W. Trappmann[1], K. Schellander[1], [1]University of Bonn, Institute of Animal Breeding Science,Endenicher Allee 15, 53115 Bonn, Germany, [2]Landwirtschafts-kammer Westfalen-Lippe, 59505 Bad Sassendorf, Germany*

Our objective was to investigate the genetic foundation of daily dry matter feed intake (FI) and daily weight gain (WG) recorded in subsequent testing periods of 1405 station tested (1995-2002) Holstein Frisian bulls. The young bulls were tested between 130kg to 450kg live weight (LW). FI was recorded daily, WG every four weeks. REML genetic parameters were estimated using a multi trait animal model (MT) including WG and FI measured in 3 equally spaced weight intervals or single trait random regression models (RR) comprising on average 11 WG or 290 FI measurements. RR-models contain a 4th order orthogonal polynoms for LW as a fixed trajectory and as covariance functions for the random effects animal and permanent environment. Estimated h^2 using the MT model for FI were around 0.4; whereas for DG a slight increase from 0.2 (130-250kg LW) to 0.4 (350-450kg LW) was observed. Almost all genetic correlations between the different periods for FI and DG were above 0.7. The genetic correlations between FI and WG were between 0.2 and 0.4. Using the RR-models h^2 were peaked at 130kg and 350kg LW, whereas relative low h^2 were found at 160kg LW and above 420 kg. In contrast to WG the h^2 for FI increased with increasing testing duration.

Poster G3.43

An additional information on the value of the breeding bulls with the metabolic traits

L. Panicke[1], E. Fischer[2], Z. Reklewski[3], K. Schlettwein[1] and R. Staufenbiel[4], [1] Research Institute for the Biology of Farm Animals, Dummerstorf, Germany, [2]Agric. and Environmental Faculty of the University Rostock, [3] Institute of Genetics of Animal Breeding, Jastrzebiec, Poland, [4]Free University Berlin, Clinic of Cattle and Pigs, Berlin, Germany,*

The glucose tolerance test (GTT) represents a possible quantification of the metabolic capacity of the cattle. The aim was to get reliable physiological indicators. The examination of the physiological capability and its relation to the milk performance of cows gets the great importance. The GTT can give an additional recommendation for the early evaluation of the young breeding bulls. In the test is grasped the insulin and glucose reaction during an induced metabolism burden. 28 bulls were examined in the third life half-year. The metabolic parameters of the glucose tolerance test are suitable for an additional evaluation of the breeding bulls before the offspring's test starts. The variation s%=7, the genetic determination h^2=0,5 and the mean correlations to the estimated breeding values by 0.4 argue for the involvement of the physiological parameter. The test parameters depend on the age and experimental conditions. Their combination with the pedigree breeding value seem to increase the amount of information. The informativness for the protein yield rises to r=0.68 with not-linear evaluation, that could be utilised in the selection of improper bulls if the present results will be confirmed.

Poster G3.44

Relationship of the enzyme activities in blood and liver of growing cattle

L. Panicke[1], M. Schmidt[2], L. Czegledi[3], U. Lendeckel[4], J. Wegner[1], K. Schlettwein[1] and R. Staufenbiel[5], [1]Research Institute for the Biology of Farm Animals, Dummerstorf, Germany, [2]Inst. for the Biology, St. Cross Academy Kielce, ul. Konopnickiej 15, 25-406 Kielce, Polen, [3]University of Debrecen, Depart. of Animal Husbandry and Nutrition, Debrecen, Hungary, [4]Otto-von-Guericke-University, Inst. of Exp. Internal Medicine, Magdeburg, Germany, [5]Free University Berlin, Clinic of Cattle and Pigs, Berlin, Germany*

The proteolytic activities of lysosomal enzymes as well as their performance are influenced by systematic environmental factors The aim of the study was to determine the correlation between the individual lysosomal enzyme activities in serum, leucocytes, liver, and muscle with different stages of cattle development. High correlations also were calculated between 9 and 16 month old heifers for enzyme activity in liver by r= 0.6 - 0.9. This has been taken into account by the simultaneity, the same age, and by the same proportion in the groups of young German-Holstein heifers. There were altogether 39 investigations, 19 in the 9 months old, and 20 in the 16 months old female young cattle. Lysosomal enzymes in leucocytes were proven inappropriate for investigation because of their high variation coefficients (up to 107%). The enzymes investigated in serum, liver and muscle only had variation coefficients ranging from 20 to 40% in most cases. The closest connection between activities of individual enzymes was observed in the liver, were highly correlated with each other.

 Poster G3.45

Level of glucose of parameter by young bulls and cows

L. Panicke[1]; E. Fischer[2]; B. Fischer[3]; R. Staufenbiel[4] , [1]Research Institute for the Biology of Farm Animals, Dummerstorf, Germany; [2]Agric. and Environmental Faculty of the University Rostock; [3] Institute of Agriculture and Horticulture of Sachsen-Anhalt, Iden, Germany, [4]Free University Berlin, Clinic of Cattle and Pigs, Berlin, Germany*

The paper deals with the role of insulin in the regulation of energy metabolism of cattle in order to evaluate the genetic equipment of bulls. Methodically, the insulin function can be measured using the glucose tolerance test (GTT, Reinicke,1993). 120 cows in the stage of 8th weeks ante parturition to 36th weeks post parturition was compared with 292 young bulls in the third life half-year. The goal of the examination was, to establish a comparable test level for cows and growing young cattle. By an infusion of 1g glucose per $kg^{0,75}$ of metabolic body weight in the GTT was kept the urine threshold. By the constant glucose base concentration (G0), the glucose half-life (GHWZ) of the young bulls at 48 min is comparable with the eighth week of lactation of the cows. Exactly in this time period has been proved by Cassel (2001) the highest genetic correlation between energy balance and yield $r_g = - 0.84$ and the highest heritability for the energy balance $h^2 = 0.20$. Thus, by the infusion quantity and the expelled test time under performance the young bulls imitate the genetic equipment of their daughters for the metabolism capability.

Poster G3.46

Milkability traits recorded with flowmeters in Italian Brown Swiss

A. Bagnato[1], A. Rossoni[1], C. Maltecca[1], D. Vigo[1], S. Ghiroldi[2], [1]Dipartimento VSA, Università degli Studi di Milano, Via Celoria 10, 20133 Milano, Italy, [2]ANARB, Loc. Ferlina, Bussolengo (Verona), Italy*

Flowmeters can record milk production, milking speed (usually used as measure of milkability) and parameters describing milk release characteristics of each cow. Objectives of this study were to investigate the variations in milkability traits recorded with flowmeter across parities and to address relationship between milk emission curves shapes with milk yield (MK) and somatic cell count (SCC). Maximum milk flow (MMF, kg/min.), average milk flow (AMF; kg/min.), total milking time (TMT), increasing (IT) and decreasing (DT) flow phase duration, time at plateau (TP), MK (kg), and SCC were recorded monthly on more than 200 cows in three herds for two years. From the beginning to the end of the lactation, MMF and AMF increased in first parity (0.5 and 0.2 kg/min. respectively) and decreased in pluriparous cows (0.85 and 0.6 kg/min respectively), while TMT and TP decreased similarly across parities (1.6 and 1 min. respectively). IT, and TP did not show significant variation across parities and along the lactation. Cows with lower MMF and longer TP or TMT showed higher production and lower SCC. If results are confirmed with a large data set, parameters recorded with the flowmeter (h^2 .15 to .21 in previous studies) may be considered as selection objectives to improve milkability and related traits, as SCC.

Poster G3.47

Correction factors for lactation length, age at calving and lactation number in Nili-Ravi buffaloes of the Punjab

M. Shafiq and M. Ahmad. Livestock production research institute, Bahadurnagar, Okara, Punjab, Pakistan.

The data on 6651 lactations of Nili-Ravi buffaloes maintained at Livestock Experiment Stations, Bahadurnagar, Rahk Gulaman, Khushab, Haroonabad and Chak Katora from 1980-2001 were used to develop correction factors for length of lactation, age at calving and lactation number by regression method. The milk yield affected significantly ($P<0.01$) by herd, year, season of calving and all regression coefficients of above said traits. The linear trend was observed in milk yield for lactation length. The milk yield increased by 5.0483 Kg for each day increase in lactation length. The correction factors for length of lactation ranged from 3.1468 to 0.6585 at 51-60 and 491-500 days of lactation, respectively. A curvilinear trend was found in milk yield for age at calving and lactation number. The milk yield increased @ 1.9347 Kg then decreased @ -0.0220 Kg for each month increase in age at calving, while it increased @ 38.4889 Kg thereafter, decreased @ -8.9738 Kg for each lactation increase in lactation number. The correction factors for age at calving ranged from 1.0042 to 1.4022 at the age of 25 and 200 months, respectively. The constants were calculated as 310.2168, 1824.7520 and 1784.0750 for lactation length, age at calving and lactation number, respectively. These correction factors may be used to adjust the lactation records on 305-day mature equivalent (ME) basis for comparison in the selection of Nili-Ravi buffaloes for higher milk yield. These correction factors are also equally applicable in whole Nili-Ravi buffaloes of the Punjab.

Poster G3.48

A preliminary analysis regarding linear morphologic characteristics on Saanen and Camosciata goat breeds

I. Pernazza[1] and P. Fresi[1], ASSO.NA.PA., viale Palmiro Togliatti 1587, 00155 Roma, Italia.*

This paper has a double purpose: to estimate proportional components of variance and to process the principal component analysis. The data consist of 1684 measurements for the Saanen and 861 for the Camosciata breeds. Regarding the Saanen breed the heritability estimates for topline, rump angle, foot angle, teat placement (side view), udder shape, rear udder attachment and teat angle ranged from 0.01 to 0.10; for pastern angle, metatarsal length, teat shape, teat placement (rear view), and fore udder attachment the heritability estimates ranged from 0.10 to 0.20; for median suspensory ligament is 0.27. The breeding values, for each doe, of the four traits related to the udder and to the teats respectively were estimated by using principal component analysis. The goal was to provide an index that enables to select for more than one trait at the same time. With regard to the Camosciata breed, the heritability estimates for pastern angle, ramp angle foot angle, teat shape, teat placement (rear view) and udder shape ranged from 0.09 to 0.20; for topline, metatarsal length, teat angle, teat placement (side view) and median suspensory ligament the heritability estimates ranged from 0.20 to 0.30; for rear and fore udder attachment ranged from 0.45 to 0.53. The small dataset available produce estimates with low accuracy; for the Camosciata breed the estimates will not allow to make other analysis.

Poster G3.49

Heterogeneity of variance across classifiers for type traits in the Italian Holstein

F. Canavesi[1], P. Orlandini[1], S. Biffani[1] and A.B. Samorè[1], [1]Associazione Nazionale Allevatori Frisona Italiana (ANAFI), Via Bergamo 292, 26100 Cremona, Italy.*

Classifiers score all first parity cows every six months. Each type trait is scored on a linear scale ranging from 1 to 50 for a total of 17 traits. Final score ranges from 65 to 99. Heterogeneity of variance across classifier have been observed with SD within year ranging from 3 to 8 linear points. This heterogeneity may have an impact on the accuracy of estimated breeding values. As a possible solution a standardisation of the within classifier variance has been proposed by Van Arendonk (1993). Data from the the official genetic evaluation of november 2002 were used to test this hypotesis. Type traits scores were preadjusted for the within year classifier SD. Results of the genetic evaluation on standardised data, based on the same model as the official, were compared with the proofs of November 2002 looking at correlations and mendelian sampling. Correlations for bulls were equal to 0.99 and higher for all traits. Trends in mendelian sampling variance were non significant or very small for some traits on both original and standardised data. In all cases test on trend in mendelian sampling variance were slightly better for standardised data although not significantly different. A closer observation of bull and cow proofs will help technicians to decide whether to apply the standardisation to the official evaluation.

Poster G3.50

Genetic polymorphisms of *DGAT1* Gen in cattle

J. Citek[1], E. Fischer[2], V. Rehout[1], L. Panicke[3], [1]Southbohemian University, Dept. of Animal Breeding, Ceské Budejovice, Czech Republic, [2]Agricultural and Environmental Faculty Rostock, Germany, [3]Res Inst for the Biology of Farm Animals, 18196 Dummerstorf, W. Stahl-Allee 2, Germany*

The frequencies of *DGAT1* polymorphism at amino acid position 232 were analysed in Czech Spotted cattle, Czech Red, Czech Black and White, German Holstein, Brown Swiss, and Jersey, respectively. Around the *DGAT1* gene assigned to a bovine chromosome 14 close to the centromere, a few polymorphisms were found (Winter et al., 2002), out of which that on the position 10433-4 in exon 8 codes for alanine or lysine. The lysine coding variant is probably the original state of *DGAT1*. In the early domestication, the substitution has materialised. The enzyme coded by the *DGAT1* locus takes part on the triglyceride synthesis as a basic component of fat incl. fat of cow`s milk. Recently a few studies has been carried out to determine the influence of alanine - lysine variants on the fat content in milk. According to our results, the bulls with genotype LL possess higher breeding value for fat yield +24,0 kg, AA bulls 3,9 kg, fat (+0,29 or -0,25) and protein +0,07 or -0,13) percentage. However, the lover breeding value for milk yield +71 kg compared to the AA bulls +513 kg was found. The results are of good promise, nevertheless, they have to be confirmed repeatedly in large extent experiments.

Poster G3.51

Effect of casein haplotypes on production traits in Italian Holstein

P. Boettcher[1], E. Budelli[2], F. Canavesi[3] and G. Pagnacco[4], [1]IBBA-CNR and [2]FPTP-CERSA, via Fratelli Cervi 93, 20090 Segrate, Italy, [4]ANAFI, 26100 Cremona, Italy, [4]VSA, University of Milan, 20133 Milan, Italy.*

The objective of this study was to evaluate the effects of casein haplotypes on production traits in Italian Holstein. Data consisted of mature equivalent phenotypes and genotypes for the a_{s1}-casein, β-casein, κ-casein loci for 354 daughters of twenty Holstein sires. A Monte Carlo based method algorithm was proposed and developed for estimation of haplotype probabilities. The software uses half-sib genotypes to determine each possible combination of parent haplotype. This information is then used to reconstruct the respective daughter haplotypes. Simulated data were used to test the software. Haplotype frequencies ranged from 0.52 for BA^2A (α_{s1}-casein, β-casein, κ-casein, respectively) and 0.004 for CA^3A. Regressions on haplotype probabilities were used to estimate effects of casein genes on yields and contents of milk, fat, and protein. The model for analysis included fixed effects of herd, random effect of sire, and regression coefficients for haplotype probabilities. Significant haplotype effects were observed for only protein percentage. The largest difference between haplotypes was 0.21% between BA^2A and CA^3A.

Poster G3.52

Mapping QTL affecting milk production in Israel Holstein dairy cattle by analysis of dam marker alleles within a daughter design

E. Lipkin, R. Tal[*], M. Soller and A. Friedmann, Department of Genetics, Hebrew University of Jerusalem, Jerusalem 91904, Israel.

A relatively small number of maternal grandsires (MGS) are active in any given years, and these provide the bulk of the dams of the daughters in a sire half-sib daughter family. In addition, the dams are not in close relationship with the sire, further limiting the selection of MGS. Thus, alleles of dam origin in the daughters may derive from only one or two MGS. Consequently, daughter dam-alleles within sires, carry information similar to that obtained by analysis of the sire alleles. Densitometric data on dam allele frequency were obtained during a daughter design genome scan of milk protein% (P), milk yield (M), and protein yield (K) by selective DNA pooling. The study involved 13 sire families and 134 markers. Within each sire-marker-trait combination, alleles originating from the dams only (not including the sire alleles) were tested for significance of the allele frequency difference between high and low pools. Significant markers were generally significant for all three traits. Direction (increasing, decreasing) of marker effects for P and M were negatively correlated; effects for K and M were positively correlated; and for K and P were uncorrelated. Dam alleles thus provide a powerful addition to the power of marker-QTL analysis with selective DNA pooling, at no additional cost.

Poster G3.53

Identification of genes affecting milk production in Finnish Ayrshire cattle

S. Viitala[1], J. Szyda[2,3], N. Schulman[1] and J. Vilkki[1], [1]Animal Production Research, MTT, 31600 Jokioinen, Finland, [2]Department of Animal Genetics, Agricultural University of Wroclaw, Kozuchowska 7, 51-631 Wroclaw, Poland, [3]United Datasystems for Animal Production (VIT), Heideweg 1, 27-283 Verden, Germany.*

In previous studies QTL with major effect on milk yield and composition have been mapped to the bovine chromosome 20. Two potential candidate genes that are known to have a role in lactation have been mapped to the proximity of the QTL. The objective of our study was to find polymorphism that could explain the variation in milk production traits in Finnish Ayrshire cattle. The coding sequence of two candidate genes was sequenced from genomic DNA. To obtain flanking intronic sequence for each exon, a bovine genomic BAC library was screened with oligonucleotide probes representing the candidate genes. The information about the intronic sequence allowed us to sequence entire coding sequences. A set of pooled DNA samples from the families segregating for the QTL was used to scan for molecular variation. The analyses revealed six coding sequence polymorphisms, five of which lead to amino acid substitutions.
To study the association between the traits of interest and observed polymorphisms a total of 810 bulls with milk trait DYDs were genotyped for the five missense mutations. The results indicate that two genes on chromosome 20 have independent effects on milk production; one gene affecting mainly composition and the other kg yields.

Poster G3.54

Fitting curves of QTL-genotypic effects on protein yield over the lactation in Danish Holstein cattle

M.S. Lund, P. Madsen, and P. Sørensen. Danish Institute of Agricultural Sciences, Dept.of Animal Breeding and Genetics P.O. Box 50, DK-8830 Tjele, Denmark

QTL affecting milk-production traits are usually mapped by fitting QTL to the mean (or some other function) of the individual recordings over a lactation. However, a previous study clearly shows the potential importance of utilising the repeated measurements, and fitting a curve describing the effects of QTL genotypes over lactation to the longitudinal data. Based on these results the hypothesis is that using a model with random regressions on lactation stage will provide two advantages. First, the power of detection is increased. Second, it provides information on the pattern of expression/effect of the QTL over the lactation.
In order to test these hypotheses we compare results from scanning a single chromosome using two models. The first model fits the effects of a fixed mean, polygenic effects and a QTL effect on DYDs of mean lactation performance. The second model fits curves of a fixed mean, polygenic effects and a QTL effect on DYDs defined for a range of intervals over the lactation.

Poster G3.55

Heritability of plasma growth hormone concentration changes slightly during lactation in first parity dairy cows

P. Theilgaard[1], P. Løvendahl[1] and K.L. Ingvartsen[2], [1]Department of Animal Breeding and Genetics, [2]Department of Animal Health and Welfare, Danish Institute of Agricultural Sciences, P.O. Box 50, DK-8830 Tjele, Denmark

The aim of this study was to investigate how the heritability of growth hormone changes during lactation. Cows (n=242) included Danish Red, Danish Holstein and Jersey breeds. Cows were equally distributed across two feeding treatments, a normal and a low energy diet. Pedigrees contained 2656 records. Blood sampling was planned on day 1, 3 and 7 and taken on the actual day. In the remaining part of the lactation samples were of practical reasons taken on the Thursday nearest day 14, 21, 28, 35, 42, 49, 56, 70, 84, 126, 168, 210, 252 and 294 relative to calving. A total of 2645 samples were assayed for bovine growth hormone. Growth hormone concentrations were log-transformed before analysis. Fixed effects were fitted as third order Legendre polynomial nested within interactions between breed, diet and genetic group, in a random regression model. Genetic variation and permanent co-variance were fitted as random coefficient using second and third order Legendre polynomials. Growth hormone concentrations decreased with advancing stage of lactation. The heritability was lowest in early lactation (h^2 0.28 at 30 DIM) and highest in mid lactation (h^2 0.40 at 150 DIM). We conclude that growth hormone concentrations are heritable with highest heritability in mid lactation and slightly lower heritability in very early and late lactation.

Poster G3.56

Estimation of genetic parameters for initial milk performance of Holsteins in Saxony

W. Brade[1] and E. Groeneveld[2], [1]Chamber of Agriculture Hannover, Johannssenstr. 10, 30159 Hannover. [2]Institute of Animal Science Mariensee, 31535 Neustadt, Germany

Routine genetic evaluation requires knowledge of covariance structure of traits considered.
For current data set on 135000 dairy cows from Saxony genetic parameters were estimated on initial records using VCE 5. To estimate genotype-environment-inter-action the data set was split in two; one with records from large herds (≥ 180 cows/herd/year) and another with the rest.
The interaction component was estimated on the basis of genetic correlation (r_g) considering milk performance in the two environment as two traits. Additionally bulls were ranged on the aggregate genotype within two environments. No substantial interactions were found ($r_g \geq 0.93$).
Also, dominance variances were estimated. Its proportion of phenotypic variance is around 5 percent. For somatic cell count only negligible dominance variance were estimated.

Poster G3.57

Variance of direct and maternal genetic effects for milk yield of Friesian cows

*M.N. El-Arian *[1] , H.G. El-Awady[2] , A.S. Khattab[3] and A.S. El-Setar[4], [1]Department of Animal production, Faculty of Agriculture, Mansoura University, Egypt. [2]Department of Animal Production, Faculty of Agriculture, Kafr El-Sheikh, Tanta University. [3]Department of Animal production, Faculty of Agriculture, Tanta University, Egypt and [4]Ministry of Agriculture, Egypt.*

A total of 2135 normal lactation records of Friesian cows kept at Sakha Experimental farm, belonging to Ministry of Agriculture, during the period from 1980 to 2000 were used. Data were analyzed using single trait animal model according to Boldman et al.,(1995). Two models were used, Model 1 included month and year of calving and parity as fixed effects, days open and dry period as a covariate and direct genetic, maternal genetic, covariance between direct and maternal genetic, permanent environmental and error as random effects. Model 2 is similar to Model 1 , but excluding maternal and covariance between additive direct and maternal effects.
Estimates of heritability for 305 day milk yield were 0.17 and 0.17, for Model1 and Model 2, respectively. The genetic correlation between direct and maternal genetic effect was - 0.06. Then, The additive maternal genetic effect and covariance between direct and maternal genetic effects do not seem to make important contributions to the phenotypic variance for milk yield and these effects are probably not important for genetic evaluations.

Poster G3.58

Variance of direct and maternal genetic effects for milk yield in Egyptian buffaloes

A. Morad Kawthar[1], A.S.Khattab*[2] and S. Awad Set El - Habaeib[1]. [1]Animal Production Research, Institute, Ministry of Agriculture, Dokki, Cairo, Egypt, [2]Animal Production Department, Faculty of Agriculture, Tanta University, Egypt.

A total of 1259 normal first lactation records of Egyptian buffaloes raised at Mehallet Mousa Experimental Station , belonging to the Ministry of Agriculture were used, to estimate variances from direct and maternal genetic effects. Data were analyzed using MTDFREML. Program of Boldman et al., (1995). Two single trait animal models are used. Model 1 included month and year of calving are fixed effects, and age at first calving as a covariate, direct genetic (o^2g) , maternal genetic(o^2m), covariance between direct and maternal genetic (ogm) and errors are random effects. Model 2 is similar to Model 1, but excluding o^2g and ogm. Estimates of heritability for total milk yield were 0.30 and 0.21 for Model 1 and Model 2, respectively. The removal of o^2g and ogm from the model decreased estimates for heritability of additive genetic effects by 0.09.
Predicted breeding values of cows, sires and dams for total milk yield using the two models are calculated. The accuracy of sires breeding values are higher than the accuracy of both cows and dams breeding values for the two models.

Poster G3.59

Estimated breeding values and genetic trend for milk yield in Friesian cows in Punjab province of Pakistan

K. Javed[1] and M.A. Khan[2]. [1]Research Institute for Physiology of Animal Reproduction, Bhunikey (Pattoki) Distt. Kasur (Pakistan). [2]Women Islamic University, Islamabad (Pakistan)

Data on 937 pedigree, breeding and performance records of 567 Friesian cows maintained at Livestock Experiment Station Bhunikey (Pattoki) Distt. Kasur during the period 1982-2001 were utilized for the present study. The data were analyzed through Best Linear Unbiased Predictions (BLUP) procedure. The fixed effects (year and season of calving, lactation length and parity) found significant in preliminary analysis were included in the model. Lactation milk yield and lactation length averaged 3391.66±137.97 kg and 278.40±90.17 days, respectively. The breeding values for milk yield considering all lactations were estimated by using Restricted Maximum Likelihood (REML) procedure fitting Individual Animal Model. The estimated breeding values for milk yield from animal model evaluations ranged from -354 to 503 Kg for all the cows. The corresponding values for the standing herd ranged from -209 to 294 Kg. Phenotypic reduction in milk yield was noticed in the present herd during the period under study. The deterioration in this trait may largely be attributable to environmental factors. The genetic trend for milk yield also depicted a deteriorating trend indicating that breeding strategy proved to be inefficient during the last 20 years.

Poster G3.60

Comparative study on progeny performance between Italian Holstein and Romanian Black and White Sires

Elena Florescu, Colceri Dan, Istok Claudia, Research Institute for Bovine Breeding, Breeding cattle, Balotesti , 8113 DN Bucharest-Ploesti Km 21, Romania.

Using indigenous and imported proven sires is a common practice in Romanian Black and White dairy cattle improvement.The present study included data recorded between1987-2000 on sires imported from USA, Netherlands, Germany and Italy.Data concerning performed genetic gain for milk yield , fat and since 1997 also for protein are compared between imported and local sire progeny . Milk yield recorded by imported sires progeny was higher than local ones as follows: 9-10.7% in first lactation, 8.2-9.1 % in second and 4-5.5 % in thirth lactation. Genetic merit for milk yield was between 350-420 kg higher as compared to local ones. Average genetic merit registered between 1990-2000 for milk production confirms the expected genetic gain placing the sires from USA, followed by Netherlands, Italy and Germany, in the top of the ranking. During the period 1995-200 genetic merit for milk yield increased by 390 kg , thanks to genetic infusion and other above mentioned sources.

Poster G3.61

Genetic aspects of productive and reproductive traits in Holstein Friesian cows in Turkey

A.S. Khattab[*1] and Hulya, Atil[2]. [1]Depaertment of Animal Production, Faculty of Agriculture, Tanta, Tanta University, Egypt, [2]Department of Animal Science, Faculty of Agriculture, Ege University, Izmair, Turkey.*

This study investigated genetic and phenotypic trends of some productive and reproductive traits in Holstein Friesian cows kept at five herds in West of Turkey. A total number of records used were 6951 during the period from 1970 to 1987. Variance components for 305 day milk yield (305 d MY) , length of lactation (LL) and calving interval (CI) were estimated by the Restricted Maximum Likelihood Method, using an animal model . The model included individual, permanent environmental and errors as random effects, herd, month and year of calving and parity as fixed effects. Estimates of heritability were 0.24 , 0.21 and 0.10, respectively. Estimated repeatability values were 0.50, 0.44 and 0.20 for 305 d MY, LL and CI, respectively. Means of predicted breeding values for cows, dams and sires according to calving year and the genetic correlations were presented.

Poster G3.62

Effect of mean and variance heterogeneity on genetic evaluations of Lesbos dairy sheep

M. Nikolaou[1], A.P. Kominakis[1], E. Rogdakis[1], S. Zampitis[2] [1]Department of Animal Breeding & Husbandry, Agricultural University of Athens, Iera Odos 75, 11855, Athens, Greece, [2]Centre of Animal Genetic Improvement of Athens, Rodopis 1,11855, Athens, Greece*

Heritability (h^2) and animals' breeding values (BVs) were estimated for raw (MY), log (LMY), square root transformed (SMY), adjusted for mean (CM) and variance (CSD) heterogeneity of the herd-year-lactation (HYL) classes for milk yield in Lesbos dairy sheep. Only CSD resulted in homogenous variances. h^2 for CSD was the smallest (0.16), for MY, LMY and SMY was the same (0.19) and for CM was the highest (0.20). h^2 for low and high production level was 0.18 and 0.22, respectively and discriminated between low and high SD level (0.09 vs 0.29, respectively). Pearson and Spearman correlations of estimated BVs for MY, CM and CSD data were high (0.88 to 0.98) when all sires and ewes were considered, but lower for top sires and ewes. Herd, lactation, number of observations and production level were found to be associated with heterogeneity of variance. Results are discussed in terms of selection strategies when natural mating or AI is envisaged.

Poster G3.63

Is the estimation of genetic correlations in dairy sheep and goats necessary?

A.P. Kominakis and E. Rogdakis, Department of Animal Breeding and Husbandry, Faculty of Animal Science, Agricultural University of Athens, Iera Odos 75, 11855, Greece*

A data set of n=67 pairs of genetic and phenotypic correlation estimates for various milk traits, constructed from an exhaustive survey of published estimates in dairy sheep and goats, was used to test whether the phenotypic correlation (r_P) may be a suitable replacement of the genetic correlation (r_G). Correlations between paired genetic and phenotypic correlation estimates were generally found to be high (from 0.87 to 0.95) and not statistically different between the two species. A paired samples t-test showed that the average difference between the genetic and phenotypic correlation estimates ($d=r_G-r_P$) was statistically significantly ($p<0.05$) different from zero only for dairy goats (d=0.11). Employment of Fisher's transformation or of a non-parametric test (Kruskall-Wallis) showed that there was statistically no significant difference ($p<0.05$) between the two estimates. Differences between the two estimates were due to sampling errors of the genetic correlations. A simulation study of two correlated traits was also performed to investigate the effects of using r_P instead of r_G on the direct and indirect true selection responses and on the accuracy of the breeding values. Based on the results of the descriptive and simulation analyses it was concluded that for the species and traits cited here phenotypic correlations may be substituted for genetic ones when genetic correlations are unavailable or not precisely estimated.

Poster G3.64

Estimates of genetic parameters for fertility traits of Italian Holstein-Friesian cattle

S. Biffani[1], F. Canavesi and A.B. Samorè[1], [1]Associazione Nazionale Allevatori Frisona Italiana (ANAFI), Via Bergamo 292, 26100 Cremona, Italy.*

Data from insemination and calving events of Italian Holstein cows and heifers collected from January 1996 until December 2002 were used to estimate phenotypic and genetic parameter for some fertility traits. A validation procedure of the data based on gestation length and information on service sire was used. According to these procedure, in Italy 75.9 % of the calvings are associated to service or inseminations events. Days to first service (DTFS), calving interval (CI), number of service per conception (NSC) and non return rate at 90 days (NRR90) were the main traits analyzed. The effect of month and year of calving (or insemination), of sampling bull code, of age of cow and of herd-year-season of calving were included in the model and were significant for all the traits analyzed. A decreasing efficiency in cow fertility was observed over the last 5 years, with a longer days to first service interval and a higher proportion of cows being re-bred after 90 days. Different data sets were successively defined according to the parities (0 and 1, 1 and 2, or 2 and 3) in order to validate the hypothesis that different parities have to be considered as different traits.

Poster G3.65

Survival analysis applied to genetic evaluation for fertility in dairy cattle

M. del P. Schneider[1], E. Strandberg[1] and A. Roth[2], [1]Department of Animal Breeding and Genetics, Swedish University of Agricultural Sciences, P.O. Box 7023, SE-75007 Uppsala, Sweden, [2]Swedish Dairy Association, Box 1146, SE-63180 Eskilstuna, Sweden.*

The objective of this research was to study whether use of survival analysis results in a better genetic evaluation than conventional methods currently used for analysis of the fertility traits: interval between first to last insemination and interval between calving to last insemination. A stochastic simulation describing the reproductive cycle of first parity cows was done. True breeding values (TBVs) for pregnancy rate were created. A model containing random effects of sire and herd was used both with survival (SA) and mixed linear (LM) analysis to analyze the data and to get predicted sire breeding values (PBVs). The heritability estimates were higher for SA than for LM. Correlations between TBVs and PBVs for both traits predicted by SA were higher than corresponding correlations with PBVs predicted by LM model. The results indicate that survival analysis is an appropriate method to analyze interval between first to last insemination and interval between calving to last insemination.

Poster G3.66

Validation of two animal models for estimation of genetic trend for female fertility in Norwegian Dairy Cattle

I.M.A. Ranberg*[1,2], G. Klemetsdal[1] and B. Heringstad[1]. [1]Department of Animal Science, Agricultural University of Norway, [2]GENO Breeding and A.I. Association, Box 5025, N-1432 Ås, Norway.

Two linear animal models were used to estimate breeding values and genetic trend for 56-day non-return rate in virgin heifers. Data of 1.5 million first inseminations in the period September 1, 1978 to December 1, 1998, from daughters of 2682 sires was analysed. Both models had random effects of herd-year and animal, and fixed effects of age and double insemination. Model 1 had effect of month of first insemination, while Model 2 had fixed effect of month-year of first insemination. Both models showed favourable genetic trend for fertility, amounting to an annual genetic improvement for 56-day non-return rate of 0.16% ($P < 0.01$) and 0.07% ($P < 0.01$) for models 1 and 2, respectively. A method described by Boichard et al. (1995), based on using daughter deviation within sire by year to determine whether the deviations remain stable over time, was used to validate genetic trends. Model 2 showed significant bias ($P < 0.01$), while no bias was detected for Model 1. This suggests that Model 2 is too conservative, and that genetic trend was underestimated using this model. Correlations between observed and predicted breeding values were 0.37 and O.36, for models 1 and 2, respectively.

Poster G3.67

Prediction of UK fertility proofs for foreign bulls

E. Wall[1], V. Olori[2], M. Coffey[1] and S. Brotherstone[1], [1]Animal Biology Division, SAC, Bush Estate, Penicuik, Midlothian,EH26 0PH, Scotland [2]ICBF, Shinagh House, Bandon, Co. Cork, Ireland.*

Proofs for fertility traits (calving interval, non-return rate) were estimated for bulls that have daughters recorded in the UK. However, only half of the available bulls have recorded daughters in the UK. It would take approximately 4 years for foreign bulls being first used in the UK to have enough daughters recorded to have a reliable fertility proof. Many foreign bulls have fertility proofs in their country of first test. Common bulls were matched between UK and each foreign country. Conversion equations were derived by first deregressing UK proofs and then the regression of these proofs on the exporting country proofs was calculated. Foreign proofs were then converted to UK equivalents using these regression equations. Correlation between fertility proofs in the UK and other countries were moderate to high. Not all countries exporting semen to the UK have fertility proofs or have proofs correlated to each of the UK fertility traits and this limited the prediction of fertility proofs for every trait and bull available. Future development of fertility proofs in other countries and collection of more detailed information from these countries would allow the development of more complete and accurate conversion equations to be derived and therefore allow breeders to have UK equivalent proofs for all bulls available for selection.

Poster G3.68

Genetic correlation estimates between ultrasound measurements and age at first calving in Nelore cattle

L.G. Albuquerque[1]; H.N. Oliveira[2]; [1]Faculdade de Ciências Agrárias e Veterinárias - UNESP,Jaboticabal-SP, 14884-980, Brazil; [2]Faculdade de Medicina Veterinária e Zootecnia - UNESP, Caixa Postal 560, Botucatu-SP, 18618-000, Brazil*

Ultrasound backfat (BF, n=4510) and longissimus muscle area (REA, n=4493) and age at first calving (AFC, n=8230) records of Nelore cattle were used to estimate genetic parameters. Nelore is a Zebu breed (*Bos indicus*) which represents 80% of Brazilian beef cattle population. Ultrasound measurements were taken on average at 514 days of age for male and females. Average of AFC was 40.8 ± 6.7 months. Data were analysed by restricted maximum likelihood applied to a multi-trait animal model. For the three traits, the model included fixed effects of contemporary groups (herd, year, sex and management group) and random effects of animal. For ultrasound measurements, fixed effects of age of dam at calving and age at recording as covariable (linear and quadratic effects) were also considered. Heritability estimates from univariate analyses were 0.30 ± 0.07, 0.12 ± 0.04 and 0.10 ± 0.02 for REA, BF and AFC, respectively. Genetic correlation estimates were -0.35 between REA and AFC; -0.48 between BF and AFC and 0.26 between BF and REA. The moderate genetic correlations between ultrasound measurements and AFC, mainly with BF, suggest that these traits can be used to help the identification of early sexual maturing animals.

Poster G3.69

Genetic evaluation of age at first conception in Nellore Cattle using survival analysis

E. Pereira[1]; H.N. Oliveira[1]; J.P. Eler[2]; M.H. Van Melis[2], [1]P.O. Box 560, FMVZ-UNESP, 18.618-000, Botucatu-SP, Brazil, [2]P.O. Box 23, FZEA-USP, 13.635-900, Pirassununga-SP, Brazil.*

Age at first conception (AFC) can be a usefull trait to select animals for sexual precocity. Restricted mating seasons are used in beef cattle exploration, which leads to data censoring. Survival analysis may be the best choice when dealing with censored data. The objective of this paper was to obtain genetic parameters for AFC using a survival model and to compare the sires' rank with others obtained by two different methodologies.

The dataset contained 8,273 records (74% censored) of AFC (in days) measured in Nellore females raised in Brazil. A Weibull mixed animal survival model (SM) was used. Two other methodologies were used to compare sires' ranks: a censored linear model allowing for censoring (LM) (using the same dataset from survival analysis) and Method Â (RM) (using the binary trait heifer pregnancy).

Heritability of AFC obtained from survival analysis was 0.40. Rank correlations between sire evaluations were: 0.92 (between SM and LM), 0.82 (SM and RM) and 0.84 (LM and RM). Little change was observed between sires' ranks from SM and LM. A more consistent change in rank was observed between these last two models and RM, which can occur because heifer pregnancy (binary trait - 0 or 1) does not consider the differences between ages at conception like AFC (continuous trait) does.

Poster G3.70

Genetic parameters for stayability of Polish Black and White cows

Andrzej Zarnecki, Wojciech Jagusiak. Agricultural University, Department of Genetics and Animal Breeding, 30-059 Krakow, Al. Mickiewicza 24/28, Poland

Longevity is considered to be one of the important traits affecting the profitability of dairy herds. Different traits such as survival, length of productive life, stayability, etc., are being used to characterise longevity. In recent years these traits have not been studied in the Polish Black and White cow population, which has undergone major structural changes.

The purpose of the paper is to estimate the heritabilities for stayability, i.e., cow survival to 36, 48, 60, 72 and 84 months.

Restrictions of a minimum of 40 cows per herd-year-season of calving and 40 daughters per sire were imposed. Data consisted of 18704 first lactation, 13268 second lactation and 8735 third lactation cows calving for the first time from 1994 through 1997.

Percentages of cows surviving to ages of 36, 48, 60, 72 and 84 months were 88%, 67%, 46%, 26%, 11%, respectively.

Heritabilities were estimated by the threshold sire model including random effects of sire and error and fixed effects of herd-year-season of calving and genetic group.

The heritability estimates for 36 and 48 month stayability were 0.03. Even lower were heritabilities for 60 (0.02), 72 (0.01), and 84 months (0.02). In other studies the heritabilities for stayability to different ages were usually similar or only slightly higher.

Poster G3.71

Effect of early production and proportion of Holstein genes on days open in Swedish Black and White dairy cows

D.O. Maizon[1], P.A. Oltenacu[1], and E. Strandberg [2], [1]Department of Animal Science, Cornell University, USA, [2]Department of Animal Breeding and Genetics, SLU, Uppsala, Sweden.*

Data consisted of 231757 SLB cows with first calving between 1988 and 1995. The effects of year and season of calving, age at first calving, early milk production, and fraction of North American Holstein genes on days open in primiparous cows were assessed by survival analysis and a sire model. The follow-up period used in the analysis was from 45 to 200 days after first calving. A Weibull distribution was assumed for the hazard of conception, and the analyses were conducted using the Survival Kit. The effect of herd was integrated out during the analysis. Twenty-three percent of the cows were censored. The hazard of conception decreased with year of first calving for the period 1988 to 1995. Days open were shorter for cows calving in winter and summer relative to cows calving in autumn. Age at first calving showed an intermediate optimum with a lower hazard of conception for cows calving at an age younger than 23 or older than 27 months relative to cows with age at first calving between 23 and 27 months. The hazard of conception decreased as the early milk production increased. Days open increased as the fraction of Holstein genes from North America increased.

Poster G3.72

Lactation records adjusted for days open in breeding values

H.G. El-Awady[1], M.N. El-Arian[2] and A.S. Khattab[3]. [1]Department of Animal Production, Faculty of Agriculture, Kafr-El Sheihk, Tanta University, 33516 Egypt, [2]Department of Animal production, Faculty of Agriculture, Mansoura University, Egypt [3]Department of Animal production, Faculty of Agriculture, Tanta, Tanta university, Egypt.

A total of 2166 normal lactation records of Friesian cows raised at Sakha Experimental farm belonging to Ministry of Agriculture, Egypt during the period from 1980 to 2000 were used. Variance components for 305 day milk yield (305dMY) were estimated by the Restricted Maximum Likelihood Method, using an animal model. Two model of breeding values for cows, sires dams were used Model 1 included, individual, permanent environment and errors as random effects. Month and year of calving and lactation number as fixed effects and days open as a covariate. While, model 2 was as to Model 1, but excluding days open. Heritability and repeatability estimates for 305dMY were 0.20 and 0.37, respectively for Model 1 and were 0.15 and 0.39, respectively for model 2.

Higher rank correlations among cows, sires and dams breeding values between the two models was obtained (0.99). The correlations of deviations between the two comparisons with the original evaluation were small.

Poster G3.73

Investigation of possible preferential treatment for imported bulls in six countries

C. Maltecca[1] A.Bagnato[1] K.A.Weigel [2], [1]Dipartimento di Scienze e Tecnologie Veterinarie per la Sicurezza Alimentare, Milano, Italy, [2]Department of Dairy Science, University of Wisconsin Madison, USA.*

Potential preferential treatment for imported bulls was investigated in six countries including Australia, Canada, Germany, Italy, Netherlands and USA. Test day records of 13,316,677 first-lactation cows calving from 1990 to 1997 were analyzed. Bulls were grouped by country of birth: Local, Canadian, American, European and Other. Herds were grouped into three classes according to peak milk yield and herd size. Progeny were assigned to classes based on the year of service of each sire in each country. Daily milk yield in each country was analyzed with a RRTDM including interactions between country of origin of bull by herd level (OHL) or by herd size (OHS). A model including interaction between origin of the bull and year of service (OYS) was also tested. Sire EBV were compared with EBV from a model without interactions. Inclusion of OHL and OHS lead to an increase of the ranking of local bulls in all countries except Netherlands. Largest increase was in Australia, with 34% more of Australian bulls in the top 100. OYS solutions for USA bulls tend to decrease over time in all countries except the USA. OYS solutions for European bulls decreased over time in Canada and USA but remained stable in the other countries.

Poster G3.74

Use of the teaching of V.I.Vernadskiy on biosphere in cattle selection in Ukraine

Y.D. Ruban, Kharkov State Zooveterinary Academy, p/o Malaya Danilovka, Dergachevsky District, Kharkov region, 62341, Ukraine

In cattle selection in Ukraine the teaching of V.I.Vernadskiy has been used. It is 140 years since Vernadskiy's birthday this year. The teaching is used in the following trends: symmetry principle, nutrition autotrophity, native cattle breed genofond conservation.

The principle of symmetry in cattle selection is aimed to determine the population stability considering the interrelation "Genotype - environment", norms and pathology, body constitution condition.

The autotrophy of feeding (nutrition) is used in the selection to define the intensity of consumption and use of bulky foods and conversion ability of the body, the ability to convert nutrient substances of feeds into food.

The conservation of native cattle breeds in Ukraine is complicated by the Chernobyl catastrophe at the atomic power station, by sharp decrease in the number local breeds (Ukrainian grey, Lebedinskay, Brown Carpathian, Pintsgau) and the decrease of common breeds such as Simmental, Red Steppe. The forms of breeds conservation are: Spermobanks (semen bancs) and embriobancs; genofond farms where purebred method is used.

 Poster G3.75

The characteristic of bull-sires for gene BLAD-syndrome

I.S. Turbina, G.V. Eskin, G.S. Turbina, N.S. Marzanov*, The Central Station of Artificial Insemination, p. Bykovo, Podolsk District, Moscow Region, *P.O. Box* 142143, Russia

Since 1996 obligatory researches of bulls for a gene BLAD-syndrome have been carried out, which are included in annual catalogues. Frequency of occurrence of genotypes and alleles BLAD is investigated in 217 bull-sires Black-and-White cattle of the Central Station of Artificial Insemination of the Ministry Agriculture of the Russian Federation. Gene BLAD in the heterozygotic form was detected in 10 pedigree bulls or at 4.6%. Frequency of a mutant gene has made 2.3%. Gene BLAD was identified only in descendants of well-known American bull Osborndale Ivanhoe 1189870. A part of them inherited this gene by paternal line and others - through matrilinear. Excluding two domestic origin bulls, they were purchased in Germany, Holland, Canada and USA in 1985 - 1990 before development of a molecular-genetic method, and one bull acquired in Holland later. In view of the fact, that these bull carriers are highly prepotent, they are used in breeding facilities under the rigid genetic control according to the developed program.

Poster G3.76

Genetic parameters for growth traits in N'Dama cattle under tsetse challenge in The Gambia

N.A. Bosso[1,2], E.H. van der Waaij[3], K. Agyemang[1] and J.A.M. van Arendonk[2]. [1]International Trypanotolerance Centre, PMB 14 Banjul, The Gambia, [2]Wageningen Institute of Animal Sciences, 6700 AH Wageningen, The Netherlands, [3]Department of Farm Animal Health, Veterinary Faculty, University of Utrecht, Yalelaan 5, Utrecht, The Netherlands.*

Heritabilities (h^2) and correlations (r_g) for growth traits in N'Dama cattle were estimated using an animal model. Data originated from ITC's breeding herd. Animals are born and weaned in a low tsetse challenge area (low trypanosomosis challenge), thereafter moved to a high tsetse challenge area. Body weight recorded at birth and after weaning at three months intervals was considered in the analysis. Season was divided in rainy (WET), early dry (EDR) and late dry (LDR). Calving occurred all year round, though with peaks in WET and EDR. h^2 ranged from 0.11 for weight at 24 months (W24) to 0.4 for weight at 36 months (W36) and from 0.13 for weight during LDR to 0.27 for weight during EDR. r_g between birth weight (BW) and weight at 12 (W12), and 15 (W15) months were moderately high (0.51 and 0.6, respectively). r_g between WET and LDR was 0.63 the one between WET and EDR was 0.44. It was concluded that growths during the three seasons are different traits. The genetic trend were highest for W36 (0.88 kg/year) and for weight gain in the EDR (0.35 kg/year).

Poster G3.77

Consequences of selection on production under metabolic stress: a resource allocation approach

E.H. van der Waaij Department of Farm Animal Health, PO Box 80151, 3508 TD Utrecht, The Netherlands*

Consequences for observed production and reproduction rate, due to long-term selection on production under metabolic stress, were investigated using a stochastic model. The model describes the allocation of resources to production and fitness of an animal. Resource allocation is controlled by a factor 'c'. To account for natural selection for fitness, female reproduction rate was allowed to decrease with decreasing fitness, using a threshold approach. Resource intake, production and allocation of resources were assumed to be genetically uncorrelated and to be partly heritable, whereas reproduction rate, fitness and observed production are resulting parameters. Results show that the consequences of artificial selection for production depend on the genetic variation in resource intake versus that in 'c'. The genetic potential for production is always higher then the observed production, the latter being a result of availability of resources. For each set of parameters and environment there seems to be a defined reproduction rate at which the population stabilises. Animals that were transferred from a poor to a good environment showed an increase in survival rate when h^2_c is high, and a negative correlation between observed production and 'c' developed. Animals that were transferred from a good to a poor environment showed a considerable decrease in survival rate, and the correlation between observed production and 'c' remained positive.

Poster G3.78

Endogenous retroviruses as potential infectious risk in biomedical products of pig and sheep

N. Klymiuk[1], M. Müller[2], G. Brem[1] and B. Aigner[2], [1]ApoGene Biotechnologie, D-86567 Hilgertshausen, Germany, [2]Institute of Animal Breeding and Genetics, Veterinary University Vienna, A-1210 Vienna, Austria.*

Use of genetically modified pigs and sheep in xenotransplantation and gene farming is planned to provide biotechnological and pharmaceutical products for humans. Prevention of the cross-species transfer of pathogens with unknown consequences for the patients and the community is essential for these techniques. The potential infectious risk of endogenous retroviruses (ERV), which are retroviral genomes integrated into the germline of the host species, is of major concern. Porcine endogenous retroviruses (PERV) have previously been found to infect other species in several *in vitro* and *in vivo* studies. Therefore, we concisely examined PERV and ovine endogenous retroviruses (OERV) by studying ERV *pro/pol* sequences in different breeds. In both species, phylogenetic analyses resulted in the classification of novel ERV families. No significant variations in the crucial proviral load were observed between different breeds. New open reading frame (ORF) containing sequences as well as hybrid sequences, which were putatively caused by recombination events, were identified. As already described in pigs, ERV expression was also shown in sheep. Thus, the potential risk of infection can not be ruled out for intact and/or mutant ERV in the biotechnological products of both species.

Poster G3.79

Effect of parity number on litter size in pigs

G.L. Restelli[1], A. Stella[2], G. Pagnacco[1]. [1]Facoltà di Medicina Veterinaria, Dipartimento di Scienze e Tecnologie Veterinarie per la Sicurezza Alimentare (VSA), Via Grasselli 7, 20137 Milano, Italy, [2]FPTP - CERSA, Palazzo L.I.T.A., Via F.lli Cervi 93, 20090 Segrate (MI), Italy*

Objective of the present study was to evaluate the effect of parity number on litter size in pigs. Traits analysed were number of piglets born alive, number of stillborn piglets, and number of piglets weaned. Data consisted of farrowing records from 1991 to 2000 of three purebred lines (Large White, Landrace and Duroc) and line crosses, concerning a total of 10061 sows in three Italian herds. The pedigree file included all individuals genetically linked with the data.
Statistical analysis were performed by using a mixed model which included breed, parity, and herd-year-season as fixed effects and sow as random effect.
Results showed that number of piglets born alive increased as parity number increased from first to third where the maximum number of born alive was observed and decreased in subsequent parities
The difference between number of piglets born alive in first and third parity was 1.2 units.
The number of stillbirths decreased from first to second parity, then increased in subsequent parities, more sharply after the fifth parity.
Parity number also influenced the number of piglets weaned, which reached a maximum in second parity and decreased quickly in later parities. Positive effect of crossbreeding was observed for all traits.

Poster G3.80

Growth of live body weight and body measurements of Large White pigs gilts

*P. Flak[1], L. Kovác[2], L. Hetényi[*1], [1]Research Institute of Animal Production, Hlohovská 2, 949 92 Nitra, [2]Slovak Agricultural University, Tr. A. Hlinku 2, 949 76 Nitra, Slovak Republic*

The growth analyses of body live weight and body live measurements between 1st to 7th month of live of 36 gilts of Large White pigs showed the importance of optimal development of body as a whole and its parts. Body live weight was at 1st month 8.65 or at 7th month 113.78 kg. Body and trunk length were 48.01 and 18.06 cm at 1st month or 124.13 and 48.17 cm at 7th month. Withers height and height in hips corresponded in this months to 29.14 and 30.53 or 65.67 and 70.28 cm. Width, depth and circumference of chest were as follows: at 1st month 10.89, 11.69 and 44.86 cm, at 7th month 28.54, 35.7 and 111.04 cm. Width of pelvis and width in hips were 11.01 and 8.19 cm at 1st or 30.54 and 26.21 cm at 7th month. Metacarpus circumference was 8.65 at 1st and 17.03 cm at 7th month.. Besides trunk length and width in hips growth of all other body measurements was nonlinear. Allometry of body measurements to the body live weight except withers height, height in hips and metacarpus circumference was positive. Allometry of trunk length to the body length was isometric.Growth and development of body live weight and somatometric measurements confirmed the significance of these studies for pig breeding.

Poster G3.81

Estimates of genetic parameters for juvenile IGF-I from MSZV trial data

U. Wuensch[1]; K.L. Bunter[2], U. Mueller[3] and U. Bergfeld[3], [1]Pig Breeding Association of Middle Germany, PSF 954, 09009 Chemnitz, [2]Animal Genetics and Breeding Unit, UNE, Armidale, NSW 2351, Australia, [3]Saxonian Federal Institution of Agriculture, Am Park 3, 04886 Köllitsch, Germany.*

Estimates of genetic parameters for juvenile insulin-like growth factor (IGF-I) concentration and several performance traits were obtained using data collected from German Landrace males entering the MSZV test station during 2000/2001. After editing for outliers, record numbers ranged from 576 for juvenile IGF-I to 678 for lifetime daily gain.
The heritability estimate for juvenile IGF-I was 0.29±0.15 (common litter effect: 0.25±0.08). Genetic correlations between IGF-I and feed intake, feed conversion ratio, ultra sound backfat and backfat area were very high and positive (range: 0.66-0.81±0.26). Genetic correlations between IGF-I and belly points or back muscle area were -0.58±0.24 and -0.47±0.22, respectively. Genetic correlations were close to zero between IGF-I and pH_1_cutlet or lifetime average daily gain, and moderate between IGF-I and test period average daily gain (-0.18±0.34) or intra muscular fat (0.20±0.25). Residual correlations between IGF-I and the performance traits tended to be low, and not significantly different from zero.
Both genetic and phenotypic correlations indicate that animals with lower juvenile IGF-I should have lower feed intake, feed conversion ratio, backfat and back fat area, and higher muscle area and belly score.
Results from this trial are overall consistent with those from previous trials, and application of the patented technology, supporting a downward selection strategy for juvenile IGF-I.

Poster G3.82

Heterosis effect in crosses between Duroc and Pietrain pigs

R. Eckert, G. Zak, National Research Institute of Animal Production, 32-083 Balice-Kraków, Poland

The aim of the study was to estimate and compare the heterosis effect for traits evaluated in performance test in two groups of ♀ Pietrain × ♂ Duroc and ♀ Duroc × ♂ Pietrain hybrids in relation to the performance of Duroc and Pietrain purebreds. Data on live evaluation of young boars and gilts, carried out in 1999-2001 in a pedigree farm of Pietrain and Duroc pigs were used in the experiment. Both the Duroc boars and gilts were characterized by markedly higher daily gains than the Pietrains. Also the hybrids born from Duroc sows exhibited slightly higher daily gains than the hybrids born from Pietrain sows and achieved higher indicators of the heterosis effect for both sexes (3,37% - boars and 2,18% - gilts). The thinnest backfat was found in the Pietrains. Hybrid gilts and boars born from Pietrain sows had much thinner backfat than the hybrids born from Duroc sows. Both for boars and gilts from Pietrain sows, a beneficial negative heterosis effect was shown (-0,88% and 2,83%). The differences followed a similar pattern between the experimental groups for carcass lean percentage. The heterosis effect was very low and positive in hybrids of both sexes derived from Pietrain sows (0,43%-boars and 0,97%-gilts) and low and negative in hybrids derived from Duroc sows (-0,78%-boars and -0,26% gilts).

Poster G3.83

Progress achieved in leanness and growth rate in some herds of Duroc pigs

R. Eckert, M.Różycki, G.Zak, National Research Institute of Animal Production, 32-083 Balice-Kraków, Poland

Research was conducted to evaluate the progress achieved in productive traits of selected herds of Duroc pigs. Results of performance testing of gilts and young boars carried out in three breeding herds of Duroc pigs were used. For each herd, selection differentials were calculated as the difference between mean values of traits of animals selected for replacement from a given generation and mean values of animals tested in a given generation. For gilts, the lowest selection differentials for daily gains were found in herd A (18 g) and the highest in herd C (32 and 35 g). Likewise for percentage lean in carcass, the lowest selection differential was found in herd A (1.2-1.3%) and the highest in herd C (2.1-2.2%).With regard to boars, selection differentials for daily gains were small in all the herds in the 31-47 g range. Greater selection differentials were observed for percentage lean in carcass, especially in herd A (1.8 and 2.4%). In the analysed herds, although animals characterized by better performance than the mean for the generation were selected for replacement, the selection differential obtained proved too small to ensure greater progress. In gilts it was equal to or lower than 0.5 standard deviation for daily gains and less than 1 standard deviation for leanness. Selection differentials for boars were similar.

Poster G3.84

Correlated responses in reproductive performance of sows selected for growth rate on restricted feeding

N.H. Nguyen[1], C.P. McPhee[2]. [1]School of Veterinary Science, University of Queensland, Q4072, Australia. [2]Animal Research Institute, Department of Primary Industries, Australia*

This study aimed to evaluate the reproductive performance of Large White pigs selected for high and low growth rate under restricted feeding regime. Data were collected from four years and analyses were carried out on 913 records using the multi-trait animal model restricted maximum likelihood. After four years of the selection process, the high growth line sows had a significantly higher number of piglets born alive than the low line sows. Average and individual birth weights of the high line piglets were also significantly heavier than those of the low line piglets. There were no statistical differences in total number of piglets born, number of piglets at weaning, individual piglet weaning weight and pre-weaning mortality between the selection lines. Relative to the low line, sows of the high growth line had a significantly higher body weight pior to mating. The apparently lower food intake of the high relative to the low line sows during lactation was not significant indicating that daily food intake differences found between grower pigs in the lines on *ad libitum* feeding were not fully expressed in lactating sows.
It is concluded that selection for high growth rate on restricted feeding produced Large White pig lines with improved growth, fatness and reproduction traits.

Poster G3.85

Response to selection of weaning weight based on maternal effect in Syrian hamsters: Results from twelve generations

K. Ishii[1], M. Satoh[2], O. Sasaki[1], H. Takeda[1] and T. Furukawa[1], [1]National Institute of Livestock and Grassland Science, Tsukuba-shi 305-0901, [2]National Institute of Agrobiological Sciences, Tsukuba-shi 305-8602, Japan.*

Twelve generations of selection were conducted to study the response for weaning weight (WW) of standardized litter size in Syrian hamsters. The experiment involved four lines: selection on an estimate of direct genetic effect of WW (line A); selection on an estimate of maternal genetic effect of WW (line M); selection on estimate of an aggregate genetic value of direct and maternal effects of WW (line B); a randomly selected control (line C). Direct and maternal effects were estimated from an animal model BLUP. Two replicates in each line were propagated from the same population. Significant difference between C and each selected line for WW was found at after generation 5; linear regression of WW for each selected line as a deviation from C on generation number was significantly positive. Direct and maternal heritability estimates for WW were 0.15 and 0.18, respectively, and correlation between direct and maternal genetic effects was 0.09. Mean estimates of direct and maternal genetic effects for WW increased linearly with generation in each selected line: estimated direct effect in generation 12 was 7.9 g, 7.5 g, and 7.2 g for A, M, and B, respectively; estimated maternal effect was 3.7 g, 5.8 g, and 4.0 g for A, M, and B, respectively. Average inbreeding at generation 12 was approximately 24 % in all selected lines. Selection using maternal effect had beneficial to genetic improvement for WW.

Poster G3.86

Development of high fat diet induced obesity in growth selected mouse lines

U. Renne[1], J. Kratzsch[2], S. Kuhla[1], M. Langhammer[1], N. Reinsch[1] and G.A. Brockmann[1], [1]Forschungsinstitut für die Biologie landwirtschaftlicher Nutztiere Dummerstorf, [2]Institut für Labormedizin, Klinische Chemie und Molekulare Diagnostik, Universität Leipzig, Germany*

Growth and body composition are complex polygenic traits. It is nessesary to identify genetic and physiological as well as exogenous factors responsible for their development. We studied the 112 generations for high body weight selected mouse line DU6, its selected inbred derivate DU6i and the unselected controls DUKs and DBA/2. DU6 and DU6i differ from their controls for more than 100% in body weight and 300% in fat accumulation. In the present study 24 males and 24 females from each of the mouse lines were divided in two groups fed either with a standard breeding diet or with a 15% fat diet from weaning up to day 150. Body composition was measured at day 21, 42, 98 and 150 by the mouse densitometer PIXImus and by chemical analysis. As expected, the responses to the fat diet were line dependent, indicating a strong genetic effect on growth, fat amount and fat% of the body. This effect was observed especially in the selected lines and in DBA/2. Under same feeding conditions females became significantly fatter than males. Interestingly, high variation in fat deposition was found between inbred families within DU6i and DUKsi. This indicates a specific genotype effect on energy intake, metabolism, heat production, or energy deposition.

Poster G3.87

Food intake and body composition in lines of mice selected for growth on normal and reduced protein diets

V.H. Nielsen. Danish Institute of Agricultural Sciences, Research Centre Foulum, Department of Animal Breeding and Genetics, P.O. Box 50, DK-8830 Tjele, Denmark

Consistent genotype-environment interactions were found in lines of mice selected for growth from 3 to 9 weeks of age on diets containing a normal and a reduced protein content when tested on both diets in generation 7. This paper reports preliminary results of correlated responses for food consumption and body composition.
On each diet there were 3 lines selected for high growth, 3 lines selected for low growth and 3 control lines. In generation 7 and 9 all lines were tested on both diets. Food intake on the normal protein diet was measured in generation 7. Body composition was measured on both test diets in generation 9. The data were analysed using a linear model. For analysis of body composition, the model included selection diet, selection direction, replicate, test diet and sex as fixed effects. Test diet was eliminated in the analysis of food consumption.
No difference in food intake and body composition was observed between mice selected on the normal and the reduced protein diet but feeding mice the low protein diet resulted in animals with a higher fat percent and a lower protein, fat and water percent. Mice selected for high growth consumed more food and were fatter than mice selected for low growth. Males consumed more food and were leaner than females.

Poster G3.88

Carcass analysis in Japanese quail lines divergently selected for shape of growth curve

L. Hyánková, A. Mohsen, J. Lastovková and Z. Szebestová, Research Institute of Animal Production, Prátelství 815, P.O.Box 1, 104 01 Prague-Uhríneves, Czech Republic*

A study was conducted to determine carcass composition changes following 18 generations of divergent selection for shape of the growth curve. Males of the HG and LG lines were fed on standard diets used during selection and individually weighed at 7d intervals from hatching to 77d of age. From 7 to 42 d of age, five quail of each line were weekly sacrificed and their defeathered carcasses were analysed for dry matter, protein and total lipid contents. Carcass composition determinations revealed significant age and line effects. Both percentage of dry matter and lipid increased with age during the whole experimental period (across lines: from 27.5 to 38.3 % and from 6.0 to 13.7%, resp.). However, the percentage of protein significantly elevated only to age at inflection point of the growth curve for LG and HG lines, i.e. approximately to 2 or 3 w of age, resp., and remained nearly constant (about 19.5%) thereafter. The interline differences in carcass composition were confirmed for early growth period. The LG males exhibiting a higher growth rate than HG males immediately post-hatch were characterized by a significantly higher percentage of dry matter to 14d and lipids to 21d of age than those of HG line. Thereafter, the interline differences for both diminished.

Poster G3.89

Best linear unbiased prediction of White Holland Turkeys toms regarding body weight and conformation measures

R.Y. Nofal[*1]; A.M. Abdel-Ghany[2] and M.Y. Mostafa[3] [1]Poultry Production Dept.; Faculty of Agric.; Tanta University; Egypt, [2]Animal Production Dept.; Faculty of Agric.; Suez Canal University; Egypt, [3]Animal Production Research Institute; Ministry of Agriculture; Egypt*

Body weight and conformation measures (i.e. length of keel, KL; shank, SHL and breast width, BRW) of 907 White Holland (WH) turkey offspring were analyzed using Restricted Maximum Likelihood (REML) under Mixed Model Equations. Best Linear Unbiased Estimates (BLUE) included the effects of hatch; sex and hatch X sex (H X S) interaction along with unrelated 33 sires as a random effect. The respective 16 wk. of age BW, KL, SHL & BRW overall BLUE for WH were 4262.74 ± 27.20 g, 138.79 ± 0.55 mm, 144.67 ± 0.40 mm and 160.02 ± 0.53 mm.
Transmitting ability estimates of WH turkeys ranged from -257.60 to 151.69 g. for BW; -2.47 to 5.17 mm. for KL; -4.35 to 3.17 mm. for SHL and -3.46 to 4.59 mm. for BRW. The range for the top 30% ranked sires were 58.30 g., 4.17 mm., 2.16 mm. and 3.20 mm. for BW, KL, SHL and BRW, respectively. However, the number of sires having positive TA records reached = 45% from the tested individuals at each of the considered trait.
The Pearson and Spearman correlation coefficients were generally intermediate to high and significant. Heritability estimates were intermediate.

Poster G3.90

Identification of (in)sensitive broiler lines to Escherichia Coli and consequential variation in physiological- and immunological characteristics and production

B. Ask[*12], E.H. van der Waaij[12], J.A. Stegeman[1], [1]Department of Animal Health, PO Box 80151, 3508TD Utrecht, The Netherlands, [2]Animal Breeding and Genetics Group, PO Box 338, 6700AH Wageningen, The Netherlands.*

Colibacillosis, induced by Escherichia Coli (EC) as primary or secondary infection, causes large economic losses in broiler production due to medical expenses, mortality and (mainly) growth depression.
It is hypothesised that different broiler lines differ in susceptibility and responses to an EC infection. Expectation is that some lines will be very sensitive, judged by clinical effects, and show considerable growth depression, while others will be relatively sensitive, but still approach their growth potential. Yet other lines are expected to be relatively insensitive and consequently proximate their growth potential.
704 1 week old chicks of 8 broiler lines (including a biological line), selected for more or less extreme growth, feed conversion and breast meat yield and known to differ in mortality in general, will be intratracheal inoculated with EC or placebo bouillon solution. Variation in physiological (thyroid hormones, organ weights), immunological (antibody titers and type) and production (growth, breast meat yield, carcass, abdominal fat) responses will be measured along with clinical effects (section score). Based on this, the relative sensitivity to and coping ability with EC infection of the different lines will be investigated and characteristics with potential importance as, or for identification of, selection criteria against EC susceptibility will be identified.

Poster G3.91

The opportunity to introduce the fertility into a breeding program in a Cornish line

I. Custura, I. Van ,St. Popescu Vifor,Elena Popescu Miclosanu, Minodora Tudorache, University of Agronomical Sciences and Veterinary Medicine Bucharest, Faculty of Animal Sciences, 59 Marasti Blvd., 1 sector, Romania*

The Cornish lines, which have given the paternal simple hybrid, besides the fact they are selected by the growing speed, body conformation and feed conversion, they have a weak fecundity, and for that, into the objective of their selection, it should be included this trait, too.
The aim of this study is, on the one hand, the elaboration of a breeding program, where to include, also, the fertility in the selection objective, and on the other hand, to estimate the economical gain through the evaluation of the meat production global indicator, expressed in Euro per dam.
The study was done using the results obtained from the control of production and selection, in the cock families, where from there were taken males for the next generation.
In this way, taking into account the performances recorded into the analysed lines and the partial genetic progress which we were expected in each line, in different economical weights, the influence of fertility on the global indicator (which it is of 286.52 Euro in the non-selected sample) have been established. In the sample selected using the selection index, on three traits, the value increased to 287.90 Euro, and in the sample selected also using selection index, but on four traits, the value reached 290.08 Euro per dam, value which increased due to the increasing of number of chicks.

Poster G3.92

Estimating genetic parameters for dressage in the Belgian Warmblood Horse population

M. Brondeel[1], S. De Smet[2], S. Janssens[1], N. Buys[1] and W. Vandepitte[1], [1]Katholieke Universiteit Leuven, Centre for Animal Genetics and Selection, Kasteelpark Arenberg 30, 3001 Heverlee, Belgium, [2]Ghent University , Department of Animal Production, Proefhoevestraat 10, 9090 Melle, Belgium*

Data of dressage competitions were used to estimate genetic parameters for dressage. The dataset comprises 179364 records of 12228 competing horses for the years 1995-2000. Three different traits were defined: 1. a "BLOM standard normal score" based on rankings; 2. a "standardised score" based on judge percentage scores; 3. a lifetime highest score based on the highest competition level and standardised score ever achieved. Fixed effects included were sex, age and class.
For the BLOM and the standardised score, the rider (RI) and the permanent environmental effect (PE) accounted each for 20% and the additive-genetic effect accounted for 10% of the variance. For the lifetime highest score, heritability was 0,050 and 0,104 in the model without and with RI respectively; the RI accounting itself for 15% of the variance.
In a multiple-trait model based on levels of competition, RI and PE estimates ranged between 16-17% and 16 to 23% respectively for the trait standardised score. Heritabilities were somewhat lower (6-10%) and genetic correlations ranged from 0,54-0,93.
In conclusion, the standardised score seem to be more explaining than the other traits and the positive genetic correlations allow prediction of genetic merit for higher levels based on data from lower levels.

Poster G3.93

Use of BLUP Animal Model for estimating breeding values of sport horses in Ukraine

O.V. Bondarenko and V.A. Danshin, Istitute of Animal Science of UAAS, P/O Kulinichi, Kharkov, 62404, Ukraine.

The possibilities and advantages of use of BLUP Animal Model for estimating breeding values of sport horses under the conditions of Ukraine were studied.
The database included data on body measurements (crest height, body length, chest circumference and shank circumference) and sport workability in competitions. The sport workability was expressed in scores, given to a horse in competitions.
Linear model included effects of sex, age, trainer and combination 'environmental conditions - preliminary training'. Joint influence of these effects explaned 74.7% of variation for sport workability, 35.5% for crest height, 25.5% for body length, 40.6% for chest circumference and 35.5% for shank circumference. Heritability estimates obtained using DFREML 3.1 program were: 0.12 for sport workability, 0.52 for crest height, 0.55 for body length, 0.22 for chest circumference and 0.30 for shank circumference.
On the basis of statistical analysis of changes in estimated breeding values of horses for sport workability the averafe genetic gain for period of 1950-2000 was estimated and the expected increase in genetic gain from use of BLUP Animal Model in sport horse breeding in Ukraine was predicted.

Poster G3.94

Genetic responses for dysplasia, behavioural and conformation traits from alternative breeding schemes in a dog population

K. Mäki[1], A.-E. Liinamo[2], A.F. Groen[3], P. Bijma[3] and M. Ojala[1], [1]Dept. Animal Science, P.O. Box 28, 00014 Helsinki University, Finland, [2]Farm Animal Industrial Platform, Benedendorpsweg 98, 6862 WC Oosterbeek, The Netherlands, [3]Dept. Animal Sciences, Wageningen University, P.O. Box 338, 6700 AH Wageningen, The Netherlands.*

Aim of this study was to assess genetic responses with simultaneous selection for hip (HD) and elbow (ED) dysplasia, behavioural traits (BE) and conformation (CO). For this purpose, structure of the Finnish Rottweiler population was simulated. Realised gain in practice had been 0.03 genetic SD for both HD and ED and relative weights according these gains were 0.4 for both traits. Assumed present weights for BE and CO were 0.5 and 2.0, respectively. Increasing information sources or increasing number of selection candidates did not result in further genetic gain for HD, ED or BE. Desired genetic gain of 1.0 genetic SD for HD and ED and 0.5 to 1.0 genetic SD for BE over a period of 10 years was reached by changing the relative weights dramatically towards favouring these traits. For CO, the goal was just to keep the trait constant. Increase in the number of selection candidates resulted in further gain for the three traits, as long as the weights clearly favoured them. To preserve desired behaviour and to improve health of the dogs in the current populations, systematic breeding programs favouring these traits should be developed.

Theatre G4.1

Between- and within breed variation of farrowing length and its relationships with litter size and perinatal survival in pigs

L. Canario[*1], T. Tribout[1], J. Gruand[2], J.C. Caritez[3], J.P. Bidanel[1] - INRA, [1]Station de Génétique Quantitative et Appliquée, 78352 Jouy-en-Josas, France [2]INRA, Unité expérimentale de Sélection porcine, 86480 Rouillé, France [3]INRA, Domaine expérimental du Magneraud, Saint-Pierre d'Amilly, 17700 Surgères, France*

Between- and within-breed variation of farrowing length (FL), defined as the period of time between the first and the last piglet born in a litter, and farrowing rhythm, estimated by the average time between two successive piglets (ATSP = FL / total number born) was investigated. Four genetic types of sows, i.e. Large White, Meishan, Laconie and Duroc x Large White were compared (564, 55, 147 and 82 litters, respectively). In spite of significant differences in litter size, sow genetic type did not significantly affects FL or ATSP. Within-breed variation was estimated in a Large White population (1901 litters) using restricted maximum likelihood methodology applied to a multiple trait animal model. Both FL and AFLB appeared as lowly heritable (0.03±0.02 and 0.045±0.02, respectively). They were positively correlated on the phenotypic scale (r_p=0.58), but presented a close to zero genetic correlation. Total number born had moderate positive phenotypic (r_p=0.24) and genetic correlations (r_g=0.49) with FL, and strong negative correlations with ATSP (r_p=-0.51; r_g=-0.82). The number of stillbirths was moderately correlated with both FL (r_p =0.12; r_g=0.37) and ATSP (r_p =-0.13; r_g=-0.36). Proportion of stillbirths was almost independent of FL (r_p =0.06 r_g=0.12) and had a negative genetic correlation with ATSP (r_p =-0.02 ; r_g=-0.45).

Theatre G4.2

Heritabilities and genetic relationships between gestation length, stillbirth, size of calves, and calving problems in Danish Holstein cows

M. Hansen[1,2,3], M. S. Lund[1], J. Pedersen[2], and L. G. Christensen[3]. [1]DIAS, Dept of Animal Breeding and Genetics, P.O. Box 50 DK-8830 Tjele, Denmark. [2]Danish Cattle Federation, Udkærsvej 15, DK-8200 Aarhus N. [3]The Royal Veterinary and Agricultural University, Dept of Animal Science and Animal Health, Grønnegaardsvej 3, DK-1870 Frederiksberg C, Denmark.*

The objective of this study was to make inference about direct and maternal heritabilities of gestation lengths (GL), stillbirths (SB), size of calves (SC), and calving problems (CP) for first calving Danish Holstein cows and to examine if the genetic relationship between these traits is non-linear. A linear model for GL and a threshold model for the other traits was fitted using Bayesian methodology. The marginal posterior mean (standard deviation) of the direct heritability was 0.42 (0.02) for GL, 0.11 (0.01) for CP, 0.22 (0.02) for SC, and 0.10 (0.01) for SB. The marginal posterior mean of the maternal heritability was 0.07 (0.01) for GL, 0.07 (0.01) for CP, 0.04 (0.01) for SC, and 0.13 (0.02) for SB. The marginal posterior mean (standard deviation) of the genetic correlation between direct and maternal effects was 0.13 (0.06) for GL, 0.21 (0.08) for CP, -0.11 (0.07) for SC, and 0.05 (0.10) for SB. Linear and quadratic regressions of predicted breeding values indicated a genetic relationship between most traits, but no evidence of a non-linear genetic relationship was found.

Theatre G4.3

Genetic study of calving difficulty, stillbirth and birth weight of Charolais and Hereford

S. Eriksson, A. Näsholm, K. Johansson and J. Philipsson, Swedish University of Agricultural Sciences, Dept. of Animal Breeding and Genetics, Box 7023, 75007 Uppsala, Sweden*

Calving traits have long been recorded for purebred beef cattle in Sweden, but only birth weight has been used in the genetic evaluation to avoid calving difficulties. The aim of this study was to estimate direct and maternal genetic parameters for calving difficulty, stillbirth and birth weight at first and later parities of beef breeds. Linear animal model analyses included records on birth weight for 60,309 Charolais and 30,789 Hereford, and calving traits for 74,538 Charolais and 37,077 Hereford born 1980-2001. The frequency of difficult calvings and stillbirths were about 6% at first and 1-2% at later parities for both breeds. Less than half of the stillborn calves had difficult calvings. Direct and maternal heritabilities for birth weight were 0.44-0.51 and 0.06-0.15, respectively. Heritabilities on the visible scale for calving difficulty were 0.11-0.16 for direct and 0.07-0.12 for maternal effects at first parity, and lower at later parities. Estimated heritabilities for stillbirth were very low both at the visible (0.002-0.016) and underlying scale. Direct-maternal genetic correlations were with few exceptions negative. Genetic correlations between the traits and between parities within traits were generally moderate to high and positive. Calving difficulty should be included in the genetic evaluation, while progeny groups for beef breeds in Sweden are too small for stillbirth to be considered directly.

Theatre G4.4

Mapping of quantitative trait loci affecting fertility traits in Finnish Ayrshire

N.F. Schulman[1], S. Viitala[1], D.J. de Koning[2], A. Mäki-Tanila[1] and J. Vilkki[1], [1]MTT, Agrifood Research Finland, FIN-31600 Jokioinen, Finland, [2]Department of Genetics and Biometry, Roslin Institute, Roslin, EH25 95P UK.*

In a QTL mapping study the whole genome was searched in order to find loci affecting fertility traits. A grand daughter design with 12 half-sib families and 491 sons was applied. A total of 150 markers were typed with an average spacing of 20 cM. The analysed traits were frequency of fertility treatments, days open and non-return rate. Fertility treatments includes information about fertility treartments done by a veterinarian within 150 days after calving and information about culling due to fertility problems. Days open is calculated as the number of days from calving to the next pregnancy. Non-return rate indicates the ability of a bull to get cows pregnant. It is evaluated based on the inseminations of the bulls semen to a random set of cows. Breeding values were provided from the Finnish Animal Breeding Association. A multiple marker regression approach was used in order to estimate QTL positions and effects. QTL on other chromosomes were accounted for to increase power of QTL detection by fitting their transmission probabilities as cofactors in the analysis.. Empirical P-values were obtained by permutation. A total of 20 genome-wise significant QTL were identified, 7 affecting fertility treatments, 10 affecting days open and 3 affecting non-return rate.

Theatre G4.5

Genetic relationship among longevity, health, fertility, body condition score, type, and production traits in Swiss Holstein cattle

H.N. Kadarmideen[1,] and S. Wegmann[2], [1]Statistical Animal Genetics Group, Institute of Animal Science, ETH Zurich, CH 8092, Switzerland, [2]Holstein Switzerland, 1725 Posieux, Switzerland.*

Genetic relationship between body condition score (BCS), type, fertility, survival (SUR) and somatic cell count (SCC) traits were investigated in Swiss Holstein cattle. Genetic parameters for BCS and genetic regression coefficients (β) of regressing BCS, 27 linear type and 5 milk production traits on sire Estimated Breeding Values (EBV) for daughter's non-return rates (NRR), calving to first insemination interval (CFI), survival and SCC were estimated. Data set consisted of 25126 records and 80329 animals in pedigree. Model terms were based on literature. Heritability and permanent environmental variance for BCS were 0.23 and 0.21, respectively. Estimated β's for BCS were -0.005, 0.002 and -0.010 for CFI, NRR, and SCC, respectively. This indicates that good BCS is genetically related to shorter CFI, higher NRR, and low SCC. Estimated β's for SUR was not significant. Type traits had favorable genetic relationship with survival (-0.001 to 0.116), SCC (-0.010 to -0.260), CFI (-0.002 to 0.009) and NRR (-0.001 to 0.006). Generally, milk production traits had unfavorable genetic relationship with genetic merit for all the functional traits. (Genetic) correlations among sire EBVs showed that NRR was favorably correlated with CFI (0.12), SCC (-0.18) and SUR (0.09); CFI was favorably correlated with SCC (-0.10) and SUR (-0.12); SCC was favorably correlated with SUR (-0.29).

Theatre G4.6

Study on longevity, type traits and production in Chianina beef cattle using survival analysis

F. Forabosco[1], A.F. Groen[2], R. Bozzi[3], J.A.M. Van Arendonk[2], F. Filippini[1] and P. Bijma[2,], [1]Associazione Nazionale Allevatori Bovini Italiani da Carne, Vio Viscioloso, 07060 S. Martino in Colle, Italy, [2]Animal Breeding and Genetics Group, Wageningen University, The Netherlands and [3]Department of Animal Science, University of Florence, Via delle Cascine 5, 50144 Florence, Italy.*

Longevity is a trait increasingly important in beef cattle. Genetic improvement of longevity reduces the cost for the farmer and increases his revenue. Survival analysis was used with a model that includes the herd-year effect, herd size variation, age at first calving, production levels, type traits and the expert who scored the cows. Herd-year and age at first calving had a strong effect on the risk of being culled for a beef cow. Production traits such as number of calves born and the weight of the calves had effects on longevity, indicating that voluntary culling is important in beef cattle. Twenty-two type traits have been analysed. Muscularity traits had the largest impact on longevity followed by dimension and finesse. Udder trait had no effect on longevity.

Theatre G4.7

Weibull log-normal sire frailty models

L.H. Damgaard[1], I.R. Korsgaard[2], J. Simonsen[3], O. Dalsgaard[3] and A.H. Andersen[3], [1]Royal Veterinary and Agricultural University, DK-1870 Frederiksberg C, [2]Danish Institute of Agricultural Sciences, P.O.Box 50, DK-8830 Tjele, [3]University of Aarhus, DK-8000 Aarhus C.*

Models used worldwide for sire evaluations of longevity are known to ignore part of the additive genetic variance. The purpose of this study was to quantify some of the consequences. In two simulation studies data were generated according to a Weibull log-normal sire frailty model with genetic interpretation (Model A), and data were analysed with this model and with a Weibull log-normal sire frailty model without genetic interpretation (Model B).
In the first study four different datasets balanced in the number of daughters per sire, but differing in the level of censoring were generated. Parameter estimates obtained from Model B were strongly biased and highly influenced by the level of censoring, and from model A consistent with true values.
In the second study the data structure in dairy breeding was mimicked. With Model B estimated sire effects of proven bulls with second crop daughters were decreased (improved) when level of censoring increased from 20% to about 86%, without changing estimated sire effects of remaining bulls. This jump of sire effects was not observed with Model A. This study suggest that the problem, with unstable sire effects observed in practise, is caused by the fact that sires are ranked for longevity based on models ignoring part of the additive genetic variance.

Theatre G4.8

Effect of AI-sires on connectedness and accuracy of breeding values in Norwegian beef cattle breeding -a simulation study

S.U. Narvestad[1], E. Sehested[1,2] and G. Klemetsdal[1], [1]Department of Animal Science, Agricultural University of Norway, P.O. Box 5025, NO-1432 Aas, Norway, [2]Geno Breeding and AI Association, 2326 Hamar, Norway.*

The objective of this study was to investigate the effect of artificial insemination (AI) on connectedness and accuracy of predicted breeding values using stochastic simulation. Data from the Norwegian Hereford population was analyzed to find population structure parameters like reproductive life for males and females, number and size of herds, exchange of animals between herds, use of AI sires etc. Beef cattle production in Norway is characterized by several breeds in few and small herds. AI-sires continue as natural mating-sires (NM) after a short semen collection period. In the simulation only one NM-sire was used per year in each herd. Use of AI was varied from zero to all matings in the herds. Number of herds (125), herd size (average 11) and population size (1370 calves born each year) were kept constant throughout the simulation. To evaluate the effect of accuracy only, no selection was performed at any stage. No import was considered. The model used was a single-trait animal model for yearling weight with sex as fixed effect and herd-year as random effect. Different alternatives were run for 20 years and with 20 replicates. Correlation between true genetic values and predicted breeding values were obtained for each situation.

Theatre G4.9

Optimum design of an on-station test of bull dams in dairy cattle breeding programs

S. König[1] and H.H. Swalve[2], [1]Institute of Animal Breeding and Genetics, University of Göttingen, D-3075 Göttingen, Germany, [2]Institute of Animal Breeding and Animal Husbandry, University of Halle, D-06099 Halle, Germany.*

In dairy cattle breeding programs, the selection of bull dams in the field in general has the inherent problems of low accuracy and the possibility of preferential treatment. In an analysis of data from five breeding organizations in Germany it was revealed that around 20% of bull dams are located in herds of extreme intra-herd variances. A test of potential bull dams on station is a helpful though costly alternative to the exclusive dependency on field results. Additionally, for the Holstein breed, populations in different countries show significant differences with respect to various traits which calls for the exploitation of these differences. Considering these findings, four scenarios for an optimal selection of bull dams were developed under inclusion of a station test with a capacity of 250 bull dams per year. The results indicate that heifers should be tested in their first lactation, the optimal fraction of selected bull dams should be below 20%, the duration of the test can be limited to 180 days, and modern biotechnologies like embryo transfer and ovum pick-up are essential.

Theatre G4.10

Survey of genetic evaluations for production and functional traits in dairy cattle

Thomas Mark, Interbull Centre, P.O. Box 7023, 750 07 Uppsala, Sweden.*

Interbull currently conducts international genetic evaluations for production, conformation and udder health traits, and longevity and calving traits are expected to follow in the near future. Knowledge of the status of national genetic evaluations is needed in preparation for international genetic evaluations. The objective of this study was to review the current status of genetic evaluations for production and functional traits as practised in different Interbull member countries. A questionaire was send to all 41 Interbull member countries, and so far 26 replies covering all the six trait groups that were defined have been received. The answers showed a substantial variation in: 1) number of traits and trait-groups considered, 2) definition of traits, 3) genetic evaluation procedure within trait, and 4) number of sub-traits considered per trait-group. It was evident that many countries lack genetic evaluations for one or more economically important trait, e.g. 12 countries had genetic evaluations for female fertility and 16 for udder health. Also, improvement in the genetic evaluation models for many functional traits, such as female fertility and health, can be achieved by closing the gap between research and practice. More detailed and up to date information about national genetic evaluation systems for traits in different countries are available at www.interbull.org. Female fertility and workability traits were considered in many countries and could be next in line for international genetic evaluations.

 Theatre G4.11

Effect of uncertain economic values on efficiency of selection in dairy cattle

H.M. Nielsen[*1], A.F. Groen[2], P. Berg[1] and L.G. Christensen[3], [1]Department of Animal Breeding and Genetics, Danish Institute of Agricultural Sciences, Research Centre Foulum, P.O. Box 50, DK-8830 Tjele, Denmark, [2]Department of Animal Sciences, Wageningen University, P.O. Box 338, Wageningen, The Netherlands, [3]The Royal Veterinary and Agricultural University, Department of Animal Science and Animal Health, Grønnegårdsvej 3, DK-1870 Frederiksberg C, Denmark.*

The objective of this study was to evaluate the efficiency of selection, defined as the response in the aggregate genotype, when selecting on an index with uncertain economic values relative to selection on an index, where the economic values (EV) are known without errors. The effect of uncertain economic values in two or more traits were illustrated using different traits and standard deviations on economic values obtained from a stochastic bio-economic simulation model. With two traits with uncertain EV's, the efficiency of selection was mainly dependent on the heritabilities and the economic values, and to minor extent on the genetic correlations between traits. In a selection index including milk yield (h^2=.28, EV=148±11 € per phenotypic standard deviation) and mastitis (h^2=.04, EV=-163 ± 682 € per phenotypic standard deviation) the efficiency of selection was 84%. Preliminary results indicated that in an index including milk yield, uncertainty on EV's on traits with low heritabilities will have small effect on the efficiency of selection.

Theatre G4.12

Estimation of realised genetic trends in French Large White pigs from 1977 to 1998 for production and quality traits using frozen semen

T. Tribout[1], J.C. Caritez[2], J. Gogué[3], J. Gruand[4], M. Bouffaud[5], P. Le Roy[1], J.P. Bidanel[1], [1]I.N.R.A., Station de Génétique Quantitative et Appliquée, 78352 Jouy-en-Josas, France, [2]INRA, Unité Porcine Le Magneraud, 17700 Surgères, France, [3]INRA, Unité Porcine de Bourges, 18390 Osmoy, France, [4]INRA, Station Expérimentale de Sélection Porcine, 86480 Rouillé, France, [5]INRA, Station de Testage Porc, 35650 Le Rheu, France.*

An experiment has been implemented at INRA to estimate realised genetic trends from 1977 to 1998 in the French Large White (LW) pig breed. LW sows were inseminated with stored frozen semen of 17 LW boars born in 1977 or with semen of 23 LW boars born in 1998, producing 30 and 33 litters, respectively. Within each experimental group, 20 males and 80 females were randomly chosen and mated to produce a second generation of animals whose growth, carcass and quality traits were compared (about 2000 individuals tested). The results showed that selection resulted in a highly significant decrease of carcass fatness and in a strong increase of carcass lean content (+0.36 % per year). A negative trend was found for ultimate pH measured on several ham and loin muscles. Reflectance of *Gluteus superficialis* and *Gluteus medius* muscles tended to increase, but water holding capacity of *Gluteus superficialis* muscle was improved significantly. Finally, only a low positive trend was found for average daily gain during the commercial fattening period.

Theatre G4.13

Precise predictions of rates of gain and inbreeding under index selection in hierarchical and factorial mating schemes

A.C. Sørensen[*1,2,3], *P. Berg*[2] *and J.A. Woolliams*[1], [1]*Roslin Institute (Edinburgh), Roslin, Midlothian EH25 9PS, UK,* [2]*Department of Animal Breeding and Genetics, Danish Institute of Agricultural Science, P.O. Box 50, DK-8830 Tjele, Denmark,* [3]*Department of Animal Science and Animal Health, Royal Veterinary and Agricultural University, Grønnegårdsvej 2, DK-1870 Frederiksberg C, Denmark.*

It is possible to predict the rate of gain (ΔG) and the rate of inbreeding (ΔF) accurately for both hierarchical and partly factorial mating designs under index selection. This hypothesis is tested in this study. Prediction equations were developed using long-term genetic contributions, which take account of the inheritance of selective advantage from parent to offspring. The predictions were compared to results from stochastic simulations with varying heritability, population size, and female mating ratio. The relative prediction errors for ΔG were between -1 and 10%, with the predictions being very accurate (errors < 2%) for both mating schemes for heritabilities of 0.2 and higher, for all population sizes and female mating ratios. The relative prediction errors for ΔF were between -10 and 17%, being largest for low heritabilities ($h^2 \leq 0.1$). The critical points in the predictions are the regression of the contributions on the selective advantages, and the variance of family sizes after selection. Thus, ΔG and ΔF can be predicted accurately for a large number of breeding schemes involving both factorial and hierarchical mating schemes under index selection. The predictions are equally accurate for the two mating schemes.

Theatre G4.14

A deterministic model for the prediction of selection response accounting for genotype by environment interaction

R. Kolmodin[1] *and P. Bijma*[*2], [1]*Department of Animal Breeding and Genetics, Swedish University of Agricultural Sciences, PO Box 7023, S-750 07 Uppsala, Sweden.* [2]*Animal Breeding and Genetics Group, Wageningen Institute of Animal Sciences, Wageningen University and Research Centre, 6700 AH Wageningen, The Netherlands.*

Genotype by environment interaction is becoming increasingly important due to the globalisation of animal breeding. With G×E, the breeding goal should define not only the traits but also the environment in which those traits are to be improved. Furthermore, the utility of data recording will depend on the environment where the data is recorded.

We developed a deterministic model to predict response to selection for cases where G×E had the form of a linear reaction norm. By using selection index theory, equations were derived to predict selection response in the average level of the trait, in the environmental sensitivity of the trait (the slope of the reaction norm), and the total response in each environment. We derived the environment that maximises genetic progress, which is a function of the genetic and environmental (co)variances of level and slope of the reaction norm and of the environment of the breeding goal. The method is useful for finding the optimum distribution of selection candidates over environments, to optimise testing capacity.

Advances in computing strategies for the solution of huge mixed model equations

V. Ducrocq and T. Druet, Station de Génétique Quantitative et Appliquée, Institut National de la Recherche Agronomique (INRA), 78352 Jouy-en-Josas, France.*

The increase in computing power has made possible the solution of large systems of linear equations using standard packages taking advantage of the sparse structure inherent to mixed model equations. However, the never-ending urge for more complex, possibly multiple trait BLUP animal models in (inter)national genetic evaluations still justifies the search for more efficient solution strategies. Numerical analysts in many fields recommend Preconditioned Conjugate Gradient (PCG) algorithms for the iterative solution of sparse positive semidefinite systems, instead of the simplistic Gauss-Seidel (block) iterative approaches that have been the reference for years in animal breeding. Our experience indicates that the choice of a good preconditioner is important for a better efficiency. In univariate BLUP animal models, an approximate incomplete Cholesky decomposition of the coefficient matrix is simple enough to advantageously surpass the (block) diagonal preconditioners that have sometimes been used in our field. Then PCG can be applied to very large systems, possibly iterating on data, that is, without necessarily storing the whole coefficient matrix in core. Unfortunately, PCG is much less attractive in multiple trait settings. Nevertheless, the use of an (approximate) canonical transformation is frequently possible, even in complex situations, e.g., with missing data, with several random effects or with heterogeneous variances. As a result, only univariate systems have to be solved with PCG, often employing a unique "average" preconditioner.

Theatre G5.2

Fuzzy classification of phantom parent groups in an animal model

W.F. Fikse, Interbull Centre, P.O. Box 7023, 750 07 Uppsala, Sweden.*

Genetic evaluations often include genetic groups to account for unequal genetic level of animals with unknown parentage. The definition of phantom parent groups usually includes a time component (e.g., years). Combining several time periods to ensure sufficiently large groups may create problems since all phantom parents in a group are considered contemporaries. To avoid the downside of such distinct classification, a fuzzy logic approach is suggested. A phantom parent can be assigned to several genetic groups, with a proportion between zero and one that sum to one. Rules are presented for assigning coefficients to the inverse of the relationship matrix for fuzzy-classified genetic groups. This approach was illustrated with simulation. Data from ten generations of mass selection were used in a genetic evaluation. Observations and pedigree records were randomly deleted with a probability that decreased with generation number. Phantom parent groups were defined on the basis of gender and generation number. In the distinct classification, two generations were combined in one group. In the fuzzy classification, each phantom parent was assigned with equal proportion to two groups pertaining to the generation of birth and the generation after birth. The trend in predicted breeding values of animals with phantom parents showed a stepwise pattern when a distinct classification was used, but was linear when genetic groups were fuzzy-classified. Consequently, the representation of animals with and without phantom parents in the top 10 percent selected animals was more correct with fuzzy-classified groups.

Theatre G5.3

Comparison of methods for breeding value estimation with uncertain paternity and twins

J.B.C.H.M van Kaam[1], F.F. Cardoso[2], R.J. Tempelman[2], B. Portolano[1], [1]Dipartimento S.En.Fi.Mi.Zo-Sezione Produzione Animale, Viale delle Scienze, 90128 Palermo, Italy, [2]Department of Animal Science, Michigan State University, East-Lansing, MI-48824, USA.*

Breeding value estimation for dairy sheep and goats is complicated by uncertain paternity for offspring conceived from natural matings within flocks containing multiple males. Additionally, dams frequently give birth to twins. Simulated populations consisting of 15 flocks with 11 generations were analysed with both a Bayesian approach, which uses phenotypes to infer upon probabilities of paternity, and a model based on Henderson's average numerator relationship matrix. The Bayesian approach samples the sire of each twin jointly. In both cases, inference was based on an animal model using Markov Chain Monte Carlo methods.
Our results indicated that (1) the power of phenotypes for inferring upon posterior probabilities of parentage was low, (2) the Bayesian method always assigned the correct sire a slightly higher (1%) probability of paternity and always sampled the correct sire more frequently (2%) than the remaining sires on average, (3) the Bayesian method led to a significantly (P<0.01) lower bias in the estimated breeding values, being most significant with a small number of candidate sires and (4) no differences in rank correlation between estimated breeding values and simulated breeding values were found.

Theatre G5.4

Evaluation of a Monte Carlo EM algorithm for likelihood inference in a finite normal mixture model with random effects

Y.M. Chang[1], D. Gianola[1,2], J. Ødegård[2], J. Jensen[3], P. Madsen[3], D. Sorensen[3], G. Klemetsdal[2] and B. Heringstad[2]. [1]Department of Dairy Science, University of Wisconsin, Madison, USA, [2]Department of Animal Science, Agricultural University of Norway, Norway, [3]Department of Animal Breeding and Genetics, Danish Institute of Agricultural Sciences, Denmark*

Finite mixture models can separate a heterogeneous population into homogeneous components by classifying individuals into unknown member groups. For example, use somatic cell scores to assign cows to putative udder health statuses. A homoscedastic two-component normal mixture model, including breeding values, was simulated. Four hundred individuals were randomly assigned to two subpopulations. The mixture parameter (P) was 75%; heritability was 0.2, and the population means differed by 1.5 phenotypic standard deviations. Parameters were estimated by maximum likelihood using the EM algorithm. Alternative Monte Carlo implementations were evaluated. The number of M-steps was 3000 or 5000, and the E-step used Gibbs sampling. Burn-in (B=100 or 1000) and Gibbs sample size (G=10 or 100) were varied as well. Longer burn-in, and larger number of Gibbs samples and of M-steps reduced relative mean-squared errors. Losses in accuracy for the least intensive strategy (M=3000, B=100, G=10) relative to strategy M=5000, B=100, G=100 were: 140% for P, 82% and 61% for the group means, 15% for the residual variance and near 0% for the genetic variance, the parameter estimated with less precision.

A Bayesian mixture model for detection of mastitis in dairy cattle by simulated test-day somatic cell score

J. Ødegård[1], J. Jensen[2], P. Madsen[2], D. Gianola[3,1], D. Sorensen[2], G. Klemetsdal[1], and B. Heringstad[1]. [1]Department of Animal Science, Agricultural University of Norway, P.O. Box 5025, N-1432 Ås-NLH, [2]Department of Animal Breeding and Genetics, Danish Institute of Agricultural Sciences, [3]Department of Animal Sciences, University of Wisconsin-Madison.

Somatic cell scores (SCS) follow different distributions in cows with and without mastitis, this is ignored in standard genetic analyses. Use of mixture models may lead to more appropriate inferences and further, selection could be based on probability of mastitis given SCS, rather than predicted breeding value for SCS. A Bayesian approach using Gibbs sampling was developed for a heteroscedastic two-component normal mixture model with random effects. SCS was simulated as a mixture of observations from healthy and mastitic cows. Random effects had the same distribution across mixture components. Model adequacy was evaluated from the posterior sensitivity, specificity, and probability of misclassification. In simulations with equal residual variances for the two mixture components, input parameters were returned without bias and with high accuracy. Inclusion of random effects in the model increased the probability of correct classification. No differences were found between models using a random cow effect (ignoring relationships), and models where additive and permanent environmental effects were fitted. When mixture components had more closely overlapping distributions, the corresponding residual variances became similar due to a high degree of misclassification. This may also cause bias in estimation of other parameters.

Theatre G5.6

Estimating variance components

A.R. Gilmour[1] and R. Thompson[2], [1]NSW Agriculture, Orange Agricultural Institute, Orange, NSW, 2800, Australia, [2]Rothamsted Research, Harpenden, Hertfordshire, AL5 2JQ, United Kingdom.*

Strategies for estimating variance components have developed over the last 30 years from equating mean squares to their expectations (e.g. Searle, 1971). The method of Residual Maximum Likelihood (Patterson & Thompson, 1971) has increased in use as computer power and computing strategies have developed. The derivative free strategy of Smith and Graser (1986) allowed widespread estimation of variance components under the animal model, predominantly in univariate settings. Development of software incorporating the Average Information (AI) algorithm (Johnson and Thompson, 1994, Gilmour, *et al.*, 1995, Jensen *et al.*, 1997) has made it easier to estimate variance parameters in multivariate settings for quite large data sets and complex genetic models. However, each frontier crossed reveals another as we move from basic models for additive gene effects to models that more accurately describe the genetic variation in ever larger sets of data. Strategies for accommodating large data sets range from acquiring bigger computers and using smarter programming to devising alternative approaches such as imputation (Clayton and Rasbash, 1999). On the other side, there is considerable interest in methods for constraining variance matrices to be positive definite and in structured variance models. These include covariance function models (Kirkpatrick *et al.*, 1994), structured antedependence models (Jaffrezic *et al.*, 2002) and factor analytic and reduced rank models (Thompson *et al.*, 2003).

Theatre G5.7

Estimates of genetic covariance functions for growth of Australian Angus cattle from random regression models fitting different orders of polynomials

K. Meyer, Animal Genetics and Breeding Unit, University of New England, Armidale, NSW 2351, Australia

The effect polynomials fit on estimates of covariance functions and the resulting variances and genetic parameters is examined. Data consisted of 80,981 weights from birth to 820 days of age for 23,640 Australian Angus cattle. The model of analysis fitted random regressions on polynomials of age at recording for direct and maternal effects, both genetic and permanent environmental. Cubic, quartic and quintic polynomials were considered for direct effects while maternal effects were modelled through quadratic or cubic polynomials. Fixed effects fitted included contemporary groups, defined as herd-sex-management group-date of weighing subclasses, with an 'age slicing' of 45 days up to 300 days and 60 days thereafter. Fixed, cubic regressions accounted for mean trends, dam age and birth type effects. Measurement error variances were considered heterogeneous with 19 classes. In total, 9 models involving 43 to 67 variance components were examined. Estimates were obtained by Bayesian analyses using Gibbs sampling. Estimates of direct variance components from different models agreed well for ages with most records, up to 650 days of age. Problems with erratically large estimates of variances for the latest ages were reduced by fitting higher order Legendre polynomials for direct environmental effects, or by a low order fractional polynomial model. Ages at which the importance of maternal effects peaked depended on the model fitted, with a quadratic polynomial yielding most plausible results. Strategies for choosing the most appropriate model are discussed.

Theatre G5.8

Estimation of genetic parameters of test-day records for milk yield for the first three lactations of French Holstein cows

T. Druet, F. Jaffrézic and V. Ducrocq, Station de Génétique Quantitative et Appliquée, Institut National de la Recherche Agronomique (INRA), 78352 Jouy-en-Josas, France.*

Genetic parameters were estimated on 1,503,359 test-day records of 96,657 French Holstein cows. In total, 152,630 animals were included in pedigree files. Variance components were estimated with an Average-Information REML algorithm and a pooling strategy to handle large data sets: the average information matrix and the first derivatives of the likelihood functions were pooled over 10 samples. Some fixed effects of the model and the residual variances were modeled with regression splines varying with days in milk. Traits defined by eigenvectors previously obtained for first lactation records were used to estimate (co)variances of random effects. Genetic variances were highest in the middle of the lactation while the environmental variances (residual and permanent environment variances) were decreasing during the lactation with, however, a slight increase at the end of the lactation. Genetic effects for production levels (first eigenvector) were highly correlated across lactations (around 0.90). For persistency (second eigenvector), genetic effects of second and third lactation were also highly correlated (around 0.90) while the genetic effect of first lactation was less correlated to the other two (close to 0.60). Finally, random herd by year of calving effects for the second and the third lactations showed a high correlation.

Theatre G5.9

Genetic correlations between production traits and resistance to clinical and sub-clinical disease in growing pigs

M. Henryon[1], P. Berg[1] and T. Ebbesen[2], [1]DIAS, Department of Animal Breeding and Genetics, Research Centre Foulum, P.O. Box 50, 8830 Tjele, Denmark, [2]National Committee for Pig Breeding, Danish Bacon and Meat Council, Vinkelvej 11, 8620 Kjellerup, Denmark.*

This study tested the premise that negative genetic correlations exist between production traits and resistance to clinical and sub-clinical disease in growing pigs. Approximately 26000 male growing pigs were assessed for three production traits (i.e., daily gain, feed conversion efficiency, percentage lean) and resistance to five categories of clinical and sub-clinical disease (i.e., any clinical or sub-clinical disease, lameness, respiratory diseases, diarrhoea, other diseases). Genetic correlations between the production traits and resistance to each disease category will be estimated by fitting multitrait linear animal models, formulated in a Bayesian context, to the production traits and incidences of disease (i.e., not diagnosed/diagnosed once/diagnosed twice or more). The production traits will be assumed normally distributed, while the incidence of disease will be assumed to follow a categorical threshold liability model. The results will have two implications for pig breeding programs. First, they will indicate whether current breeding programs, which concentrate on the improvement of production traits, are likely to have adverse effects on resistance to clinical and sub-clinical disease. Second, the genetic correlation estimates should provide a basis upon which to develop breeding programs for the simultaneous improvement of growing pigs for production traits and resistance to disease.

Theatre G5.10

Strategies to control inbreeding in dairy cattle breeding programmes in New Zealand

J.E. Pryce, B.L. Harris, W.H. McMillan and M.D. Sellars, Livestock Improvement, Private Bag 3016, Hamilton, New Zealand*

Two strategies to optimise genetic progress, while constraining inbreeding have been developed taking into account rate of inbreeding in NZ Jersey and Holstein-Friesian dairy cow populations. The first is to control the rate of inbreeding in the commercial population. While the second is to control inbreeding in the elite population. Liquid semen is used in the NZ breeding season (Spring) and most farmers opt to use bulls that are rostered for use each day (generally a team of three bulls per breed per three day dispatch). Each AI technician has a hand-held digital device loaded with pedigree information. A warning is generated on this if the bull and cow being considered for a mating have relatives in common. Software has been developed to roster teams of bulls, so that the chances of inbreeding warnings for more than one bull in a three day dispatch team are minimised. In the nucleus breeding scheme we have developed software to optimise selection for our breeding objectives while controlling inbreeding and thus make better decisions about choice of sires and dams to be parents of future progeny test bulls. The software is based on a multiple goal integer program, which enables us to place priorities on goals and place restrictions on other parameters, such as number of matings acceptable per sire and future inbreeding impact.

Poster G5.11

A comparison of models for genetic evaluation of mastitis data: Heritabilities, repeatabilities and genetic correlation with milk production traits

D. Hinrichs, E. Stamer, W. Junge and E. Kalm, Institute of Animal Breeding and Husbandry, Christian-Albrechts-University, D-24098 Kiel

The aim of the present study was to compare different models for estimating genetic parameters for mastitis. Lactation models (LM) for the first 50, 100 or 300 days of lactation (LM50, LM100, LM300), or test day models (TDM) for the first 50, 100 or 300 days of lactation (TDM50, TDM100, TDM300) were used.
Data were collected on three commercial milk farms from 1998 to 2001. Mastitis information from 6974 cows with 13324 different lactations were available. This resulted in 2937986 lactation days with mastitis information.
The heritabilities estimated with the TDM (0.09 TDM50, 0.07 TDM100, 0.06 TDM300) were higher compared to the estimates of the LM (0.05 LM50, 0.06 LM100, 0.06 LM300). The repeatabilities were significantly increased for the estimates from the TDM (e.g.73% for the TDM50 compared to 12% LM50). The reason was that the TDM used all available mastitis information. Multiple mastitis for a single cow were treated as distinct observations. This was not possible with the LM.
Genetic correlation between mastitis and milk production traits were estimated with a TDM. The correlation was r_g=0.29 (milk yield), r_g=0.30 (fat yield), r_g=0.20 (fat percentage), r_g=0.34 (protein yield) and r_g=0.20 (protein percentage). The estimated genetic correlation between mastitis and somatic cell score was r_g=0.84. The estimated correlations are in agreement with literature reports.

Poster G5.12

Definition of subgroups for fixed regression in test-day animal model for milk production of Czech Holstein cattle

L Dedková, E. Nemcová, J. Pribyl and J. Wolf, Research Institute of Animal Production, Prátelství 815, CZ 104 01 Prague-Uhríneves, Czech Republic.*

Test-day data for milk production of Czech Holstein breed were used to find the appropriate way of definition of subgroups for fixed regression according to age at calving, year and season of calving, days open and calving interval. The data included roughly 4.0, 2.7 and 1.7 millions records for first, second and third lactation, respectively, sampled from 596 200 cows from 1991 to 2002. Random regression test-day models were applied for the estimation of breeding values. The models employed differed in the definition of the subgroups. Beyond the fixed regression subgroups, the model equations contained fixed effects of herd-test-date and random effects of animal and permanent environmental effects. Third order Legendre polynomials (with four coefficients) were used for both the fixed and random regressions. The (co)variance parameters were estimated by Gibbs sampling on a sample of data. The predicted lactation curves were different according to defined groups. Preliminary results showed rank correlations over 0.95 between breeding values for sires. The changes in the definition of subgroups caused some difference in the ranking of breeding values.

Poster G5.13

Test day model of daily milk yield predication across days within months of lactation of mixed and separate parities in Egyptian buffaloes

A.A. Amin[1], A.M. Abdel-Samee[2], T. Gere[3], 1.Animal Prod.Dept., Fac.of Agri., Suez Canal Uni.,Egypt, 2. Animal Prod.Dept., Fac.Environmental Agri.Sci., Suez Canal Uni., Egypt., 3: Animal Breeding and Genetics Dept, Szent Istevan Uni., Hungary.*

Predicated daily milk yield equations were generated for multiple lactations, separate lactations, and age at calving groups of ≤32, >32-<36, and ≥36 months within the 1st parity. Polynomial regression were fatted to study the effect of stage of lactation on test-day milk yield. Test-day animal model was used to avoid statistical biases due length of lactation. Animals are presented through at least five successive sample test day through therein months of lactation. The studies showed that influences of fixed effects on test day yield observations were significant. Variations in test day yield due to effect of age at calving within the first parity were significant and accounted 25.7 % approximately relatively to the total variance. The overall least square means of test day yields were 4.9 Kg per day. Prediction equation (intercept and partial regression) of mixed parities across the first 30 days of lactation (1st month) was A=4.034, X1=-0.007432, X2=0.000195, X3= 0.000000275. Prediction equation of mixed parities across the last 30 days of lactation (13th month) was A=-134.523, X1=0.736286, X2=-0.000976. Estimates for constructing test-day milk yield predicated equations across days of lactation of the mixed parities and age at calving groups of the first parity were tabulated.

Poster G5.14

Utilization of shorter lactations in cattle and buffaloes

M.S. Khan[1], I.R. Bajwa[1] and S.A. Bhatti[2], [1]Department of Animal Breeding and Genetics, University of Agriculture, Faisalabad, [2]Livestock Services Training Centre, Bahadurnagar, Okara, Pakistan.*

Progeny testing program in Sahiwal cattle and Nili-Ravi buffaloes in Pakistan is in its inception. Program is important both for conservation and improved utilization of these valuable indigenous genetic resources. Most of the recorded cows/buffaloes (60-70%) have lactations shorter than 10 months. Currently, lactations shorter than 180 days are deleted from the data sets while others are extended using linear extrapolation. Present study presents an improved procedure of extending shorter lactations. Weekly recorded lactations (n= 4743) of >8 weeks from an institutional herd were used. Lactation milk yield averaged 1475±14 and 1984±15 kg for Sahiwal and Nili-Ravi. Lactation curves were different for first and later parities with different days in milk, in both breeds. Lactations were short mostly due to reproductive problems, mastitis or culling because of poor production, old age and repeat breeding. However, in most cases animals with shorter lactations dried gradually. Heritability estimates of unadjusted lactation milk yield using an animal model were 0.15±.04 and 0.09±.05 for Sahiwal and Nili-Ravi, respectively. Yields adjusted by linear regression had heritability of 0.13±0.04 and 0.081±0.04 for the two breeds, which improved to 0.20±0.04 and 0.11±0.05 for yields adjusted using the improved procedure. New procedure is suggested for adjusting milk yield data in Sahiwal cattle and Nili-Ravi buffaloes in Pakistan.

Poster G5.15

Estimation of breeding values for milk traits by using an animal model of Friesian cattle in Egypt

A.S. Khattab[1], E.A. Omer [2]and E, A. Gohnem[1]. [1] Department of Animal production, Faculty of Agriculture, Tanta University, Egypt, [2]Animal production Research, Egypt.*

A total of 2169 normal lactation records of Friesian cows kept at Sakha Farm, in Egypt, during 1981 to 2000 were used. Data were analysis using multivariate analysis. The model includes, month and year of calving and parity as a fixed effects, days open as covariate, individuals, permanent environmental and errors as random effects. Traits studies are 305 day milk yield (305 d MY), lactation period (LP) and dry period (DP). Heritability estimates were 0.17, 0.10 and 0.01 for 305 d MY, LP and DP, respectively. Repeatability values 0.41, 0.43 and 0.11, respectively for the same traits. Estimates of predicted breeding values for cows ranged from -324 + 18 to 632 + 19 for 305 d MY, from -37 + 12 to 38 + 13 d for LP and from -16 + 13 to 18 +13 d for DP. Predicted sire breeding values were - 360 + 19 to 489 + 16 kg, - 12+ 11 to 19 + 9 d ,-17 + 10 to 18 + 10 d for the same traits, respectively. Estimates of predicted breeding values from dams ranged from -190 + 21 to 260 + 20 kg, from -16 + 14 to 29 + 14 d, and from -9 + 14 to 11 + 14 d for the above mentioned traits.

Poster G5.16

Genetic and phenotypic correlations between three times milking monthly test day milk yields in Iranian Holstein heifers

H. Farhangfar and H. Rezaie, Animal Science Department, Agriculture Faculty, Birjand University, Birjand, P.O. Box 97175-331, Iran.*

A total of 179,610 monthly test day milk records from 17,961 Iranian Holstein heifers calved between 1986 and 2001 and distributed in 287 herds located at different climatic regions of Iran was analysed by a covariance function model to estimate genetic parameters of monthly-sampled milk yields over the lactation course. Theoritically, covariance function allows fitting random regressions (as sub-model) to take account of the variation of monthly test day records during the lactation at two genetic and permanent environment levels for individual cows. The results obtained from the present study showed that the heritability estimates of monthly test day milk yields ranged between 0.055 and 0.300. The lowest and highest heritabilites were observed for the first and eight month of lactation. It was also revealed that the average heritability estimates of monthly test day milk yields during the first half of lactation was lower than that of the second half of lactation. Phenotypic, genetic and permanent environment correlations between monthly test day milk yields were positive. Genetic correlations between adjacent monthly test day milk yields were high but dropped as the number of test days in between increased. Phenotypic correlations between monthly test day milk yields had the analogous pattern to the one observed for genetic correlations although on a lower magnitude of estimates.

Poster G5.17

Heritability of milk coagulation parameters in Italian Friesian dairy cows

R. Leotta[1], *F. Cecchi*[1*], *A. Summer*[2], [1]Dipartimento di Produzioni Animali, Viale delle Piagge 2, 56124 Pisa, Italy, 2Dipartimento di Produzioni Animali, Biotecnologie Veterinarie, Qualità e Sicurezza degli Alimenti, Via del Taglio 8, 43100 Parma, Italy

A trial was carried out on 137 Italian Friesian cows reared in an herd of the province of Pisa (Tuscany) with the aim to estimate the heritability of coagulation parameters, somatic cell count (SCC) and titratable acidity. One sample was taken from the morning milking from each cow during 1 year. The following analyses were carried out on each sample of fresh milk: SCC, titratable acidity and coagulation parameters (r, clotting time; k_{20}, curd firming time; a_{30} and a_{45}, curd firmness measured at 30 and 45 minutes after rennet addition, respectively).
The heritability coefficients were estimated using paternal half sib analysis. It has been tested using a mixed model: parity and season as fixed effects, bull as random effect and days in milk as covariate. The heritability coefficient of the clotting time (r) was 0.23 (± 0.18), while for the other technological parameters the coefficient was rather low (0.02 ± 0.21 for k_{20}, 0.06 ± 0.25 for a_{30} and 0.10 ± 0.24 for a_{45}); our results are similar than previously described on other breeds. Also the heritability coefficient of the SCC was low (h^2= 0.03 ± 0.13) but not different from values reported elsewhere, as for titratable acidity (h^2= 0.01 ± 0.22) too.

Poster G5.18

The repeatability of morphometric characteristics of milk fat globules from Massese ewes during lactation

F. Cecchi, M. Martini, C. Scolozzi. Dipartimento di Produzioni Animali, Università degli Studi di Pisa, Viale delle Piagge 2, 56124, Pisa, Italy.*

The aim of this research was to estimate the repeatability of morphometric characteristics of milk fat globules [number of globules/ml, average diameter, frequency distribution of globules according to size: small (from <1 to 2µm), medium (>2 to 5µm) and large globules (>5µm)] analyzed in three different phases of lactation (10, 30 and 90 days from parity). Milk samples were taken from twenty-five Massese ewes homogeneous for age and diet; all animals came from a single herd located in the province of Pisa (Tuscany). The repeatability of morphometric characteristics of milk fat globules tested in the three phases of lactation was estimated by Pearson's correlation coefficient (r) while the average repeatability was tested following the method of intra-correlation-class.
Small globules gave results that were highly repeatable (r=0.83), while average diameter and medium and large globules showed a low repeatability (r= 0.18, 0.18, 0.19, respectively). The lowest value was observed for the total number of globules/ ml (r= 0.04).
Since the percentage of small milk fat globules represents a minor portion of the fat measured, the results of this research indicate that a morphometric analysis of the globules in one phase of the lactation provides little indication of the variability of such parameters in the other lactation phases.

Poster G5.19

Genetic evaluation of beef cattle in the Czech Republic

J. Pribyl[1], I. Misztal[2], J. Pribylová[1], K. Seba[3], [1]Res.Inst.Anim.Prod., P.O.Box 1, Uhríneves 10401, Czech Rep., [2]Univ. of Georgia, Athens, GA 30602, USA, [3]Czech Beef Cattle Assoc. Tesnov 17, 11705 Praha 1, Czech Rep.*

The objective of this study was to estimate breeding values for 12 beef breeds (Angus, Belgian Blue, Blond D`Aquitaine, Charolais, Galloway, Gasconne, Hereford, Highland, Limousin, Piedmontese, Salers and Simmental) and their crosses with Czech Spotted (dual purpose) and dairy breeds. Data collected in recent 12 years consisted of 126 608 records on calving ease and birth weight, 57 906 records on weight at 120 and 210 days of age, and 22 467 records on yearling weight. The complete pedigree included 183 754 animals. Evaluation is with Multiple-breed Multiple-traits Animal Model with Maternal effect. Fixed effects included in model were sex, dam age and regressions on calf and maternal heterosis. Random effects were herd x year x season, direct and maternal genetic and maternal environmental effects. Direct effects were largest for all traits in Charolais followed by Simmental. Maternal effects were largest for weight at 120 and 210 days of age in Czech Spotted followed by Salers and Simmental, and for yearling weight in Salers followed by Simmental. Lowest effects were for all traits in Highland followed by Galloway.

Poster G5.20

Breeding value for growth curve of performance tested dual-purpose bulls

H. Krejcová[1], J. Pribyl[1], I. Misztal[2], [1]Res.Inst.Anim.Prod., P.O.Box 1, Uhríneves 10401, Czech Rep., [2]Univ. Georgia, Athens, GA 30602, USA,*

Before the selection to insemination are bulls of Czech Spotted cattle performance tested for growth. Weighting is monthly from the birth till the age of 420 days. Each bull has 26 half-sibs in the stations in average. 6599 bulls with total of 70615 measurements are used. Gain and cumulative growth are evaluated by the 6th grade of the orthogonal Legendre polynomial (LP). Together the fixed effects of station-test-day of weighting (STD) and LP explained 96% of variability in growth and 39% in gain. Variance components were calculated by REML (programme REMLF90) taking in account the heterogeneous variance during the growth. Effects in models: STD (fixed), LP_F (fixed), animal (random with relationship matrix) and permanent environment of the animal (random). Animal and permanent environment are included as an additive constant or random regression LP. Estimated genetic parameters differ depending on trait (growth, gain) and selected model. Genetic variability of growth increases with the age of the animal, but it is almost equal for the gain, except for the beginning and the end of growth period. Heritability is 0.80 in average for growth, and 0.16 for the gain if only the additive constant is used, or 0.47 for the gain if random polynomial is used for the animal. Heritability for growth is affected by multiple counting of values in cumulative function.

Poster G5.21

The genetic resistance to gastrointestinal parasites in Massese sheep breed: Heritability and Repeatability of faecal egg counts (FEC)

M.N. Benvenuti, F. Cecchi, D. Cianci. Dipartimento di Produzioni Animali, Università degli Studi di Pisa, Viale delle Piagge 2, 56124, Pisa, Italy.*

The gastrointestinal parasitosis in sheep represents, with the mastitis, a severe limit to the productiveness of the animals and also to the effective definition of the food desk.
Resistance to parasites is usually estimated by means of FEC still considered to be the easier and most efficient method due to its phenotypic relations to the total parasite burden.
The lack of information available in bibliography on the topic, encouraged to carry out a preliminary research to identify the genetic fraction of the resistance to the gastrointestinal helminths in Massese breed, estimating the heritability and the repeatability of FEC.
In a farm of Massese sheep breed, 50 daughter-mother pairs has been considered; they were tested monthly (November 2001-December 2002), and one fecal sample per animal was collected. The samples were processed in order to determine the FEC using the modified McMaster tecnique recommended by Hansen and Perry.
FEC's were trasformed to the natural logarithm ln(FEC+1). The repeatability of monthly FEC was estimated by Pearson's correlations while the average repeatability between the monthly values has been tested with the method of intra-correlation-class.
The heritability coefficients of FEC using daughter-mother regression were 0.15; this value is rather low but not different from values reported elsewhere. Repeatability is resulted instead high (r= 0.66).

Poster G5.22

A method of computing restricted best linear unbiased prediction of breeding values for a part of animals in the population and application to computer program

M. Satoh and M. Takeya, National Institute of Agrobiological Sciences, Tsukuba-shi 305-8602, Japan.*

Restricted best linear unbiased prediction (RBLUP) is derived by imposing restrictions directly within a multiple trait mixed model. If restrictions are imposed on only a part of animals in the population, computing a large sub-matrix of additive relationship matrix (**A**) and **A** to the second power are required for writing RBLUP equations. As a result, the RBLUP procedure requires large memory and computing time. In the present study, a new method for computing RBLUP of breeding values using animal model was presented, when the constraints of no change and (or) proportional change were imposed on the additive genetic values of a part of animals in the population. The solver techniques consist of two steps: First, the original RBLUP equations derived by Quaas and Henderson (1976) are reordered to simpler equations without $\mathbf{A}^2$. Secondly, new linear equations in each trait are written using the first-step solutions. Every coefficient matrix of the second equations is $\mathbf{A}^{-1}$; they are solved separately for each trait. The new and original methods were implemented in programs using preconditioned conjugate gradient iteration. Comparison of the programs was based on memory requirement and central processing unit time for the solver. The new technique resulted in less than memory requirement and computing time than the original technique; at best the memory requirement was reduced to less than five percent and the computing time was reduced to less than ten percent.

Theatre G6.1

Animal breeding and product quality

P.W. Knap, R.E. Klont, A. Diestre, PIC, POBox 1630, D-24826 Schleswig, Germany

Product quality has always been an important issue for many categories of animal production (meat, milk, eggs, wool, fur). The current rapid increase of consumer affluence and awareness has led to a focus on an increasing range of product characteristics that influence "quality" as it is experienced by an increasing range of societal parties: product composition (proportion of high-value components), processing quality (chemical and physical features), organoleptic quality (flavour, colour, texture), nutritious quality (presence of specific proteins or fatty acids; low cholesterol levels etc.), food safety (absence of microbial and chemical contaminants), animal welfare (reproduction, housing, nutrition, transport and slaughter as they influence animal health, behaviour and comfort), ecological impact (pollution, biodiversity). An important feature of this development for the animal breeding sector is that breeders have less and less control over these issues in the order they are listed here. This has five consequences for practical animal breeding: (i) strategic alliances with the production sector become more important, (ii) the design of consistent and stable breeding objectives becomes more complicated, (iii) the inclusion of field data into selection criteria becomes more important, (iv) the generation lag between those field data and the nucleus must be reduced to make this inclusion genetically worthwhile, (v) techniques such as marker-assisted selection become more relevant. These points combined lead logically to customised breeding programs that cater for specific series of QTL alleles integrated with specific process control techniques.

Theatre G6.2

Some statistical tools for meat quality analysis

A. Blasco, Departamento de Ciencia Animal, Universidad Politécnica de Valencia, P.O. Box 22012, 46071 Valencia, Spain.

Some statistical tools for meat quality analyses are reviewed. The first part of the paper is dedicated to exploratory data analyses. First, univariate exploratory data analyses are exposed focusing on checking data distribution and detecting outliers. Some multivariate procedures, Principal Component Analysis and related methods (Generalised canonical analysis, Three way Factor analysis), and also Procustes analysis are discussed.
The second part of the paper showS the advantages of the Bayesian approach to analyze meat quality data. The different ways in which uncertainty is expressed in Bayesian and classical analysis is compared, focusing the discussion in analyses with a reduced number of data, since meat quality data are often obtained in small samples. Bayesian hypothesis tests and model choice are briefly discussed stressing the advantages of the Bayesian approach when a large number of traits is analysed.

 Theatre G6.3

A genome scan to detect QTL for CLA content in the milk fat of dairy sheep

A. Carta[1], M. Fiori[1], G. Piredda[1], C. Leroux[2], F. Barillet[2]. [1]IZCS, Loc. Bonassai, I-07040 Olmedo,Italy.2 INRA URH Theix and SAGA Toulouse, France.*

Fatty acid composition of milk fat was determined on a Sarda x Lacaune backcross population two times in the middle of 2nd (847 records) and 3rd lactation (795 records). The ewes were daughters of 10 F1 sires, corresponding to a classical daughter design for QTL detection. Main attention was given to CLA for its possible role on human health. A large part of CLA in milk is produced in the mammary gland where the vaccenic acid is desaturated by delta 9-desaturase. Thus QTL detection was carried out for CLA and the ratio between CLA and vaccenic acid. A repeated measure model including the fixed effect year*group of management and the random effects individual and sire ws applied. The individual solutions of the 727 ewes with two records were used as phenotypes for QTL analysis. 132 microsatellite markers spread all over the genome were available. An across family single trait QTL analysis was carried out by within family linear regression. Locations either close or significant at the chromosome-wise level of 5 % were found on OAR 4, OAR 14 and OAR 19 for CLA content in the milk fat and on OAR 3, OAR 4, OAR 6, OAR 14 and OAR 22 for the ratio between CLA and vaccenic acid. Particularly interesting is the QTL found for the ratio on OAR 22 where the SCD gene encoding for delta 9-desaturase is located. Simultaneously, a candidate gene approach for 5 genes, including SCD gene, is carried out on the same resource population.

Theatre G6.4

Effects of the IGF2 gene region and the HAL locus on body composition and meat quality traits in a F2 Pietrain x Large White population

*M.P. Sanchez[1], J. Riquet[2], K. Fève[2], H. Gilbert[1], P. Le Roy[1], N. Iannuccelli[2], J. Gogué[3], C. Péry[3], J.P. Bidanel[*1] and D. Milan[2] - INRA, [1]Station de Génétique Quantitative et Appliquée, 78352 Jouy-en-Josas Cedex, [2]Laboratoire de Génétique Cellulaire, 31326 Castanet-Tolosan Cedex, [3]Domaine expérimental de Galle, 18520 Avord, France*

Effects of the IGF2 locus region (SSC2), of the HAL locus and their interaction were tested on 39 growth, carcass and meat quality traits in 593 F2 Pietrain x Large White (PI x LW) pigs. Analyses of variance, single and multitrait interval mapping analyses testing Mendelian or imprinted QTL were applied.

Large effects of the HAL locus were detected for most body composition traits, growth and water holding capacity. The IGF2 region significantly affected carcass lean content, fat content and compactness, meat quality (ultimate pH and lightness) and teat number, but did not explain more than 3% of F2 phenotypic variance. Limited imprinting effects of the IGF2 region and no interaction between IGF2 and HAL regions were evidenced.

Additional statistical analyses revealed heterogeneous effects of the IGF2 region between sire families. SNP analyses showed that PI favourable haplotypes were highly frequent in the LW population and that all but one F1 sires might be homozygous at the QTL locus.

Theatre G6.5

A candidate gene approach to identify DNA markers for muscle glycolytic potential and meat quality traits in pigs

L. Fontanesi, R. Davoli, L. Nanni Costa, E. Scotti and V. Russo, DIPROVAL, Sezione di Allevamenti Zootecnici, University of Bologna, Via F.lli Rosselli 107, 42100 Reggio Emilia, Italy.*

Meat quality traits in pigs are correlated to glycolytic potential (GP) values of skeletal muscles. As this measure is related to the energy metabolism of this tissue, we selected 25 genes, involved in the glycogen metabolism and glycolysis and in their regulation, that were considered candidates for GP. For some of these genes we identified new DNA markers (*GAA*; *LDHA*; *PGAM2*; *PKM2*; *PRKAB1*; *PYGM*) or analysed the polymorphisms already described in literature (*GPI*; *PRKAG3*, mutations T30N, G52S, I199V, R200Q). Eleven genes were physically mapped using a somatic cell hybrid panel (*PYGM*, chr. 2; *ALDOA*, chr. 3; *AGL* and *PRKAB2*, chr. 4; *PFKM*, chr. 5; *GYS1*, chr. 6; *PKM2*, chr. 7; *GAA* and *ENO3*, chr 12; *PRKAB1*, chr. 14; *PGAM2*, chr. 18) and four (*GAA*, *PKM2*, *PRKAB1*, *PGAM2*) were also linkage mapped genotyping the reference populations of the PiGMaP Consortium. Allele frequencies of the polymorphisms analysed were studied in seven pig breeds (Large White, Landrace, Duroc, Belgian Landrace, Hampshire, Piétrain and Meishan). The markers at the candidate genes were analysed in commercial pigs for which GP and other meat quality traits were measured. Association analyses indicated that *GPI*, *PGAM2*, *PKM2*, *PRKAB1* and *PRKAG3* G52S have significant effects ($P<0.05$) on some of these meat quality parameters.

Theatre G6.6

QualityPorkGENES: Variation in phenotypic traits for functional genomic analysis of meat quality

M. Gil[1], M. Gispert[1], D.C. Carrion[2], J.A. Garcia[1], P. Mormede[3], A. Foury[3], M. Cairns[4], G. Davey[4], R. Tilley[5], M. Delday[5], C. Maltin[5], R. Klont[2], A. Sosnicki[2], G.S. Plastow[2] and S.C. Blott[2], [1]IRTA, Spain, [2]PIC/Sygen International, [3]INRA, Bordeaux, [4]NUI Galway, [5]Rowett Institute.*

Data on 250 pigs from five different breed types (Landrace, Large White, Duroc, Pietrain and Meishan Synthetic) were measured for 116 traits representing growth, stress response, carcass composition and meat quality. Summary statistics were calculated and "trait maps" and Principle Component Analyses developed. Samples were also collected from *Longissimus dorsi* and *Semimembranosus* for subsequent analysis of fibre type and gene expression at the transcriptome and proteome level.

Most traits showed a significant breed effect. However, variation in all traits was as large within as between breeds. Between breed differences reflect the diverse genotypes in the project. For example, breed means for backfat ranged from 11.5 to 21.2mm and corresponding loin depth from 66.5 to 52.6mm at carcass weight of approximately 90kg. Stress responses, determined by endocrine levels in plasma and urine also differed significantly between breed. Interestingly, the Meishan and Duroc breeds appear to return more quickly to basal levels than the other breeds, suggesting that they may be more resistant to environmental stressors. A total of 100 pigs per line will eventually be collected and the variation exploited by utilising gene expression approaches in order to identify potential candidate genes associated with variation in the traits.

 Theatre G6.7

Relationships between intramuscular, abdominal and subcutaneous fat in broiler chickens

S. Zerehdaran[1], A.L.J. Vereijken[2], J. A. M. van Arendonk[1] and E.H. van der Waaij[1,3], [1]Wageningen University, PO Box 338, 6700 AH Wageningen, The Netherlands; [2]Nutreco research Center, P.O. Box 220, 5830 AE, Boxmeer, The Netherlands, [3] Department of Animal Health, Yalelaan 7, Utrecht The Netherlands.

Genetic parameters of carcass- related traits were estimated in an experimental meat-type chicken line including 3278 birds: 1752 females and 1526 males. Estimated heritabilities of body weight at 5 (BW5) and 7 weeks (BW7), carcass weight (CW), carcass percentage (CP), abdominal fat weight (AFW), abdominal fat percentage (AFP), breast muscle weight (BMW), breast muscle percentage (BMP), skin weight (SW, indicator for subcutaneous fat), skin percentage (SP) and femoral head necrosis (FHN) were moderate to high (from 0.24 to 0.73) whereas the heritability of intramuscular fat percentage (IFP) was low (0.08).
BW7 showed positive genetic correlations (rg) with fat production traits, which were high for IFP (0.87) and moderate to low for SP (0.17) and AFP (0.13). There was high rg between AFW and SW (0.54) whereas rg between AFW and IFP was low (0.02). There was no rg between BW7 and FHN (0.01) whereas, FHN showed an unfavorable rg with BMP (0.31). Two important conclusions were: 1. Selection for BW not only increases abdominal and subcutaneous fat but also increases intramuscular fat. 2. Selection for reduced AFW doesn't result in a change on IFP and probably meat quality.

Theatre G6.8

Biallelic markers as a tool for the traceability of bovine breeds

R. Negrini[1], E. Milanesi[1], F. Chegdani[1], J. Bernardi[1], F. Filippini[2], A. Valentini[3], P. Ajmone Marsan[1], [1]Istituto di Zootecnica, Università Cattolica del Sacro Cuore, 29100 Piacenza, Italy, [2]ANABIC, S. Martino in Colle, 06070 Perugia, Italy, [3]Dipartimento di Produzioni Animali, Università della Tuscia, 01100 Viterbo, Italy.*

Tracing the origin of animal products contributes to food safety, consumers confidence and sustainable conservation of genetic resources through the valorisation of typical products. We have used a Bayesian approach to evaluate the ability of AFLP biallelic markers to assign field meat samples to their breed of origin. A reference breed database was constructed typing 416 individuals from 16 Italian cattle breeds with 132 AFLP markers. These were clustered using the software "STRUCTURE", including breed origin as prior information. Overall. 98% of the individuals of the reference dataset were clustered correctly (p>90%). In particular, all (20 out of 20) reference Romagnola individuals were grouped in a single cluster. A total of 44 field samples from Romagnola were blindly assigned to these clusters. In the blind test, 40 out of 44 individuals of Romagnola were correctly assigned to the Romagnola cluster (p>90%), 3 were assigned to different clusters and one remained unassigned. The results obtained indicate that biallelic markers can be used in assigning individuals to breeds or populations, in this sense AFLPs represent a good model for SNPs that are being developed in most animal species.

Theatre G6.9

Meat traceability of cattle breed: a likelihood ratio approach applied to STR genotypes

R. Ciampolini[1], E. Ciani[1], V. Cetica[1], E. Mazzanti[1], C. Sebastiani[2], M. Biagetti[2], S. Presciuttini[3], and D. Cianci[1], [1]Dipartimento di Produzioni Animali (DPA) Viale delle Piagge 2, 56100 Pisa, [2]Istituto Zooprofilattico Umbria Marche (IZSUM), via Salvemini 1, 64126 Perugia, [3]Centro di Genetica Molecolare e Clinica (CGMC), S.S. Abetone e Brennero 2, 56127 Pisa, Italy.*

An increasingly concerning commercial problem is the difficulty in tracing back the breed origin of individual beef cuts. Current methods, being based on paper certifications, are vulnerable to fraud. We report the use of DNA profiles from STR loci for inferring the breed of given specimens, using both our published IGM (individual multilocus genotype) method, and a novel approach based on likelihood ratio statistics. We first analyzed 134 unrelated individuals from Limousine and Chianina breeds (67 animals each) for 19 STR. Hardy-Weinberg genotype probabilities were multiplied over loci, separately for the two breeds, in the end obtaining the likelihood ratio (LR) that a given animal originated from one breed rather than the other. The two breeds were perfectly separated ($P < 0.001$). We then extended the analysis to common breeds available in the Italian market, and generalized the methodology by defining a likelihood function that a given specimen originated from a specific breed. The present work will be useful in defining a set of informative markers to be used in routine analyses to discriminate between beef cattle breeds.

Poster G6.10

The effect of selection for growth rate on lipolytic and proteolytic enzyme activities in rabbit meat

B. Arino[1], P. Hernández[2], A. Blasco[1], [1]Dpto. Ciencia Animal, Universidad Politécnica de Valencia, P. O. Box 22012, 46071 Valencia, Spain, [2]Dpto. Producción Animal y Ciencia y Tecnología de los Alimentos, Universidad Cardenal Herrera-CEU, 46113 Moncada, Spain.*

Two groups of rabbits belonging to different generations of a selection experiment were compared. Embryos belonging to generation 7 of selection were frozen and after several selection generations were thawed and transfer to females. A control group (C), formed from the offspring of these embryos, was contemporary to offspring of 21 generation of selection, chosen at random, constituted the selected group (S). Animals were slaughtered at 63-days-old. At 24h *pm*, *Longissimus dorsi* and the set of muscles of a hind leg were dissected from the carcasses and frozen at -20ºC. Cathepsins, cystein proteinase inhibitor and lipolytic enzymes activities were measured. Our objective was to study the effect of selection for growth rate on the activity of these enzymes in rabbit meat.

There were no differences between selection and control group on the activity of the enzymes measured. The main values for the activity of cathepsin B, B+L, H and cystein proteinase inhibitor were 0.608, 2.03, 0.549 and 1.70 (U/g muscle), respectively. Acid lipase, acid phospholipase and neutral lipase activities were 0.51, 1.05 and 0.456 (U/g muscle), respectively. According to our results, we can not conclude that selection for growth rate affect the activity of these enzymes.

Poster G6.11

Liver androstenone metabolism in relation to boar taint

E. Doran[1], F.M. Whittington[1], J.D. McGivan[2], J.D. Wood[1], [1]Department of Clinical Veterinary Science, University of Bristol, Langford, Bristol, BS40 5DU, UK. [2]Department of Biochemistry, University of Bristol, University Walk, Bristol, BS8 1TD, UK.*

Androstenone is produced in the testis as a by-product of testosterone synthesis. Excessive accumulation of androstenone in adipose tissue of some pigs is one of the characteristics of "boar taint". The genetic basis of this phenomenon is not yet understood. We have tested a hypothesis that excessive deposition of androstenone in adipose tissue of some pigs is related to defective hepatic androstenone metabolism. Androstenone metabolism was investigated in isolated microsomes from liver of two breeds of pig exhibiting different levels of androstenone in backfat - Large White (LW) and Meishan (M) (both crossed with Landrace). The major product of liver androstenone metabolism in both breeds was β-androstenol and the reaction of androstenone reduction required NADH as a co-factor. For LW pigs the rate of androstenone metabolism was six fold higher compare to M. The enzyme 3β-hydroxysteroid dehydrogenase (3β-HSD) was suggested to be involved in hepatic androstenone metabolism. No sequence difference in the coding region of liver 3β-HSD for LW and M pigs was found. However, the expression of 3β-HSD mRNA was twelve fold higher for LW compared with M. It was concluded that defective expression of 3β-HSD in liver of M pigs could affect the rate of hepatic androstenone metabolism and thus could lead to excessive accumulation of androstenone in adipose tissue.

Poster G6.12

Effects of breed, diet and muscle on fat deposition and eating quality in pigs

J.D. Wood[1], G.R. Nute[1], R.I. Richardson[1], F.M. Whittington[1], O. Southwood[2] and K.C. Chang[3], [1]Division of Farm Animal Science, University of Bristol, Langford, Bristol BS40 5DU, UK, [2]Sygen International, Fyfield Wick,Oxfordshire OX13 5NA, UK, [3]Department of Veterinary Pathology, University of Glasgow,Glasgow G61 1QH, UK.*

The study compared 4 breeds (Berkshire B, Duroc D, Large White LW and Tamworth T), 2 diets (lysine 1%H and 0.7%L) and 2 muscles ('white' *longissimus* and 'red' *psoas*) in terms of fat deposition and eating quality. The 2 traditional breeds (B and T) had more subcutaneous fat than the 2 modern breeds (D and LW). Intramuscular (marbling) fat was much higher in B and D than LW and T (results not in line with subcutaneous fat), especially in *longissimus*. Diet L increased fat deposition, particularly marbling fat in *longissimus*, this effect being more pronounced in D and LW. *Longissimus* contained more marbling fat than *psoas*, due mainly to neutral lipid. Intramuscular fatty acid composition was affected by diet and breed, partly through differences in the amount of marbling fat. Muscle was also important, with *psoas* neutral lipids and phospholipids having higher concentrations of linoleic acid (18:2) than *longissimus*. Muscle had the biggest effect on sensory characteristics in griddled steaks, *psoas* being more tender and juicy than *longissimus*, with higher scores for pork flavour and overall liking. Breed effects were relatively small and diet L produced higher scores for juiciness than diet H.

Poster G6.13

Effect of CSN1A^G allele on milk mineral composition in Italian Brown dairy cows

M. Malacarne[1], A. Summer[1], P. Franceschi[1], A. Sabbioni[1], A. Rando[2], P. Mariani[1]. Dip. PABVQSA, Università degli Studi, via del Taglio 8, 43100 Parma, Italy. [2]Dip. SPA, Università degli Studi, via Nazario Sauro 85, 85100 Potenza, Italy.*

The CSN1A^G allele affects milk composition with reference to casein content. Aim of this research was to study its effect on content and distribution of the main milk mineral components. The study was carried out on individual milk samples collected from 8 pairs of Italian Brown cows in three herds in Parma province. Each pair within herd was formed by a "low α_{s1}-casein" cow (L) (7 CSN1A^{BG} and 1 CSN1A^{CG}) and a "normal α_{s1}-casein" cow (N) (7 CSN1A^{BB} and 1 CSN1A^{BC}). The cows of each pair were healthy and comparable for management conditions and physiological state. Statistical significance of differences was analysed by two way ANOVA (G_i: presence/absence of CSN1A^G allele; H_j: herd effect). Milk from heterozygous CSN1A^G cows was characterised by lower α_{s1}-casein percentage proportion on total casein (27.30L *vs* 35.73N; $P<0.0001$) and lower casein content (2.17L *vs* 2.38N, g/100g; $P<0.05$). Compared to N cows milk, colloidal calcium content from L cows milk was about 2% lower (75.97L *vs* 77.13N mg/100g; $P>0.05$) and colloidal phosphorus content was about 4% lower (43.64L *vs* 45.31N mg/100g; $P>0.05$). Differences between groups are mainly due to casein phosphorus content (17.57L *vs* 20.24N mg/100g; $P<0.05$): compared to N cows milk, casein from L cows milk was characterised by a significant lower prosthetic phosphorus content (0.81L *vs* 0.85N g/100g of casein; $P<0.05$).

Poster G6.14

Identification of SNPs in candidate genes which may affect meat quality in cattle

H. Levéziel[1], V. Amarger[1], M.L. Checa[2], A. Crisà[3], D Delourme[1], S. Dunner[2], F. Grandjean[1], C. Marchitelli[3], M.E. Miranda[2], N. Razzaq[4], A. Valentini[3], J.L. Williams[4], [1]UMR1061, INRA/Université de Limoges, 123 Avenue Albert Thomas 87060 Limoges, France, [2]Facultad de Veterinaria, Universidad Complutense de Madrid, Madrid 28040 Spain, [3]Universita della Tuscia, via de Lellis, 01100 Viterbo, Italy, [4]Roslin Institute (Edinburgh), Roslin Midlothian EH25 9PS Scotland.

Within the context of an EC funded project (GeMQual, QLRT-CT2000-0147, www.gemqual.org), a list of 459 candidate genes, that may be expected to have an influence on muscle development, composition, metabolism or meat ageing and hence affect the quality of meat, was established from knowledge of their physiological role. About 200 of the candidates have been assigned to laboratories for SNP detection. For each gene, PCR primers were designed to give about 3 fragments. Several strategies to reveal polymorphisms have been followed (direct sequencing of PCR products or sequencing after SSCP, RFLP-SSCP or DHPLC analysis). So far a total of 179 SNPs have been identified in 74 genes (ranging from 1 to 12 for a given gene), 22 of them corresponding to amino-acids substitutions. A variety of SNP genotyping methods are being evaluated in preparation for typing of the 480 bulls (30 x 16 breeds) that have been measured for meat characteristics in the project. The ultimate objective is to examine up to 300 candidate genes and to test associations with variation in meat quality.

Poster G6.15

Milk of some autochthonous Zackel types in Serbia and Montenegro

N. Adzic[1], M. Savic[2], S. Jovanovic[2] and R .Trailovic[2], [1]Institute of Biotechnology, Podgorica, [2]Faculty of Veterinary Medicine, Belgrade, Bulevar JA 18, 11000 Belgrade, Serbia and Montenegro*

Zackel (Pramenka) sheep is native breed inhabiting different regions of Serbia and Montenegro. Special bigeographic conditions of separate habitats are reflected in specific character of different types of Zackel. Therefore, types differ in fleece (coarse or less coarse, or wavy), color (particularly face color), horning, tail length, body size and milk yield. Mutual characteristics of different Zackel types are good adaptability to severe environments and exceptional disease resistance.
All native Zackel types are endangered, some critically reduced to small herds, less than 100 individuals. Monitoring of endangered types of Zackel concerning morphological, productive and genetic characteristics was performed in aim to establish conservatory program.
Estimation of milk yields and milk composition of the following Zackel types: Bardoka, Zetska Zuja, Piva and Sjenicka revealed significant difference between types. Highest milk yield was established in Bardoka (109.82 kg) and Piva (106.79 kg) comparing to Sjenicka (93.27 kg) and Zuja (77.72 kg). Percentage of fat was 7.50, 6.92 and 5.54 in Zetska zuja, Sjenicka and Piva types, respectively. Milk composition of autochthonous Zackel types allows manufacturing of traditional cheeses and skorup (collected and traditionally processed milk fat).

Poster G6.16

Casein haplotype effects on milk traits in the Reggiana cattle

G. Gandini[1], P. Bolla[1], E. Budelli[2], S. Chessa[1] and A. Caroli[3] [1] Dept. VSA, University of Milan, Via Celoria 10, 20133 Milano, Italy, [2]CERSA, Segrate, Milano, Italy, [3]Dept. SBA, Veterinary Faculty, Bari, Italy.*

The Reggiana is a local Italian dairy cattle traditionally linked to the production of the parmigiano reggiano cheese. From 40,000 cows in the 1940's, a severe numerical reduction occurred up to 500 cows in the early eighties. Since the late eighties a conservation programme was started, including the production of a specific brand of parmigiano reggiano and selection under controlled inbreeding, leading to a progressive increase of population size.
From a genetic point of view, the breed is characterised by rather high frequencies of milk protein alleles which are usually uncommon in Bos taurus cattle. At the casein cluster, particular haplotypes occur with relevant frequencies, allowing the study of their effects on production traits. The aim of this study was to evaluate the effect of particular casein haplotypes on milk traits. A total of 432 Reggiana cows were typed at the casein loci by milk isolectrofocusing, revealing in particular the remarkable frequency of some casein alleles. At the αs1-casein (CSN1S1) locus, the C variant showed a frequency of 25%, while the B allele at β-casein (CSN2) locus was found with a frequency as high as 29 %. Informative genotypic combinations were considered to estimate the effects of particular casein haplotypes on milk traits. Significant relationships were detected, mainly with milk protein percentage and yield.

Poster G6.17

Source of variation of milk rennet-coagulation ability of five dairy cattle breeds reared in Trento province

M. Povinelli[1], D. Marcomin[1], R. Dal Zotto[3], G. Gaiarin[2], L. Gallo[1], P. Carnier[1], M. Cassandro[1]
Department of Animal Science, University of Padova, Viale dell'Università 16, 35020 Legnaro, Padova, Italy, [2]Consorzio Trentingrana - Concast, Segno di Taio, 38100 Trento, [3]Consortium Superbrown of Bolzano and Trento, Via Lavisotto, 125, 38100, Trento, Italy.

A total of 506 samples of bulk tank milk from morning and evening milkings were analyzed to assess the milk rennet-coagulation ability. Data from the following dairy breeds reared in 55 herds of Trento province, were available: Holstein Friesian (8 herds), Brown (16 herds), Simmental (10 herds), Rendena (13 herds) and Alpine Grey (8 herds). Minimum and maximum number of samples per herd was 4 and 12, respectively. Traits analyzed were: coagulation time in minutes (R), curd-firming time in minutes (K_{20}) and curd firmness in millimeters (A_{30}). Mean and standard deviation for R, K_{20} and A_{30} was: 15.90 ± 3.26, 6.13 ± 2.52 and 24.03 ± 6.95, respectively. Analysis of variance was performed using a GLM procedure (SAS package) in order to study the effect of the following sources of variation: breed, herd, recording season, class of milk yield, fat and protein percentage, acidity, urea, bacterial count, clostridia contamination, somatic cell count, herd average days in milk and herd average age at calving. Breed resulted one of the most important sources of variation analysed; other results will be discussed.

Poster G6.18

Genotyping of the double-muscling locus (mh) in Piedmontese cattle

G. Bongioni, A. Pozzi and A.Galli, Istituto Sperimentale Italiano "Lazzaro Spallanzani", Localita' La Quercia 26027 Rivolta d'Adda, Cremona, Italy

Muscolar hypertrophy is a recessive trait presents in some European beef breeds: Belgian Blue, Charollais and Piedmontese. The Piedmontese bovine is one of the most important and finest Italian beef breed. Its interest is determined by the exceptional development of muscle mass, known as "double-muscled".The autosomal recessive mh locus causing double-muscling condition maps to bovine chromosome 2 within the same interval as myostatin, a member of the TGF-β superfamily of genes. The Piedmontese myostatin sequence contains a missense mutation in exon 3, resulting in a substitution of G-A at position 941.This mutation predicts the replacement of the cysteina at amino acid 314 with tyrosine. The aim of this work was to genotype 324 samples of Piedmontese animals: 304 sires "double muscled" phenotype and 20 animals "not double muscled" phenotype (15 males and 5 females). DNA was isolated by kit Genomix-Talent and amplyfied by specific labelled primers for wild type and mutated condition to obtain specific fragments. The PCR products were separated by electrophoresis on 377 DNA Sequencer.The results obtained confirm the high incidence of the mutation: only 9 heterozygotes (5 females and 4 males) in comparison with 315 homozygotes for the mutated gene were found. All the heterozygotes belonged to the "not double muscled" phenotype animals group.

Poster G6.19

Research on the performances in breeding, raising and slaughtering of some strains of Mollards with different paternal origin

Elena Popescu-Miclosanu, Consuela Roibu, I. Van, I. Custura, Minodora Tudorache, University of Agronomical Sciences and Veterinary Medicine 59 Marasti Blvd., 1 Sector, 71331 Bucharest, Romania*

Studies were made on 4 hatches of Muskovy grandparents of 4 different strains, the same number of hatches of parents formed of Muskovy drakes of the same strains and Pekin ducks and finally 4 groups of Mollards with the anterior presented paternal origin. Determinations were performed of eggs production, fertility and hatching percentage of grandparents and parents and body weight, viability, plumage colour and slaughtering yield in Mollards.

The best breeding results were obtained by the grandparents of B_1 strain (87,6 eggs/female in 20 laying weeks) and in the interspecific hybridization the parents of B_1 and Pekin (P) who achieved a fertility of over 52% and hatching results of 83%.

The highest average daily gain of Mollards, both in 10 and 12 weeks and the best carcass weight were obtained by the Mollards B_1P and B_4P.The B_1P ducklings are distinguished by the greatest weight of the carcass and breast, the best weight and proportion of the liver. They have plumage of lighter colour than the B_4P hybrid, predominantly light grey with white belly, making a superior commercial aspect of the carcass and white skin.

B_4P Mollards have the best slaughtering efficiency in carcass of 81,56%, the greatest weight of shanks and skin of grey colour.

Poster G6.20

Analysis of milk protein polymorphisms and casein haplotypes in Italian Friesian, Italian Brown Swiss and Reggiana cattle

A. Caroli[1], S. Chessa[2], G. Vivona[2], P. Bolla[2] and G. Pagnacco[2], [1]Dept. SBA, Veterinary Faculty, Strada Prov. per Casamassima km 3, 70010 Valenzano, Bari, Italy, [2]Dept. VSA, Veterinary Faculty, Via Trentacoste 2, 20134 Milano, Italy.*

The importance of milk protein genetic polymorphisms is well know in cattle since the second half of the last century. A total of 1135 individual milk samples from three cattle breeds, Italian Friesian (n = 311), Italian Brown Swiss (n = 392) and Reggiana (n = 432), were typed by isoelectrofocusing for a screening of the actual milk protein genetic variability of the breeds. Polymorphism was found at α_{s1}-casein (*CSN1S1*), β-casein (*CSN2*), κ-casein (*CSN3*), and β-lactoglobulin (*LGB*) *loci*. *CSN*E* allele was found only in Italian Friesian with a frequency higher than 10%. A great variability among the genetic structure of the breeds was found, mainly considering the occurrence of the different casein haplotypes. A strong linkage *disequilibrium* was detected at the three polymorphic casein *loci CSN1S1 - CSN2 - CSN3.* Only nine haplotypes were present at a frequency higher than 0.05 in at least one breed. The most common haplotypes were BA^2A (frequency = 0.48) in Italian Friesian, BA^2B (0.51) in Italian Brown Swiss, and CA^2B (=0.23) in Reggiana cattle. In Italian Friesian and Italian Brown Swiss a large difference was found between the most common haplotypes and the others, while in Reggiana breed, where selection has been much less intensive, a more shaded variability was evident among casein haplotype frequencies. Particular attention should be paid at rare haplotypes for the biodiversity conservation.

Poster G6.21

Casein genetic variability in five Italian goat breeds

P Sacchi[1], E. Budelli[2], G. Ceriotti[3], S. Chessa[3], S. Maione[1], S. Sartore[1], A. Caroli[4] and E. Cauvin[1], Dipartimento di Produzioni Animali Epidemiologia ed Ecologia, via Leonardo da Vinci 44, Grugliasco, Italy, [2] CERSA, Via Fratelli Cervi 9, 20090 Segrate, Milano, Italy, [3]Dept. VSA, Veterinary Faculty, Via Trentacoste 2, 20134 Milano, Italy, [4]Dept. SBA, Veterinary Faculty, Strada Prov. per Casamassima km 3, 70010 Valenzano, Bari, Italy.*

Within a national research project (COFIN 2001), five Italian goat breeds were analysed for an accuarate screening of the genetic structure at the whole casein cluster. Vallesana and Roccaverano are two local goat endangered populations reared in Northern Italy (Piedmont), while Jonica, Garganica and Maltese are Southern Italian breeds. Genomic analysis was performed by means of AS-PCR, PCR-RFLP, PCR-SSCP on 430 goats from different flocks, aiming to identify polymorphisms at αs1-casein (CSN1S1), αs2-casein, (CSN1S2), β-casein (CSN2) and κ-casein (CSN3) loci. The allelic distribution at CSN1S1 locus showed a high frequency of the alleles associated with a low content of αs1-casein (F and 0) mainly in the Northern populations, while the Southern goats presented a higher frequecy of the strong alleles. At the CSN1S2 locus, alleles associated with a normal content of αs2-casein were predominant, with interesting differences among breeds. CSN2 was less polymorphic, while a remarkable variability was found at CSN3 locus, in agreement with the recent literature on the subject. Particular attention was paid to the definition of casein haplotypes, which can be of great interest for the future development of goat breeding.

Poster G6.22

Genetic characterisation at the CSN1S1 locus of a goat population reared in Basilicata (Italy)

C. Senese1, M. Blasi2, A. Lanza2, A. Rosati2, M. Urciuoli1, P. Di Gregorio1, A. Rando1, P. Masina1,1Dipartimento di Scienze delle Produzioni Animali, Via N. Sauro 85, 85100 Potenza, Italy, 2Laboratorio Gruppi Sanguigni, Potenza, Via dell'Edilizia, 85100 Potenza, Italy.*

In the last years the study of the genetic structure of autochthonous goat populations is assuming a strong relevance since these populations represent both a source of genetic variability and a source of typical dairy products. We analysed the genetic structure of the αs1-Cn locus (CSN1S1) of an autochthonous goat population reared in Basilicata. This analysis has been accomplished since this locus shows a strong variability in several breeds with alleles correlated with qualitative and quantitative differences of milk produced by carrier goats and will be extended to the other three casein loci. Results of genomic DNA typing (PCR and RFLP-PCR) show that goats belonging to this population are characterised by a high frequency of alleles associated with high and low content of αs1 casein. Therefore, the genetic structure of this population is similar to that of Malta breed and different from those of Saanen and Alpine breeds, characterised by a high frequency of alleles associated with mean and low content of αs1 casein.

Poster G6.23

Gene expression profiling of sheep mammary tissue using oligo-array: comparison of two Italian breeds

M. Graziano[1,2], M. D'Andrea[1], C. Martin[2], E. Petit[2], R. Rubino[3], F. Pilla[1] and P. Martin[2], [1]Dip. S.A.V.A. Università degli Studi del Molise, 86100 Campobasso, Italy, [2]INRA Laboratoire de Génétique biochimique et de Cytogénétique, 78352 Jouy-en-Josas, France, [3]Istituto Sperimentale per la Zootecnia, 85054 Muro Lucano, Italy.

DNA array technology has been used to compare gene expression profiling of the mammary tissue within two Italian sheep breeds: Sarda and Gentile di Puglia. Differences in phenotypic characteristics (milk production level, lactation length and milk composition) as well as differences in selection and breeding programs in those breeds have triggered a growing interest for this kind of approach. Meaningful pieces of information were expected to explain some genetic traits as well as physiological mechanisms responsible for the qualitative and the quantitative variabilities in milk synthesis. A biopsy of the mammary gland has been taken at three different stages of lactation: beginning, middle and ending from which RNA were extracted in order to make comparison of gene expression pattern both between breeds and, within the same breed, between different physiological stages. For this purpose, 656 oligonucleotides (50-mer) have been designed to be specific for genes or EST relevant for the mammary gland function, synthesized and spotted in duplicate on glass slides by MWG-Biotech AG. Hybridizations, performed for comparing gene expression patterns in both sheep breeds, allowed to identify differentially expressed genes, putatively involved in milk production traits.

Poster G6.24

Genetic relationship between ultrasonic and carcass real measures for marbling score, longissimus muscle area and fat thickness in Korean steers

D.H. Lee[1], H.C. Kim[2] and S. Islam[1]. [1]Hankyong National University, Anseong, Keonggi-Do, Korea, National Livestock Research Institute, R.D.A., Seonghwan, Kyonggi-Do, Korea

Real time ultrasonic and carcass measurements of 13th rib fat thickness (LBF & BF), longissimus muscle area (LEMA & EMA), marbling score (LMS & MS), as well as body weight of live animal at preharvest, carcass weight (CW), and dressing percentage (DP) on 755 Korean beef steers were analyzed to estimate genetic parameters. Data were analyzed using multivariate animal models with an EM-REML algorithm. The heritability estimates for LEMA, LBF, and LMS on RTU scans were 0.17, 0.41, and 0.55 in the age-adjusted model (Model 1) and 0.20, 0.52, and 0.55 in the weight-adjusted model (Model 2), respectively. The Heritability estimates for subsequent traits on carcass measures were 0.20, 0.38, and 0.54 in Model 1 and 0.23, 0.46, and 0.55 in Model 2, respectively. Genetic correlation estimate between LEMA and EMA was 0.81 and 0.79 in Model 1 and Model 2, respectively. Genetic correlation estimate between LBF and BF were high as 0.97 in Model 1 and 0.98 in Model 2. Real time ultrasonic MS were highly genetically correlated to carcass MS of 0.89 in Model 1 and 0.92 in Model 2. These results indicate that RTU scans would be alterative to carcass measurement for genetic evaluation of meat quality in a designed progeny-testing program in Korean beef cattle.

Poster G6.25

A single nucleotide polymorphism in the k-casein (CSN3) coding region

M. Feligini[1], V. Cubric-Curik[2], P. Parma[1], G.F. Greppi[1,3] G. Enne[1,4], Istituto Sperimentale Italiano "Lazzaro Spallanzani", Viale Giovanni XXIII 7, I-26900 Lodi, Italy, Dairy Science Department, Faculty of Agriculture University of Zagreb, Svetosimunska 25, HR-10000 Zagreb, Croatia, [3]Dipartimento di Clinica Medica Veterinaria Università degli Studi, Milano, Italy, [4]Dipartimento di Scienze Zootecniche, Facoltà di Agraria Università di Sassari, Via de Nicola, Sassari, Italy.*

Genetic polymorphism at CSN3 in 80 unrelated sheep from Sarda and Paska breeds was investigated. Primers (K-casF and K-casR) were designed on the available sequence in order to amplify the genomic region encoding the mayor part of the mature protein. A SNP was detected at bp 290 of the sheep κ-CN mRNA where a cytosine was substituted with a tymine. For sheep genotyping we chose LightCycler-based Real Time PCR with product detection using generic SYBR Green I dye. Allelic discrimination was performed using second set of primers wich combine one forward (SNP-F) primer with two reverse primers (SNP-Rt and SNP-Rc), the specificity of the reaction is monitored by determination of the product melting temperature (T_m). The annealing temperature was optimised until the T_m of the specific product and that of the primer-dimers were separated by at least 3-4°C.The amplicons were analyzed on agarose gel to verify that the product of interest was reproduced to obtain the correlation between the gel and fluorescence data. The new SNP was faund both in Sarda (22%) and in Paska (12%) sheep.

Poster G6.26

Study of governing liquid from buffalo and bovine Mozzarella cheese by chromatographic and electrophoretic methods

A. Brambilla, S. Frati, M. Feligini and R. Aleandri, Istituto Sperimentale Italiano "Lazzaro Spallanzani", Viale Giovanni XXIII 7, 26900 Lodi, Italy

Capillary zone electrophoresis (CZE), isoelectric focusing (IEF) and reverse phase-high performance liquid chromatography (RP-HPLC) to identify bovine proteins in water buffalo mozzarella were reported. Calibration curve was performed by mixtures of governing liquid from bovine and water buffalo mozzarella. CZE-urea analysis of samples, performed at pH 3.0 with a coated capillary, gave typical electrophoretic profiles due to the species-specific products of casein proteolysis.

The characterization of mozzarella governing liquid by IEF in a pH gradient 2.5-6.5 and 3.5-8 was achieved because of differences in the isoelectric points from bovine and water buffalo proteins. The quantitative analysis of electrophoretic profiles were carried out by a molecular imager system.

The chromatographic analysis of individual profiles of bovine and water buffalo proteins was performed by RP-HPLC on the basis of the different retention time. This method was able to separate protein components present in mixtures of the governing liquids and allowed a quantitative analysis of peaks of interest.

Limits, advantages and repeatability of each technique were investigated.

Poster G6.27

Study of casein and whey fractions in Algerian dromedary (*Camelus dromedarius*): a preliminary approach

N. Alim[1], S. Frati[2], M. Feligini[2], R. Teniou[1], A. Bouhbel[1] and G. Enne[2], [1]Institut National de la Médecine Vétérinaire (IMNV), Alger, Algery, [2]Istituto Sperimentale Italiano "Lazzaro Spallanzani", Viale Giovanni XXIII 7, 26900 Lodi, Italy

Dromedary (Camelus Dromedarius) casein and whey fractions from Algerian breeds were investigated by electrophoretic and chromatographic analysis. The individual caseins were precipitated at its isoelectric pH. Alpha s1-, alpha s2-, beta and kappa-casein were separated by a sensitive and reliable reversed-phase HPLC method using C_4 column. Whey fraction was separated to casein fraction by centrifugation. Serum albumin, alpha-lactalbumin, beta-lactoglobulin and lactoferrin were separated by PAGE and compared to bovine whey. Chromatographic and electrophoretic patterns showed a marked heterogeneity in protein fractions from different breeds. Further investigations are required to verify the presence of protein polymorphism in dromedary milk.

Poster G6.28

The application of prolactin to reduce pigs' reaction to stress during transportation to slaughterhouse

G. Zak and M.Tyra, National Research Institute of Animal Production, 32-083 Balice-Kraków, Poland

One method of softening the reaction to stress factors is to administer prolactin, which shows anti-stress and adaptogenic action by inhibiting adrenaline secretion. The studies were carried out with 82 fattening pigs that were the offspring of F1 boars with Pietrain inheritance. Animals from the experimental group (37 pigs) were administered intramuscularly with prolactin prior to slaughterhouse transportation, which took 45 minutes. pH and electric conductivity (EC) measurements were performed in the loin of experimental and control pigs 45 minutes postmortem. Tissue sections were taken and PCR tests for the presence of RYR1 gene were performed according to genotype. Significantly higher values of pH45 were observed in the experimental group (6.41) than in the control group (6.21). There were no significant differences between the groups for EC. Genotype analysis of the RYR1 gene showed that within the control and experimental groups, homozygous (NN) animals achieved higher pH45 values compared to the heterozygous ones (Nn) (differences were not significant). A highly significant difference was shown for pH45 between the Nn genotype of the control (6.11) and NN genotype of the experimental group (6.51) and a significant one between Nn genotype of the control group and Nn genotype of the experimental group. These correlations validate the use of prolactin especially when the presence of animals with Nn genotype of the RYR1 gene is suspected.

Poster G6.29

Study of candidate genes for carcass traits in heavy pigs

R. Floris[1], S. Braglia[2], B. Stefanon[3], R. Davoli[2], L. Fontanesi[2], S. Dall'Olio[2], V. Russo[2] and P. Susmel[3], [1]Dipartimento di Biologia, University of Trieste, 34100 Trieste, Italy, [2]DIPROVAL, Sezione di Allevamenti Zootecnici, University of Bologna, 42100 Reggio Emilia, Italy, [3]Dipartimento di Scienze della Produzione Animale, University of Udine, 33100 Udine, Italy.*

Six commercial hybrids of heavy pigs, reared for the production of Italian dry-cured hams, were identified for having homogeneous feeding and farm conditions. For a total of 235 pigs, slaughtered in the same slaughterhouse, the following phenotypic traits were measured: carcass weight, lean percentage, back fat thickness, back muscle thickness, ham weight and ham fat thickness. These data were initially used in a multivariate model to cluster the animals in 100 "lean" and 135 "fat". Furthermore, a similar partitioning of "lean" and "fat" pigs within each hybrid was verified. The pigs were genotyped for single nucleotide polymorphisms (SNPs) already described in the following genes: Na^+, K^+-ATPase subunit alpha 2 (*ATP1A2*), cystatin B (*CSTB*), mitochondrial 2,4-dienoyl-CoA reductase 1 (*DECR1*), leptin (*LEP;* 4 SNPs), melanocortin receptor 4 (*MC4R*), melanocortin receptor 5 (*MC5R*), sarcolipin (*SLN*) and titin (*TTN*). To evaluate if these SNPs could be used to correctly assign the pigs to the two identified groups a logistic regression was applied. The inclusion of *ATP1A2*, *LEP* and *MC4*R in the regression model yielded a correct classification of 71% of the animals in the two clusters.

Poster G6.30

Meat composition of chicken after first, second and third production cycle

*Zia-Ur-Rahman**, *N. Shah, K. Almas, N. Abbas and M.A. Sandhu, Department of Physiology and Pharmacology, University of Agriculture, Faisalabad, Pakistan*

Broilers are mostly used as poultry meat but the layers are also used for meat purpose after completing their production cycle. In the present study 288 commercial layers who have completed their first production cycle were molted for second and third production cycle. Meat was taken from the chest, legs and thigh regions of layers after first, second and third molting for proximate and electrolytes analysis. Moisture, protein, ash and sodium contents were not significantly different but the fat and potassium contents were significantly different among three production cycles. Fat content of meat were significantly higher during second production cycle. A non-significant differences for protein, ash, sodium and potassium while the moisture contents showed significant differences among body parts. Potassium concentration was significantly higher in the right chest and left thigh during first and second production cycle respectively. During first production cycle overall protein and potassium concentration, moisture and ash contents in the second production cycle and sodium concentration in the third production were higher.

Theatre CSN2.1

Consumer perception of meat quality and safety

K. Brunsø, K. Grunert and L. Bredahl, The MAPP Centre, The Aarhus School of Business, Haslegaardsvej 10, DK-8210 Aarhus V, Denmark.*

An understanding of how consumers perceive meat quality and safety is important for the development of products and quality labels that corresponds to consumer demands. In this presentation, the Total Food Quality Model will be used as a framework for analysing the way in which consumers perceive meat quality, and a number of European studies dealing with consumer perception of beef and pork will be presented. The way in which consumers form expectations about quality at the point of purchase, based on own experience and informational cues available in the shopping environment, is described, as well as the way in which quality is experienced in the home during and after meal preparation. Furthermore, the relationship between quality expectations and quality experience and its implication for consumer satisfaction and repeat purchase is analysed. Results show that consumers have difficulty in evaluating meat quality, resulting in uncertainty and dissatisfaction, and reveal a need for taking consumer perception more into account in the development of meat products and quality labels.

Theatre CSN2.2

Desirable characteristics of animal products from a human health perspective

P.J. Morgan, J.C. MacRae and L. O'Reilly, Rowett Research Institute, Bucksburn, Aberdeen, AB21 9SB, Scotland, UK

Animal products, contribute a significant proportion of the food intake in Western societies. Since meat and milk are good sources of bioavailable nutrients they provide numerous benefits to human health.

Meat is an excellent source of protein, which may be important in weight management. It is also a source of key vitamins and micronutrients (Fe, Zn and Cu), which required for optimal immune and cell function. Iron deficiency is associated with increased mortality and morbidity for mothers and their offspring. Diets low in iron are associated with lower birth weights, and epidemiological studies have linked these with increased risk of developing obesity, stroke, type II diabetes, immune function and cardiovascular disease in adulthood.

Milk and milk products are also of benefit to human health. Probiotics, based on gut commensal microflora, is an emerging area of nutrition with potential health benefits. Milk is also an important source of calcium, and recent evidence suggests that this micronutrient may influence the risk of colorectal cancer.

Numerous health benefits have been attributed to conjugated linoleic acids (CLAs), which are lipids present in both meat and milk derived from ruminant animals. Animal studies have shown that CLAs can reduce adiposity, improve plasma lipoprotein profiles and significantly modulate humoral and cellular immunity. However, the findings in humans have been varied and need to be examined in more detail.

Theatre CSN2.3

Potential quality control tools in the production of fresh meat demanded by the European society

H.J. Andersen, N. Oksbjerg and M. Therkildsen, Danish Institute of Agricultural Sciences, Department of Food Science, Research Centre Foulum, P.O.Box 50, DK-8830 Tjele, Denmark.

The market conditions for fresh meat have never faced bigger challenges than today, which is a result of the rapid changes in the market situation for foods. Ever increasing consumer demands and subsequent retail claims from the retail trades combined with political ideas and increasing competitiveness are all issues which set new framework conditions for the present and future food production. This combined with e.g. incidences of Salmonella outbreaks, use of antibiotic, BSE and Foot and Mouth Disease in the production of meat animals have confronted fresh meat marketing of today and the future with enormous challenges to expand or even maintain present market shares of the total food production.
This presentation outlines potential tools that can be implemented in the production of meat animals to control fresh meat quality and hereby fulfil some of the customer demands expected to dominate the market in the years to come. The quality control tools in question cover the whole chain from conception to consumption and include selection of genotype, feeding strategy, production system, pre-slaughter handling, stunning method and slaughter procedure, which separately or in combination can be used to meet customer demands for technological quality, eating quality and nutritional quality together with sustainable and ethic quality aspects.

Theatre CSN2.4

Primary production factors as tools for optimization of milk quality

J.H. Nielsen, Dept of Food Science, Danish Institute of Agricultural Sciences, P.O. Box 50, 8830 Tjele, Denmark

During the last decade, consumers have increased their attention on food quality and demand well-tasting and healthy food. Normally dairies develop new products through modification in the processing of the milk or improvement of the packaging. However, modification of the milk through changes in feeding strategy for the dairy cow affects milk flavour, nutritional value as well as shelf life of the processed milk.
Examples of the influence of the roughage (maize vs grass silage) on the milk flavour will be presented. Furthermore the relation between feed composition and the oxidative stability of milk and dairy products will be given in relatin to the content of polyunsaturated fat in the milk and the antioxidant content with special emphasis on the effect of uric acid and α–tocopherol.

Theatre CSN2.5

Effect of stress at slaughter on meat quality

Claudia Terlouw, Meat Research Station, INRA de Theix - France

Meat quality is influenced by stress responses of the animal before and at slaughter. Behavioural, physiological and metabolic responses to slaughter or to other stress-inducing situations depend on the animal's genetic background and prior experience. For example, Duroc pigs were more reactive to humans than Large Whites. Concerning prior experience, pigs used to reciprocal physical interactions with a human, touch familiar and unfamiliar humans more often. Behavioural and physiological reactivity, determined by genetic background and prior experience, often influences the effect of slaughter conditions on meat quality. For handled pigs, presence of the familiar human during slaughter limited muscle glycogen catabolism, as shown by higher muscle glycogen levels. Pigs showing a stronger cardiac response to transport and handling conditions had lower initial muscle pH. However, reactivity to stress and meat quality are not necessarily correlated. Despite their increased reactivity to humans, meat quality of Duroc pigs was less sensitive to slaughter conditions than that of Large Whites. Various mechanisms may explain relative insensitivity of muscle cells to stress-induced physiological changes. For example, the effect of physiological changes on muscle metabolism depends amongst others on adrenergic receptor density on muscle cells. In cattle, this density varies according to genetic background. Summarising, we have some knowledge on factors influencing stress reactivity at slaughter. Further studies are needed to extend this knowledge and to elucidate physiological and metabolic mechanisms underlying the relationship between stress responses and meat quality, or to understand its absence.

Theatre CSN2.6

Alternative production systems. Do they augment quality, safety and healthiness of animal products?

A.J. van der Zijpp, Animal production Systems Group, Wageningen University and Research Centre, P.O.Box 338, 6700 AH Wageningen, The Netherlands

Alternative systems are developing in response to societal concerns like animal welfare and health, food quality and safety. Organic, outdoor and group housing systems are examples of new developments. Consumers assume that food from alternative systems is healthy and safe, being an important attribute for purchasing. Recent inventories by WUR and Expertisecentrum LNV regarding food safety, quality and health (including risk of zoonoses) reveal that few experimental research results are available from alternative systems or from comparisons with conventional sysems. These inventories are based on literature reviews and expert opinions. Organic systems excell in low levels of residues and antibiotics in foods. Outdoor housing provides more opportunities for infection with Salmonella and Campylobacter, Toxoplasma gondii and Taenia species, helminths and avian influenza (see recent outbreaks in the Netherlands). Monitoring of food safety is not yet general practice in the alternative sector characterised by many small farms and processors. Basic questions have to be addressed like: Do natural behaviour, better nutrition, adapted breeds and less stress promote healthy animals? Does organic manure application lead to pathogen reservoirs? Sound comparitive data of alternative systems are needed that replace expert opinions on health and safety now dominating the debate. For sustainability assessment of alternative systems this knowledge is crucial.

Poster CSN2.7

Integration to produce quality beef in Hungary

Zs. Wagenhoffer, F. Szabó, University of Veszprem, Georgikon Faculty, Keszthely, Hungary*

Looking back after more than one decade, it is clear that livestock production is one of the victim sectors of Hungary's transition. It is particularly true for beef cattle farming, that had been since very long time one of the most important exporter sectors of the country. Not only has its output decreased but also per capita consumption of beef has been dropped to 50%. Because of financial reasons (lack of current assets) fattening sector is practically missing in Hungary, calves are exported right after calving. In consequence of that, there is a lack of quality beef products on the market. In order to move beef cattle sector away from the present nadir, a project had been developed under the leadership of the Georgikon Faculty. The aim of that project is to set a direction for the development of beef cattle production, to provide the sector with substantial assistance and to set it on a new track of growth. Our project integrates stakeholders of beef production as well as representatives of basic and applied research and technological development, being the key factors of a potential progress. When identifying our objectives, we must take into account Hungary's ecological faculties and thereby give a preference to grassland-based livestock production systems. By working out a specific alternative for potential development scenarios on a scientific basis our project will promote all these concepts by vertically integrating the sector's stakeholders in order to provide consumers with quality beef products.

Poster CSN2.8

Animal food quality and human health - general considerations

K.J. Peters and C. Kijora, Institute of Animal Sciences, Humboldt-University Berlin, Philippstr. 13, Building No.9, 10115 Berlin*

The content of valuable nutrients, undesirable substances, hygienic aspects, requirements of humans for animal products and problems of malnutrition (over- and undernourishment) are parameters that must be considered in connection with food quality and human health. A further aspect is the possibility to improve the quality by feeding and breeding practices.
The composition of amino acids, the content of some essential fatty acids (EPA, DHA), specific vitamins and minerals make animal products indispensible for children and valuable for adults.
Adverse effects of a high consumption of animal products in developed countries and hygienic aspects, pollutants and contaminants in developing and developed countries are the main reasons for a negative impact of animal products on human health.
Changing the nutrient content of meat through means of feeding is possible, but seems to be not the way of choice. Milk and eggs are influenced easier by feeding practices.
Breeding activities focus on 3 main issues which are all correlated with product quality, i.e.
- alteration in product composition
- improving stress resistance and
- improving disease resistance.

Maintaining the balance between product quality and quantity and functional efficiency, fitness and welfare should be the prime breeding goal.

Poster CSN2.9

Frabosana sheep breeding in NW Italian Alps: livestock farming systems and milk characteristics

L. Battaglini, M. Bianchi, A. Mimosi, A. Ighina and Carola Lussiana, Dipartimento Scienze Zootecniche, via Leonardo da Vinci 44, 10095 Grugliasco, Italy*

The Frabosana sheep, original breed from the NW Italian Alps valleys, threatened of extinction in the 80's, has currently become the more diffused dairy sheep breed in Piedmont (approximately 7500 heads), thanks to the EC regulations. Its prevailing milk attitude allows several typical cheese productions. The more traditional breeding systems adopt the transhumance, i.e. transfer from the stables at the bottom of the alpine valleys progressively to the alpine pastures in spring and summer. Such breeding technique has demonstrated to be particularly suitable for this sheep breed, being characterized by a remarkable rusticity. Feeding is based on pasture in the vegetative season, while it is almost exclusively made up of hay in wintertime. From the analysis of the milk characteristics in the passage from the stabled period to alpine pastures, an increase of the fat percentage and an improvement of cheese making properties can be observed; this last feature is to be put in relation with the significant parallel reduction of somatic cells content. Such results would indicate the exigencies to improve the breeding techniques in winter period, often conditioned by poor hygienic-sanitary conditions, and to enhance the milk yield on summer pastures, also by better managing the frequently too late utilised swards.

Poster CSN2.10

Comparaison de l'activité fermentaire chez les camélidés, les caprins et les ovins nourris à base de foin de vesce-avoine

A. Boubaker-Gasmi [1], C. Kayouli[1], H. Rouissi[2] et D. Demeyer[3], [1]Institut National Agronomique, Tunis, Tunisie, [2]Ecole Supérieure d'Agriculture Mateur, Tunisie, [3]Université de Gent, Belgique.*

Quatre dromadaires, 4 béliers et 2 boucs, tous porteurs de fistules au niveau du rumen ont été nourris à base de foin de vesce-avoine en vue de comparer le faciès fermentaire, la population des protozoaires ciliés et le taux de disparition de la matière sèche (MS) du foin incubé *in situ* pendant 120 h. Les valeurs du pH étaient plus élevées et plus stables chez les camélidés que chez les petits ruminants malgré des concentrations en acides gras volatils (AGV) significativement plus importantes ($P<0,05$) chez les camélidés. Les caprins et les ovins ont présenté des concentrations en AGV statistiquement comparables ($P>0,05$). Alors que les plus faibles concentrations en azote ammoniacal ont été enregistrées chez les camélidés, les concentrations les plus élevées ont été observées chez les caprins. Les ciliés dénombrés sur le contenu de rumen prélevé 2 heures après la distribution du repas du matin étaient moins nombreux chez les camélidés que chez les caprins et les ovins (2,7; 4,6 et 4,1 * 10^5 / ml, respectivement). Les ovins n'ont hébergé que des ciliés du type A (*Polyplastron*). Ceux du type B (*Epidinium spp et Eudiplodinium spp*) ont été observés chez les caprins et les camélidés. Ces derniers ont mieux digéré le foin que les caprins et les ovins (57,4 ; 52 et 48,3%, respectivement). Ces résultats pourraient expliquer l'aptitude des camélidés à mieux utiliser les aliments fibreux que les petits ruminants.

Staphylococcus species prevalence in cows'raw milk from dairy farms in Latvia

A. Jemeljanovs, I.H. Konosonoka and J. Bluzmanis, Research Centre "Sigra" of the Latvia University of Agriculture, Instituta Street 1, Sigulda LV-2150, Latvia

Milk is most important food during early childhood and remains an important dietary component through life. At the same time milk is first rate medium, which permit the growth of microorganisms, some of which may cause undesirable changes. Occasionally, dairy products serve as the vehicle for the transmission of pathogenic microorganisms such *Staphylococcus aureus*, which is a major bovine mastitis agent and primary human pathogen.
Raw milk samples from different dairy farms were analysed. Coagulase positive *Staphylococcus aureus (S.aureus)* (39.5%), coagulase negative staphylococci (CNS) (49.4%) and associations of *S.aureus* and CNS (7.4%) were determined. *Staphylococcus* strains have not been isolated from milk samples in 3.7% of cases. When average *S.aureus* count is 210.3±64.9, average somatic cell count (SCC) is 148 710.5±17 139.3, when average *S.aureus* count is 1 667.1±572.8, average SCC is 539 357.1±28 546.6, but when average *S.aureus* count is 4 301.6±1 300.1, average SCC is 1 607 480±223 661.2. The results show that higher *S.aureus* count in the milk of dairy farms is correlated to increasing SCC (r=0.58).
The high prevalence of *S.aureus* and CNS in raw milk testifies that hygienic conditions in dairy farms are not observed enough. Farmers are not aware of the sources of microbial contamination and do not understand how they can be controlled.

Poster CSN2.12

Some carcass/meat quality traits relation to the measurements of novel (CT, MR) techniques

G. Holló, J. Seregi, I. Holló and I. Repa, University of Kaposvár Guba S. 40 H-7400 Kaposvár, Hungary*

The aim of the study is to analyse the carcass/meat quality traits using non-invasive techniques. Young bulls (n=40) from Holstein-Friesian, Hungarian Grey were used. Besides slaughter data the right half carcasses were dissected samples taken between the 11-13th rib of which tissue composition were measured by X-ray computer tomography (CT). The crude fat, the intramuscular fat content and the relaxation times of longissimus were determined according to Hungarian Standard, Magnetic Resonance Imaging (MRI) and $^{+}$H NMR spectroscopy, respectively. Correlation coefficients were calculated among parameters (SPSS 10.0). Closest correlation was found for amount and percentage of carcass fat and fat content of rib samples using CT (r=0.93. r=0.86 P<0.001). Coefficients of amount of bone and muscle in carcass and that of in rib samples were r=0.81, r=0.88 (P<0.001). The relationship of the fat of longissimus determined by MRI to crude fat of longissimus showed r=0.52, and to fat amount of rib samples analysed by CT r=0.53. Based on the results of multiexponencial analysis of relaxation times obtained by spectroscopy a negative relationship between biexponencial T_2 fast (%) component and pH_{45} as well as colour (a*) r=-0.37, r=-0.39 (P<0.01) was established. Contrary tendencies were presented in case of T_2 slow (%) component. In conclusion, these novel techniques can be used for the slaughter value estimation and determination of some beef quality traits.

Poster CSN2.13

Shear force value in meat of slaughter bulls of various breeds

J. Mojto, K. Zaujec and K. Novotná, Research Institute of Animal Production, Hlohovská 2, 949 92 Nitra, Slovak Republic

The aim of the work was to evaluate and compare the shear force value in meat (tenderness) of slaugter bulls of various breeds in the conditions of Slovakia for the national audit of beef quality.The group of meat breeds (Piemont, Blond d'Aquitaine, Limousine and Belgian Blue) was evaluated together, the further evaluated breeds were the Slovak Spotted (SS), Slovak Pinzgau (SP) and Holstein (H). A sample was taken from mns.long.dorsi between the 9th-11th rib during the carcass dissection 24 hrs post mortem. The samples were stored in a refrigerator. On 7th day were the 2.5 cm thick slices cooked 20 min., and after 5 min. cooling the shear force value was measured by Warner-Bratzler system.

The average values of shear force value were 4.69 kg in the group of meat breeds, 3.87 kg in SS, 3.96 in SP, and 3.85 in H breeds. The differences were statistically nonsignificant.

In case the meat samples were ordered according to the selected span (< 4.0 kg tender meat, 4.0-7.0 kg still acceptable, > 7.0 kg tough meat) most of the samples in all breeds were of the tender meat (53.1 - 56.6 %). Most samples of tough meat were with the meat breeds (23.9 %) and the least ones (4.5 %) with the SS breed.

Poster CSN2.14

The effect of excessive selenium intake on selenium concentration in cow`s milk

J. Trinácty[1], M. Sustala[1], P. Homolka[2], V. Kudrna[2], K. Sustová[3], [1]Research Institute of Animal Nutrition, Ltd. Pohorelice, Vídenská 699, Czech republic, [2]Research Institute of Animal Production, Praha-Uhrineves,Czech republic, [3]Mendel Agricultural and Forestry University Brno, Czech republic.

The effect of selenium feed supplement on milk selenium concentration and milk selenium production was studied in a feeding periodic trial on dairy cows. Cows of the Czech Red Pied breed yielding 21±2.1kg of milk per day were fed twice daily on a basal diet (maize silage 33 % DM and alfalfa hay) plus concentrate feed mixture. The eight cows were arranged in two groups, experimental group received concentrate feed mixture enriched with selenized yeast (average daily selenium intake 6.8 mg, correspond to 200 % of its recommended requirement for dairy cows), the control group was not supplemented. Each of two experimental periods lasted 21 days. The highest milk selenium concentration was 59.51 μg/l. Selenized yeast supplement significantly increased milk selenium concentration (44.04 μg/l vs. control 15.29 μg/l; $P<0.01$). 24-hours milk selenium production was calculated, the highest milk selenium production was 1.440 mg/day. Experimental group showed increased milk selenium production in 24-hours (+0.6087 mg; $P<0.01$) in comparsion to control.

This study was supported by GACR (523/02/0164) and NAZV (QD0176).

Poster CSN2.15

Effects of the extensive culture system as finishing production strategy on biometric and chemical parameters in rainbow trout

Giovanni M. Turchini, Vittorio M. Moretti and Franco Valfrè. Dipartimento di Scienze e Tecnologie Veterinarie per la Sicurezza Alimentare, Università degli Studi di Milano, Via Trentacoste 2, 20134 Milano, Italy.*

The efficacy of an extensive farming period, as a finishing production strategy to reduce fat content and also ameliorate the fatty acid profile of fish muscle, was evaluated in rainbow trout. Fish were stocked in an artificial lake, in which fish feed only on naturally available nutrients with no supply of artificial feed, for different length of time from 0 to 120 days. No weight loss was noted during the whole finishing period while total length increased from 227.8 ± 6.9mm to 268.7±3.3mm and the condition factor decreased from 1.41±0.04 to 0.89± 0.02. Total fat of the fillets decreased considerably from 4.7±0.65% at the beginning to 2.4±0.41% and 0.7±0.17% after 45 and 120 days, respectively. Fillets fatty acid composition were largely affected by the time of stocking in the extensive farm and, against the reduction of C18:1n-9, C18:2n-6, MUFA% and n-6% values, it was evident an increase in the C20:5n-3, C22:6n-3, PUFA% and n-3% values. Summing up it was showed that while other finishing strategies for salmonids have some disadvantages, the extensive culture system seems to be a potential useful tool for increasing the general quality of end product with no effects on fish weight and on the total outlay costs for feeding.

Poster CSN2.16

Changes in proteolysis in beef meat during ageing

J. Oprzadek, A. Józwik, A. Oprzadek, A. Sliwa-Józwik, A.Kolataj Institute of Genetics and Animal Breeding Polish Academy of Sciences, Jastrzebiec, 05-552 Wólka Kosowska, Poland*

During the ageing process many proteolytic enzymes are released and their products are studied in relation to bovine meat tenderness. The study was performed on 16 beef bulls. At 15 months of age the animals were slaughtered after 24 hours of fasting. Approximately 10 min, 24 hours, 7 days and 14 days post-mortem 10g samples of longissimus dorsi muscle at the 12th rib were obtained from right side of each animal for analysis of lysosomal activity. Muscle samples were subjected to perfusion in 0.9 % NaCl solution at +5° C. In the lysosomal fraction, basing on substrates from SIGMA-ALDRICH Co., the activities of dipeptidyl peptidase (DP II, EC. 3.4.14.4.) and DP IV (EC. 3.4.14.5), arginyl aminopeptidase (ARG, EC. 3.4.11.6) were estimated. The activity of ARG, DPII and DPIV was determined spectrophotometrically as Fast Blue BB salt derivatives at 520 nm according to the method of McDonald and Barret (1986). The activity of the enzymes was expressed as nMol/mg of protein/hour. The pH was measured at 1 h, 24 h, 7 days and 14 days post-mortem on the muscle *L.dorsi*. Significant differences in the activity of DPIV and ARG during ageing were observed. There were no significant differences in the activity of DPII during ageing. The highest activity of DPIV 24 hours post-mortem and the lowest activity of ARG 10 minutes after slaughter in the *LD* muscle were observed.

Poster CSN2.17

Effect of grazing on chemical composition and CLA content of suckling kid

A. Caputi Jambrenghi, F. Giannico, G. Di Martino, A. Di Luccia, A. Vicenti, G. Vonghia, Dipartimento di Produzione Animale, University of Bari, Via G. Amendola 165/A, 70126 Bari, Italy.*

The study evaluated the chemical composition and CLA content of the meat of kids suckled by grazing and non-grazing nannies. 20 female Ionica goats were divided into homogeneous groups of 10 immediately after giving birth. Goats in the control group (Group C) were fed on hay and concentrated feed; those in the experimental group (Group P) grazed, with supplementary hay and concentrated feed in the shed. Single kids born to the goats in the two groups were suckled *ad libitum* directly by their mothers, and slaughtered at the age of 46 days. Productive performances of the kids were evaluated, both live and after slaughtering. Samples of raw and cooked meat were tested. Statistical differences ($P<0.05$) between the kids in Group C and Group P were evident only for raw meat, regarding saturation (13.45 *vs* 14.92), shear force (3.58 *vs* 2.86 kg/cm^2), water content (74.41 *vs* 75.46%) and ash (1.12 *vs* 0.98%), and for cooked meat, regarding cooking loss (26.89 *vs* 31.51%). In any case, a higher CLA content in the raw meat from Group P (2.57 *vs* 2.25%) and a higher isomer cis9-trans11 content in the cooked meat (1.52 *vs* 1.10%) were an indication of the increased CLA level in the meat of suckling kid due to the mother grazing.

Poster CSN2.18

Measurement of the total oxidative stability of beef of Belgian Blue bulls fed rations differing in a-tocopherolacetate content

K. Raes[1], I. Vermander[1], A. Balcaen[1], S.K. Lee[2], E. Claeys[1], D. Demeyer[1], S. De Smet[1], [1]Department of Animal Production, Faculty of Agricultural and Applied Biological Sciences, Ghent University, Proefhoevestraat 10, 9090 Melle, Belgium, [2]Department of Animal Food Science and Technology, Kangwon National University, Chunchon, 200-701, South Korea*

Increasing the n-3 polyunsaturated fatty acid content of meat may compromise oxidative stability, if not accompanied by an appropriate supply of antioxidants. Aiming at a comparison of several methods for measuring total oxidative stability of meat, two groups of six Belgian Blue bulls were finished on a concentrate/maize silage diet with linseed as the main source of linolenic acid, and either or not supplemented with 200 ppm α-tocopherolacetate. No differences in fatty acid profile of the intramuscular fat of the *longissimus thoracis* was measured between the two groups. No effect of dietary α-tocopherolacetate was observed on colour stability evaluated by CIELAB measurements, even after display of the meat for 14 days under continous light. However, clear differences were found between the two groups for lipid stability, measured by the ferrous oxidation-xylenol orange and thiobarbituric acid reactive substances method, and for the a-tocopherol content of the meat. On the other hand, the total reducing activity of the meat following the method described by Lee et al. (1981) was not different between the two groups. It is suggested not to rely on one method when evaluating oxidative stability of meat.

Poster CSN2.19

Effect of environment and cow genotype on milk quality of black-and-white cattle

R. Zieminski, A. Cwikla, P. Nowakowski, A. Hibner, Institute of Animal Breeding, Agricultural University, Chelmonskiego 38, 51-630 Wroclaw, Poland

The aim of research was to describe the effect of environment and genotype on milk quality in high yielding cows. Research was performed in the herd of Black-and-White cattle (n=283) yielding ca 10.000 kg of milk per cow during two consecutive years. Model of analysis of variance was used where effects of: genotype (<87.5 or >87.5% of HF blood), the year of testing (1 or 2), feeding season (summer or winter), lactation (1-st, 2-nd or 3-rd), level of daily milk yield (<20.0 kg, 20.1-25.0 or >25.0 kg) on milk yield (305 days) and somatic cells count in milk (SCC) were analysed. Better milk production performance was stated for cows with >87.5% of HF blood when compared to contemporaries with HF blood share <87,5%. Influence of the year was stated ($P<0.01$) on share of test milkings with low level of SCC (<400.000 cells/ml) in cows with low daily milk yield (<20,0 kg). Group of cows with the lowest daily milk yield showed statistically significant ($P<0,01$) higher share of milkings with low SCC in the 3-rd lactation when compared to their 1-st lactation.

Poster CSN2.20

Comparative spectroscopy of dried cattle muscles

G. Masoero[1], G. Bergoglio[1], G. Destefanis[2], A. Brugiapaglia[2], C. Lindeman[3], D. Pavino[4], M.C. Abete[4], V.Di Carlo[5]. [1]Istituto Sperimentale per la Zootecnia, Via Pianezza 115, 10151-Torino, Italy, [2]Dipartimento di Scienze Zootecniche, Agraria, Via L. da Vinci 34, Torino, 10100-Grugliasco, Italy, [3]DELTA, Hjortekaersvej 99, DK-2800, Lyngby, DK, [4]Istituto Zooprofilattico Sperimentale, Via Bologna 148, 10154-Torino, Italy, [5]Istituto per la Nutrizione delle Piante, Via della Navicella 2/4, 00184-Roma, Italy*

Five comparative spectroscopies collecting 6.677 overall points: Fluorescence (F, 310-590nm), Near Infra Red reflectance (NIR, 1308-2393nm), Fourier Transformed Near Infra Red reflectance (FT-NIR, 1000-2500nm), Fourier Transformed Near Infra Red reflectance Microscopy (FT-NIRM, 1250-2500nm), Fourier Transformed Medium Infra Red reflectance (FT-MIR, 2500-25000nm) Spectroscopies were applied to 82 freeze-dried meat samples derived from well distinguished categories of Valdostana cattle (A-Veal, B-Young-cattle, C-Cow). Averages of R^2c results were: 13_{LAB}values multivariate=0.914, F=0.836, NIR=0.654, FT-NIR=0.985, FT-NIRM= 0.792, FT-MIR=0.474. FT-NIR gave better results than 13_{LAB}values in separating all the individuals, while FT-NIRM gave low separation of B vs C samples. F spectroscopy performed well as FT-NIR except for the B vs C classes. The NIR spectroscopy appeared useful, while not so powerful as FT-NIR.

Poster CSN2.21

Retraceability and classification of some Piedmont and mountain cheeses by NIR method

G. Masoero[1,2], G. Bergoglio[2], F. Abeni[2], G. Zeppa[3]. [1]Consorzio Vezzani, 10050-Sauze d'Oulx, Italy [2]Istituto Sperimentale Zootecnia, Via Pianezza 115, 10151-Torino, Italy, [3]DIVAPRA, Agraria, Via Leonardo da Vinci 44, 10095-Grugliasco, Italy*

Retraceabilty was intended as ability of recovering a twin of the sample among a number of the others in a spectra database. Classification ability was intended to verify a label or to separate specific experimental effect studied on dairy animals. The Near Infrared Reflectance (NIR) Spectroscopy method was tested in 14 experiments comprising a wide variability in types and species (N=1373). The NIRS were very well able to recover the twin samples with average recovery rate 73% (63-100%) vs prior probability 1/1228. Regarding classification of the types in a first database, results were positive because Toma cheeses from Piedmont and mountain were 97% recovered, Fontina 88%, Fromadzo 85%, Pecorino 95%, tipo Sbrinz 96%, Murianeng 73%, Gruyere-Etivaz 98% and Goat cheeses 100%. Other types of cheeses were misclassified and intended as Toma, because of strong unbalance in categories and great variability inside Toma. Separation of experimental treatment was possible in a feeding experiment (R^2=0.88) and in geographic origin (R^2=0.50, mountain vs plain). In a further database (N=99) with chemically analysed seven DOP cheeses NIR classification averaged 77%, the types chemically nearer to Toma being misclassified.

This technique could improve promotion of mountain cheeses because ready information about cheese characteristics.

Poster CSN2.22

Antimicrobial activity of green tea extract on rabbit caecum microflora

D. Tedesco, S. Stella, S. Galletti, S. Rossetti, Department of Veterinary Sciences and Technologies for Food Safety, Via Celoria 10, 20133, Milano, Italy.*

This research will examine the potential of using plant extracts not considered harmful for human and animal health as alternatives to antimicrobials, including antibiotics, used as prophylactic and growth promoting agents in livestock.

The inhibitory activity of green tea extract (Greenselect, Indena S.p.A.) towards the development and growth of bacteria isolated from rabbit caecum was evaluated. *Escherichia coli*, *Staphylococcus aureus*, *Clostridium* spp., *Enterococcus* spp., total coliforms, anaerobic bacteria, *Lactobacillus* spp, aerobic mesophilic bacteria. were cultured in plates added with tea polyphenols solution. Bacteriostatic effect on *E. coli* has also been tested using a broth medium. Inhibiting activity of green tea extract has been observed on total aerobic mesophilic and total anaerobical count. The colony development of *E.coli* in the medium containing 50 μg/mL green tea extract was 20-fold lower than in control medium; at 100 μg/mL the development was completely inhibited. On the other hand, green tea extract did not inhibit or promote growth of all other bacteria tested.

In conclusion, our results showed a strong activity of green tea extract against *Escherichia coli*. Tea extract is worth further investigations as a possible natural antimicrobial additive.

Poster CSN2.23

Effects of fructo-oligosaccharides, lactic acid bacteria or antibiotics on performances of weaned piglets

M. Morlacchini[1], M.L. Callegari[2], F. Rossi[3], G. Piva.[3], CERZOO[1], CRB[2], Istituto di Scienze degli Alimenti e della Nutrizione[3], Facoltà di Agraria, Via Emilia Parmense 84, Piacenza, Italy.

Development of alternatives to antibiotics for prevention of enteric diseases is an important topic in livestock. 96 piglets weighting 6.0 ± 0.94 kg were allotted to three treatments: control diet; control diet supplemented with chlortetracycline and spyramicine (1000 e 400 mg/kg of mixed feed respectively); control diet supplemented with fructo-oligosaccharides (FOS) (0.5%; degree of polymerization 2-7) and lactic acid bacteria (LAB) (10 ml of a $2x10^9$ CFU/ml suspension of *Lactobacillus amylovorus*, *Lactobacillus brevis*, *Bifidobacterium boum*). Experiment lasted for 35 days, antibiotics were given only in the first 14 days, while FOS and LAB were fed for the whole experimental period. After 14 d animals fed FOS+LAB shown (P<0,01) a average daily gain (ADG) (141 g/d) lower than control group (184 g/d) and antibiotics treated group (186 g/d). Supplementing diet with FOS+LAB determined, in the second period, a better ADG (380 g/d) compared to antibiotics supplemented diet (331 g/d; P<0,01). No differences were observed towards control group (360 g/d). Feed intake and feed efficiency were not significantly different between groups. Use of antibiotics or pre- and probiotics have shown a similar effect on animal performances, but these last treatments are not associated with spreading of antibiotics resistance and consequently could be more acceptable for the consumers.

Poster CSN2.24

***N-3* fatty acids, C18:1*trans* isomers and CLA*cis-9,trans-11* in subcutaneous and intramuscular fat of lambs**

Karin Nuernberg[1], D. Dannenberger[1], W. Zupp[2], G. Nuernberg[1] and K. Ender[1], [1]Research Institute for the Biology of Farm Animals, [2]Research Institute of Agriculture and Fishery Mecklenburg-Vorpommern, 18196 Dummerstorf, W.-Stahl Allee 2, Germany.

The objective of the study was to increase the concentration of *n-3* fatty acids and CLA*cis-9,trans-11* in lamb muscle by feeding on grass. Thirteen male crossbred lambs (Schwarzköpfiges Fleischschaf x Gotland) were kept on a salt grass pasture until the beginning of the experiment at 24 kg live weight. The lambs were randomly divided in two feeding groups (1. feeding concentrate indoor; 2. feeding grass on pasture). The concentration of total *n-3* fatty acids in *longissimus* muscle was significantly ($p < 0.05$) increased up to 119.6 mg/100 g muscle in lambs fed grass compared to 65.6 mg/100 g in lambs fed concentrate. The total saturated fatty acid percentage of muscle lipids was unaffected by the diet. Keeping lambs on pasture increased the concentration of C18:1*trans-11* to 5.7 % *vs.* 3.75 % in lambs fed concentrate. The relative content of CLA*cis-9,trans-11* (1.94 %) in grazing lamb muscle was significantly ($p < 0.05$) higher than in concentrate fed animals (1.08 %). The relative percentage of *n-3* fatty acids, C18:1*trans-11* and CLA*cis-9,trans-11* was significantly higher in subcutaneous fat of grass fed lambs compared to concentrate feeding (1.7 % vs 0.85 %, 7.4 % vs 4.7 %, 2.5 % vs 1.35 %, respectively).

Poster CSN2.25

Identification of critical points in monitoring the origin of beef

H.-J. Rösler[*1], S. Jäsert[1], S. Maak[2] and L. Döring[1], [1]MRA of Saxony-Anhalt, Angerstraße 6, D-06118 Halle; [2]Institute of Animal Breeding, University Halle, A.-Kuckhoff-Str.35, D-06108 Halle, Germany*

We have recently described the implementation of a tissue bank for beef cattle within a monitoring system for the origin of beef in Saxony-Anhalt. In order to identify critical points in this system we took multiple tissue samples at different time points in the slaughterhouse. More than 400 samples were characterized at molecular level with a set of 11 microsatellites (Stockmarks cattle paternity PCR typing kit; Applied Biosystems). A total of 4.6% of the samples taken at the cold-storage depot were not identical with the respective samples from the ear tag although, each two further samples per animal from the slaughterhouse matched the ear tag result. This identifies the transfer of the carcasses from the slaughter line to the cold-storage depot as the major source for loss of identification. Analysis of tissue samples from 75 additional carcasses confirmed this result since the only discrepancy was again observed at this point. Another major obstacle was the poor sample quality obtained from the slaughterhouse. Twenty five samples (5.9%) were not suitable for obtaining DNA in sufficient quality for marker analysis due to strong degradation. A total of 4 samples indicated contamination with other samples as revealed by the occurrence of more than two alleles in some markers. All of those samples were again taken at the cold-storage depot. Our results clearly identify critical points and provide a basis for optimization of the sampling procedure.

Poster CSN2.26

Comparison of three supplements high in linseeds or linseed oil in dairy cows

J.F. Cabaraux[1], C. Marche[2], J.L. Hornick[1], O. Dotreppe[1], L. Istasse[1] and I. Dufrasne[3], [1]Nutrition Unit, [3]Experimental Station, Animal Production Department, Veterinary Medicine Faculty, Liege University;[2]Centre de technologie agronomique, Stree, Belgium.*

Dairy cows, offered a diet based on maize silage and grass silage, were supplemented with either linseeds or linseed oil. The linseeds were steam treated with barley as support or were ground with sugar beet pulp. The inclusion of linseeds was 0.5 kg/d and that of linseed oil 0.180 kg/d. The supplementation lasted for three weeks.
Milk yield was maintained to a larger extent in the supplemented groups with no difference between groups than in the non-supplemented animals. Fat concentration and yield were decreased when linseeds were steam treated and when linseed oil was added while ground linseed increased milk fat concentration and maintained fat yield. Both treatments of linseeds significantly reduced the concentration of short chain fatty acids (C6-C14: 21.41 and 22.52 *vs* 23.37 weight%) and of C16 (36.19 and 36.19 *vs* 38.42%) while there was an increase in the C18 group (41.50 and 40.37 *vs* 36.75%) (steam treatment and grounding *vs* control period before supplementation). There were increases in the C18:3 n-3 group (0.73 and 0.79 *vs* 0.58%, $P<0.05$) and a tendency for larger concentrations in C18:2 n-6 and in C18:1 n-9. There were also corresponding increases in daily fatty acid yields. By contrast linseed oil supplementation did not affect the fatty acid composition.

Poster CSN2.27

Diet effect on the concentration of n-3 polyunsaturated fatty acids of ovine muscle and subcutaneous adipose tissue

E. Kasapidou[1], J.D. Wood[1], L.A. Sinclair[2], R.G. Wilkinson[2] and M. Enser[1], [1]Division of Farm Animal Science, University of Bristol, Langford, Bristol BS40 5DU, UK [2]ASRC, School of Agriculture, Harper Adams University College, Edgmond, Newport, Shropshire, TF10 8NB, UK.*

Polyunsaturated fatty acids (PUFA) particularly the ones from the n-3 series are important in the maintenance of healthy life. We investigated the effect of diet on the PUFA levels of *m. semimembranosus* and adipose tissue. Two groups of eight Suffolk × Charollais lambs were finished on concentrates or on a mixed diet (grass silage plus concentrates, 65:35, DM basis) to similar live weight. The concentrate consisted of wheat, soya hulls, soya bean meal, rapeseed meal, oatfeed, molasses and Megalac®. Diets were supplemented with 500mg/kg DM vitamin E for optimum meat quality. The concentration of a-linolenic acid (18:3 n-3) was 69% and 87% higher in the muscle and adipose tissue respectively from the lambs fed the mixed diet. The concentration of linoleic acid (18:2 n-6) was 48% and 80% lower in the muscle and adipose tissue respectively from the mixed diet group. The linoleic:a-linolenic acid ratio exceeded the recommended value of 4.0 in both tissues from the concentrate group compared with the more desirable values in the mixed diet group (2.5 and 1.6 in muscle and adipose tissue respectively). Inclusion of grass silage in the diet resulted in beneficial changes in the PUFA composition of both tissues but the effect was greater in adipose tissue.

Poster CSN2.28

Can strategies for feeding and cooling of milk in automatic milking systems improve milk quality?

L. Wiking and J.H. Nielsen, Department of Food Science, Danish Institute of Agricultural Sciences, Research Centre Foulum, P.O. Box 50, 8830 Tjele, Denmark.*

The implementation of automatic milking systems in the dairy production has caused an increased lipolysis in bulk milk. Free fatty acids accumulated from lipolysis result in appearance of rancid flavour in dairy products. With the continuously increasing number of automatic milking systems the quality of drinking milk could be impaired. However, if a more stable milk fat globule could be achieved by feeding it could increase raw milk quality in automatic milking systems.

The fat content and the fatty acid composition in raw milk can be manipulated through feeding. Together with temperature and pumping flow these attributes influence the degree of damage to the milk fat globules. The current study examines how the pumping stability of raw milk can be improved by the diet of the cow. Furthermore, cooling strategies for milk in automatic milking systems are evaluated. Results of formation of free fatty acids and the particle size distribution of milk fat globules in pumped milk from cows fed concentrates with a high amount of lipid supplement vs. a low fat diet will be presented.

Poster CSN2.29

Chemical composition of meat from fattened beef bulls

J. Krzyzewski, N. Strzalkowska, J. Oprzadek, E. Dymnicki, A. Oprzadek, Istitute of Genetics and Animal Breeding, Jastrzebiec, 05-552 Wólka Kosowska, Poland*

The objective of this study was to compare chemical composition of muscle of young fattened bulls. The experiment was carried out on 71 bulls, belonging to the following different 5 beef breeds: Red Angus, Charolais, Hereford, Limousine, Simental and Friesian. Between the age of 9 and 15 months all the animals were fed ad libitum complete diet (TMR), consisting of corn silage (75%), concentrates (20%) and meadow hay (5%). All the bulls were slaughtered at the age of 15 months. The right carcass-side was dissected separating lean, bones and fat. In samples of 3 muscles, i.e. *m. longissimus dorsi*, iliopsoas and semimembranosus, the concentrations of dry matter, ash, total protein, intramuscular fat and cholesterol were estimated. At the slaughter time the body weight of bulls was ranging between 465 kg and 540 kg. Also the concentration of total protein in the muscles of these two breeds was the highest. Slight differences were observed in the content of intramuscular fat in the m. longissimus dorsi between the breeds examined (3.43-4.98%). The lowest cholesterol content in the m. longissimus dorsi was recorded for Simental and Black-and-White bulls (39.6 and 42.3 mg/100 g meat), whereas the highest for Red and Limousine (53.6 and 48.4 mg/100 g). Generally, the protein concentration in m. longissimus dorsi was about 1-1.5 percent unit higher than in iliopsoas and semimembranosus. Small differences were achieved in the ash concentration in the three muscles examined.

Poster CSN2.30

Colour and sensory characteristics of grass-fed beef: Effect of duration of grazing prior to slaughter

A.P. Moloney[1,2], F. Noci[1], B. Murray[2] and D.J. Troy[2], [1]Teagasc, Grange Research Centre, Dunsany, County Meath, Ireland, [2]Teagasc, The National Food Centre, Ashtown, Dublin 15, Ireland.*

The objective was to determine the impact on meat quality when heifers grazed grass for different periods before slaughter. Sixty crossbred continental heifers (initial live weight 338 (sd = 39.7) kg) were offered before slaughter : *ad libitum* unwilted grass silage and concentrates (SC) for 158 days, grazed grass (G158) for 158 days, SC for 118 days followed by grazed grass for 40 (G40) days or SC for 68 days followed by grazed grass for 90 days (G90). Carcass weight averaged 258, 247, 248, 258, (sed=8.1) kg (P=0.07), for SC, G40, G98 and G158, respectively. An increase in the duration of grazing before slaughter increased subcutaneous fat yellowness (Hunter b value) (linear (P=0.08) and cubic (P<0.05), 16.5, 17.4, 16.7 and 17.5, (sed=0.43)) and decreased (P<0.05) *longissimus* muscle colour saturation (linear and quadratic, 14.9, 12.7, 12.4 and 12.1, (sed=0.55)) and drip loss (linear, 2.8, 2.1, 1.7 and 1.8, (sed=0.28) %). There was no treatment effect on *longissimus* muscle composition, on pH or hue at 48h post-slaughter or on tenderness, flavour, firmness, texture, chewiness or overall acceptability when aged for 14 days. It is concluded that grazing influenced beef colour in a duration-dependent manner but that it had little effect on the eating quality of beef.

Poster CSN2.31

Intramuscular fatty acid composition in lambs fed green sulla (*Hedysarum coronarium*) or concentrates

A. Priolo, M. Bella, M. Lanza, V. Galofaro, D. Barbagallo, L. Biondi, P. Pennisi. University of Catania, DACPA Sez. Scienze delle Produzioni Animali, Via Valdisavoia 5 - 95123 Catania, Italy*

Sixteen male Comisana lambs, divided into two groups at age 85 days, were penned in two collective boxes. One group (Control) received concentrates, while the other (Sulla) was fed green sulla. The concentrate given to the Control animals was regulated to have similar growth rates between groups. Animals were slaughtered at 30 kg live weight. Fatty acids were determined on the *longissimus* muscle ($g*100g^{-1}$ fatty acid methylesters). C18:2*n*-6 was higher in the Control group (17.43 *vs* 11.52; $P < 0.001$) compared to Sulla animals. These latter animals had a proportion of C18:3*n*-3 four times higher than the Control lambs (4.98 *vs* 1.18; $P < 0.001$). *Cis*-9, *trans*-11 conjugated linoleic acid was higher in the fat from sulla-fed animals compared to Control lambs (0.91 *vs* 0.46; $P < 0.001$). Both C20:5*n*-3 and C22:5*n*-3 were higher in the sulla-fed lambs ($P < 0.001$). Overall, the saturated fatty acids were higher in the Control group (39.37 *vs* 34.90; $P < 0.001$); the monounsaturated fatty acids were higher in the fat from Sulla lambs (29.69 *vs* 25.55; $P < 0.001$) and the polyunsaturated fatty acids were unaffected by the diet treatments. However the *n*-6:*n*-3 ratio was decidedly higher in the Control lambs compared to the sulla-fed animals (7.21 *vs* 2.09; $P < 0.001$).

Poster CSN2.32

Carcass characteristics in lambs fed green sulla (*Hedysarum coronarium*) or concentrates

M. Bella, M. Lanza, V. Galofaro, D. Barbagallo, L. Biondi, P. Pennisi, A. Priolo. University of Catania, DACPA Sez. Scienze delle Produzioni Animali, Via Valdisavoia 5 - 95123 Catania, Italy*

Sixteen male Comisana lambs, divided into two groups at age 85 days, were penned in two collective boxes. One group (Control) received concentrates, while the other (Sulla) was fed green sulla. The concentrate given to the Control animals was regulated to have similar growth rates between groups. Animals were slaughtered at 30 kg live weight and carcass characteristics were then registered.

Despite a similar growth rate, animals fed sulla showed a lower net dressing percentage (47.9 *vs* 51.6; $P < 0.05$). No differences were found on muscular conformation or fatness as assessed by the European carcass classification system. These results were confirmed by the hind leg dissection. Perirenal fat of sulla fed animals had a higher concentration (91 *vs* 25 $ng*g^{-1}$ fat; $P < 0.001$) of 3-methylindole (skatole), a compound considered extremely unpleasant odorant. Perirenal fat was also different in colour between groups. The Hue angle was higher (51.13 *vs* 39.54; $P < 0.001$) for the Sulla group compared to the Control lambs. This difference is probably due to a different content in carotenoid pigments between the animals fed grass and those fed concentrates.

Poster CSN2.33

Utilization of extruded linseed cakes to modify fatty acid composition and increase CLA content in goat milk

A. Nudda, M.G. Usai, S. Mulas and G. Pulina, Università di Sassari, Dipartimento di Scienze Zootecniche, Via E. De Nicola 9, 07100 Sassari

The objective of this experiment was to evaluate the effects of feeding additional fat through supplementation in the diets of integral extruded linseed cakes (Linopiù - CortalÒ) on cis-9, trans-11 conjugated linoleic acid (CLA) content in goat milk. Thirty goats were randomly assigned to three groups fed TMR diets supplemented with 10% (DM basis, group high, H), 5% (group low, L) or 0% (control group, C) integral extruded linseed cakes, which supplied 40 g/d (group H), 20 g/d (group L) and 0 g/d (group C) of linseed fat. The trial lasted 3 weeks: 2 of adaptations and 1 of sampling. Milk yield, fat, and protein concentration were not influenced by treatments. Linseed supplementation increased unsaturated fatty acids (FA) and decreased saturated FA in comparison with control group. CLA content in the control group was lower (3.6 mg/g of fat; $P<0.01$) than in treated groups (6.8 and 5.8 mg/g of fat in H and L, respectively). The same trend was observed for trans-11 C18:1 (8.5, 7.4 and 4.3 mg/g of fat in group H, L and C, respectively). No differences were observed between the two treated groups for most important FA. A linear relationship was found between CLA and trans11 C18:1 in milk fat (CLA, mg/g = 1.79 + 0.54 x trans-11 C18:1, mg/g; r2 = 0.77). Research supported by National Strategic Dietolat Project (Mipaf).

Poster CSN2.34

Interactions between nature of forage and oil supplementation on cow milk yield and composition. 1. Effects on fatty acids (FA) except 18:0, isomers of 18:1 and CLA

A. Ferlay, A. Ollier, P. Capitan, Y. Chilliard, INRA-Theix, 63122, France.*

Twelve primiparous mid-lactation Holstein cows used in 2 replicated 3 x 3 Latin Square designs were fed diets based on either grass hay (H, 60 % of DM intake) or maize silage (M, 69% of DM intake) with 5% sunflower oil (SO), 5% linseed oil (LO), or 2.5% fish oil (FO). Milk yield ranked by oil was FO or LO (21.4 kg/d) < SO (23.4 kg/d). For M diets, milk fat percent was greater ($P<0.05$) for FO (3.1) than for LO (2.6) whereas for H diets, it was greater for LO (2.9) than for FO (2.4). M diets, compared to H diets, decreased *anteiso*15, *iso*18, *cis*9-14:1, *trans*11,*cis*15-18:2 (an intermediate of 18:3*n*-3 hydrogenation), 18:3*n*-3, 20:5*n*-3, 22:5*n*-3. FO, compared to LO or SO, increased 4:0 to 16:1. Percentage of branched-chain (BC) plus odd-numbered (OD) FA ranked by oil was SO (2.7 % of total FA)<LO (3.0%)<FO (4.1%). Percentage of 18:2*n*-6 ranked by oil was FO (1.1%)<LO (1.2%)<SO (1.7%). Percentage of 18:3*n*-3 and *trans*11,*cis*15-18:2 ranked by oil was LO (0.5 and 2.5%) > FO (0.4 and 2.1%) > SO (0.3 and 0.1%). FO, compared to LO or SO, increased FA with 20 or 22 atoms. Several significant oil-forage interactions were observed with *trans*11,*cis*15-18:2, 20:4*n*-6, 20:5*n*-3, and 22:5*n*-3. In conclusion, oil supplemented H diets, compared to oil supplemented M diets, increased some BC and *n*-3 polyunsaturated FA. FO, compared to LO or SO, increased sharply 4:0 to 16:0, and long-chain (>20 atoms) FA, and decreased 18:2*n*-6. SO or LO increased slightly 18:2*n*-6 or 18:3*n*-3, respectively.

Poster CSN2.35

Interactions between nature of forage and oil supplementation on cow milk composition. 2. Effects on 18:0, isomers of 18:1 and CLA

Y. Chilliard, A. Ollier, P. Capitan, A. Ferlay, INRA-Theix, 63122, France.*

Twelve primiparous mid-lactation Holstein cows used in 2 replicated 3 x 3 Latin Square designs were fed diets based on either grass hay (H, 60 % of DM intake) or maize silage (M, 69% of DM intake) with 5% sunflower oil (SO), 5% linseed oil (LO), or 2.5% fish oil (FO). Percentage of milk 18:0 or *cis*9-18:1 was higher ($P<0.05$) for M (9.0 or 17.0% of total fatty acids) than for H (7.4 or 14.6%) diets. In contrast, percentage of *cis*12-, *cis*-13, *trans*11-18:1 (7.0 *vs* 3.6%) and *cis*9,*trans*11-18:2 (3.2 *vs* 1.5%) was higher for H than for M diets. Percentage of 18:0 ranked by oil was FO (2.6%) <LO (9.8%) < SO (12.6%). Percentage of *cis*9-18:1 was much lower for FO (6.6%) than for LO or SO (20.4%). Percentage of *trans*4- to *trans*9-18:1, and *cis*12-18:1 ranked by oil was FO<LO<SO. LO compared to SO, decreased *trans*10-18:1 (3.5% *vs* 5.4%), the value was intermediate with FO (4.1%). Percentage of *trans*12-, *cis*10-, *cis*13-18:1 ranked by oil was FO<SO<LO. Percentage of *cis*11-18:1 ranked by oil was SO<LO<FO. In conclusion, oil supplemented H diets, compared to oil supplemented M diets, increased *trans*11-18:1 and *cis*9,*trans*11-18:2, and decreased 18:0 and *cis*9-18:1. FO, compared to LO or SO, decreased strongly 18:0, *cis*9-18:1 and several other isomers of 18:1. *Trans*11-18:1 and *cis*9,*trans*11-18:2 did not differ between the 3 oil supplementations studied here.

Poster CSN2.36

Interactions between nature of forage and oil supplementation on cow milk composition. 3. Effects on kinetics of percentages of milk CLA and *trans*-fatty acids

A. Ferlay, P. Capitan, A. Ollier, Y. Chilliard, INRA-Theix, 63122, France.*

Twelve primiparous mid-lactation Holstein cows, divided into 2 groups, received diets based on either grass hay (H, 60 % of DM intake) or maize silage (M, 69% of DM intake) during 3 weeks. Then, the cows were fed these basal diets (2 per block) with either 5% sunflower oil (SO), 5% linseed oil (LO), or 2.5% fish oil (FO) during 3 weeks. Milk samples were collected at -4, -2, +3, +5, +7, +9, +13 and +20 days (d) relative to the addition of oil into the diet. Milk *trans*10-18:1 increased ($P<0.05$) slightly until +13 d, then it enhanced strongly between +13 and +20 d (up to 2.0 or 4.5% of total fatty acids for H and M diets). The kinetics of *trans*11-18:1 and CLA percentages were curvilinear ($P<0.05$) for the 3 oils. The values with basal diets were 0.7 and 0.4 % for *trans*11-18:1 and CLA. The maximal response (MR) of *trans*11-18:1 and CLA to LO was at +13 d (11.7 and 5.3%) or +7 d (8.3 and 3.2%) for H or M diets, respectively. The *trans*11-18:1 MR to SO was at +7 d (13.5 %) or +13 d (11.8%) for H or M diets. The MR to FO was at +13 d (6.6 and 9.6%) for H and M diets. The CLA MR to SO and FO was at +13 d (5.9, 5.1, 3.4 and 3.7% for HSO, MSO, HFO and MFO diets). In conclusion, the kinetics of appearance of *trans*10-, *trans*11-18:1 and CLA in milk fat depend on interactions between nature of forage and oil supplementation.

Poster CSN2.37

Minimal dietary structural value for a maximum performance in Belgian Blue double-muscled bulls

A. Van Herck, S. De Campeneere*, L.O. Fiems and D.L. De Brabander, Agricultural Research Centre, Department Animal Nutrition and Husbandry, Scheldeweg 68, 9090 Melle, Belgium.*

The structural value (SV) is the unit in the physical structure evaluation system for dairy cattle used in Belgium and other European countries. For beef cattle, only empirical recommendations for a minimal level of physical structure in the diet are available. The minimal SV of a concentrate/maize silage diet was investigated during 5 years. One hundred and fifty-six Belgian Blue double-muscled bulls, with a live weight interval from 350 kg to 650 kg were divided over 12 diets, with a SV ranging from 0.97 to 0.34/kg DM. All diets were fed ad libitum as a total mixed ration. Different SV between treatments were obtained by changing the roughage/concentrate ratio and/or by changing the SV of the concentrate. Within each year the diets were iso-energetic and iso-nitrogenous. Animals were loose-housed in pens with wood shavings on the bedding. No straw was available in the rack.
Regression analysis was applied to determine the breakpoint. From these results we found no negative effect on feed intake, growth and feed conversion when the SV of the diet is 0.5/kg DM or more, but research is still continuing.

Poster CSN2.38

Influence of feeding strategy (pasture vs TMR) on proteolysis in Ragusano cheese during ripening

V. Fallico[1], L. Chianese[2], J. Horne[1], S. Carpino[1], G. Licitra[13], [1]CoRFiLaC, Regione Siciliana, s.p. 25 km5, 97100 Ragusa, Italy, [2]Food Science Department, Naples University, 80055 Portici, Italy, [3]D.A.C.P.A., Università di Catania, Italy.*

Pasture contributes to aromatic profiles of milk and derived-cheese as odor compounds were found in the milk and cheese of grazing ewes, but not in those of sheep fed TMR. Proteolysis contributes to cheese flavour, producing low MW aromatic compounds and amino acids acting as flavour precursors. The effect of feeding strategy (pasture vs TMR) on Ragusano cheese proteolysis was then evaluated throught a 210-days ripening time. Primary proteolysis was monitored by urea-PAGE, isoelectrofocusing and immunoblotting. RP-HPLC was used to assess secondary proteolysis. Urea-PAGE and IEF profiles of pasture and TMR cheeses showed similar proteolytic patterns, indicating that diet had no effect on primary proteolysis. Densitometry of urea-PAGE profiles revealed slightly higher proteolysis levels in TMR cheeses and similar but not significant ($P>0.05$) trends were found in chemical analyses. Immunostained patterns were useful in identifying the origin of primary peptides. In vitro hydrolyses with chymosin and plasmin clarified their potential role in primary proteolysis. Different feeds had a qualitative impact on secondary proteolysis. Peptide patterns resolved better in pasture HPLC profiles suggesting a more defined and balanced action of microbial peptidases involved in oligopeptide and amino acid production. Chemical analyses revealed a nonsignificant ($P>0.05$) trend showing larger 12% TCA-soluble peptide fractions in TMR profiles.

Poster CSN2.39

Influence of brine temperature on lipolysis and proteolysis within blocks of Ragusano

C. Melilli[1], D. M. Barbano[2], M. Manenti[1], J. M. Lynch[2], S. Carpino[1], and G. Licitra[13]. [1]CoRFiLaC, Regione Siciliana, s.p. 25 km 5, 97100 Ragusa, Italy, [2]Northeast Dairy Food Research Center, Department of Food Science, Cornell University, Ithaca, NY, [3]D.A.C.P.A., Università di Catania, Italy.

Cheeses (26) were made on each of 3 d. A block was analyzed prior to brine salting, the others were split into 5 saturated brines at 12, 15, 18, 21, and 24°C and analyzed after 1, 4, 8, 16, and 24 d of brining. Each block was divided into four portions from outermost to innermost. Total, individual free fatty acids, pH 4.6 and 12% TCA soluble nitrogen (SN) were measured. The SN as a percent of Total N at 24 d increased with brine temperature and was higher in the block center and lower at the surface at all temperatures. Total FFA content increased with increasing brine temperature for all portions and the total FFA content across all temperatures was higher at the exterior of the block than the interior at 24 d. Higher total FFA content at the surface of the block was the opposite of the behavior of the SN content. This may be due to a different direct effect of salt on enzyme and substrate interaction during lipolysis or a combination of this effect and movement of low molecular weight water-soluble FFA from the interior to the surface of the block.

Poster CSN2.40

Effects of brining time on sensory profiles of Ragusano cheese produced from pasture-fed animals

J. Horne[1], C. Melilli[1], S. Carpino[1] and G. Licitra[1,2], [1]CoRFiLaC, Regione Siciliana, s.p. 25 km 5, 97100 Ragusa, Italy. [2]D.A.C.P.A., Università di Catania, Italy.*

This study was undertaken to determine some of the important sensory changes in Ragusano cheeses brined 0 to 24 days. Mini-cheeses produced using traditional manufacturing techniques were brined for 0-24 days and evaluated by a trained QDA panel at the time of removal from brine and at 30,45 and 60days. Cheeses were evaluated in three sections from outermost to innermost. Perceived saltiness decreased from external to internal portions of the cheeses ($P<0.05$). A non-significant increase ($P=0.07$) in perceived saltiness as age increased was observed, the largest of which occurred between 0 and 30 days. This result agreed with instrumental data. Perceived saltiness likewise increased with brine time, but reached an asymptote at 10days. A significant second-order function of brine time was the best predictor of saltiness ratings ($R^2=0.73$). Other characteristics related to saltiness and the concurrent moisture loss showed similar trends. PCA on the sensory attributes and selected instrumental measures resulted in two varimax-rotated factors explaining more than 50% of the total variance. The first factor contained high positive loadings for saltiness, roughness, astringency, hardness, percents salt and salt-in-moisture, and high negatives for sensory characteristics related to moisture and percent moisture. The second factor contained high positives for butter, milk and sweet odours and tastes and high negatives for colour and butyric-pungent odours and tastes.

Poster CSN2.41

Hygiene protocols for pathogens in farmhouse dairy products

B.A. Slaghuis[1] and M.C. van der Haven[2], [1]Research Institute for Animal Husbandry, P.O.Box 2176, 8203 AD Lelystad, The Netherlands, [2]Omni-Kaas u.a., Bennekomseweg 126, 6704 AJ Wageningen, The Netherlands*

In the Netherlands about 600 dairy farms process their own milk into dairy products. About 380 of these farms produce farmhouse "Boerenkaas", a raw milk cheese mainly from the Gouda type. Product quality and food safety is of utmost importance.

Absence of harmful bacteria before and during preparation of raw milk into farmhouse dairy products is very important. Especially pathogenic bacteria are undesirable. Therefore hygiene protocols were developed, to be used during the milking process and processing of raw milk at the dairy farm. The aim of using these protocols is to decrease the contamination and/or growth of these for humans harmful bacteria. Seven different pathogenic bacteria have been described by using an HACCP approach. Per process step the chance at high numbers, the risk for the milk to get contaminated, preventive measures to control, some targets, action at defects and way and frequency of control are given.

Also relationships between farm and processing characteristics and presence of pathogens and/or indicator bacteria were investigated by modelling based on results of monthly sampling of cheeses. Use of an active starter is very important for good quality cheeses.

The use of the hygiene protocols is preferably for people working for farmhouse dairy producers and dairy farmers.

Poster CSN2.42

Use of Cobalt as tracer for detection of chemical residues during the milking and cleaning process

B.A. Slaghuis[1], R.T. Ferwerda-van Zonneveld[1], M.C. te Giffel[2] and G. Ellen[2], [1]Research Institute for Animal Husbandry, P.O.Box 2176, 8203 AD Lelystad, The Netherlands, [2]NIZO Food Research, PO Box 20, 6710 BA Ede, The Netherlands.*

Before, during and after milking of cows chemical agents are used for cleaning and disinfection of the milking machine. It is known that some problems occurred with residues in milk and dairy products, originating from the use of combined cleaning and disinfection products at the farm. Also higher levels of iodine are reported, due to the use of teat dips. To investigate the importance of possible residues in raw milk, a tracer was used to overcome different chemical agents used at different farms. As tracer a cobalt solution was used and milking equipment and teats of cows were treated with this solution. Milk was sampled and cobalt was detected. Results show that residues were detectable in all samples at low levels, but the interpretation is difficult. Behaviour of the tracer (e.g. adherence to walls and release from these walls by water or milk) may be different from the chemical agents employed. However, the level of tracer in milk is comparable for conventional systems and automatic milking systems. Also the level of cobalt is comparable with levels of chlorine derived residues found in earlier studies. The tracer should not be mixed with reactive materials, because of reactions of cobalt with these materials.

Poster CSN2.43

Valorisation of typical products by the study of the most significant qualitative parameters of sheep and goat milk

E. Duranti[1*], A. Caroli[2], E. Cauvin[3], L. Chianese[4] and M. Martini[5], [1]Dept. Sci Zoot., Borgo XX Giugno 74, 06100 Perugia, [2]Dept. SBA, Strada Prov. per Casamassima km 3, 70010 Valenzano, Bari, [3]Dept. Prod. Anim. Epidem. ed Ecol., V.L. da Vinci, 44, 10095 Grugliasco (TO), [4]Dept. Sci. Alim., V. Università 100, 80055 Portici (NA), [5]Dept. Prod. Anim., V. delle Piagge, 2, 56100 Pisa, Italy.

The valorisation of typical sheep and goat cheeses presents a double interest, first for the tight relation with the culture and tradition of the country where they are produced, secondly in order to efficiently safeguard the consumer's health in all the steps of production. Moreover, the organoleptic and nutritional quality differentiates these cheeses from cattle industrial products which, although assuring the microbiological health by heat treatments, show less organoleptic variability and less nutritional value. Within a national research project (Cofin 2001: prot. 2001077279) particular attention was paid to the following biochemical and genetic aspects closely related to the technological quality of sheep and goat milk: plasmin-plasminogen system; lactodynamographic parameters; fat globule dimension; genetic polymorphisms of milk protein loci and MUC1. The research project has been developped in different Italian sheep (Comisana, Sarda, Massese, Laticauda, Bagnolese, Polimeticcia) and goat (Garganica, Jonica, Maltese, Roccaverano, Vallesana) populations or breeds. The variability of the measured objective parameters has been analysed, and relevant indications have been drawn from the data for the safeguard of typicalness of dairy products and for the traceability of milk origin.

Poster CSN2.44

Effect of somatic cell count and plasmin activity on sheep milk quality

E. Duranti[1], M. Pauselli[1], L. Bianchi[1], A. Bolla[2], C. Casoli[1], [1]Dipartimento di Scienze Zootecniche, Borgo XX giugno, 74, 06121 Perugia, [2]Petrini Institute, Via IV Novembre, 2/4, 06083 Bastia Umbra (PG) Italy*

Aim of the work was to evaluate the effect of different mammary health status on ewe milk qualitative characteristics and plasmin-plasminogen activity. 213 milk samples were collected monthly from 40 primiparous Sardinia ewes during lactation (beginning, middle and late lactation). Physico-chemical characteristics, somatic cell count (SCC), cheese making properties and plasmin-plasminogen activity were determined on each sample. The different level of SCC is used to asses the presence of subclinical mastitis in the dairy flock. An udder was considered "health" (H) if every month control SCC was below 500,000 cells/ml, "infected" (I) when at least two SCC were over one million per ml and "doubtful" (D) in other cases. To evaluate the influence of mammary health status and period of lactation, a mixed model was performed using the ewe as random effect. All milk physico-chemical parameters were influenced by SCC level. Plasmin activity was higher in "infected" group than in the others, (16.11 *vs* 11.77 and 11.21 U/ml in "I", "D" and "H"; $P<0.001$). Samples reactive to rennet were 92.73%, 70.65% and 64.6% in "H", "D" and "I". Curd rennet time and curd firmness were better in "H" group (16'55" and 41,26 mm; $P<0.001$) respect to the samples of the others groups. Milk from udders characterized by involution process or with inflammation process, is worst for cheese making.

Poster CSN2.45

Milk quality and yield in ewes from Central Italy

E. Duranti[1], L. Bianchi[1], C. Casoli[1], L. Chianese[2], S. De Pascale[2], M. Martini[3], M. Pauselli[1], [1]Dipartimento di Scienze Zootecniche, Borgo XX giugno, 74, 06121 Perugia, [2]Dipartimento di Scienza degli Alimenti, Via Università,110, 80055 Portici (NA), Dipartimento di Produzioni Animali, Via delle Piagge 2, 56100 Pisa, Italy*

Aim of the work was to evaluate the major factors affecting milk quality and yield in Massese and crossbred ewes reared in Central Italy. Milk samples from 25 Massese and 20 crossbred ewes from two commercial flock were collected thrice during lactation, in order to assess: physico-chemical, lactodynamographic and fat globule morphometric carachteristics; plasmin activity; phenotypic characterization of αs1-casein. In Massese breed, αs1-CN phenotypic frequency was: CC 76%, BC 12%, AC 8% and BB 4%, while in crossbred ewes: CC 40%, AC 35%, AA 15% and BB 10%; αs1-CN D wasn't found. Production and SCC levels were higher in Massese ewes than in crossbred ones (1,510 *vs* 389 g/d; 1,014,000 *vs* 793,000/ml). In Massese sheep, milk quality parameters could be mostly affected by the udder health status, while in crossbred ewes by an enhanced mammary gland involution process, as showed by the marked yield decrease (from 573 to 267 g/d). The mean number of fat globules/ml of milk was about 2.30×10^9, with a mean diameter of 5.75 and 4.31 mm in Massese and crossbred ewes respectively. During lactation, both flocks showed a decrease in fat globule diameter, which could affect milk and cheese fat composition and quality.

Theatre N4.1

Testing of mass-produced farm animal housing systems with regard to animal welfare

B. Wechsler, Swiss Federal Veterinary Office, Centre for proper housing of ruminants and pigs, FAT, 8356 Taenikon, Switzerland.

In 1981, an authorisation procedure regarding animal welfare was introduced in Switzerland for mass-produced housing systems and equipment for farm animals. When asking for an authorisation, the manufacturer or importer of a housing system or equipment must send detailed documentation (plans, measures, technical data) to the Federal Veterinary Office. The authorisation can only be given if the housing system or equipment is in accordance with the requirements of the Swiss animal welfare legislation. Whenever possible, a decision is made on the basis of literature or experience with similar equipment. In some cases, however, practical tests are required. Such tests may include veterinary, physiological and behavioural measurements to assess animal welfare.

Authorisations are given by the Federal Veterinary Office. It may consult an advisory board which consists of experts in animal husbandry, animal housing construction, and animal protection. Over the last 20 years, more than 1300 authorisations were given, and 13 applications were rejected. The manufacturers may appeal against a decision of the Federal Veterinary Office. To illustrate the authorisation procedure and the indicators used to assess animal welfare, examples of current testing of housing systems are given.

In conclusion, pretesting of farm animal housing systems that are intended to be mass-produced is a promising way to increase and ensure product quality from livestock systems.

Theatre N4.2

Food safety and 'animal friendly' production: is there a conflict of interests?

G. Regula, J. Danuser, U. Ledergerber and B. Bissig-Choisat, Federal Veterinary Office, Schwarzenburgstr. 161, CH-3003 Bern, Switzerland.*

'Animal friendly' production systems differ from traditional production in the use of bedding, more contact among animals, and outdoor access. However, there is a potential of these properties to impair the safety of foods from animal origin. For the milk, pork and poultry, microbiological quality was compared among traditional production and products labelled as 'animal friendly' production.

Bulk milk bacteria counts were recorded monthly from 129 dairy farms over 24 months. Seventy-eight milk samples were cultured bacteriologically and results compared among traditional tie stalls, tie stalls providing regular exercise in an outdoor yard, and freestalls with regular exercise outdoors. Total bacteria counts were slightly lower in loose housing systems than in tie stalls, whereas spores from anaerobic bacteria were more frequent in farms with outdoor access. Faecal samples from 88 swine fattening farms and 865 pork samples were cultured for Campylobacter, Salmonella, and Yersinia. There was no difference in the prevalence of these zoonotic bacteria among traditional indoor farms with slatted floor pens, and farms providing straw bedding and an outdoor yard. Samples from 98 poultry farms and 415 poultry meat samples showed a higher prevalence of Campylobacter in free range production compared to traditional indoor farms.

Overall, it could be shown that except for poultry production, there was no negative impact of 'animal friendly' production on microbiological food quality.

Theatre N4.3

Use of somatic cell count patterns for udder health management and improvement of genetic resistance against pathogen-specific clinical mastitis

Y. de Haas[1], H.W. Barkema[2], Y.H. Schukken[3] and R.F. Veerkamp[1], [1]ID-Lelystad, P.O. Box 65, 8200 AB Lelystad, The Netherlands, [2]University of Prince Edward Island, Charlottetown, PEI, Canada C1A 4P3, [3]Cornell University, Ithaca, NY 14853, United States of America

In this study was investigated whether defining patterns of peaks in somatic cell count (SCC) from individual test-day records, rather than using average lactation values for SCC, would improve the prediction of pathogen-specific clinical mastitis (CM). Patterns differentiated between short or longer periods of increased SCC, with or without recovery. Test-day records on SCC were available from January 1990 to December 1999, and pathogen-specific CM was monitored from December 1992 till June 1994. Genetic associations were estimated between pathogen-specific CM, lactational average of somatic cell score (LACSCS), and patterns of peaks in SCC. Generally, genetic correlations between pathogen-specific CM and patterns of peaks in SCC were stronger than the correlations with LACSCS. This suggests that genetic selection purely on diminishing presence of peaks in SCC would decrease the incidence of pathogen-specific CM more effectively than selecting purely on lower LACSCS. The possible use of the peak patterns in SCC for udder health management on dairy farms was investigated by determining the associations between the incidence of CM and the occurrence of peak patterns in SCC on herd level. Large differences in the incidence of specific patterns existed between farms. Herds with predominantly short peaks had higher incidences of cases of CM associated with environmental pathogens, whereas a predominance of long increased SCC can be associated with high incidences of contagious pathogens.

Theatre N4.4

Hepatoprotective effects of silymarin in veterinary medicine

D. Tedesco and S. Galletti, Department of Veterinary Sciences and Technologies for Food Safety, Via Celoria 10, 20133 Milano, Italy.*

The use of herbs as feed additives in livestock instead of other chemical compounds, e.g. antibiotics, could be a new goal in livestock production, as a consequence of the increased demand of safe products for human consumption. This work describes recent advances of our research into effects of silymarin in animals. Silymarin, the bioactive extract of Silybum marianum (milk thistle), has documented hepatoprotective properties. Silymarin stimulates hepatocyte protein biosynthesis and cell regeneration in the damaged liver. It has also been reported to possess antitoxic, antioxidant and anti-inflammatory properties. Clinical trials in humans have shown that silymarin exerts hepatoprotective effects in cirrhosis, chronic hepatitis, and environmental toxins exposure. Dairy cows experience moderate to severe fatty liver during the peripartum. In our study, we found that silymarin as hepatoprotector can be usefully used in periparturient dairy cows to prevent metabolic disorders. Milk quality and safety parameters were maintained and no residue was detected. According with silymarin action against toxin exposure, in dairy cows and poultry we found an effect against aflatoxin B1 (AFB1) intoxication. In broilers, silymarin provided a protection against the AFB1 negative effects on performance. In dairy cows it contributed to reduce AFM1 excretion in milk. These studies illustrate that silymarin has a great potential in veterinary medicine as feed additive or medicinal. A major concern in the development of new remedies is their legal status.

Theatre N4.5

Aroma compounds and sensory characteristics of Sicilian traditional cheeses from cows on pasture

S. Carpino[1], S. Mallia[1], J. Horne[1] and G. Licitra[1,2], [1] CoRFiLaC, Regione Siciliana, s.p. 25 km 5, 97100 Ragusa, Italy. [2] D.A.C.P.A., Università di Catania, Italy.*

Odor active volatiles in cheeses may be important markers of both quality and diversity. Five traditional Sicilian cheeses were evaluated for their odor active volatiles by HSPME and GCO dilution analysis (Charm Analysis). These methods seek to both identify odor active compounds in the cheeses and rank the same compounds in terms of relative odor potencies. The same cheeses were evaluated sensorially using QDA by a panel of trained individuals. Cheeses evaluated included Maiorchino, Pecorino, Provola dei Nebrodi, Ragusano, and Ricotta infornata. A total of 31 odor active compounds were detected in the cheeses by GCO analysis; 26 of these were identified by GC/MS, published retention index matches and authentication standards. Ragusano, Pecorino Siciliano and Maiorchino had the most diversified odor profiles which included odor active terpenoids. These terpenoids were not found in Provola dei Nebrodi and Ricotta infornata. Sensory analysis of these same cheeses revealed some of the same trends. The impact of green/herbaceous, mushroom/earthy, fruit and floral aromas were all more pronounced in the Ragusano, Maiorchino and Pecorino Siciliano cheeses than they were in Provola dei Nebrodi and Ricotta Infornata. These results are in keeping with the GCO results showing the terpenoid compounds having these aromas to be present in the former group of cheeses but not the latter.

Theatre N4.6

Fatty acid composition of milk fat in relation to roughage type

D.L. De Brabander[1], K. Raes[2], N.E. Geerts[1] and S. De Smet[2]. [1]Agricultural Research Centre, Department Animal Nutrition and Husbandry, Scheldeweg 68, B-9090 Melle, Belgium; [2]Department of Animal Production, Ghent University, Proefhoevestraat 10, B-9090 Melle, Belgium*

Nutritional guidelines recommend a higher proportion of n-3 polyunsaturated fatty acids in the human diet. Besides, a lot of attention is nowadays paid to the conjugated linoleic acids (CLA), being naturally present in ruminant products.
In a trial with 3 x 4 Holstein cows, 3 diets were compared in a 4 week period (May-June). Roughages were: 1) maize silage (MS), 2) normally managed perennial grass (NG) and 3) extensively managed grass (EG). No fertiliser or herbicides were used in the EG for 12 years, resulting in a considerable diversity of species. The grass was mown daily and fed indoors. Crude fibre content of both grasses indicated an advanced growth stage. The mean roughage/concentrate ratios (DM basis) were 61/39, 54/46 and 56/44, respectively. Mean daily milk yield amounted to 25.2 kg.
The proportion of c9t11CLA in total milk fatty acids (FA) was 0.51, 0.61 and 0.75 % for the MS, NG and EG diets, respectively, whereas the C18:3n-3 proportion amounted to 0.27, 0.53 and 0.61 %. Both parameters were significantly different between the 3 diets ($P < 0.001$). The C18:2n-6/C18:3n-3 ratio was 5.5, 2.6 and 2.5, while a significantly higher C18:1t11 proportion was observed for the EG diet. The grass based diets resulted in significantly less saturated FA and more branched chain FA.

Theatre N4.7

Grazing on Mountain pastures - does it affect Meat quality in lambs?

T. Ådnøy[1], A. Haug[1], O. Sørheim[2], M.S. Thomassen[1], Z. Varszegi[3] and L.O. Eik[1], [1]Department of Animal Science, P.O. Box 5025, N-1432 Ås, [2]MATFORSK - Norwegian Food Research Institute, [3]University of Debrecen, Hungary*

Meat from lambs raised on mountain pastures without any supplementary feeding or treatments is often considered to be of superior quality. Hence, the objective of this study was to compare quality and flavour of meat from lambs grazing unimproved mountain range (1000 m above sea level) with meat from lambs grazed on cultivated lowland pastures.
The experiment was undertaken in Hardanger on the Western Coast with 150 Norwegian Cross Bred Sheep (Norsk Kvitsau) randomly allocated to "Lowland -" and "Mountain Pasture Groups". Slaughtering and grading were undertaken at a commercial slaughterhouse. Thereafter, loin samples of *m. longissimus dorsi* were analysed for sensory traits and meat quality. For further comparisons, loin samples were also taken from lambs slaughtered at two other locations in Norway. Significant differences between locations were found in grading, fat content and fatty acid concentration, meat colour and flavour. Differences were in general small and most likely not noticed by the typical consumer. Still the results suggest that meat from lambs raised in extensive systems on mountain range have certain qualities that might be used in promotion of local and regional products.

Theatre N4.8

Effect of breed and feeding system on sensory and chemical characteristics of goat's ricotta cheese

M. Pizzillo, S. Claps, R. Rubino, Istituto Sperimentale per la Zootecnia, Via Appia - Bella Scalo; I - 85054 Muro Lucano

The aim of the present study was to evaluate the effect of goat breeds (Girgentana, Siriana, Maltese and local breed) and feeding system (grazing and zero grazing) on the chemical and organoleptic properties of ricotta cheese. The protein, non-protein N, lactose, ash and free fatty acid contents were not affected by breed. The ricotta cheese from milk of Siriana breed showed higher fat content than other breeds. In general, breed did not influence the rheological parameters such as firmness and hardness; only the ricotta cheese from Girgentana breed showed a greater adhesineveness than that of other breeds. Sensory assessment evidenced better differences among ricotta cheese samples than chemical and rheological analysis. Sensory attributes of ricotta cheese such as softness, fattiness, grain size and goat-like odour were significantly different ($P<0.001$) between breeds. The feeding system influenced mostly free fatty acid content. Caprinic acid (C6:0), capric acid (C10:0) and lauric acid (C12:0) contents were higher in ricotta cheeses from milk of grazing goats.

Theatre N4.9

***N-3* fatty acids and conjugated linoleic acids of *longissimus* muscle in different cattle breeds**

K. Nuernberg[1]; D. Dannenberger[1], G. Nuernberg[1], K. Ender[1], N. Scollan[2], [1] Research Institute for Biology of Farm Animals, Wilhelm-Stahl-Allee 2, D-18196 Dummerstorf, Germany, [2] Institut of Grassland and Environmental Research, Aberystwyth, SY23 3EB, UK.

The objective of this study was to enhance the content of beneficial fatty acids in beef muscle, namely *n-3* polyunsaturated fatty acids (PUFA) and conjugated linoleic acid (CLA*cis-9,trans-11*). German Simmental (GS; n=33) bulls and German Holstein (GH; n=31) bulls were produced on either an indoor concentrate system or a period of summer pasture feeding on grass following by a indoor finishing period on a concentrate containing linseed. All animals were slaughtered at 620 kg. Linolenic acid contained in grass was absorbed and deposited into the lipids of muscle. Feeding grass with a finishing period increased significantly the concentration of long chain *n-3* fatty acids in the muscle lipids of grazing bulls (GS 57.3 *vs.* 20.5 mg/100 g; GH 65.1 *vs.* 28.1 mg/100 g). The *n-6* fatty acids (C18:2 and C20:4) were decreased in GS and GH muscle fat by keeping on pasture. Therefore the *n-6/n-3* ratio of grazing Simmental bulls was 2.0 and of GH 1.9 in contrast to 8.3 and 6.5 of bulls fed concentrate in stable. Grass feeding resulted in a higher relative content of C18:1*trans* isomers in both breeds. The relative concentration of CLA*cis-9,trans-11* in muscle of both breeds was significantly higher by grazing on pasture.

Theatre N4.10

Fatty acids in hen eggs from different sources

S.P. Marelli, V .Ferrante, D. Baroli, M.G. Mangiagalli, L. Guidobono Cavalchini, Istituto di Zootecnica, Facoltà di Medicina Veterinaria Università degli Studi di Milano, Via Celoria 10, 20133 Milano, Italy.*

Hen egg is one of the most common foods all over the world; it is a rich source of lipids and proteins. Food function is nowadays not merely limited to nourishment supplying. Human health and nutritional value, animal welfare, traceability, environment and organic production standard side are attracting consumer's interest. The aim of this study was to compare physical parameters and fatty acids profiles of eggs from 4 different sources (marketing labels: standard, litter-floor1, litter-floor2, ω-3 enriched). Statistic analysis was conducted applying a GLM procedure. There were significant ($P<0.01$) differences in Palmitic and Stearic acid content. Eggs from the different sources had significantly different profiles concerning Oleic acid, Linoleic acid and Linolenic acid ($P<0.001$). Designer ω-3 enriched eggs showed the lowest content in Arachidonic acid ($P<0.001$). Nutritionally important fatty acids like EPA and DHA underline the differences ($P<0.001$) between ω-3 enriched eggs and eggs from different sources: this group of egg is the only one supplying EPA. DHA percent content in ω-3 eggs is three times higher then DHA level of the other three groups. Physical parameters like egg weight, albumen weight and shell weight are not significantly influenced by the production-feeding method; otherwise egg yolk weight and total lipids content revealed significant differences ($P<0.001$).

Theatre N4.11

Effect of diet and added antioxidants on meat quality of beef

F.J. Schwarz[1], S. Linden[2], C. Augustini[3] and H. Steinhart[2], [1]Department of Animal Sciences, Division of Animal Nutrition, Technical University of Munich, D-85350 Freising-Weihenstephan, [2]Institute of Food Chemistry, University of Hamburg, D-20146 Hamburg, [3]Institute for Meat Production and Market Research, Federal Centre for Meat Research, D-95326 Kulmbach, Germany*

Consumers of beef show increasing interest in healthy, natural products. In Central Europe beef is mainly produced with bulls kept and fed in intensive indoor housing. Therefore, a two-factorial experiment with 72 Simmental bulls ($n=9$ per treatment) was carried out with a ration of either maize silage + 2.3kg concentrates (M) or grass silage + 3.2kg concentrates (G). Daily supplementation per animal was either none (control), 1000mg α-tocopheryl-acetate, 15g ascorbic acid, or 700mg β-carotene. The trial lasted 144d on average with final live weights of 575kg (G) and 618kg (M). Besides measuring standardized meat quality parameters the experiment was focused on colour stability of muscles, the tocopherol and β-carotene content in tissues and the fatty acid composition of the meat. Forage type had a major effect across all treatments. All bulls fed grass silage had higher tocopherol and β-carotene contents and higher PUFA concentrations in the tissues and muscles. Vitamin E or β-carotene addition primarily increased their retention in treatments M. After 6 days storage, redness (a*) of meat from G bulls had decreased less than of meat from M bulls. All supplemented antioxidants had slight effects, but major improvements could be recognized in rations M.

Poster N4.12

The influence of grinding and pelleting on the physical structure value of concentrates for dairy cows

N.E. Geerts, D.L. De Brabander, J.M. Vanacker and J.L. De Boever, Agricultural Research Centre, Department Animal Nutrition and Husbandry, Scheldeweg 68, B-9090 Melle, Belgium*

The effect of the physical properties of concentrates on their physical structure value (SV) was investigated in two experiments with dairy cows. Pelleted concentrates of ground ingredients (6 mm sieve) were compared in experiment 1 to a mixture of the same unground concentrate ingredients and in experiment 2 to a mixture of ground ingredients but not pelleted. The starch content of the concentrates in experiment 2 was higher to increase the effect of pelleting. Maize silage and grass silage were fed as the sole roughage in experiment 1 and 2 respectively. Each diet was fed to 16 Holstein cows. To derive the SV of the concentrates, the tolerable concentrate proportion in the ration was determined by decreasing weekly the roughage part of the diet until symptoms of physical structure deficiency appeared (decreased milk fat content, decreased milk yield, off feed). The results showed that grinding as well as pelleting lowered the physical SV of concentrates. Both effects depend on type of concentrate (starch content) and particle size and vary between 0.05 and 0.15 as expressed in SV per kg DM. The lowest pH values in rumen fluid of fistulated cows were measured for the pelleted concentrates with ground ingredients.

Poster N4.13

Optimal standardised ileal digestible (SID) dietary lysine level in hybrid meat pigs (40-70 kg)

N. Warnants, M.J. Van Oeckel and M. De Paepe, Agricultural Research Centre, Department Animal Nutrition and Husbandry, Scheldeweg 68, 9090 Melle, Belgium.*

A trial was performed with Pietrain x Hybrid pigs between 40 and 70 kg live weight (age 13-18 weeks). Six diets with SID lysine levels from 0.70 to 1.34% were fed to 60 barrows and 60 gilts per treatment. Barrows and gilts were housed separately in pens of 5. Diets were based on cereals and soybean meal and were balanced in threonine, methionine + cystine and tryptophan relative to lysine, according to the ideal protein. The net energy content was calculated at 9.2 MJ/kg feed. Daily feed intake, average daily gain (ADG) and feed conversion ratio (FCR) were recorded as a function of dietary lysine level. The SID amino acid content of the diets was verified in an ileal digestion trial with 4 pigs. The ADG and FCR data of both barrows and gilts as a function of %SID dietary lysine were described by quadratic curves. The optimum SID lysine levels, derived from the ADG and FCR curves were respectively 0.88 and 0.96% for barrows and 1.08 and 1.12% for gilts. The lysine requirements in the present study are elevated compared to other recommendations, probably because of the limited feed intake capacity of the used pig genotype. Hence, a diet more concentrated in essential amino acids seems to be necessary.

Poster N4.14

Effects of fumarate on *in vitro* rumen fermentation of two diets with variable proportion of concentrate

M.J. Ranilla, R. García Martínez, M.L. Tejido and M.D. Carro. Dpto. de Producción Animal I, Universidad de León, 24071 León, Spain*

Batch cultures of mixed ruminal microorganisms were used to study the effects of disodium fumarate on the *in vitro* fermentation of two diets with different forage to concentrate ratio. Diets consisted of forage (alfalfa hay:corn silage, 50:50) and concentrate (corn:barley:soybean meal, 35:50:15) in the proportions of 80:20 (C20 diet) and 20:80 (C80 diet). Samples were incubated for 16 h at 39°C with buffered ruminal fluid from sheep. Disodium fumarate was added to the incubation bottles to achieve final concentrations of 0 (control) and 8 mM fumarate. For both diets, volatile fatty acids production increased ($P<0.05$) when fumarate was aded to the cultures (1.25 vs 1.54 mmol and 1.43 vs 1.70 mmol for C20 and C80, respectively). Final pH was also higher ($P<0.05$) when diets were incubated with fumarate (6.34 vs 6.41 and 6.27 vs 6.32 for diets C20 and C80, respectively). Fumarate supplementation decreased ($P<0.05$) the acetate:propionate ratio from 2.77 to 2.17 for diet C20 and from 2.71 to 2.10 for diet C80. Addition of fumarate did not affect ($P>0.05$) either the methane production or the organic matter apparent disappearance for any of the diets. The results show that fumarate stimulated the *in vitro* rumen fermentation of both diets by increasing the production of total volatile fatty acids and had a beneficial effect on the final pH.

Poster N4.15

Effect of forage type on the efficiency of utilization of energy for milk production in dairy cows

E. Kebreab, J. France, J.A.N. Mills, D.E. Beever and L.A. Crompton, The University of Reading, School of Agriculture, Policy and Development, Reading RG6 6AT, UK*

The objective of the study was to investigate the effect of forage type on the efficiency of utilization of metabolisable energy intake (MEI, MJ/kg $W^{0.75}$/d) for milk production (k_l). A database containing 243 dairy cow observations was assembled from calorimetry studies. The dataset was subdivided into four sets containing diets with grass silage (GS), maize silage (MS), fresh grass (FG) or mixed silage (MX) as forage types. The following equation was fitted to the dataset:

$E_l = a + b\,[\mathrm{MEI} - (T_g/k_g)] - (T_l \times k_t) + \varepsilon$,

where E_l is milk energy (MJ/kg $W^{0.75}$/d), a is the intercept and b is k_l. T_g and T_l (both MJ/kg $W^{0.75}$/d) are tissue energy gain or loss, respectively, k_g and k_t are efficiencies of utilization of energy for growth and of body stores for milk production, respectively, and ε is an error term. Meta-analysis of the data estimated the values of k_g and k_t to be 0.83 and 0.65, respectively. k_l was estimated to be 0.56 (SE 0.0051), 0.57 (SE 0.0049), 0.44 (SE 0.0027) and 0.60 (SE 0.034) for GS, MS, FG and MX, respectively. Dietary energy consumption was converted to milk energy with an efficiency of about 60% in cows consuming MX diets, decreasing to 44% with FG diets.

Poster N4.16

Effect of DHA and vitamin E enriched diets on the fatty acid content and quality of rabbit semen

T.M. Gliozzi[1], A. Maldjian[2], S. Cerolini[2], F.M.G. Luzi[3], L. Parodi[2], L. Zaniboni[2], L. Maertens[4].* [1]*I.B.B.A.-C.N.R. Milano, Italy* [2]*Dipartimento VSA, Università di Milano, Italy;* [3]*Istituto di Zootecnica, Università di Milano, Italy* [4]*Dep. Animal Nutrition Husbandry, Merelbeke, Belgium.*

The effect of supplementing the feed with Docosahexaenoic acid (DHA, 22:6*n-3*) and/or vitamin E to bucks was studied on semen quality and biochemical parameters. 52 rabbits were allocated to 4 groups fed diets as follows: A: control; B: A+200mg/kg Vit.E; C: A+1.5% fish oil (FO); D: A+1.5% FO+200mg/kg Vit.E. Semen was analysed at various time-points: volume, concentration, motility, viability were recorded. The spermatozoa lipids were separated in their various classes: phospholipids (PL), free cholesterol (Chol), free fatty acids and triacylglycerols; the fatty acid profile of these classes was determined. PL was the main lipid class present in spermatozoa, followed by Chol. PL displayed a high content of 22:5*n-6* (~30% of total fatty acids) and low content of 22:6*n-3* (~1%) in the control. At the end of the experiment, the proportion of DHA in groups C and D increased by 10-fold (8% against 0.8 % in the control). This was followed by a slight decrease of 22:5*n-6*, suggesting an increase of unsaturation of PL for animals receiving FO. Ejaculate volume was reduced when extra vitamin E was present in the feed. More work is required to understand the role of specific long chain polyunsaturated fatty acids on sperm functions.

Poster N4.17

Milk production of dairy cows given diets with increasing amounts of solvent extracted palm kernel meal

L.F.P.F. Carvalho[1,2], A.J.M. Fonseca[1,2], A.R.J. Cabrita[1,3], M.F. Miranda[4], Z. Lopes[4] and R.J. Dewhurst[5],* [1]*CECA-ICETA,* [2]*ICBAS,* [3]*FC, Universidade do Porto, Rua Padre Armando Quintas, 4485-661 Vairão, Portugal,* [4]*DLL-DRAEDM, Av. dos Templários 421, Ap 156, 4590-909 Paços de Ferreira, Portugal,* [5]*IGER, Plas Gogerddan, Aberystwyth, SY23 3EB, UK.*

Twenty Holstein cows (100±61.5 DIM) were used in an 11-wk randomised block design experiment to evaluate the effects of increasing dietary content of solvent extracted palm kernel meal (PKM) on intake and milk yield and composition. Cows were blocked by energy-corrected milk yield and randomly assigned to four complete diets with equal effective rumen degradable protein (RDP) to fermentable metabolizable energy ratios, based on maize silage, wheat straw and concentrates. The increasing dietary levels of PKM were achieved by replacing RDP sources with PKM and urea in concentrates (0, 90, 180 and 270 g PKM/kg; and 1, 4, 7, 10 g urea/kg; for PKM0, PKM9, PKM18, PKM27, respectively). Neither dry matter (DM) intake nor milk yield (20.7, 22.2, 21.0 and 21.6 kg DM/day; sem 0.68; and 33.2, 32.4, 33.5 and 33.3 kg/day; sem 1.50; for PKM0, PKM9, PKM18, and PKM27, respectively) was significantly affected by dietary treatments. Milk composition was also not significantly affected (mean milk fat and protein contents were 33.0 and 31.5 g/kg). This study confirms the assumptions used in formulating the diets that PKM is a reasonable source of both RDP and rumen undegradable protein for dairy cows.

Poster N4.18

Relationship between nutrition and reproductive efficiency in ostrich: yolk fatty acid content and fertility

C. Sussi, P. Superchi, A. Sabbioni, E.M. Zambini, V. Beretti and A. Zanon, DPABVQSA, Università degli Studi, via del Taglio 8, 43100 Parma, Italy.*

N-3 fatty acids deficiency affects embryo development and great emphasis has to be placed on α-linolenic acid role in ostrich (Noble et al., 1996, Comp. Biochem. Physiol., 113B, 775). The aim of the work was to modulate yolk fatty acid composition of ostrich egg by feeding, increasing linolenic acid content, and to evaluate the effect on reproductive performance. Thirty two ostrich females, divided into 3 groups, were fed a diet without (group 0: CP 17%; E.E. 3.5%; EM 2678 Kcal/kg feed as fed), with 3% (group 3) or 6% (group 6) of linseed oil, from 1 month before laying beginning until its end. The 1st, 20th, 40th and 60th egg of each female were collected. Number of laid eggs, fertility and hatchability were recorded. Yolk fatty acid content was analysed by gas chromatography on capillary column. Data were processed by ANOVA. Linseed oil supplementation significantly affected α-linolenic acid (3.86, 5.57, 7.08% for group 0, 3 and 6, respectively; $P<0.05$), n-3 fatty acids content (4.12, 6.24, 7.81%, respectively; $P<0.05$) and n-6/n-3 ratio (3.70, 2.83, 1.88%, respectively; $P<0.05$). Reproductive efficiency parameters showed no significant variations. In conclusion, under our farm conditions it was possible to modulate yolk fatty acid content of ostrich egg by feeding, but reproductive performance were not positively affected.

Poster N4.19

Antimicrobial effect of medium - chain fatty acids and their derivatives in mixed cultures of rumen microorganisms

M. Marounek[1,2], E. Skrivanová[1], R. Snep[3]; [1]Research Institute of Animal Production, 104 01 Prague 10; [2]Institute of Animal Physiology and Genetics, 104 00 Prague 10; [3]Faculty of Veterinary Medicine, University of Veterinary and Pharmaceutical Sciences, 612 42 Brno, Czech Republic*

The aim of our study was to compare antimicrobial effects of caprylic (C 8), capric (C 10), lauric (C 12) and myristic acid (C 14), monolaurin, laurylsulphate and triglycerides of medium-chain fatty acids (MCFA). These compounds were added at 2 and 5 mg/ml of the rumen contents of a cow, diluted with buffer. Cultures were incubated anaerobically at 39°C for 8h, then production of fermentation gas, volatile fatty acids (VFA) and lactate was measured. Capric acid at 2 mg/ml and laurylsuphate at 5 mg/ml almost completely inhibited the *in vitro* fermentation. Antimicrobial activities of C 8, C 12 acids and monolaurin were less pronounced. Caprylic acid, however, was highly efficient at 5 mg/ml. Triglycerides of MCFA (Akomed R, coconut oil) and myristic acid had no effect. The combination of Akomed R and a fungal lipase was as efficient as free C 8 and C 10 fatty acids. The decrease of VFA in treated cultures was accompanied by increase of lactate production. It can be concluded that some MCFA and their derivatives are very efficient antimicrobials.

Poster N4.20

The gas production technique: a possible laboratory tool for the estimation of TDN?

M. Antongiovanni[*1], A. Buccioni[1], A. Cappio Borlino[2], N. Macciotta[2], F. Petacchi[1] and S. Rapaccini[1], [1]Dipartimento di Scienze Zootecniche, via delle Cascine 5, 50144 Firenze, Italy, [2]Dipartimento di Scienze Zootecniche, via De Nicola 9, 07100 Sassari, Italy.*

The aim of the work was to test the suitability of the gas production technique as a possible tool for the prediction of TDN of ruminant feeds.
A multiphasic function was fitted to data of over time gas production of 4 simple feeds and of 9 mixed diets, measured by means of a laboratory fermenter, by using a non linear procedure. Moreover, relationships between the total amount of gas and TDN, NDF, tdNDF (calculated according to NRC 2001) were analysed by linear or quadratic regressions.
The different samples were classified either as "monophasic"or as "biphasic" according to the pattern of their over time gas production curves. Best fits were linear regressions for monophasic samples and quadratic regressions for biphasic ones. The highest R^2 values were found between gas and TDN (0.82 for monophasic samples; 0.71 for biphasic samples). If only the 9 mixed diets were considered, R^2 values were higher (0.97 for monophasic diets; 0.92 for biphasic diets).
Even if the number of the tested feed samples is indeed quite low, yet the attempt to predict the nutritive value of ruminant feeds in terms of TDN content from the amount of gas produced at the asymptote appears a promising approach. Further measurements on a wider range of feeds and diets are needed.

Poster N4.21

The in vitro gas production method to evaluate feed blocks and polyethylene glycol effects on *Acacia cyanophylla* Lindl. based diets

N. Moujahed and C. Kayouli. Institut National Agronomique de Tunisie, 43 Avenue Charles Nicolle, 1082 Tunis, Tunisia.

The in vitro gas production method was used to determine the effect of feed blocks supply and polyethylene glycol 4000 (PEG) on *Acacia cyanophylla* based diets fermentation. Diets consisted on mixtures of oat-vetch hay and acacia foliage (D1), with urea-molasses-minerals blocks, without (D2) or with 10% of PEG (D3). Incubations were carried out in glass syringes using rumen liquid from three fistulated sheep. Gas production during 72 hours of fermentation, volatile fatty acids (VFA) concentrations and fermented organic matter (FOM) were determined. Statistical analysis was carried out using GLM procedure.
Both feed blocks and PEG increased ($P<0.001$) potential gas production (29.5, 40.9 and 45.4 ml. 200mg^{-1}, respectively in D1, D2 and D3), but reduced ($P<0.001$) the rate of production (0.074, 0.045 and 0.048 h^{-1} for D1, D2 and D3 respectively). Concentration of total VFA was the highest in PEG diet and the lowest in control ($P<0.001$). Neither feed blocks nor PEG had basically modified VFA composition. Calculated FOM increased ($P<0.001$) both with feed blocks and PEG. It was concluded that blocks supply enhances in vitro fermentation of acacia based diet and that PEG is likely to reduce adverse effects of acacia condensed tannins on microbial activity. The cumulative gas production technique appeared to be an excellent previous stage for laborious in vivo measurements.

Poster N4.22

Measure of effective protein degradability of five protein supplements, with or without correction for microbial contamination

Ch. Milis[1*], *D. Liamadis*[2] *and* D. Nitas[3]. [1]*Ministry of Agriculture.* [2]*Department of Animal Nutrition, Aristotle University of Thessaloniki 540 06.* [3]*Technological Institution of Thessaloniki. Greece.*

Soy bean meal (SBM), corn gluten meal (CGM), wheat bran (WB), corn gluten feed (CGF) and cotton seed cake (CSC), were weighed into dacron bags for incubation in three ruminally cannulated chiou breed ewes for 0, 2, 4, 8, 16, 24, and 48 h. SBM, WB and CGF were degraded the most extensively in the rumen (EPD; 64, 50 and 48%, respectively) and, CGM and CSC was degraded the least extensively (EPD; 38 and 40%, respectively), at a fractional passage rate of 5%/h. Correction for microbial contamination was made by the use of two bags containing 4g of milled potato (0 % N). These bags were incubated in the same time with each feed and every incubation time, by subtracting the g of CP measured in N free potato, for each incubation time, from the g of CP measured in feeds. After correction for microbial contamination EPD of SBM, CGM, CSC, WB, and CGF, was 72, 45, 55, 58, and 65%, respectively. Microbial contamination was increased by time and resulted in an approximately 7-17% underestimate of EPD. This substantial overestimation of rumen undegradable protein (RUP) of all protein supplements suggest that correction for microbial contamination should be made at every *in situ* degradability trial in order to measure the real RUP of protein supplements, improve *in situ* technique and, in consequence, to have comparable values between different laboratories.

Poster N4.23

Milk odd chain fatty acids as predictors of microbial protein supply in dairy cattle

B. Vlaeminck[1*], *V. Fievez*[1], *W. Peirtsegaele*[1], *H. Vandewoude*[1], *A.M. van Vuuren*[2] *and D. Demeyer*[1], *Department of Animal Production, Ghent University, Proefhoevestraat 10, 9090 Melle, Belgium,* [2] *ID TNO Animal Nutrition, Edelhertweg 15, 8200 AB Lelystad, The Netherlands.*

Four Holstein cows in early lactation were fed grass silage/concentrate diets (55/45, DM-basis) in a 4 X 4 Latin square. The 4 concentrates differed in amount of (protected) starch and fat (13 to 54 g crude fat/kg DM). After a 2 week adaptation period, milk samples were collected from 8 milkings and OBCFA were determined by GLC. Urine, in which allantoin was determined by HPLC, was collected during 6 consecutive days. Duodenal supply of microbial N, estimated from daily allantoin excretion, varied between 274 and 650 g N/d ($N_{allantoin}$) and showed no correlation ($r_{pearson}$ = 0,166) with the amount of digestible microbial protein as estimated from the Dutch-Belgian protein evaluation system (DMVE). $N_{allantoin}$ tended to be related with the excretion of OBCFA in the milk (mg/g milk) ($r_{pearson}$ = 0,434, p=0.093) and this correlation reached significance when controlling for differences in the dietary fat content ($r_{partial}$ = 0,599, p=0.018). This could be explained by the preferential use of preformed long-chain fatty acids by rumen bacteria. As different groups of rumen bacteria show distinctive patterns and amounts of OBCFA, we are currently evaluating possibilities to further improve the latter correlation by taking into account changes in the milk OBCFA pattern.

Poster N4.24

Effect of aflatoxins on growth of some lactic bacteria strains isolated from dry fermented sausages

R. Rullo[1], D.Balzarano[1]. A.L. Basso[2], L. Ferrara[1] and G. Maglione[1], [1]ISPAAM- CNR Via Argine 1085, 80147 Naples, Italy, [2]Ist. di Biol. Cellulare -CNR Via Ramarini, 32, 00016 Monterotondo Scalo, Rome

The aflatoxins, are secondary metabolites of some strains of *Aspergillus flavus* and *parasiticus*. They are very toxic worldwide contaminants, like other xenobiotics, particularly to the liver. Four aflatoxins commonly occur in pre- and post-harvest contamination of food and feed and these are: AFB_1, AFB_2, AFG_1 and AFG_2. AFM_1, a hydroxylated metabolite of AFB_1, has been found associated to the casein in cheese where it achieves a concentration 5 fold greater than in milk. Many strategies are under investigation to eliminate or inactivate the aflatoxin contaminants from animal feed and human food chain. In this study we show how the growth parameters of some lactic bacteria strains change by adding different amount (1 to 7 μg/ml) of aflatoxin. All strains were cultured with and without toxins for 24 h in MRS broth under aerobic conditions at 37° C. The amount of toxins in the media were significantly reduced after 12 hours of incubation. Reverse-phase HPLC was used to quantify the aflatoxins remaining in the supernatant incubated with toxins. Detoxification by using bacteria can be considered a useful and more appropriate method to remove or inactivate these contaminants from feed. Only little is known about the naturally occurring microflora of Italian traditional sausages. The identification of strains typical of a geographic area and bacterial species harbouring relevant probiotic activity against aflatoxins is a further feature which valorise and enhance the typicality of these products.

Poster N4.25

Effect of dietary energy density on growth performance and slaughtering characteristics of Awassi lambs

S. Haddad and M. Husein, Department of Animal Production, Jordan University of Science and Technology, P.O. Box 3030, Irbid 22110, Jordan*

Eighteen Awassi lambs (16.7 ± 1.5 kg) were offered two isonitrogenous finishing diets that contained 60:40 (HF) and 15: 85 (HC) forage: concentrate ratio. Feed was offered ad libitum as totally mixed diets for 62 days. At the end of the experiment, lambs were sacrificed to obtain slaughtering data. DM, OM, and CP intakes were not affected ($P > 0.05$) by the dietary treatment. Metabolizable energy intake was higher ($P < 0.05$) for lambs fed the HC diet compared with lambs fed the HF diet. Average daily gain (ADG) for lambs fed the HC diet was higher ($P < 0.05$) as compared with lambs fed the HF diet (258 versus 178 g d^{-1} for HC and HF diets, respectively). Feed to gain ratio was improved ($P < 0.05$) with the HC diet (3.8) as compared to HF diet (5.4). Lambs fed the HC diet had higher ($P < 0.05$) dressing percentage (48.5 %) compared with the HF diet (43.5 %). Lambs fed the HC diet had a lower ($P < 0.05$) GI tract weight (6.0 kg) compared with lambs fed the HF diet (6.8 kg). Regardless of the dietary treatment, a high positive correlation ($P < 0.05$) was observed between digestible OM and ADG for all lambs. These results demonstrate that finishing Awassi lambs on high-energy diets improve DM intake, feed efficiency, ADG and slaughtering characteristics.

Poster N4.26

The effect of protected fat inclusion in finishing diets for Awassi Lambs on nutrient intake and growth performance

S. Haddad and H. Younis, Department of Animal Production, Jordan University of Science and Technology, P.O. Box 3030, Irbid 22110, Jordan*

Twenty-one Awassi lambs (20.4 ± 0.4 kg) were used in a complete randomized design to evaluate the effects of adding ruminally protected fat (Ultralac(tm) 100) to fattening Awassi lamb diets on nutrient intake and digestibility and production responses. Lambs were fed three isonitrogenous diets for 72 days (7 lambs/treatment). Diets contained 1) no added fat (CON); 2) 2.5% added fat (LF); 3) 5% added fat (HF). Dry matter intake was higher ($P < 0.05$) for lambs fed CON diet compared with lambs fed HF diet. However, there was no difference ($P > 0.05$) in DM intake in LF diet as compared with either CON or HF diets. Similar results were observed for CP and ADF intake. Neutral detergent fiber intake was higher ($P < 0.05$) for lambs fed CON diet as compared with lambs fed LF and HF diets. Ether extract intake was higher ($P < 0.05$) for lambs fed HF (66.7 g/d) diet as compared with LF and CON diets. Organic matter and ME intake were not affected by the dietary treatments. There was no difference ($P > 0.05$) in weight change for lambs fed the three experimental diets and the same results were obtained for final body weight (Avg. = 34.8 kg), ADG (Avg. = 201.4 g/d) and feed to gain ratio (Avg. = 4.59). Dry matter digestibility was higher ($P < 0.05$) for lambs fed HF and LF diets as compared with lambs fed CON diet. Digestibility results of OM, CP, NDF, ADF and energy followed similar patterns for DM digestibility. It seems that there are no advantages for using protected fat in high concentrate finishing diets for Awassi lambs.

Poster N4.27

Feeding frequency of ensiled pressed beet pulp in relation to physical structure supply

N.E. Geerts, D.L. De Brabander, J.L. De Boever and J.M. Vanacker, Agricultural Research Centre, Department Animal Nutrition and Husbandry, Scheldeweg 68, B-9090 Melle, Belgium*

When concentrates are fed more frequently, a larger proportion of concentrates in the diet can be tolerated. One may ask if this effect also applies when high-moisture concentrates like ensiled pressed beet pulp (PBP) are fed. In ration 1, PBP was fed twice a day, each time 2 h before a mixture of maize silage and concentrates was fed. Ration 2 was a complete mixed ration fed 3 times a day. The PBP part was held constant at 32 % of DM during the whole trial. Both rations were administered to 15 Holstein cows. The minimum roughage proportion in the ration was determined by decreasing the maize silage part of the diet weekly until symptoms of physical structure deficiency appeared (decreased milk fat content, decreased milk yield, off feed). The minimum maize silage parts in the diets were not significantly different (resp. 17.6 and 19.0 % of DM) indicating that more frequent feeding of PBP was not effective. However, a more stable pH pattern in rumen fluid of fistulated cows suggested that more frequent feeding was safer for the rumen function.

Poster N4.28

Comparative *in vitro* and *in vivo* investigation of plant origin fat sources

H. Fébel H.[*1], I. Várhegyi[1], E. Andrásofszky[2] and Sz. Huszár[1], [1]Research Institute for Animal Breeding and Nutrition, Herceghalom, [2]Szent István University, Gödöllő-Budapest, Hungary.*

This study was designed to determine the effects of calcium salt of palm oil fatty acids (CS, 3.9%), hydroxyethylsoyamide (HESA, 5%), butylsoyamide (BSA, 3.6%) and soybean oil (SO, 3.2%) on degradation of crude protein (CP) and fibre *in vitro*, and on rumen fluid parameters (VFA, ammonia and pH) *in vivo*. Five diets were fed to the sheep in a 5x5 Latin square design with 17-d periods. The diets consisted of 50% meadow hay and 50% concentrate. In contrast to effect of other treatments, CP degradation was greatest in the test tubes with inocula obtained from sheep fed diet with HESA. Fat supplements equally inhibited the fibre breakdown of alfalfa pellet. CS and HESA seemed to be less detrimental to *in vitro* fermentation of NDF than BSA and SO. Different fat sources reduced acetate:propionate ratios and mean ruminal ammonia concentration. The proportion of acetate to propionate was higher for CS than for BSA, HESA and SO diets. This order indicates the protection degree of fat sources against ruminal degradation. *In vitro* fibre degradation data correspond with the *in vivo* results of ruminal fermentation considering the direction of changes, however they are not suitable to establish the smaller differences between treatments. *In vitro* results of protein degradation do not indicate the *in vivo* changes unambiguously.

Poster N4.29

Study of the nutritional value of Hedychium gardnerianum (Roscoe, 1828) and its influence on the rumen fermentation

A.E.S. Borba, M. Alexandra Oliveira, C.F.M. Vouzela, O.A. Rego, J.P. Barreiros and A.F.R.S. Borba, Departamento de Ciências Agrárias da Universidade dos Açores, 9700 Angra do Heroísmo, Açores, Portugal*

The objective of this work was to characterize the plant *Hedychium gardnerianum* (Roscoe, 1828), in order to determine its nutritional value and its influence on the gas production, and define its potential use as ruminant food. *H. gardnerianum* is an exotic and invading common plant in the Açores that, in some of the islands, is used as animal food at times of low grass production (Autumn - Winter). The analysis of its chemical composition showed that it is a poor fodder plant in terms of crude protein (CP) - 8,55 % of the DM, and the coefficients of in vivo digestibility are low for dry matter (DM) and for organic matter (OM) (57,39% and 55,25%, respectively). The values of gas production, at 24h, increased by 57.42ml, in the samples with 100% hay, and 74.75 ml, in the samples with 100% *H. gardnerianum*. When gas production values were corrected by Menke's et al. (1979) equation, they changed from 62.28ml to 59.12ml, respectively. Thus, it is possible to say that *H. gardnerianum* is a poor fodder plant that can, however, be of use as a voluminous complement in the feeding of ruminants, as traditionally made in the Açores, during the periods of grass scarcity.

Poster N4.30

Differences in growth intensity, slaughter parameters, and meat quality in bulls, fattened with corn and alfalfa silages

V. Kudrna, P. Lang, P. Mlázovská, K. Runová, Research Inst. of Anim. Prod., Praha 10-Uhríneves, Prátelství 815, 10401, Czech Republic*

The main aim of an experiment with 24 bulls was to find out an effect of two basic kinds of roughage - corn and alfalfa silages - on growth intensity and meat quality, including contents of meat fatty acids. The bulls were divided into two well-balanced groups. Animals of the control group (C) were given alfalfa silage, wheat meal and wheat straw, whereas in the diet of the experimental group (E) corn feeds (corn silage, silage of ground corn cobs + bracts mixture - LKS) dominated. Both feeding rations used were isonitrogenous and isocaloric. When the bulls were slaughtered at the live weight of 550 kg, sensoric analysis of their meat quality and carcass analysis were done. Higher DMI was achieved in the E-group. Bulls of this group also had insignificantly higher growth intensity, and considering chemical analysis of *musculus longissimus dorsi* - they had higher fat contents (6.43 g/kg), higher proportion of ?-3 fatty acids, and statistically significant higher ($P < 0.01$) contents of oleic acid. On the contrary, statistically significant higher urea concentration and higher concentration of cholesterol at sampling 5 hrs after feeding were found in blood plasma of the C-group, as well as statistically significant higher linolic, a-linolenic and ?-linolenic acids contents ($P < 0.05$) and $C_{22:5}$ acid contents ($P < 0.01$).

Project No. M02-99-04 was supported by NAZV (Ministry of Agriculture, The Czech Republic).

Poster N4.31

Prediction of urinary and blood pH in non-lactating dairy cows fed anionic diets

M. Spanghero, Dipartimento Scienze Produzione Animale, Università di Udine, Via S. Mauro 2, 33010 Pagnacco, Udine, Italy

Anionic diets are fed to non-lactating (dry) cows to produce a negative DCAD (dietary cation/anion difference) thereby reducing their risk of milk fever, and other associated metabolic diseases, in early stage lactation. Data from 20 studies (84 dietary treatments) with dry dairy cows, and published in referred scientific journals, were identified for meta-analysis to predict urinary and blood pH (pHu and pHb) in response to feeding anionic diets. All studies reported pHu, while only 12 (43 treatments) reported pHb.The pHu was predicted by the DCAD, as calculated from three combinations of dietary ions (i.e., $DCAD_1$: Na, K,Cl; $DCAD_2$: Na, K,Cl, S; $DCAD_3$: Ca, Mg, Na, K,Cl, S), and expressed as mEq/kg of diet DM, or as amounts consumed in Eq/d. The best prediction of pHu (R^2=.867), adjusted for the trial effect, was: pHu=5.848(±.154) + .0908(±.0077)*(DCAD1) -.00074(±.00011)*($DCAD1)^2$. Poorer predictions occurred with $DCAD_2$ and $DCAD_3$ (R^2=0.829 and 0.739, respectively), while use of daily equivalent intake in place of DCAD did not improve the predictions. The smaller data set of 43 dietary treatments was used to predict pHb on the basis of pHu. A significant linear regression (R^2=.786), after adjusting data for the trial effect, was found to be: pHb=7.275(±.026) +.0193(±.0031)*(pHu). These predictive equations quantitate the impact of DCAD on pHu and pHb thereby allowing accurate decisions on anionic salts supplementation.

Poster N4.32

Model of fat and protein deposition in supermeat type pigs

L. Zeman[1], P. Hodbod[1], P. Novak[2], L. Novak[2], P. Dolezal[1], P. Mares[1], [1]Mendel university of agriculture and Forestry, Brno, [2]University of Veterinary and Pharmaceutical Sciences, Brno, Czech Republic.

The aim of our work was to verify standard specifications of nutrient requirements by use of an existing model for nutrient requirements and to suggest modifications for modern pig genotypes. From data of our experiments or the data published by other authors we calculated equations of protein and fat retention in growing pigs. In our experiments we used for deposition of protein and fat in the meat type pigs the following eqations (H - weight kg):

Protein $= 0{,}1694 * H^{0{,}9889}$ [kg] $(R^2 = 0{,}9962)$

Fat $= 0{,}0154 * H^{1{,}603}$ [kg] $(R^2 = 0{,}9298)$

The data calculated by the above equations for growing pigs were compared with real data determined in university farm Zabcice. The results calculated by our optimization model were applied to results gained from 50 best growing pigs selected out of 31000 pigs in the field experiments accomplished during the years 2000-2001. From the following equations is evident the higher protein deposition and lowered value of the fat deposition:

Protein $= 0{,}1694 * H^{1{,}006}$ [kg]

Fat $= 0{,}0154 * H^{1{,}496}$ [kg]

The detailed analysis has shown that the second group of equations describe better the state of protein and fat deposition for the supermeat type of pigs. Other methodical approaches of protein and fat deposition models are discussed.

Poster N4.33

The influence of different intakes of metabolisable energy and lysine in pregnant sows and during lactation period on weight of piglets

L. Zeman, P. Hodbod, P. Dolezal and D. Klecker, Mendel University of Agriculture and Forestry, Brno, Czech Republic*

In 136 groups of sows fed during pregnancy and lactation period with experimental mixtures different in content of Metabolisable energy (MEp MJ/kg) and level of lysine (g/kg), the differences of body weights of new born piglets and of the weaned piglets were evaluated.

The following equations for the weight of litter and of the weaned piglets were correlated with amount of MEp and lysine content in the feed of sows.

Weight New Born Piglets = 12,0187 + 0,0008 * MEp intake [kg] $(R^2=0.9997)$

Weight New Born Piglets = 13,1031 + 1,0068 * Lys intake [kg] $(R^2=0.9998)$

Weight New Born Piglets = 27,7821 + 0,0153 * MEp intake [kg] $(R^2=0.9964)$

Weight Weaned Piglets = 36,4538 + 18,0387 * Lys intake [kg] $(R^2=0.9964)$

Weight Weaned Piglets =30,1096+0,0082*MEp intake +10,1563*Lys intake [kg] $(R^2=0.9961)$

The data gained indicate the need to install the estimated specifications of ME and lysine in the new models of nutrient requirements based on comparison of the real and theoretical requirements. The new standard specifications of nutrient requirement for the meat sows are recommended to be developed.

Poster N4.34

Nylon bag degradability and mobile nylon bag digestibility of crude protein in rapeseed, barley and maize

J. Harazim[1], P. Homolka[2]. [1]Central Institute for supervising and testing in Agriculture, Opava, [2]Research Institute of Animal Production, Uhríneves, Czech Republic.*

Samples of rapeseed, barley and maize were incubated in situ to evaluate rumen effective degradability of crude protein (CP). The diet of the fistulated animals was composed of maize silage (10 kg), clover silage (7 kg), meadow hay (5 kg) and mixture. Nylon bags containing tested samples were suspended in the rumen of three cannulated steers for 2, 4, 8, 16, 24 and 48 h. In each steer, two repetitions were done in each time interval (the nylon bags were made of nylon with pore size 42 μm). The rumen effective degradability was calculated at rumen outflow rate 5 % and no correction for microbial contamination was included. The contents of CP in samples of rapeseed, barley and maize were as follows: 213.6, 111.9 and 100.5 g per kg DM, respectively. Effective degradability values for these feeds were 73.9, 83.6 and 56.6 %, respectively.
The mobile bag technique with dry cows fitted with the large ruminal cannulas and the T-piece cannulas in the proximal duodenum was used to measure the intestinal digestibility.
Intestinal digestibility of rumen undegraded protein was 30.0 % for rapeseed, 72.8 % for barley and 94.7 % for maize. The study was supported by the the Ministry of Agriculture of the Czech Republic (NAZV, project No. QD 0211).

Poster N4.35

Effect of malate on digestibility and rumen microbial protein synthesis in growing lambs fed a high-concentrate diet

M.D. Carro[1], M.J. Ranilla[1], F.J. Giráldez[2], A.R. Mantecón[2] and J. Balcells[3]. [1]Dpto. Producción Animal I. Universidad de León. 24071 León, Spain. [2]EAE (CSIC). Apdo. 788, 24080 León, Spain. [3]Dpto. Producción Animal y Ciencia de los Alimentos, Miguel Servet 177, 50013 Zaragoza, Spain.*

Twenty-four Merino lambs (initial weight 15.3±1.27 kg) were divided into three homogenous groups. Each group was randomly allocated to three malate (disodium malate:calcium malate; 0.16:0.84) levels: 0 (C), 4 g/kg concentrate (M4) and 8 g/kg concentrate (M8). Lambs were fed concentrate (based on barley, corn and soyabean meal) and barley straw *ad libitum*. After a period of 19 days, digestibility was determined by total faecal collection and microbial nitrogen flow at the duodenum (MNDF) was estimated from the urinary excretion of purine derivatives. There were no effects ($P>0.05$) of malate either on diet intake or on organic matter digestibility, and consequently digestible organic matter intake (DOMI) did not differ ($P>0.05$) among treatments (1024, 1102 and 1014 g DOMI/d for C, M4 and M8, respectively). Malate treatment did not affect ($P>0.05$) the daily urinary excretion of total purine derivatives (9844, 9711 and 10500 μmol/d for C, M4 and M8, respectively). As a consequence, both the estimated MNDF and the efficiency of microbial yield were not affected ($P>0.05$) by malate supplementation (9.85, 9.99 and 10.62 g microbial N/d, and 9.68, 9.12 and 10.61 g microbial N/kg DOMI for C, M4 and M8, respectively).

Poster N4.36

The effect of the number of foil layers on the pH and lactic acid content in clover-grass silage in wrapped round bale

P. Dolezal, L. Zeman, J. Trinacty, P. Mares, Department of Animal Nutrition, Mendel University of Agriculture and Forestry Brno, Zemedelska 1, 613 00 Brno, Czech Republic*

The influence of the number of foil layers in ensilaged wilted clover-grass crops on the quality of fermentation processes was studied. Silage with 3 foil layers and 6 foil layers was prepared. Dry matter of the silaged clover-grass was higher than 400 g/kg. Statistical differences were tested at the significant level ($P<0.05$). Sensorial quality of silages with different numbers of foil layers was compared. The occurrence of fungi was not confirmed visually.
The most intensive decrease ($P<0.05$) of pH value in silage was observed after application of 3 foil layers as compared with the variant of 6 layers (5.18 ± 0.13 vs 5.56 ± 0.22). The silage wrapped with a higher number of foil layers had the statistically insignificantly ($P>0.05$) lower content of fermenting acids, including lactic acid, than that analysed with the lower (3) number of foil layers. Statistical differences were also found between both variants in the titration acidity content in favour of the silage wrapped with 3 foil layers. Between individual indices, no statistically significant ($P>0.05$) differences were ascertained.
This study was supported by NAZV (Project No. QD 0211), and MSM 432100001.

Poster N4.37

Use of stinging nettle and buckthorn in poultry diets

D. Grossu, Institute of Biology and Animal Nutrition, Calea Bucuresti nr. 1, 8113 Balotesti, Romania*

The investigation was conducted on 72 heavy breed cocks with an initial weight of 3300±100 g assigned to three groups. The birds received a corn, soybean meal and fish meal-based control diet and an experimental diet in which stinging nettle and buckthorn accounted for 20% of the total diet. The diet control had 159 g CP/kg DM and 17.73 J GE/kg DM, while the experimental diets had 160.4 g CP/kg DM and 17.94 J GE/kg DM (stinging nettle group) and 155 g CP/kg DM and 19.5 J GE/kg DM (buckthorn group). Digestibility trials were conducted according to Burlacu (1993). Total excreta was collected and analyzed with standard methods. The digestibility coefficients of the analyzed feeds, the biological value of the dietary amino acids, the energy spent for deamination, the digestible protein, the available protein and the retained protein were used to calculate the corrected metabolisable energy (ME_c). Stinging nettle gave the following results: 15.98 MJ GE/kg DM, 7.25 MJ ME_c/kg DM and 143 g DCP/kg DM, while buckthorn yielded 17.78 MJ GE/kg DM, 15.54 MJ ME_c/kg DM and 99 g DCP/kg DM. Stinging nettle and buckthorn can be used in poultry diets, this study ascertaining their nutritive value for diet optimization.

Poster N4.38

Performance, digestibility of nutrients and clinical pattern of cryptosporidiosis in experimentally infected calves treated with halofuginon-lactate

P. Klein[1], A. Fineo[2], V. Skrivanová[1], [1]Research Institute of Animal Production, Prátelství 815, Praha-Uhríneves, 104 01, Czech Republic, [2]Clinic of Infectious Diseases, Ospedale Regionale Torrette, Via Conca, 600 20, Ancona, Italy.*

Halofuginon-lactate (HFL) administration is considered as the effective prevention and therapy of bovine cryptosporidiosis, but no information about the effects of treatment on animal performance are available. In this study, total 24 neonatal Holstein calves were divided into four groups, six in each: untreated/uninfected, treated/uninfected, untreated/infected and treated/infected, and the effects of infection and/or treatment were studied in three successive 6-days digestibility trials. Infected calves received 6.10^6 oocysts of *Cryptosporidium parvum*. HFL was administered perorally from 4th day p.i. at 120 mg/kg of body weight for 7 consecutive days. Cryptosporidiosis had a typical clinical pattern in untreated calves (4-days prepatent period, oocysts shedded for 6-10 days with peak at 5-9 days p.i.). Administration of HFL significantly reduced counts of oocysts in faeces, intensity of diarrhea, and patent period in infected animals. Digestibility of nutrients and live body gain in treated animals were significantly higher in the 1st and 2nd digestibility trial in comparsion with those untreated. HFL did not affected performance in uninfected calves. (Support: Project QD-0176; Intervet, Czech Republic).

Poster N4.39

Diets with fresh Sudan grass for average yielding dairy cows

A. Dihoru, S. Pop, I. Voicu, M. Nicolae, A. Dumitru, Institute of Biology and Animal Nutrition, Calea Bucuresti nr. 1, 8113 Balotesti, Romania*

In the non-irrigated areas from the Romanian Plain it is difficult to feed dairy cows profitably during summer. The crops of drought resistant Sudan grass yield 2-3 cuts per year. It was shown experimentally that diets with fresh Sudan grass, beer mark and concentrate feeds (diet 1) or with Sudan grass and alfalfa hay (diet 2) support daily milk yields up to 15-19 kg. To prolong the period of harvesting at the same growth stage, two indigenous Sudan grass cultivars with different precocity (Silviu and Sonet) were grown. The experiment used 26 multiparous Romanian Black Spotted dairy cows in full lactation, weighing on average 550 kg, assigned to two groups (according to diet), each with 2 blocks corresponding to their yield. All animals received the same compound feed with protein-vitamin-mineral concentrate (PVMC) (33%) and energy feed, ear corn (67%). PVMC consisted of 85% sunflower meal, 2% monocalcium phosphate, 6% feed grade limestone, 3% salt and 4% vitamin-mineral premix. Sudan grass had 1.03 MFU, 101 g IDPN, 83 g IDPE, 4.5 g Ca and 2.5 g P at harvesting. Average feed intake (kg DM/cow/day) was 14.41 and 13.14 for block 1, respectively 12.39 and 11.65 for block 2. Average milk yield (kg/day) was 18.99(±1.61) and 19.62(±1.31) for block 1; 14.94(±0.82) and 14.65(±1.24) for block 2, respectively.

Poster N4.40

Omega-3 veal enrichment using suckling feed

G. Marsico[1], S. Dimatteo[1], A. Vicenti[1], F. Zezza[2] and A. D. Marsico[2]. [1]Dipartimento di Produzione Animale, Via Amendola, 165/A, 70126 Bari, Italy. [2]Collaboratore esterrno.

The aim of the research was to evaluate the possibility of using suckling feed to increase omega-3 fatty acid levels in veal. Twelve Bruna di Puglia calves were divided into two groups and fed for 150 days, using suckling feed at 10%. The first suckling feed was supplemented with 1% of coconut oil; the second with 1% of an oil mixture rich in omega-3 fatty acids. Statistical analysis was conducted using GLM procedure of SAS. The results showed a significant increase in unsaturated fatty acids (60.83% *vs* 62.03%, $P<0.05$), particularly of the omega-3 series (1.10% *vs* 2.13%, $P<0.01$), in the second group of animals (omega-3 diet). They also showed a significant increase in the healthiness indicators such as: atherogenicity index (0.62 *vs* 0.57, $P<0.01$), thrombogenicity index (1.09 *vs* 0.96, $P<0.01$) and Plasma Cholesterol Lowering/Plasma Cholesterol Elevating ratio (1.26 *vs* 1.39, $P<0.01$). The results suggest that the research ought to continue, also using varying levels of w3 supplementation.

Poster N4.41

Effects of two high energy content diets on buffalo rumen microbial counts

S. Puppo, A. Chiariotti, S. Lucioli and F. Grandoni, Istituto Sperimentale per la Zootecnia, Via Salaria, 31. 00016 Monterotondo scalo, Roma, Italy*

An investigation of the rumen ecosystem of Buffaloes in relation to the administred diet could optimize the ration and improve production and quality of milk and mozzarella cheese.

Four cannulated Buffalo females were fed two different diets characterized by a very high energy content: BF1 (alfalfa hay 10%, corn silage 38%. concentrate 52%) and BF2 (alfalfa hay 22%, corn silage 33%. Conc 45%) according to a factorial plan.

Chemical composition of the diets and total viable (T), cellulolytic (C) and xylanolytic (X) bacteria, fungi and protozoa were determined. pH and VFA of rumen samples were also scored.

No differences were found in pH, T or X between the two diets. Significantly more Fungi grew as a result of diet BF2, while C were higher as a result of diet BF1. These findings could be due to the different percentage of fiber (long and chopped).

Significantly higher proportions of propionic and butyric acids in total VFA were found on diet BF1.

In general a better growth of all microrganisms was observed in this trial when compared with our previous trials carried out in our laboratory with either high fiber content or silage + concentrate content.

Poster N4.42

The feeding strategy of the growing rabbits receiving diet with potato pulp as a main source of digestible fibre

Z. Volek[*1], M. Marounek[1,2], V. Skrivanová[1] [1]Research Institute of Animal Production, Prague 10-Uhríneves, Czech Republic, [2]Institute of Animal Physiology and Genetic, Prague 10-Uhríneves, Czech Republic*

A total of 108 Hyplus rabbits, weaned at the age of 35 days, were divided into 3 groups. Three diets were formulated. The control diet (18.5% starch; 16.3% ADF) contains no potato pulp and was fed to rabbits of the 1st group from weaning to 77 days of age. Another two diets contained no potato pulp and were formulated for the weaning (W:14.4% starch, 22.1% ADF) and fattening (F:18.6% starch, 21.0% ADF). The rabbits of the 2nd group received the diet "W" from 35 to 56 days of age and those of the 3rd group from 35 to 49 days of age. Then all rabbits were fed with diet "F" until 77 days of age. Weight gain averaged 36 g/day and did not vary significantly among groups. The feed intake was significantly lower in the 2nd and 3rd groups, compared to the 1st group (116, 109 and 126 g/day, respectively). Significantly better feed conversion (3.15 g/kg) was recorded in the 3rd group, compared to the 1st group (3.41 g/kg). The morbidity was significantly lower in the 2nd group than in other groups ($P<10^{-3}$). Caecal concentrations of volatile fatty acids were higher in the 2nd and 3rd group than in the 1st group ($P<0.05$). It can be concluded that potato pulp is a suitable source of digestible fibre for the partial replacement of starch without a major impairment of growth performance. A favourable time for a change of diet seems to be the third week after weaning with regard to health of rabbits. (Project MZE-MO2-99-04).

Poster N4.43

Alfalfa organic matter true digestibility: correlation between in vitro and NRC 2001 calculated values

F. Masoero, A. Pulimeno, M. Moschini , Istituto di Scienze degli Alimenti e della Nutrizione, Facoltà di Agraria, Università cattolica del Sacro Cuore, Piacenza, Italy

The in vitro organic matter (IVTD) and NDF ruminal true digestibilities of fifty alfalfa hay samples from the Po valley were evaluated. Samples were incubated 48 hours with the Ankom Daisy system. The rumen fluid was collected from two non lactating cows after 3 hours from the morning meal. Cows were feeding on a corn silage, concentrate and hay based diet with 14% crude protein, 32% NSC and 65:35 forage to concentrate ratio. The objective of the work was to compare the IVTD with the estimated digestible organic matter obtained either with the NRC 2001 full equations or with equations in which the NDF digestibility was replaced by the in vitro value. In addition, the IVTD was compared to calculated values obtained according to the Mertens equation and based on the ADF or NDF contents. The IVTD was correlated ($r = 0.76$) with calculated data, however, the higher in vitro values could suggest shorter incubating time (30 hours) as already in use by other authors. The obtained equation for the in vitro organic matter digestibility is $IVTD48 = 83.16 + 0.29*CP - 0.49*ADF - 2.79*ADFIP - 0.24*NDFIP - 0.91*ADL$ ($r^2 = 0.87$). No correlation was found between in vitro and calculated NDF digestibility for the tested samples.

Poster N4.44

Effect of two different diets during the dry-off period on the metabolism in dairy cows

K. Holtenius, and M.O. Odensten, Department of Animal Nurition and Management, Kungsangen Research Centre, SE 753 23 Uppsala, Swedish University of Agricultural Sciences, Sweden

Drying-off (DO) can be stressful due to ration changes and cessation of milking. The objective of this study was to investigate the effects on the metabolism of two diets during DO in dairy cows. Twenty cows, divided into two equal groups, were investigated. The daily milk yield immediately prior to DO averaged 19 kg energy corrected milk in both groups. One group of cows were only fed straw *ad libitum* (STRAW) during the 5 days DO period. The cows in the second group (SILAGE) were fed 4 kg DM/day of silage and straw *ad libitum* during the DO period. All cows were milked twice during the 5 days DO period, in the mornings of day 3 and day 5. The plasma concentration of NEFA was markedly elevated during the DO period in H cows but in SILAGE cows the increase was less pronounced. The glucose level in plasma was not significantly affected by DO. Both the β-hydroxybutyrate and urea concentration in plasma were significantly reduced during DO. Preliminary results also show that insulin was markedly reduced. The diurnal profile of cortisol was monitored prior to DO and during the third day of DO. The cortisol level was significanly elevated during DO in STRAW cows but not in SILAGE cows. Our results indicate that DO markedly affected the metabolism of the cows, and that those cows which were only given straw were most affected.

Poster N4.45

Effect of various origin of starch on its ruminal digestibility

P. Homolka, Research Institute of Animal Production, Uhríneves, 104 00 Prague, Czech Republic

The objective of this study was to determine *in sacco* ruminal starch digestibility of oat meal, wheat meal and barley meal. Starch is the major energy component of cereal grains. The main part of starch in the diet of high yielding cows originates from grains. Optimal fermentation in the rumen is very important, because excessive by-pass of starch, higher then 1.5 kg/d to the intestine, decreases its utilization.

The starch and nitrogen degradation were determined using *in sacco* method in three dry cows with a large ruminal cannula. The bags containing feed samples were attached to a cylindrical carrier and incubated in the rumen for 2, 4, 8, 16 and 24 hours. The content of starch was 453 g per kg dry matter (DM) in oat, 646 g per kg DM in wheat and 622 g per kg DM in barley. The highest degradation of starch was in oat (after 2 hours in rumen was in sample 64 g starch per kg DM; after 16 hours 9 g). Slower degradation of starch was in wheat (after 2 hours in rumen was in sample 310 g starch per kg DM; after 16 hours 107g). The slowest degradation of starch was in barley (after 2 hours in rumen was in sample 538 g starch per kg DM; after 16 hours 48 g).

This work was supported by the Ministry of Agriculture of the Czech Republic (project MZE-MO2-99-04 and QD 0176).

Poster N4.46

Intake and digestibility of *Atriplex nummularia* in rabbits

D. Camacho-Morfin, L.L. Morfin and M. Moreno-Castelazo, Faculty of Superior Studies Cuautitlan. UNAM.Campo 4. km 2.5 Carretera Cuautitlán-Teoloyucan, Edo. de Méx. México.*

In order to evaluate the intake and digestibility of *Atriplex nummularia* leaves in rabbits, 12 female New Zealand White rabbits were randomly allocated in a complete randomized design to 3 treatment: the first one was fed a concentrated diet only, the second was fed 75 % of *A. nummularia* and 25 % concentrate, the last one was fed with *Atriplex* and concentrate *ad libitum*. The trial lasted 15 days: 10 days as preliminary period and five days as a collection period. Chemical composition (dry matter (DM), crude protein (CP) and detergent neutral fiber (DNF)) of the ration, refusals and feces was analyzed. The total intake was 79.2, 81.1 and 100.1 g/day, the DM digestibility were 66.5, 66.6 and 68.4%; CP digestibility: 79.2, 80.1 and 81.7 %; DNF digestibility: 35.6, 40.1 and 44 %, respectively. There were not significative differences between DM, CP and DNF digestibilities with increasing the level of *Atriplex* forage and the intake was similar between treatments. In conclusion Atriplex could replace 20 % of the concentrate without affecting intake and DM, CP and DNF digestibilities.

Poster N4.47

Effects of main protein source and non-forage fibre source on nutrient digestibility of sheep rations

D. Liamadis[1], Ch. Milis[2] and D. Kallias[1], [1]Aristotle University of Thessaloniki, [2]Ministry of Agriculture, Greece

An in vivo digestibility trial was conducted using 4 castrated rams, in a 4x4 latin square design. The purpose of the study was to examine the effects on digestibility of the substitution of Cottonseed Cake (CSC) and Wheat Bran (WB) by Corn Gluten Meal
(CGM) and Corn Gluten Feed (CGF), respectively. Four isoenergetic-isonitrogenous-isofiberous rations were used, as follows: (A) CSC and WB, (B) CSC and CGF, (C) CGM and WB and finally (D) CGM and CGF. Statistical analysis was performed by the use of SPSS, and significance was declared at $P<0.05$. The results of this trial revealed that rations C and D had increased digestibility of DM (73.4; 74.8; 76.5 and 76.5, for rations A, B, C, and D, respectively), OM (76.5; 77.7; 79.7 and 79.6, for rations A, B, C and D, respectively) and CP (72.2; 73.5; 83.5 and 79.9, for rations A, B, C, and D, respectively) in comparison with rations A and B. These results suggest that CGM is increasing digestibility of those nutrients when replacing CSC, in ewes rations. Also, ration B had higher digestibility of CF than ration A (39.5 vs 32.6) as though as did ration D compared with ration C (37.9 vs 25.9), suggesting that CGF exceeded in CF digestibility in comparison to WB. The conclusion is that CGM increases OM and CP digestibility of the ration when it substitutes CSC, whilst CGF increases CF digestibility of the ration when it substitutes WB.

Poster N4.48

Effect of addition of plant feed CCM to milk diet on cholesterol and fatty acid of calves meat

V. Skrivanová, Y. Tyrolová , Z. Volek*, Res. Inst. Anim. Prod., Prátelství 815, 104 01, Praha 10, Uhríneves, Czech Republic

Fatty acids are the most important lipid components. Fourteen Holstein bulls of average age of 19 days at the beginning of the trial were used. The calves were divided into two groups. The 1st group was given milk replacer only. The 2nd group was given milk replacer (5 % less than 1st group), and given *ad libitum* maize silaged by method CCM (Corn Cob Mix). The calves were slaughtered at the age of 4 months. The *m. longissimus dorsi* was sampled in all animals and analysed. Contents of cholesterol in the meat was 513 vs. 532 mg/kg. The differences were not significant. Contents of cholesterol and fatty acids were determined by gas chromatography. We aimed at fatty acids with long chains: n-3 and n-6 of PUFA. The most important PUFA are linolenic acid 18:3n-3, arachidonic acid 20:4n-6, and linoleic 18:2n-6. It was found out that contents of PUFA was 33.72 % in the 1st group and 35.46 % in the 2nd group. Differences between groups were not significant. Differences in contents of linolenic acid (0.46 vs. 0.41 %), arachidonic acid (5.84 vs. 6.25 %), and linoleic acid (23.59 vs. 24.67 %) were not significant either between both groups. These results suggest that the plant food addition (CCM) to veal calves does not have any influence on profile of meat lipids PUFA.

(The project of Ntl. Acad. Agr. Sci. (NAZV) No. QD 0176)

Poster N4.49

Effect of addition of plant feeds CCM to milk diet of calves on digestibility of nutrients and quality parameters of meat

Y. Tyrolová[1], V. Skrivanová[1], M. Houska[2], [1]P. Lang[1], [1]Res. Inst. Anim. Prod., Prátelství 815, 104 01, Praha 10, Uhríneves, Czech Republic, [2]Food Res. Inst. Prague, Radiová 7,102 31, Praha 10, Hostivar*

The experiment was conducted on 14 Holstein bulls of average age of 19 days and weight of 46 kg. The animals were divided into two groups: 1) fed only milk replacer (1st group), 2) fed milk replacer with addition of maize silaged by the method CCM (Corn Cob Mix) (2nd group). The amount of milk replacer of the 2nd group was reduced by 5 % in comparison with 1st group. The animals consumed the CCM *ad libitum*. The nutrient digestibility was investigated at the age of 12 weeks in 5 days balance period using the chromic oxide indicator method. Differences of digestibility of DM (82.2 vs. 85.4 %), crude protein (67.3 vs. 76.8 %) and ash (65.7 vs. 72.2 %) were significant ($P<0.05$). Daily weight gains of calves were not significantly different. The calves were slaughtered at the age of 4 months. The slaughter weight was 131.9 and 129.0 kg. The *m. longissimus dorsi* was sampled. The pH of meat was measured after 24 and 48 h. The values of both groups (1st group pH 24 h 5.65; pH 48 h 5.62; 2nd group pH 24 h 5.65; pH 48 h 5.61) were in the optimum range. The differences were not significant. Shear force of the meat was determined with the Warner-Bratzler apparatus. The contents of vitamin B1, B6, B12 in the meat and the colour meat expressed by parameters L*, a* b* were also assayed. Differences were not significant. It can be concluded that the effect of plant feed addition as CCM on the meat quality was not found. (The project of Ntl. Acad. Agr. Sci. (NAZV) No. QD 0176)

Poster N4.50

Influence of Aspergillus oryzae administration on milk yield and quality of Italian River Buffalo

F. Sarubbi[1], F. Polimeno[1], R. Baculo[1], G. Maglione[1] and L. Ferrara[1], [1]ISPAAM- CNR Via Argine 1085, 80147 Naples, Italy.

The administration of *Aspergillus oryzae* (AO) in bovine gave contradictory results related to its effect on the yields. In order to verify the AO administration effect on lactating buffaloes were established two experimental groups each of 14 buffaloes multiparous homogeneous for yield level and milk composition (pH, DM, fat, proteins, lactose and urea). The treated group (T) received, besides the unifeed, a mix containing an AO fermentation extract, while the untreated group (C) received only the unifeed. The period of lactation was divided in 5 intervals (A, B, C, D and E). During the first 100 days the yields of group T was lower than C group even if not significantly. In the third interval there were no differences between the two groups and in the intervals D and E the yield was overlapping. Only significant differences ($P<0.05$) were observed related to urea concentration higher for the T group. This behaviour could be due to the decrease proteins degradability consequently to the AO administration. The higher value in fat contents for the T group gave no significant difference as well as the contents of lactose and proteins.
The AO administration implied a decrease of yield, even if no significant, in the first 100 days likely ascribed to a modification of food retention time into the intestinal tract.

Poster N4.51

Comparison of the blood urea recycling in sheep and goat

J-L. Tisserand, établissement national d'enseignement Supérieur Agronomique de Dijon BP 87999 21079 Dijon France

Microbial digestion is less diminished by nitrogen deficiency in goat than in sheep. To try to explain the observation we compare nitrogen balances on three castrated rain and three castrated male goat nourished with sodium hydroxide treated straw only or with 100 g lactose by head and by day in order to have a better urea recycling. The addition of lactose is withoot effect in sheep but in goat reduce uraemia and level of urinary urea (52 % and 32 % respectively).
In conclusion goat recycle better blood urea than sheep.

Poster N4.52

State of european ped nutrition research

J-L. Tisserand, établissement national d'enseignement supérieur agronomique de Dijon BP 87999, 21079 Dijon Cedex France

On request of European Association for Animal Production Council a survey is realized on ped nutrition in Europe with the ains to create a working groop on this topic.
Veterinarians are the main colleagues concerned. Some specialists are identified in most EAAP Countries in connection with ped-food industry.
We have many international work and in particular one European net-work in connection with American colleague is very efficient. A list of concerned colleagues is draw up.

Poster N4.53

Effect of a biological additive on silage fermentation, intake, milk quality and performance of lactating dairy cows

J. Jatkauskas and V. Vrotniakiene, Lithuanian Institute of Animal Science, R. Zebenkos 12, LT-5125Baisogala, Radviliskio raj., Lithuania*

Additive-free and AIV Bioprofit (*Lactobacillus rhamnosus* and *Propionibacterium freudenreichii* ssp.) inoculated silages were made from grass(clover 64%, timothy 12%, meadow fescue 8%) in two trenches of 120 tons each and at the same time under laboratory conditions. The inoculated treatment gave a silage with lower ammonia-N and pH and higher lactic acid compared to the untreated silage and without butyric acid. The aerobic stability of silage and rumen metabolism of cows were investigated in the course of the trial. AIV Bioprofit inoculated silage had lower crude fiber and increased dry matter, crude protein and WSC contents. Nutrients losses were lower by 1.0%, organic matter digestibility by 1.5% and energy values were higher by 0.2MJ/kg^{-1}DM for the inoculated silage in comparison with the ordinary made silage. A feeding trial with lactating dairy cows lasted for 100 days. The cows fed AIV Bioprofit treated silage had higher intake (on average 2.09 kgDM/day/cow forage; equivalent to 16.6 MJ metabolizable energy) and as a result milk yield (FCM) of these cows was higher (+1.0 kg/day/cow) compared with cows fed untreated silage. Fat and protein contents of milk tended to be higher for the AIV Bioprofit silage fed cows.

Poster N4.54

Improved utilization of rice processing waste in growing pig feeding

Mihaela Habeanu, Veronica Hebean, I. Moldovan, Al. Lionide, *Institute of Biology and Animal Nutrition- Balotesti: Calea Bucuresti nr.1; 8113; Romania*

The purpose of this paper was to establish the data for a better utilization of rice wastes, while decreasing the antinutritive effect of some factors contained by the wastes using an phytase enzyme produced from natural microorganisms. The bioproductive test was conducted on 85 hybrid (Large White x Peris Synthetic) piglets weaned at 28 days, with an average initial weight of 8 kg, assigned to six groups, a control group M and five experimental groups MF,V1, V1F, V2, V2F. The control group received no dietary rice meal, while the experimental groups received 5 and 10% rice meal Phytase enzyme was also included in the vitamin-mineral premix of groups MF, V1F, V2F.The compound feed formulations were izoenergetic and izoproteic. The average daily gain was influenced positively by phytase supplementation: 2.9% higher in group MF compared to group M, 3.6% higher in group V1F compared to group V1 and 4.3% higher in group V2F compared to group V2. The differences were not significant, however (P>0.05- test Student).Feed conversion ratio was reduced by 3.38% in MF compared to M, by 2.3% in V1F compared to V1 and by 2.6%in V2F compared to V2. The performance of animals did not differ significantly (P>0.05) between the groups, while it was better in the animals treated with phytase.

Poster N4.55

Improved nitrogen utilisation by dairy cows fed low crude-protein diets containing grass/clover silage and hay as only forages

E. Nadeau[1], A.H. Gustafsson[2], E. Forsberg[3] and A. Lundgren[4], [1]Dept. of Agricultural Research Skara, The Swedish University of Agricultural Sciences, Box 234, 532 23 Skara, [2]Div. of Research and Development, The Swedish Dairy Association, Kungsängen Research Centre, 753 23 Uppsala, [3]Svenska Foder, [4]Svenska Lantmännen, 531 87 Lidköping, Sweden.*

Life-Ammonia, a project financed by EU and national organisations, demonstrates different techniques to minimise ammonia emission from the Research farm Brogården, Skara, The Swedish University of Agricultural Sciences. Objective for the feeding task of the programme was to improve nitrogen efficiency of the dairy cows by formulating rations for decreased crude protein concentrations and recommended levels of degradable/undegradable proteins, without decreasing milk yield. During the reference period (October 1999-April 2000), no adjustments were made to the diets, containing grass/clover silage, hay and small grains. During the following two winter seasons (October-April 00/01, 01/02), average dietary crude protein concentrations were decreased from 170 to 160 g/kg of DM, by adding dried sugar-beet pulp to diets of high-producing cows and increasing the average dietary proportion of small grains from 53 to 59% of DM. Total feed intake increased from 18.6 to 19.9 kg DM/day and milk yield increased from 30.6 to 32.4 kg energy-corrected milk (ECM)/day, resulting in an average constant nitrogen efficiency of 31% for lactating cows. For cows producing > 35 kg ECM/day, nitrogen efficiency increased from 32 to 33%. When dry cows were included, nitrogen efficiency increased from 27 to 29%. Consequently, increasing milk yield, while controlling nitrogen intake, has the potential to improve nitrogen efficiency.

Poster N4.56

Effects of two different diets during the dry-off period on rumen metabolism and milk production in dairy cows

M.O. Odensten, A. Odelstrom and K. Holtenius, Department of Animal Nutrition and Management, Kungsangen Research Centre, SE-75323 Uppsala, Swedish University of Agriculture Sciences, Sweden.

With a short calving interval and an increasing milk yield, metabolic and health problems during the drying-off (DO) period will rise. The objectives of this study was to investigate different feeding strategies of high yielding dairy cows during DO. Twenty dairy cows were divided into two groups. At DO the cows had an average milk yield of 19.2 kg of energy corrected milk. At the DO period group one (STRAW) were fed straw *ab libitum* and group two (SILAGE) were fed 4 kg of DM silage per day and straw *ab libitum*. All cows were milked twice during the DO period, which lasted for 5 days. Milk production decreased at DO, but milk fat percentage increased. Rumen fluid was sampled with an esophageal tube; one week prior to DO, at DO and two weeks post DO. VFA, pH, ammonium nitrogen (Am-N) were measured and protozoa were counted. Total VFA production decreased at DO in both groups ($P<0.001$) and the drop was most pronounced among STRAW cows. Rumen pH increased significantly ($P<0.001$) in both groups and STRAW cows had significantly higher pH at DO compared with SILAGE cows. Am-N in rumen decreased significantly at DO and there were a tendency of lower Am-N in STRAW at DO. The number of protozoa decreased in both groups signficantly ($P<0.001$). The results indicates a marked change in rumen environment at DO and the STRAW cows were most affected.

Poster N4.57

Investigation of different levels of RDP in the ration of lactating cows and their effects on MUN, BUN, and urinary N excretion

Ali Moharrery, Anim. Sci. Dept., Agricultural college, Shahrekord University, Iran

Twenty-one multiparous Holstein cows were used in complete randomized design to investigate the effect of rumen degradable protein on milk urea nitrogen (MUN) and some blood metabolites. Experimental periods were 6 wk in length, with d 1 to 14 used for adjustment and wk 2 to wk 6 used for a sampling (urine, blood, and milk). Three concentration of a rumen-degradable protein (RDP) supplement according to National Research Council recommendations (9.3, 11.4, and 14% of dry matter intake) were treatments. Estimations for microbial protein yield were compared with the measured excretion of purine derivative as yeast RNA equivalent, in urine. No significant effect of concentration of RDP supplement was detected on the excretion of purine derivative as yeast RNA equivalent in urine (mean, 10.87 mg/ml). For better prediction of urinary nitrogen (UN) excretion, body weight (BW) was included in the model. Result showed that milk urea N is a simple and noninvasive measurement that can be used to monitor N excretion from lactating dairy cows.

Poster N4.58

Biochemical parameters of rumen fluid when feeding silages with different acidity

P. Dolezal, L. Zeman, J. Trinacty, Department of Animal Nutrition, Mendel University of Agriculture and Forestry Brno, Zemedelska 1, 613 00 Brno, Czech Republic*

Twenty dairy cows were used in experiment at which studied the influence of silages with different content of acids on the rumen fermentation. Animals were divided in to experimental and control groups, each of them 10 cows. The feeding ration consisted of maize silage (26 kg), lucerne silage (13 kg), meadow hay (1 kg) and feeding mixture (8.5 kg). Dairy cows in experimental group received different (higher) quantity of total acids per 1 kg live weight (1.98 g vs. 1.48 g/kg weight) from inoculated silage.

Mean value of pH of rumen fluid significantly ($P<0.05$) reduced in experimental group (5.8 ± 0.08), vs. control (6.2 ± 0.06).

The most intensive increase ($P<0.01$) of VFA (125 ± 5.2 mmol/l) and lactic acid (4.8 ± 0.2 mmol/l) content in rumen fluid of experimental group was observed. Statistical differences ($P<0.05$) were also found in rumen fluid in experimental group of cow´s in the propionic and butyric acid content. The content of acetic acid had the no statistically significant ($P>0.05$) lower differences in fluid of experimental group. Statistically significant ($P<0.01$) differences were ascertained by the content of infusoria value in experimental group (175.76 ± 12.54 thousand/ml vs. 288.1 ± 13.73 thousand/ml.

This study was supported by Project MSM 432100001.

Poster N4.59

Natural antioxidants in traditional Sicilian cheeses obtained from pasture-fed animals

M. Rosato[1], G. Di Rosa[1] S. Carpino[1], G. Licitra[12], CoRFiLaC, Regione Siciliana, s.p. 25 km 5, 97100 Ragusa, Italy, .[2]D.A.C.P.A., Università di Catania, Italy.*

Milk and its derivatives from pasture-fed animals contains higher levels of antioxidants compared to those obtained from more controlled feeding systems. Epidemiological studies have indicated the existence of a negative correlation between diets rich in fruits, vegetables and dairy products, and therefore antioxidants, and incidence of cancer.

In the present work, several natural antioxidants in traditional Sicilian cheeses were studied. Cheeses were obtained from pasture-fed animals. Categories of antioxidants included fat-soluble vitamins (vitamins E, A and its precursors, β-carotene) and lipids (squalene).

Samples were extracted according to the modified Ueda and Igarashi method, and antioxidant contents were determined from the extracts by HPLC/UV-Vis. Vitamins A, E and squalene varied quantitatively in each sample according to the type and degree of maturation of the cheeses. β-carotene, however, was found only in cow's milk cheeses. Ragusano and Palermitano cheeses were found to be particularly rich in this compound. This latter result, regarding cow's milk cheeses but not the specific cheeses studied here, has also been reported in the literature. Finally, Fiore Sicano was found to contain higher mean levels of squalene and Pecorino Siciliano along with other cheeses obtained from sheep's milk were found to contain higher mean levels of vitamins A and E than other cheeses studied.

Theatre NP6.1

The growing-fattening Iberian pig: Metabolic profile and nutrition

J.F. Aguilera and R. Nieto, Unidad de Nutrición Animal, Estación Experimental del Zaidín (CSIC), Camino del Jueves s/n, 18100 Armilla, Granada, Spain*

Extensive systems encourage the production of native pig breeds and the use of local feed resources, what helps maintaining genetic diversity and facilitates the provision of niche products to the market. The production of the Iberian pig complies with these prospects. The Iberian pig has a low genetic potential for lean tissue deposition. Protein and energy requirements for this breed have been recently determined at different stages of its productive cycle, based on the assessments of maximum daily rate of protein accretion, marginal efficiency of body protein deposition, energy required for maintenance and efficiency of utilization of metabolizable energy for production.

The final fattening phase of the Iberian pig (100-160 kg BW) takes place at the 'dehesa', the Mediterranean forest, which supplies mainly acorn and pasture and stimulates physical activity. Acorn (the *Quercus* fruit) is very palatable for the pig and provides a characteristic fatty acid profile to the lipid tissue of the animal and special flavour to cured products. It contains a low amount of protein of poor biological quality due to a marked lysine deficiency, but it is a rich source of available energy. Therefore, acorn consumption favours fat deposition and constrains protein accretion.

Muscular activity seems more energetically efficient in this native breed which is probably related to a comparatively higher abundance of oxidative muscle fibers.

Theatre NP6.2

The production of the heavy pig high quality processed products

P. Bosi and V. Russo, DIPROVAL, University of Bologna, via Rosselli 107, 42100 Reggio Emilia, Italy.

To obtain high quality processed pig products, heavy pig production in Italy is subjected to rules fixed by Consortia, on the base of empirical and scientific experience. First of all, slaughtering animals of at least 9 months of age and 160 kg live weight are required, to provide heavy cuts with excellent meat. Breeds are limited to Italian Large White and Landrace, selected for specific parameters such as loss at 1st salting of the ham, and to their crosses. Crosses with Duroc and hybrids can be used if obtained from selection and crossing schemes that fit the objectives of Italian selection. Backfat thickness must be "sufficient" to obtain retailed fresh hams with fat cover ranging from 20 to 30 mm, depending on ham weight, and the content of linoleic acid in ham fat cover must be lower than 15%. Fat quantity and quality in feeds should be carefully controlled to satisfy the quality of fat in the ham. The feeding level is also relevant, due to the imposed minimum age at slaughter. Feed restriction is a necessary practice to respect the rules for ham production. For castrate males of medium genetic value, the restriction should reduce fat deposition, but the diet composition can be adapted to maintain the maximum growth of protein. For strains with high lean deposition potential and particularly for gilts, also protein deposition should be limited to maintain a sufficient fat cover of ham.

Theatre NP6.3

Pig keeping over a fattening period of 14 (standard) or 20 weeks (heavy): effect on growth performances

N. Quiniou[1], Y. Le Cozler[2] and A. Aubry[1], [1]ITP, BP3, 35650 Le Rheu cedex, [2]EDE de Bretagne, Avenue Borgnis Desbordes, 56002 Vannes cedex, France*

Two trials were carried out in two French research stations to quantify growth performances of group-housed barrows or gilts over two fattening durations corresponding to production of French standard pigs (S, 14 weeks) or heavy (H, 20 weeks) ones. Average daily gain (ADG) and feed conversion ratio (FCR) were calculated from 28 kg body weight (BW) to slaughter (total), over the first 14 weeks (0-14) for all pigs (H + S), and over the following 6 weeks (14-20) for H pigs. Barrows were fed ad libitum below 70 kg BW, 2.7 kg/d from 70 to 110 kg BW, and 2.9 kg/d thereafter in both trials. Gilts were fed ad libitum from 28 kg to slaughter in trial 1 and restrictively fed like barrows in trial 2. The H pigs were slaughtered at 151 and 142 kg BW in trial 1 and 2, respectively. Corresponding values were 112 and 108 kg BW for S pigs. Differences in gilts' feeding level between trials 1 and 2 resulted in sex effect on ADG_{14-20} (significantly higher in trial 1: 967 vs. 785 g/d for barrows, but not different in trial 2: 770 g/d). Total FCR increased by 0.06 unit per additional 10 kg BW at slaughter in trials 1 and 2. Growth and feed intake curves were also obtained.

Theatre NP6.4

Pigs keeping over a fattening period of 14 (standard) or 20 weeks (heavy): effect on carcass quality and chemical composition of raw muscles and cured-cooked hams

B. Minvielle[1], G. Alviset[2], J.L. Martin[3], J. Boulard[1], Y. Le Cozler[4] and N. Quiniou[1], [1]ITP, BP3, 35650 Le Rheu cedex, [2]Fleury Michon, ZI Montifaut, 85700 Pouzauges, [3]CTSCCV, 7 av. du Général Leclerc, 94704 Maisons-Alfort Cedex, [4]EDE de Bretagne, av. Borgnis Desbordes, 56002 Vannes cedex, France*

Two trials were carried out in two French research stations to quantify performances of group-housed barrows or gilts over two fattening durations corresponding to production of French standard pigs (S, 14 weeks) or heavy (H, 20 weeks) ones (Quiniou et al., EAAP 2003). Carcass quality of S and H pigs was evaluated from muscle (M2) and subcutaneous fat depths at the 3-4th rib and from early and ultimate pH. Chemical analyses were performed on the left *Semimembranosus* muscle and on slices of the right cured-cooked hams processed according to the rules laid down by the high French standard quality 'Label Rouge'. Muscle and subcutaneous fat depths were higher for H than for S pigs (more than 5 additional mm for M2 on average). The H hams were 3 kg heavier on average, but their anatomic yield after deboning was not different. Ultimate pH was higher for H than for S pigs, that partly explained the slightly better cooking yields, lower slicing losses and higher global processing yields of H hams. Fat content of raw ham muscle and cure-cooked ham was higher for H pigs.

Genetic parameters for quality traits of raw and dry-cured hams

C. Romani[1], E. Sturaro[1], R.J. Tempelman[2], L. Gallo[1] and P. Carnier[1]. [1]Department of Animal Science, University of Padova. [2]Department of Animal Science, Michigan State University.*

Data on 1425 typical Italian dry-cured hams were analysed. Pigs were progeny of 74 Gorzagri C21 Large White boars and of 221 Large White-derived crossbred sows. Marbling (MB), fat thickness (FTS), ham firmness (HF) and fat quality (FQ, color, oiliness, firmness) were scored on both raw and cured hams. Total area, fat eye area (FEA) and fat thickness (FTM) of the cross section of dry cured hams were measured using computer image analysis (CIA). Records were analyzed with Bayesian methodology via Gibbs sampling using a univariate linear model for continuous traits, a univariate threshold model for scores and a bivariate threshold linear model to estimate genetic correlations between raw and cured ham traits. Besides animal effects, the effects of batch, gender, weight of carcass and interactions were included in the statistical models. For cured ham traits, heritabilities were 0.35 for MB, 0.07 for HF, 0.45 for FTS, 0.20 for FQ, 0.15 for FEA, 0.34 for FTM. Heritability of MB, FQ, and FTS of raw hams was similar to that of cured hams. Genetic correlations between quality traits of cured hams and corresponding traits of raw hams were greater than 0.80 with the exception of FQ. FQ of raw hams was positively related to FTS. Correlations between FEA and other raw ham traits were small.

Theatre NP6.6

Quality of subcutaneous fat of raw hams for dry-curing: nongenetic effects and genetic parameters for iodine number and linoleic acid content

P. Carnier, E. Sturaro, M. Noventa and L. Gallo, Department of Animal Science, University of Padova, Agripolis, 35020 Legnaro (PD), Italy*

Subcutaneous fat from 930 raw hams was sampled with the aim of investigating sources of variation and genetic parameters of iodine number (IN) and linoleic acid content (LA%). Pigs, offspring of 25 Gorzagri Large White C21 line boars and 123 Large White-derived crossbred sows, were slaughtered in 14 monthly batches at 166±15 kg of liveweight. Herd, management and feeding regime were the same throughout the trial. IN and LA% were determined using Wijs and gas-chromatography procedures, respectively, and mean±SD was 68.8±3.3 for IN and 12.7±1.7% for LA%. Batch and sire were the most important sources of variation. R2 of models was > 60% for both traits and all effects included in the model were significant. IN and LA% decreased at increasing carcass weight, and were higher in barrows than in gilts. Variance components were estimated using an univariate bayesian via Gibbs sampling. Estimated h2 was 0.414 for IN and 0.378 for LA%, and the lowest values of h2 delimiting the 90% posterior probability density region were 0.321 and 0.251, respectively. Genetic correlation between IN and LA% was 0.837. Selection for reducing IN and LA% of subcutaneous fat of hams is feasible and can be achieved by focusing on IN only, which is cheaper to determine than LA%.

Theatre NP6.7

Effect of bacterial protein on performance, carcass traits and sensory quality of pigs

N.P. Kjos[1], M. Øverland[2], H. Müller[1] and A. Skrede[1], [1]AUN, N-1432 Aas, Norway, [2]Norsk Hydro, N-0240 Oslo, Norway.*

Bacterial protein (BioProtein) is produced by mainly *Methylococcus capsulatus* but also *Alcaligenes acidovorans, Bacillus brevis* and *Bacillus firmus*, by using natural gas (99% methane), ammonia and salts. BioProtein contains 95% DM, 70% CP and 10% lipids. The lipid fraction consists mainly of phosphatidyl-glycerol and phosphatidyl-etanolamine with predominantly 16:0 and 16:1 fatty acids, and no poly-unsaturated fatty acids.
Three studies were conducted to evaluate BioProtein in diets for growing-finishing pigs (26 to 102 kg), on performance, carcass traits, and sensory quality. In Exp. 1 (18 pigs), adding 0, 6, and 12% BioProtein had no effect on performance or carcass quality, but tended to increase fat firmness. In Exp. 2 (24 pigs) and Exp. 3 (48 pigs), three levels were used, replacing 0, 50 and 100% of lysine in soybean meal with BioProtein. In Exp. 2, both levels of BioProtein tended to improve performance. Both BioProtein levels also improved P2-backfat thickness, fat firmness and colour, and tended to improve backfat flavour. In Exp. 3, BioProtein did not affect performance, but improved fat firmness and colour. BioProtein also tended to increase P2-backfat thickness, and to improve backfat flavour. In conclusion, BioProtein had no adverse effect on performance, but improved sensory quality of backfat. Due to its specific lipid characteristics, feeding BioProtein might be a means to improve sensory quality of heavy pigs.

Theatre NP6.8

Digestibility and energy utilization of high fibre diets in the heavy pig

G.M. Crovetto, G. Galassi and L. Rapetti, Istituto di Zootecnia Generale, Università degli Studi, via Celoria 2, 20133 Milano, Italy*

Eight Landrace x Large White fattening pigs were fed 3 high fibre (on average 17.8% NDF on DM) diets and a traditional (C) diet (13.5% NDF) in a Latin Square design. Feeding was restricted. Each of the 4 periods included 21 days adaptation and 7 days digestibility/calorimetry. The high fibre (HF) diets included wheat bran (coarse or milled) or beet pulp. In periods 1, 2, 3 and 4 the pigs weighed, on average, 105, 124, 140 and 158 kg.
Fibre digestibility (%) of diets HF increased from period 1 to period 4: 56.2, 56.6, 58.8, 62.2 for NDF and 46.0, 47.1, 49.0, 53.4 for ADF. A similar trend was registered for the digestibility of DM, OM, CP, EE and energy. Comparing the digestibility of diet C with HF diets, independently of the periods, diet C had always significantly higher digestibilities (e.g. DM=87.5 *vs* 84.9%) except for fibre which gave similar coefficients. Methane energy losses increased significantly from period 1 to period 4 for both diets C and HF, while heat production and retained energy, (% of the intake energy, IE), did not differ significantly between periods. Retained energy of C diet (37.1% IE) and of HF diets (35.3%) considered as the average of the four periods were similar, confirming that the heavy pig can utilize fibre to a good extent.

Theatre NP6.9

Hog farmer feeding strategies under animal disease quarantine

J.K. Niemi and K. Pietola, MTT Economic Research, Luutnantintie 13, 00410 Helsinki, Finland.*

Animal movement restrictions applied in eradicating a contagious animal disease may lead to a situation where hog farmers are forced to keep ready-to-slaughter animals on the farm. Farmers need to consider adjusted feeding strategies, because feeding heavy animals may cause income losses. The problem is interesting also from society's point of view, since a large number of farms can be affected by the quarantine measures related to a single infected farm.
A dynamic programming model is developed to estimate optimal feeding strategies and farmer's income losses under animal movement restrictions in Finland. The model takes into account carcass quality in terms of red meat percentage and carcass weight, increased animal density in the pen and optimal slaughter time under specific prices. Income losses are compared to preventive slaughter option that allows to cull the hog and keep the capacity unit empty until the quarantine is lifted.
The results suggest that the optimal feeding policy under animal movement restrictions is characterised by reduced energy feeding that decreases daily weight gain. Through adjusted feeding farmer can significantly affect quality adjusted price of meat. A long remaining feeding period implies smaller financial losses and adjustments as well as better animal welfare than a short period. In addition, a long quarantine increases farmer incentives to avoid costly maintenance feeding of animals by having his herd culled preventively or due to an infection.

Poster NP6.10

High linoleic acid diets for growing-finishing heavy pigs: performances, carcass and "Pancetta Piacentina D.O.P." quality

A. Prandini[1], G. Della Casa[2], M.T. Pacchioli[3], A. Rossi[3], F.Conti[1], P. Baldini[4] and G. Piva[1], [1]ISAN, 29100 Piacenza, Italy, [2]Istituto Sperimentale per la Zootecnia, 41018 Modena, Italy, [3]C.R.P.A., 42100 Reggio Emilia, Italy, [4] SSCIA, 43100 Parma, Italy.

The aim of the trial was to study the effect of heavy pigs diets with high level of linoleic acid on the quality of "Pancetta Piacentina D.O.P." (PP). Forty Duroc x Large White pigs (39.94+ 1.52 kg initial l.w.; half females and half castrated males), were randomly assigned to two dietary treatments and housed in 4 pens (replicates)/dietary treatment. Experimental diets were: 1) Linoleic acid level of the diets according to Parma and S. Daniele Ham Consortium rules (<2%), control diet (C); 2) High linoleic acid diet (>3%) (HL) using soya oil (3%) added to the diets. Animals consumed the experimental diets for 168 d (175 kg l.w.). No statistical differences were recorded for growth parameters but HL diet had lower feed/gain than C diet. Slaughtering and FOM parameters did not statistically differ between treatments. PP were seasoned according to the Consortium Rules up to 90 d (minimum seasoning time) and 200 d. PP from HL animals had higher unsaturated fatty acids and did not differ for oxidation parameters (peroxide, acidity, MTB); panel test showed that PP from HL had softer and higher oil fat content, but the over-all sensory evaluation was similar between dietary treatments.

Poster NP6.11

Meat quality of pigs in Basilicata assessed by conventional variables or by NIR

G. Masoero, R. Rubino, G. Morone. Istituto Sperimentale Zootecnia, Via Pianezza 115, 10151, Torino, Italy*

Thyrthy-two pigs from six experimental groups grew under different conditions in two herds, according to the confinement vs open air, the disposable surfaces and the feedstuffes. One seventh control group was constituted by pigs on pasture. A body of 40 variables from slaughtering, L.D. muscle and backfat were analysed. NIR spectra was recorded on freeze-dried L.D. muscle. Binary contrast matrices were builded on NIR by stepwise regression or on LAB40 variates by Modified Partial Least Squares chemometric methods. Clusters of these matrices indicate the relative position of the seven groups. In general between-group variability was high, the most relevant being: C14:0_backfat (Miristic, R2=0.51), free lipids in muscle (R2=0.49), C20:1(ω9)_backfat (Eicosenoic, R2=0.49), C18:1(ω9) _backfat (Oleic, R2=0.47) and other 15 variables with R2>0.30. The NIR was fitted to lipids (R2=0.98), C18:3(ω3)_muscle (Alfa-Linolenic, R2=089), C18:3(ω6) *backfat (Gamma-Linolenic,* R^2*=0.79), C20:1(ω9)*_backfat (Eicosenoic, R^2=0.78), C22:4(ω6)_backfat (Docosatetraenoic, DTA,R^2=0.75).In four cases LAB and NIR evaluations agreed in confirming that the cycle within herd was the most important factor than the management of the available space. On the contrary in another herd with byproducts the available space was a dominant factor, whole appreciated by NIR and by LAB. Pigs on pasture where clusterized near a conventional product by NIR or relatively discarded from another cycle of the same herd.

Poster NP6.12

Meat quality of Lithuanian wattle pigs slaughtered at different live weight

V. Razmaite, Lithuanian Institute of Animal Science, R. Zebenkos 12, LT-5125 Baisogala, Radviliskis distr., Lithuania.

According to the sequence of conservation and research of the critical Lithuanian indigenous wattle pigs after the formation of the closed herd, investigation of biological, farming qualities and preparation of evaluation standards, the next step should be the search for possibilities of their wider use in pork production. In order to have leaner carcasses the most likely use of these fat pigs should be in crossbreeding, organic production or slaughter at lower live weight. If the average weight of indigenous pigs was increase from 57 to 102 kg, the lean meat content of carcass has decrease by 9.5% (P<0.001). At the same time the chemical composition and analytical meat characteristics have improved. Significant differences were determined between dry matter (P<0.001) and fat (P<0.025) in the meat of pigs slaughtered at 55-60 and 97-102 kg weight. When the weight of pigs at slaughter was increased, the ratio of tryptophane and oxyproline (P<0.005) and fat melting temperature (P<0.025 - P<0.010) have also increased, but cooking losses (P<0.005) decreased. Pigs of 97-102 kg weight were found to have poorer quality of carcasses but the highest quality of meat. Feed intake (including the feed intake to obtain a piglet) was the lowest when indigenous wattle pigs were grown up to 80 kg weight.

Poster NP6.13

Comparison of the performances of Nero Siciliano pigs reared indoors and outdoors: chemical- physical traits of fresh meat and fat

C. Pugliese[1], G. Gandini[2], G. Madonia[3], A. D'Amico[3], V. Chiofalo[4] and O. Franci[1]. [1]Università di Firenze, Italy, [2]Università di Milano, Italy, [3]Istituto Sperimentale Zootecnico per la Sicilia, Palermo, Italy, [4]Polo Universitario Annunziata, Messina, Italy.

A total of 78 Nero Siciliano pigs were used. Forty-one pigs were reared on natural pastures, which included woods, mainly composed of *Quercus* and Fagus *genus,* grasslands and Mediterranean bush. Thirty-seven pigs were reared in pens and fed to appetite using commercial rations. The slaughter weigth was 101.9 and 88.2 kg for indoor and outdoor pigs respectively. As regard ham dissection, outdoor-pig showed the highest percentages of lean (58 vs 55 %) and the lowest of subcutaneous fat (31 vs 134 %). Analysis were carried out on the *Longissimus lomborum.* Outdoor-pigs showed higher intramuscular fat percentage (4.3 vs 3.3 %), lower protein content (22.2 vs. 23.4 %), lower pH_{45} (5.89 vs. 6.32) and higher free water (9.6 vs 7.9 cm^2). As regard colour parameters, outdoor pigs produced more reflecting (50 vs. 46.7 L*) and more coloured (0.368 vs 0.310 Hue) meat. Concerning the fatty acid composition of subcutaneous fat, outdoor-pig showed higher percentage of MUFA (53.3 vs. 47.2 %) and lower of PUFA (10.85 vs. 14.45 %), because of the lowest percentage of PUFA *n-6*, indeed no differences were found for PUFA *n-3*. Finally, outdoor-pigs had lower indexes of atherogenicity (0.48 vs 0.53) and thrombogenicity (1.03 vs 1.21).

Poster NP6.14

Carcass and meat traits of Cinta Senese pigs fed diets with different levels of protein

F. Sirtori, C. Pugliese, R. Bozzi, L. Pianaccioli, M. Badii. Dipartimento di Scienze Zootecniche, Università di Firenze, Via delle Cascine 5, 50144 Firenze, Italy.

The aim of the work was to identify the level of crude protein that optimise the performance of Cinta senese breed. Sixty pigs, females and barrows, were reared indoor in four groups balanced for sex. Initial live weight was on average 45 kg. Each group received one of four diets characterised by different levels of protein, 8, 10, 13 and 16 % (D8, D10, D13, D16) and the same energy level. D8 showed the lowest ADG (at 300 days from trial start: 137 kg for diet 8% vs 150 kg on average for others) while no differences were found among the other diets. Fat thickness evolution was no strictly affect by protein level. D8 only discriminated carcass composition with lower percentage of lean cuts than D10, D13, D16 (56.9, 61.1, 60.7, 60.9 % respectively), and higher fat cuts (37.5, 33.2, 33.9, 33.7 %). Sample joint dissection reflects the carcass composition with D8 showing the lowest value of meat percentage (35.4, 41.3, 39.9, 39.5 %) and highest of fat percentage (55, 48, 49.5, 50.3 %).

Poster NP6.15

Low levels of N, P vitamins and minerals in the diets of heavy pigs: effect on performance, carcass characteristics and excretions of N, P and trace elements

M. Morlacchini[1], A. Prandini[2], C. Cerioli[2] and G. Piva[2], [1]CERZOO, 29100 Piacenza, Italy, [2]ISAN, Agricultural Faculty, 29100 Piacenza, Italy.

A trial was carried out using 240 pigs D x (LW x L). Animals were fed from 40 to 160 kg l.w. with 4 diets: 1) basal diet (CTR) without synthetic amino acid added; 2) lower levels of nitrogen (-20%), lysine (-10%) *vs* CTR but according to I.N.R.A. ideal protein adding synthetic lysine, and Ca (-50% from 80 kg l.w. *vs* CTR diet); 3) as diet 2) without mineral premix and only A, D and E vitamins added from 80 to 160 kg l.w.; 4) as diet 3) but with 700 U/kg feed of microbial phytase added. Pigs were fed with a wet diet (2.5:1 water:meal) at 9% of the metabolic weight. The reduction of N and lysine levels and the depletion of inorganic P and trace elements in the diets did not reduce growing performances and feed efficiency of animals *vs* CTR. Slaughtering parameters and fresh ham quality did not differ among dietary treatments. Diets 4 from 40 to 160 kg l.w. reduced nitrogen and P excretions and nitrogen and lysine intake of 20.2%, 30.7%, 20.3% and 9.5%/kg weight gain *vs* CTR, respectively. Using diets 3 and 4 trace elements excretions were significantly decreased.

Poster NP6.16

Effect of genotype and feeding on parameters of fattening, slaughter and meat quality of pigs slaughtered

J.Gundel[1], Hermán A. Ms.[1], Szelényi M. Ms.[1], A.Király[1], Regius Á. Ms.[1], P.Szabó[2], I.Bodó[2], S.Mihók[2], [1]Research Institute for Animal Breeding and Nutrition, 2053 Herceghalom, Hungary, [2]University of Debrecen, Centre of Agricultural Science, P.O. Box 36, 4032 Debrecen, Hungary*

Presently there are significant differences in most of the quality parameters of pig carcasses. Unfortunately, so far only few pig breeders and experts of pork industry have realized this problem. Only lean meat content was in focus. This paper summarizes and briefly introduces an experiment which was carried out with Large White x Landrace and Mangalica genotypes. Current and traditional feeding system was used, and animals were kept until 130 kg slaughter weight. The effect of genotypes, feeding systems and slaughter weight was studied. Traditional slaughtering age at 130 kg was prolonged by 7 % at LWxL and by 6 % at Mangalicas with diet as compared to current diet. The age-difference of the two breeds at reaching the slaughter weight was 26-28 %. Proportion of valuable lean meat, the quantity of lean meat and lard was slightly influenced by the higher slaughtering weight. Results of this experiment support that a traditional genotype can not utilize more nutrients than its requirement determined in empirical way. If slaughter weight was increased to 130 kg in LWxL then daily weight gain decreased significantly (by 7-10%). The effect of slaughter weight was less dramatic (4% decrease) on daily weight gain in Mangalica breed.

Poster NP6.17

Meat quality and pigs growth duration correlative connections

A. Jemeljanovs[1], R. Kaugers[1], E. Ramins[1], A. Stira[1], I. Jansons[1] and J. Zutis[2], [1]Research Centre "Sigra" of the Latvia University of Agriculture, Instituta Street 1, Sigulda LV-2150, Latvia, [2]Latvian Association of Meat Producers and Meat Processors, Dzirnavu Street 42, Riga LV-1010, Latvia

In Latvia 189 pigs carcasses were tested in different meat processing enterprises. Remarkable pigs realization weight range has been ascertained and connection with pigs growth duration. Live weight was positively correlated with the day mass increase (r=0.38; P<0.01) and with animals growth time (r=0.35; P<0.01). With the increase of realization weight and growth duration were several coherences established: protein content was reduced in muscle *longissimus dorsi* (r=-0.27; P<0.01), but intramuscular fat content increased (r=0.23, P<0.01). In case of heavier animals was changed ratio of amino acids in protein. With growth of realization weight enlarged oxyproline content (r=0.44; P<0.001), according to it narrowed the ratio limit of triptophane/oxyproline and reduced the value of protein. But intramuscular fat (marbling fat) content enlargement in *m.longissimus dorsi*, indicator of muscle tissue quality, can by regarded as improvement of production sensor qualities. For younger pigs - with smaller realization weight was ascertained intramuscular fat content lower than 2%, that is regarded as neutral for flavour, or flavour less. Supplementary was established rather norrow, but essential connection of intramuscular fat and triptophane quantities (r=-0.20; P<0.05), and direct positive correlative coherency of intramuscular fat and phosphorus amounts, too (r=0.63; P<0.01). For meat quality evaluation essential is genetic origin, too.

Poster NP6.18

Quality of "Zampone Modena PGI" and "Mortadella Bologna PGI" produced with meat and fat of heavy pigs fed with high linoleic acid diets

A. Pizza[1], G. Barbieri[1], R. Pedrielli[1], M. Bergamaschi[1], G. Della Casa[2], A. Rossi[3], [1]Stazione Sperimentale per l'Industria delle Conserve Alimentari, 43100 Parma, Italy, [2]Istituto Sperimentale per la Zootecnia S.O.P. di Modena, 41018 S.Cesario, Italy, [3]Fondazione CRPA-Studi e Ricerche ONLUS, 42100 Reggio Emilia, Italy.*

"Zampone Modena" (ZM) and "Mortadella Bologna"(MB) are produced by PGI disciplinary with frozen heavy pigs meat and fat, whose origin and quality largely influence the characteristics of final products.

Forty Duroc x Large White pigs were randomly assigned to two dietary treatments:

1) Moderate linoleic acid diets (<2% on dry matter), control diet (C); 2) High linoleic acid diets (<3% on dry matter) (HL) with added soy oil (3%).

After slaughtering, meat and fat cuts were selected according to ZM and MB production rules, frozen at -15°C and stored for 13,208 or 322 days at -15°C or -30°C.

ZM and MB produced with HL meat showed a poorer quality at all the production times. Since the first test it is found for MB HL poorer smell (5.25±0.89) and taste (5.50±0.53), lower hardness (1.54±0.28 N) and resistance to chewing (6.75±0.89). The defects of raw meat increase ordinary mistakes of processing conditions, such as the fluctuation of temperature during frozen storage. Prolonged storage resulted in an increase in the TBAR's values (0.24±0.003 ppm) and oiliness of the slice and a reduction in adhesiveness of fat cubes.

Predicting feed intake from body measurements on heavy pigs

S. Schiavon[1], L. Gallo[1], P. Carnier[1], F. Tagliapietra[1], A. Piva[2], A. Prandini[3], M. Morlacchini[4], A. Mordenti[2], G. Piva[3], [1]Department of Animal Science, Agripolis, 35020 Legnaro (PD), Italy, [2]DIMORFIPA, I-40064 Ozzano Emilia (BO), Italy, [3] ISAN, Agricultural Faculty, 29100 Piacenza, Italy, [4]CERZOO, 29100 Piacenza, Italy.*

A set of functions to estimate feed intake from body measurements was evaluated. Over 3 years, 920 Goland boars were fed *ad lib.*, for 54±2 d, a diet containing 12.4 MJ/kg of effective energy (EE). Individual feed intakes, initial and final live weight (77.4±7.4 and 136.6±12.8 kg, LW) and backfat thickness (8.3±1.3 and 13.5±2.4 mm, BCK), were recorded. Body lipid percentage was estimated as: 4.44+0.69*BCK; equation developed on heavy pig. Fat free mass was partitioned into protein (P), water and ash by using literature relationships. EE used for maintenance was computed as $1.63*P^{0.73}$, that used for protein (Pr) and lipid (Lr) retention was assumed to be 50 and 56 MJ EE/kg. Measured (MFI) and predicted (PFI) feed intakes were on average 2.803 and 2.784 kg/d. MFI was analysed for batch, initial and final LW and BCK, $LW^{0.73}$, eating time, number of meals. In another model body measurements were replaced by PFI. The two models had the same R^2 (0.83), similar variance composition and rsd (0.196 and 0.202 kg/d). Correlation between residues was 0.97. The set of functions used provided good estimates of feed intake and body composition changes. Average Pr and Lr were 198±35 and 204±59 g/d.

 Theatre CMNS1.1

Product quality attributes associated with outdoor pig production

S.A. Edwards, University of Newcastle, School of Agriculture Food and Rural Development, King George VI Building, Newcastle upon Tyne NE1 7RU, UK.

Outdoor pig production offers animals increased environmental diversity and behavioural freedom but imposes challenges for breed adaptation, management control, biosecurity, and environmental protection. Each of these issues has potential implications for the real and perceived quality of the product. In most conventional Northern European production systems, only adult and suckling animals are at pasture. However, in traditional Mediterranean systems and in organic production systems, meat animals may be maintained outdoors throughout their lives. Major influences on organoleptic quality of product derive from the choice of breeds most appropriate to outdoor systems, modifications to growth rate and the increased proportion of forage in the diet. Indirect consequences may also result from both positive and negative influences on physiological stress responses in the pre-slaughter period. Whilst some aspects of animal health and hygiene may be improved in more extensive conditions, exposure to parasites and to contact with wildlife may increase zoonotic infection risk. Perceptual attributes of product quality may be either positively or negatively influenced, depending on the ethical attitudes of consumers and the quality of management and husbandry in outdoor pig units which are visible to the public. The extent to which real and perceived differences in product quality are reflected in changed economic value is more a function of marketing than production system.

Theatre CMNS1.2

Extensive bedded indoor and outdoor pig production systems in USA: Current trends and effects on animal care and product quality

M.S. Honeyman, Iowa State University, Department of Animal Science, B1 Curtiss Hall, Ames, IA USA*

Extensive bedded indoor and outdoor pig production in USA has expanded due to growing niche markets for natural and organic pork. Bedded hoop (tent-like) barns and bedded converted poultry barns are used for finishing pigs and gestating sows. Seasonal outdoor farrowing and some indoor bedded farrowing systems coupled with group lactation are also used. Most niche markets require outdoor or bedded settings, no sub-therapeutic antibiotics or growth promotants, no animal by-products in feed, and a family farm production setting. Finishing pigs in hoop barns consume some bedding, have more backfat and smaller loin area, and lower carcass yield compared with confinement-fed pigs. Hoop-fed pigs had fewer aberrant behaviors and handled easier than confinement pigs. Health differences were minor except for an increased incidence of internal parasites in hoop-fed pigs. Pigs in hoops are in larger groups than in confinement, thus husbandry skills are distinct. Biosecurity in hoops is more difficult due to incoming bedding and open access for birds and feral animals. Hoop-fed pig growth performance varies depending on thermal environment, which is closely related to season and climate. Bedded hoop barns with individual feeding stalls provide an acceptable environment for gestating sows. Overall, product quality differences are relatively minor compared with wide variations in rearing environment for extensively-reared pigs.

Sustaining animal health and food safety in European organic livestock farming

M.Vaarst[*1], M.Hovi[2], A. Sundrum[3], D.Younie[4] and S.Padel[5], [1]DIAS, P.O.Box 50, DK-8830 Tjele, [2]VEERU, The University of Reading, POBox 237, UK-RG6 6AR-Reading, [3]University of Kassel, Nordbahnhofstr. 1a, D-37213 Witzenhausen [4]SAC, Craibstone Estate, AB219YA, Aberdeen, [5]IRS University of Wales, Llanbardarn Campus, Llanbardarn Fawr, SY233AL, Aberystwyth*

In Europe, organic livestock production has experienced rapid growth in the past decade, and not without problems. Whilst emphasising the importance of a systems approach to animal health and welfare protection, organic livestock production standards place considerable restrictions on the use of many animal health inputs that are routinely used in conventional production systems. Recommended practices in the European Organic Livestock Standards (EU Regulation 1804/1999) such as closed herds and flocks and improved health security on farms, also include extensive production systems that expose livestock to increased disease challenge. Organic livestock production faces major challenges with regard to harmonisation and successful integration of organic animal husbandry into the organic production system. Major questions about food quality and safety exist. Significant diversity between farming systems between European countries including candidate countries, should be taken into account in developing farming systems that comply with common EU standards, but are in harmony with their geographic and cultural localities. A newly initiated EU network project (SAFO) with 26 partners in Europe focuses on the integration of animal health and welfare issues with food safety aspects. Important key questions of this network project will be presented, and suggestions to future improvements will be discussed.

Theatre CMNS1.4

Improvement of health and welfare of dairy cows and fattening pigs in 'animal friendly' housing systems

G. Regula, J. Danuser, B. Spycher and A. Cagienard, Federal Veterinary Office, Schwarzenburgstr. 161, CH-3003 Bern, Switzerland.*

Indicators for the assessment of health and welfare on farms were established and validated. These indicators were used to evaluate the impact of 'animal friendly' housing on dairy cows and fattening pigs.

Health and welfare were compared among 136 dairy farms with three different production systems: traditional tie stalls, tie stalls providing regular exercise in an outdoor yard, and freestalls with regular exercise outdoors. Gait abnormalities, skin lesions at the tarsal joints and teat injuries were found less frequently in freestalls compared to tie stalls. Fewer treatments with antibiotics were recorded in freestalls than in tie stalls. Tie stalls with regular exercise differed from traditional tie stalls in a lower prevalence of gait abnormalities and teat injuries.

On 84 swine fattening farms, health and welfare of pigs was compared among traditional indoor farms with slatted floor pens, and farms providing straw bedding and an outdoor yard. 'Animal friendly' farms had a lower prevalence of recumbent pigs, tail biting, skin injuries at carpal and tarsal joints, and skin alterations at the snout. Pigs were also found to be dog sitting less frequently in 'animal friendly' farms. Sunburn was observed in a few 'animal friendly' farms only.

Overall, it could be shown that the 'animal friendly' systems had a substantial positive effect on health and welfare of the animals.

Quality control on dairy farms, with emphasis on food safety, animal health and animal welfare

J.P.T.M.Noordhuizen[1] and J.H.M. Metz[2], [1]Dept. of Farm Animal Health, Faculty of Veterinary Medicine, Utrecht University, PO Box 80151, 3508 TD Utrecht, The Netherlands; [2]Dept. of Agrotechnology & Food Sciences, Farm Technology Group, Wageningen University, PO Box 43, 6700 AH Wageningen, The Netherlands*

BSE and chronic wasting in cattle have alarmed the consumer with regard to the way animal production takes place. This has given way to the "EU white book" on food safety and consumer protection, next to new regulations and directives on hygiene related to food production. Consumers show increasing influence on animal production. This is reflected in demands of retailers for on-farm production. Farm status monitoring should be based on biological needs regarding welfare and health, while attention should be given to risks in the animals' surroundings. Animal health has impact on herd performance but also affects public health because some disease agents can be transferred to man. Because food safety impacts on both market share and public image of dairy companies, the latter counteracted by chain-based integrated quality assurance programmes. Since recently those programmes comprise the dairy farm too. Examples of the latter can be found in EU-member states. Animal health and welfare, and public health and food safety can be considered to be features of quality in its broadest sense, concerning product and production process. In this presentation these issues are addressed and components of an integrated quality control programme highlighted by means of the Dutch example.

Theatre CMNS1.6

Herd health in dairy farming systems in Pays de la Loire (France)

C. Fourichon, H. Seegers, N. Bareille and F. Beaudeau, Veterinary School - INRA, Unit of Animal Health Management, BP 40706, 44307 Nantes, France*

Influence of farming system on herd health is often questionned and could result from different risks and different health management options in different systems. The objective of this study was to compare the herd health in farming systems classified according to intensification of the dairy production. Herd health was assessed through overall economic impact of production diseases (called disease costs), i.e. the sum of losses consecutive to disease effects and disease control expenditures. Diseases cases and expenditures were recorded in 197 farms during two years. Losses were calculated by partial budgeting for 21 health and reproduction disorders. Farms were classified into 8 categories of intensification according to breed, age at 1st calving, concentrates, maize silage, and average milk yield. Few differences were evidenced for each disease incidence between farming systems. Average expenditures, losses and total costs varied from 62 to 94, 125 to 184, and 204 to 278 €/cow-year between categories, respectively. Intensification was not systematically associated with higher disease costs. On average, the two most intensive categories had the highest expenditures but one had the highest losses whereas the other one had the lowest ones. Higher expenditures in intensive systems probably resulted from different health management options (wider use of preventive measures or systematic treatments) rather than from poorer health status.

Organic beef production with emphasis on welfare, health and product quality

B.K. Nielsen, Organic Animal Husbandry, Department of Animal Science and Animal Health, Royal Veterinary and Agricultural University, Groennegårdsvej 2, 1870 Frederiksberg C, Denmark.

This paper gives an overview of organic beef production in Denmark with emphasis on welfare, health and product quality of organic dairy bred steers. Organic beef production is based on grazing in the summertime, feeding of minimum 60% of roughage during whole the year and the ban of GMO and hormones. However, problems with parasites and periodically feeding with high amounts of cereals results in reduced welfare and health problems. The feeding strategies as well as systems used in organic steer production seem to assure general healthy animals. However several issues should be mentioned. Finishing conditions can mean metabolic disorders, summer grazing can result in parasite infections, especially on marginal areas. Management strategies in relation to turn-out and to prevent parasite infections are important tools to secure healthy animals. Increased attention should be given to product quality of organic beef. Feeding with high amounts of roughage and usage of feedstuffs with bioactive forages seems to improve product quality by among others increasing the content of CLA, that are expected to have healthy effect in humans.

Poster CMNS1.8

Microbial quality of silages produced in Portugal : contamination with *Listeria monocytogenes*

M.M. Guerra, and F.A. Bernardo, Laboratório de Inspecçao Sanitária/CIISA, Faculdade de Medicina Veterinária, Universidade Técnica de Lisboa. Rua Prof. Cid dos Santos, Polo Universitário da Ajuda, 1300-247 Lisboa, Portugal.

Silage consumption has been frequently associated to listeriosis in ruminants and considered to be the main way which leads to milk contamination in farms. Many cases result from the consumption of low-quality, improperly fermented silage having a pH of >4.0, where *L. monocytogenes* can proliferate reaching levels >10^6 cfu/g. To assess the microbiological quality of silages produced in Portugal, 71 samples were investigated for the presence of *Listeria spp.* by conventional bacteriological methods. Samples with 25 g were suspended and pre-enriched on Peptone Buffer Water and a selective enrichment on UVM I was performed during 48h at 30°C followed by plating on Palcam agar and incubated at 30°C for 48h. Four or five presumptive *Listeria* colonies were subcultured for purity on Triptone-Soya Agar with 0,6% of Yeast-Extract and were biochemically identified. Enumeration of *Listeria* spp. on Palcam agar was also determined in 43 samples and a quantitative assessment of the lactic acid microflora and moulds was determined in 18 samples, using MRS and CRB. Twenty samples were contaminated (28%), 10 with *L. monocytogenes* (14%) and 10 with *L. innocua* (14%). Only *L. innocua* was isolated from two of the enumerated samples with numbers of 10^6 cfu/g. Levels of lactic acid microflora were from 9,9x10^4 to 5,5x10^8 cfu/g and for the moulds, from <100 to > 1x10^7 cfu/g. These preliminary results presented here, indicate a possible risk of *Listeria* transmission from silages in Portugal.

 Poster CMNS1.9

Animal husbandry and animal health - Knowledge transfer via Internet

M. Andres. German Centre for Documentation and Information in Agriculture (ZADI), Villichgasse 17, 53177 Bonn, Germany

Effective animal husbandry depends on management methods which consider all aspects of animal behaviour and animal health. Veterinarians, administrators, and farmers need up-to-date information on legal conditions in animal husbandry and veterinary medicine as well as information on the production and use of feedstuffs and veterinary drugs. Alternative farming methods influence techniques and procedures in animal husbandry and veterinary control and lead to an increasing demand for up-to-date information. Meanwhile, a lot of official responsible institutions are publishing these information on the Internet. Portals and systems offer access to various kinds of information resources as documents, articles, reports, descriptions of projects, factual data, figures and discussion platforms. Agricultural information systems as the German Agricultural Information Network (dainet) allow a central overview on subject-related portals for animal husbandry, health control and animal welfare. Online searchable databases, integrated in this network, contain information on animal diseases and details on farming enterprises which are controlled by the veterinary administration. In addition, information about institutions responsible for veterinary tasks and disease control can be found. Important examples of information resources, databases and institutional Internet sites are described.

Poster CMNS1.10

Genetic parameters of preweaning growth traits of Egyptian Zaraibi kids

E.Z.M. Oudah[1]; Z.M.K. Ibrahim[1]; A.I. Haider[2] and M. Helmy[1], [1]Department of Animal Production, Faculty of Agriculture, Mansoura University, 35516, Egypt [2]Sheep and Goats Research Division, APRI, Egypt.

Records of biweekly live weight (LBW) from birth to 12 wk of 562 Egyptian Zaraibi kids progeny of 17 sires and 296 dams born during the period from 1999 to 2000 were used. The overall mean of LBW at birth, 2, 4, 6, 8, 10 and 12 wk of age were 2.2, 4.6, 5.9, 7.4, 8.9, 10.8 and 11.3 kg, respectively. Hertiabilty estimates of LBWs were medium to high ranged 0.273 to 0.422. Average daily gains (ADG) from 0-4, 0-8, 0-12, 4-8, 4-12 and 8-12 wk of age were 110, 109, 100, 98, 90 and 80 g/d, respectively. Heritability estimates of ADGs were low to high ranged 0.138 to 0.352. The effect of sire (as random effect) on LBWs was significant on at all studied traits and on ADGs were significant on all traits except 0-8 and 4-8 wk of age. The effects of season and type of kidding, sex of kid (as fixed effects) and dam weight and birth weight (as covariates) on LBWs and ADGs during different ages were also studied. Ranges of transmitting ability estimated using Best Linear Unbiased Predictor method (BLUP) were 0.330, 1.20, 1.18,1.30, 1.68, 1.89 and 1.32 kg for LBWs, respectively and 34.1, 25.7, 12.7, 21.3 and 27.6 g/d for ADGs, respectively.

Monitoring herd performance in dairy farms using Test-Day models

J. Vasconcelos[*,1] and J. Carvalheira[1,2], [1]Centro de Investigação em Biodiversidade e Recursos Genéticos (CIBIO-ICETA) - Universidade do Porto, Rua Padre Armando Quintas-Crasto, 4485-661 Vairão, PORTUGAL, [2]Instituto de Ciências Biomédicas de Abel Salazar (ICBAS) - Universidade do Porto*

The objectives of this study were to analyse the ability of an autoregressive test-day (TD) animal model to monitor management factors affecting herd performance in a monthly basis. TD data were used to estimate systematic environmental effects to evaluate schemes of herd management and individual cow productivity on a farm basis. Management curves, lactation curves and predictions of daily and cumulative yields were updated every month, showing the dynamics of each herd and were translated into a series of tables and graphics for further analysis. Management curves indicate the within-year variation in average daily yield and seasonal effects on quality, availability and cost of feed. These estimates are adjusted to a common age, stage of lactation, genetic differences and random environmental residuals. They represent herd production as if all cows were at the same age, stage of lactation, etc., on every TD. As an indicator of the farmer's feeding and management program, management curves shows what the cows would have produced if they were all the same. An example with the performance of a farm for a period of one year is discussed. This information may provide farmers and consultants with a better understanding of the dairy farm enterprise and contribute for a greater efficiency.

Poster CMNS1.12

Effects of parity on physiology and production performance of Comisana ewes exposed to solar radiation under high ambient temperature

A. Sevi[1], L. Taibi[2], M. Albenzio[1], G. Annicchiarico[2], P. Centoducati[3], A. Muscio[1], [1]Dipartimento PRIME. Facoltà di Agraria, 71100 Foggia, Italy, [2]Istituto Sperimentale per la Zootecnia; Segezia-Foggia, Italy; [3]Dipartimento di Sanità, Patologia, Farmaco-Tossicologia e Benessere degli Animali, 70010 Valenzano-Bari, Italy.

Thirty-two Comisana ewes were included in this study, with eight ewes each in parities 2 (P2), 3 (P3), 4 (P4) and 5 (P5). Groups were separately penned in a prefabricated building during a 7-day period and then exposed to solar radiation in unshaded pens for other 21 days. Rectal temperatures (RT), respiration rates (RR), cell-mediated immune response, concentrations of plasma metabolites and enzyme were monitored during the trial. Ewe milk yield was recorded daily and were analysed weekly for milk composition, coagulating properties and somatic cell count. The P5 ewes had significantly lower ($P < 0.001$) respiration rates than the P2 and P3 ewes. The P2 ewes displayed higher plasma concentrations of LDH and of AST/GOT than did the ewes in the three other groups and higher levels of ALT/GPT ($P < 0.01$) than the P4 and P5 ewes. The plasma concentration of magnesium was higher ($P < 0.01$) in the P5 than in the P2 group. Results suggest that exposure to solar radiation under high ambient temperatures has a stronger impact on the metabolism and production performance of ewes lower in parity.

 Poster CMNS1.13

Influence of ventilation regimen on air quality and on ewe milk yield in summer

A. Sevi[1], L. Taibi[2], M. Albenzio[1], G. Annicchiarico[2], R. Marino[1], M. Caroprese[1], [1]Dipartimento PRIME. Università di Foggia, Via Napoli25, 71100 Foggia, Italy, [2]Istituto Sperimentale per la Zootecnia. Sezione Operativa di Segezia-Foggia (Italy).

The effects of ventilation regimen (summer 2002) were assessed on 36 Comisana ewes subjected to the following treatments: low ventilation regimen (LOV) providing a mean ventilation rate (VR) of 35 m^3/h per ewe (30 min ventilation cycles; air speed 2 m/s); two moderate ventilation regimen MOV-SH = 70 m^3/h per ewe; 30 min ventilation cycles; air speed 4 m/s and MOV-LN = 70 m^3/h per ewe; 60 min ventilation cycles; air speed 2 m/s. During the trial were monitored: air concentrations of microorganisms, dust, and gaseous pollutants; respiration rate, rectal temperature, behavioral traits, cell-mediated immune response and humoral response to ovalbumin of the ewes. Individual milk samples were analyzed weekly for composition, renneting parameters and somatic cell count, and fortnightly for bacteriological characteristics. Significant interactions of treatment x time ($P < 0.05$) were found for respiration rate, and for the time the ewes spent lying, idling and eating in the afternoon. Significant effects of ventilation regimen x time ($P < 0.05$) were also observed for milk yield and milk renneting parameters. Results show firstly that ventilation regimen had a very moderate impact on ewe behavior, physiology and production performance, and secondly that the length of ventilation cycles and air speed, together with ventilation rate, are critical for efficient ventilation regimens.

Poster CMNS1.14

Effect of breed and nutrition on carcass and beef quality traits

G. Holló[1], Z. Andrássy[1], Cs. Ábrahám[2], J. Seenger[2], R. Zándoki[2], J. Seregi[1], I. Repa[1] and I. Holló[1], University of Kaposvár, Kaposvár 7401, [2]St István University, Gödöllö 2103, Hungary.*

The effect of feeding extensive (E) vs. intensive (I) diets on carcass and meat quality was compared using Holstein-Friesian (HF) and Hungarian Grey (HG) growing-finishing bulls (N=40) in this study. Means of initial weight and age of HF and HG were 293±36 kg and 321±69 day, resp. Half of the breed groups were fed either grass silage/grass and low concentrate (E) or maize silage and high concentrate (I) based rations. Higher slaughter weights were recorded in I groups in comparison with that of measured in groups E ($P<0.001$). After a 24hr chilling longissimus samples were taken from the right half carcasses. Data processing made by SPSS 10.0. Carcass weight and length, amount of perinephric and trimmed fat were higher in groups I ($P<0.01$). Higher lean meat content in carcass was recorded in HG breed (E: 71.0 and I: 67.5%, respectively). The dry matter and crude fat content of the longissimus of the E groups are significantly lower, and contain from the minerals less Na, Cu, but more Fe, P, than the I groups. In conclusion, the different feeding methods have a significant effect on the slaughter value and beef quality. The utilization of the native HG breed on development of novel beef cattle production systems especially on roughage-based diets seems to be justified.

 Poster CMNS1.15

Use of oil extracts from *Callendula oficinalis* and *Medicago sativa* in broiler feeding

Rodica Criste, Doina Grossu, Manuela Chetea, Ionelia Taranu, Institute of Biology & Animal Nutrition, 8113 Balotesti, Romania*

The experiment used 3 groups of Cobb500 broilers raised for 6 weeks in metabolic cages. The broilers received the same diet consisting of corn, soybean meal and fish meal, but theyreceived different amounts of vitamin-mineral premix. The control group (C) received 1% premix developed by IBNA, while in group E1, 50% of the premix of group C was replaced by the oil extract of *Callendula oficinalis*, and in group E2, 50% of the premix of group C was replaced by the oil extract of *Medicago sativa*. The oil extracts (stabilised by addition of vitamin E) were put on sunflower oil carrier obtained by cool pressing. the oil/plant ratio being 5/1.
Broiler performance, A, E, B1 and B2 vitamin level, fatty acids and cholesterol level in the extracts, feeds, serum and liver were monitored.
Broiler performance (gain, intake) didn't differ among groups; serum vitamin A level, sampled in the end of the experiment, was higher in the experimental groups (525 IU/100ml in E1 and 467 IU/ 100ml in E2) than in the control group (371.33 IU/100ml), which shows diet balancing in vitamin A content by oil extracts treatment. Saturated vs. unsaturated fatty acids ratio was slightly favourable to the unsaturated fatty acids in the experimental groups, with no significant difference between groups; blood cholesterol was significantly lower in the treated groups.

Poster CMNS1.16

Effect of *Helmox* antioxidant on protecting the water-soluble vitamins (A and E) from poultry feed ingredients

M. Chetea[1], D.V. Grossu[1], R. D. Criste[1], A. Bercaru[1], D.I. Holban[2], J. Neculce[2], M. Bejenaru[2], [1]Institute of Biology and Animal Nutrition, Balotesti, Romania; [2]Faculty of Veterinary Medicine Chisinau, Republic Moldova*

The following categories of samples were used to assess the effect of *Helmox* antioxidant on protecting the water-soluble vitamins from poultry feed ingredients: compound feeds, formula 21-1 and 21-2, supplemented with fats, treated and not treated with 125 ppm and 250 ppm *Helmox*. The relative loss of vitamins A and E was monitored through out 90 days of storage, with determination every 15 days.
The effect of *Helmox* on vitamin A is evident -vitamin level remained constant 45 days for the 125 ppm treatment and 60 days for the 250 ppm treatment, the differences between treatments not being significant; we therefore recommend using the 125 ppm dose.
The level of vitamin E from the compound feed not treated with *Helmox* displayed a drastic decrease after 90 days, while in the treated compound feeds the relative loss of vitamin E was up to 19% for the 125 ppm treatment and 9.5% for the 250 ppm treatment.
This significant decrease may be accounted for by the involvement of the vitamin in the reactions inhibiting selfoxidation, because it is a natural antioxidant protecting both vitamin A and the fat. The dose of 250 ppm *Helmox* was the most efficient in protecting the level of vitamin E.

Poster CMNS1.17

Alleviation of physical and chemical agents' action on poultry feed ingredients

M. Olteanu[1], D.V. Grossu[1], R.D. Criste[1], A. Bercaru[1], D.I. Holban[2], J. Neculce[2], M. Bejenaru[2], [1]Institute of Biology and Animal Nutrition, Balotesti, Romania; [2]Faculty of Veterinary Medicine Chisinau, Republic Moldova*

The alleviation of physical and chemical agents' action on feeds is done with antioxidants. The following categories of samples were used to assess the effect of *Helmox* antioxidant on poultry feed ingredients: plant fat (sunflower oil, sunflower + soybean oil) and compound feed, formula 21-1 and 21-2, supplemented with fats, treated and not treated with 125 ppm and 250 ppm *Helmox*.

The rate of fat degradation indices (acidity and peroxide) increase was monitored through out 90 days of storage. The oils treated with *Helmox* were protected for a period of 30 days from getting rancid, while the non-treated oils displayed changes after 15 days. The oil mixture (sunflower + soybean) displayed significantly ($p<0.05$) different results compared to the sunflower oil. The differences between the oils treated with 125 ppm and with 250 ppm antioxidant were not significant; therefore we don't recommend using the 250 ppm dose.

The rate of acidity and peroxide indices increase in the compound feed was significantly lower ($p<0.05$) in all the samples treated with 125 and 250 ppm *Helmox* compared to the untreated samples. However, there were no significant differences between the results obtained with the dose of 125 and 250 ppm respectively; therefore we don't recommend using the 250 ppm dose.

Poster CMNS1.18

Pathomorphological pattern of the liver in Pomeranian lambs and crossbreeds of Pomeranian ewes with Berrichion-du-Cher rams

J. Szarek[1], H. Brzostowski[2], Z. Tanski[2], A. Andrzejewska[3], J. Lipinska[1] and J. Sowinska[2], [1]Faculty of Veterinary Medicine, [2]Faculty of Animal Bioengineering, University of Warmia and Mazury in Olsztyn, 10-717 Olsztyn, Poland, 3Medical Academy, 15-269 Bialystok, Poland*

The production of good quality lamb meat can be obtained, among others, by various crossbreeding. The aim of this study was to examine the effect of the breeds used for crossbreeding on liver pathomorphological pattern in the resulting crossbreeds. The investigations were carried out on 50- and 100-day old young rams of meat and wool sheep line origin (Pomorska - P) and young rams at the same age ($n = 8$) that are crossbreeds of P breed lamb and meat breed lamb - Berrichion-du-Cher (BCH). After macroscopic evaluation, the liver was sampled for microscopical and ultrastructural examination. According to the observed microscopic and ultrastructural lesions (particularly retrogressive changes and circulation disturbances), the most pathological alterations of the liver were observed in young rams of F_1 P x BCH and statistically significantly less lesions (approximately two) were seen in purebred lambs of P breed. The number of lesions and their intensity increased with the age of young rams, particularly in the crossbreeds. This study has shown that breed growth-rate differences influences the pathomorphological pattern of the liver in lambs. It is known that crossbred lambs have higher productivity in comparison to the purebreds, and this could be the main reason why the liver of the crossbreds is more susceptible to morphological lesions than the liver of the purebreds.

 Poster CMNS1.19

The quality of lamb meat stored in modified gas atmosphere

Z. Tanski, H. Brzostowski, J. Sowinska, K. Majewska, J. Szarek. Uniwersity of Warmia and Mazury, 10-718 Olsztyn, ul. Oczapowskiego 5, Poland*

The meat quality of 50-days-old ram lambs singles of Pomeranian breed and their crossbreeds F_1 with meat breed rams: Ile de France, Suffolk and Teksel, was studied. The meat quality: chemical content, physicochemical, sensory properties as well as the intramuscular fatty acids composition of fresh and stored in modified gas atmosphere
(80% N_2 / 20% CO_2) during 10, 20 and 30 days-long period quadriceps tight muscle was evaluated in the present study.
The used for crossbreeding meat breed ram lambs improved the dry mass, crude protein and fat content, increased the unsaturated fatty acids content and decreased caloric value with the similar sensory parameters of the studied samples.
The storage of lamb meat in modified gas atmosphere (80% N_2 / 20% CO_2) influenced the increase of dry mass, crude protein, fat and ash content. Prolongation of storage period caused lightening of meat color, decrease of pH as well as worsening of intensity and desirability of taste and juiciness. Storage of lamb meat in modified gas atmosphere improved also intramuscular fatty acids composition.

Poster CMNS1.20

The meat quality of Pomeranian breed lambs and their crossbreeds F_1 with the meat breed rams

*H. Brzostowski *, J. Sowinska , Z. Tanski, K. Majewska, J. Dzida, University of Warmia and Mazury, 10-718 Olsztyn, ul. Oczapowskiego 5, Poland.*

The selected indexes of the meat quality in 100-days-old ram lambs singles of Pomeranian breed (P) and their crossbreeds F_1 of Berrichon du Cher (PB) and Charolaise (PCH) breed were evaluated in the present study. The chemical content, physical and sensory properties, energetic value, collagen and cholesterol content as well as the aminoacids composition was evaluated in samples of quadriceps tight muscle.
The meat obtained from P lambs had higher cholesterol content than the meat from PB and PCH and higher caloric value than the meat from PCH. The highest collagen content in the studied samples was observed in PCH ram lambs. The meat from P lambs had higher egzogenic aminoacids content, especially treonin, metionin and tryptophane than in the other genetic groups. The highest content of endogenic acids as prolin, glycin, and lizin was observed in meat from PB ram lambs. The meat obtained from PB ram lambs had the worst juiciness and tenderness, what may be the effect of low intramuscular fat content.

Study on influences of nutraceuticals dietary addition on some milk and blood immune parameters and intarmammary infections in organic dairy goats

*V. Bronzo[1], P. Moroni[1], G. Pisoni[1], A. Casula[1], D. Cattaneo[2] and *G. Savoini[2], [1]Dipartimento di Patologia Animale, Igiene e Sanità Pubblica Veterinaria, [2]Dipartimento di Scienze e Tecnologie Veterinarie per la Sicurezza Alimentare, via Celoria 10, 20133 Milano*

Increasing in organic animal foods demand (following UE guidelines 2092/91 e 1804/99), pay attention on use of some dietary substances, defined as nutraceuticals, as traditional therapy alternative to prevent some diseases. Study was performed in an organic dairy goat farm using dietary integration with panax ginseng and rosemary dry extract, goats were shared in three experimental groups sampled for a whole lactation: group HD (High Dose), group LD (Low Dose) and no treated control group for both treatments. Results show a decrease in leukocytes count and in neutrophils in blood in both treatments than an increase in neutrophils milk fraction and a decrease in intramammary infections in both treatments. Result suggest as nutraceuticals dietary integration with panax ginseng and rosemary dry extract could be helpful in control of intramammary infections in organic dairy goat farms.

Poster CMNS1.22

Meat quality of Mangalica and LWxDL pigs

Lugasi Andrea[1], K. Neszlényi[1], Gergely Anna[1], Hóvári Judit[1], Barna Éva[1], Kontraszti Mariann[1], Hermán Istvánné[2], J. Gundel[2], I. Bodó[3], S. Mihók [1], [1]Institute of Food Hygiene and Nutrition, P.O. Box 52. 1097 Budapest, Hungary, [2]Research Institute for Animal Breeding and Nutrition, 2053 Herceghalom, Hungary, [3]University of Debrecen, Centre of Agricultural Science, P.O. Box 36, 4032 Debrecen, Hungary*

Te quality and nutritional value of meat are influenced by the genotype of the animals and the keeping practice, as well. Composition of nutrients such as DM, EE and CP, fatty acids, and lipid peroxidation characteristics were investigated in ham of pigs from two different breeds. (Hungarian mangalica (MAN) and LWxDL) Animals were fed on two different mixtures of feed a "traditional" and a "modern" which contained significantly higher concentration of linoleic acid (2%) than the other one. Significantly higher level of DM, CP and fat content, were detected in meat of mangalica than in crossbreed. In relation to higher fat content the level of lipid peroxidation products especially conjugated dienes was also significantly higher in the traditional breed. At the same time the activities of antioxidant enzymes were also higher in MAN breed showing a well balanced prooxidant/antioxidant system in the animals. More mono unsaturated (palmitoleic and oleic acid) and less polyunsaturated fatty acids like linoleic, linolenic and arachidonic acids were detected in mangalica muscle tissue than in crossbreed.

 Poster CMNS1.23

EU Project "Assessment of Genetic Variation in Meat Quality and the evaluation of role of candidate genes in beef characteristics with a view to breeding for improved product quality" - First production and carcass quality results

S. Gigli[*1], P. Alberti[2], P. Ertbjerg[3], J.F. Hocquette[4], G. Nute[5], C. Sanudo[6]. [1]Animal Production Research Institute, Italy, [2]Servicio Investicacion Agroalimentaria, Spain, [3]Royal Veterinary Agricultural University, Denmark, [4]INRA Theix, France, [5]University Bristol, UK, [6]University Zaragoza, Spain.*

Some previous data on production and carcass quality results from 8 European cattle breeds (*Asturiana de la Montana, Asturiana de los Valles, Avilena-Nigra Iberica, Charolais, Limousine, Marchigiana, Piemontese, Pirenaica*) are presented. These results are part of an ongoing larger EU Project, which contains a total of 450 animals from 15 different breeds; meat quality parameters are measured in all animals. The aim of this Project is to relate quality parameters and molecular gene information of the same animals. Animals were reared intensively in the same conditions with concentrate *ad libitum* and cereal straw.
Results show variability between the European breeds studied and also important variability within the same breed, which could give good information to improve their quality.
Animals were slaughtered at about 15 months of age (from 428 d to 469 d) and at final weights varied between 444.0 and 624.7 kg kilogrammes.
Average daily gain was between 1.191 and 1.530 kilogrammes. The rustic types had longer legs and poorer conformation scores, however fatness fat percentage was higher in this type of breed.

Poster CMNS1.24

Effect of housing system on meat quality of Piemontese young bulls

G. Destefanis[1], M.T. Barge[1], A. Brugiapaglia[*1], [1]Dipartimento di Scienze Zootecniche, Via Leonardo da Vinci 44, 10095 Grugliasco, Torino, Italy.*

Thirty hypertrophied Piemontese young bulls were divided in two groups: 15 subjects were tie stalled, 15 were housed in pens. The animals were fed hay and concentrate and were slaughtered at an average weight of 560 kg. After 7 days of cooling, from the right side of each carcass, samples of *longissimus thoracis et lumborum* (LT), *semitendinosus* (St), and *supraspinatus* (Ss) were taken to perform chemical, physical and sensorial analyses. The results indicate that the housing system and muscle had a significant influence on water, hydroxyproline, haeme iron content and lightness. Moreover, there was a significant effect of housing system on collagen solubility, while the muscle affected fat content, shear force, drip and cooking losses. The meat from animals reared in pens had a higher water, hydroxyproline and haeme iron content, collagen solubility, but a lower lightness. Concerning muscles, LT showed the lowest values for water and hydroxyproline, lightness, shear force, drip and cooking losses. On the contrary, Ss had the highest fat and haeme iron content. The interaction housing system by muscle was significant for protein, redness and yellowness. Ss showed the same protein content in both the housing systems, while LT and St had a protein content lower in meat from animals reared in pens. In these latter, redness and yellowness values were higher in Ss and lower in LT and St.

 Poster CMNS1.25

Ensiled legumes for store lambs

M.H.M. Speijers[1], M.D. Fraser[1], V. Theobald[1], J. Roberts[1], R. Fychan[1] and W. Haresign[2], [1]Institute of Grassland and Environmental Research, Plas Gogerddan, Aberystwyth, SY23 3EB, Wales UK, [2]Institute of Rural Studies, University of Wales, Llanbadarn Fawr, Aberystwyth, SY23 3AL, Wales, UK.*

Indoor lamb finishing based on grass-silage diets may result in low and variable voluntary intakes, resulting in poor lamb performance and longer finishing periods. The aim of this study was to compare the effects of feeding lucerne and red clover silages on the performance of lambs of a hill breed.
After a four week adaptation period, Beulah Speckled Faced lambs were allocated on the basis of live weight and body condition score to one of three treatments (n=11); lucerne, red clover or ryegrass silages. All the diets were supplemented with molassed sugarbeet shreds to avoid energy being a limiting factor. Individual intakes were determined daily and measurements of live weight and body condition score were made weekly. Additional body composition measurements were made by scanning the lambs for depth of *Longissimus dorsi* muscle and subcutaneous fat. Over an experimental period of 7 weeks, offering red clover silage resulted in higher voluntary intakes and improved feed conversion efficiencies. This was reflected in improved growth rates and body condition of lambs. Lambs that were offered lucerne silage had variable intakes and growth rates, with no performance benefits over lambs fed ryegrass silage.

Poster CMNS1.26

Effect of a herbs tranquillizer on capture and transport stress in ostriches

S. Diverio[1], C. Federici[1], A. Barone[1], C. Canali[1] and N. Falocci[2], [1]Dpt. Scienze Biopatologiche Veterinarie, Faculty of Veterinary Medicine, Perugia University, Via S. Costanzo 4, 06126 Perugia, Italy, [2]Dpt. Scienze Statistiche, Faculty of Economy, Perugia University, Via Pascoli, 06100 Perugia, Italy*

The study was made to investigate the effect of a mixture of herbs as a tranquillizer to reduce the stress induced by transport and slaughtering on ostriches. 4 African Black Neck ostriches (2 male and 2 female) 18-36 months old, reared in the DKL Ospedalicchio farm (Perugia - Italy), were used. The experiment was conducted over a 3 week-period. During the first week the animals had no herbs treatment, which started to be daily administered, at the end of second week (6th day), in the drinking water (1.5 cm^3/l), until the end of the third week. On the 5th day of the 1st and 3rd week, the ostriches were loaded into a van and transported over a 1-hour period. During the 1st and the 3rd week ostriches behaviour was recorded by instantaneous sampling, at 3 min interval, and data recorded in an apposite ethogram. From all subjects, blood samples were collected by venipuncture before and after transport. Plasma was assayed for corticosterone, muscular and hepatic enzymes, blood urea nitrogen (BUN), total protein, glucose, triglyceride, cholesterol, Creatinina, sodium and potassium. Herbs tranquillizer treatment seemed to have an effect on some physiological parameters and animal behaviour. Treated ostriches showed a reduced or null number of "negative interactions", lower excitement and reduced plasma corticosterone and CK responses to transport stress.s

The effects of two floor space allowances on meat quality and behaviour of heavy pigs

G. Martelli[1], R. Scipioni[2], P. Parisini[1], A. Badiani[1], L. Sardi[1], [1]DIMORFIPA, Via Tolara di Sopra, 50, 40064 Ozzano Emilia (BO), Italy, [2]Dipartimento Interdisciplinare Scienze Agrarie, Via Kennedy, 17, 42100 Reggio Emilia, Italy.*

Forty male Large White pigs with an average body weight of 115 kg were homogeneously divided into two groups T1 and T2. Animals were kept on a slatted floor in collective pens containing 5 pigs each. T1 pigs had a floor space allowance of 1 m^2/head in compliance with the current EU legislation, while pigs of group T2 had, according to their body weight (160 kg at slaughtering), an individual space allowance of 1.3 m^2. The trial lasted 62 days. Pigs were fed at the rate of 9% of their metabolic live weight up to a maximum of 3.3 kg/head/day. Carcass and meat quality (lean meat yield, lean and fat cuts yields, pH, colour, thigh and loin chemical composition) were determined. Animal behaviour was videotaped every week over a 24-hour period. The two different space allowances did not modify (P>0.05) carcasses and meat quality. All pigs spent the most part of their time resting. The higher floor space allowance made T2 pigs able to lye at the same time, mainly in lateral recumbency, while T1 pigs spent more time standing. From our data it is suggested that a floor space allowance of 1.3 m^2/head, i.e. higher than presently recommended for pigs weighing more than 110 kg (1 m^2/head), may improve heavy pigs welfare (all pigs can lye at the same time) and does not modify the quality of meat.

Poster CMNS1.28

Recherches concernant a variété ALINA (*Lotus corniculatus*) utilisation par paturée en melange avec graminées

I. Scurtu and V.A. Blaj Grassland Research-Development Institute, 5, Cucului*

Dans les espaces pâturés, le pâturage joue un rôle déterminant dans la dynamique de la diversité des espé ces végétales et animales. Comme tout processus écologique, le pâturage est un processus complexes a structure hiérachique. On a utilisé les resultats optenus pendant plusieus années (2000-2002). La prairie est formue de un melange simple de: *Lolium perenne,Phleum pratense, Festuca pratensis et Lotus corniculatus* varieté Alina. Observations effectués: matiére séche (MS), proteine brute (PB), cellulose brute (Cel.B), analyses botaniques, problemes de pollutions, le gain poids vif (g/j), palatabilité de la fourage, consumation et perennité de l' herbe, résistance, quantité de la refus.

L' interpretation statistique a été l' analise de la variance, corelations et regretions. La année 2000 a été tres séche et la varieté Alina a eu une production tres bonne. Pourcentage de leguminéuses a été plus élevée, en moyenne 32. Le gain de poids vif moyen par jour a été 825 g/jour/animal. Le contenu en PB a été plus élevée 21,33 (%MS). La quéntité d' herbe données aux animaux durant toute la periode a été de 8,7 t/MS/ha. La mise en relation des fonctionnements écologiques avec les structures de la végétation, et les caractéristiques des sols permettra l' élaboration d'indicateurs des valeurs d'usages et des propriétés des prairies, et par la, des modalités d' interventions techniques qui devront etre testées expérimentalement pour etre intérgrées dans les sistémes de pâturage.

 Poster CMNS1.29

Hygienic characteristics of the Hungarian sheep and goat milk

S. Kukovics, A. Abrahám, Research Institute for Animal Breeding and Nutrition, Gesztenyés u. 1. 2053 Herceghalom Hungary*

There are significant breed and species differences in the characteristics of the sheep and goat milk. The characteristics of sheep- (773, 373, 486) and goat milk (446, 801, 689) bulk samples were studied in 2000, 2001, and 2002, representing different quantities of milk (1.48; 1.34 and 1.51 million litres of sheep milk, as well as 0.71; 1.23 and 2.10 million litres of goat milk, respectively). The following traits were studied based on the regulations: physical cleaning, degree of acidity, pH, freezing point, total bacterial count, somatic cell count, antibacterial inhibitory matter, extraneous water in milk, (and in 2000) fat %, protein %, fat free dry matter %. According to the results the samples were classified (first class quality or not) following the orders of regulations. In the year 2000, the biggest part of the samples did not reach the first class quality; only the smaller part was accepted. In 2001 the situation was improved: only 23% of the sheep and 18% of the goat milk samples could not reach level of the first class classification. In 2002, 12.96 % of the sheep milk-, and 13.79 % of the goat milk samples were refused to get the first class quality certification. The main limiting trait was the total bacterial count, followed by the freezing point, pH value, acidity degree in the classification. The somatic cell count (included in the study of the year 2000) also caused some problems. Details of regulations are presented in the paper.

Poster CMNS1.30

NIR spectroscopy of freeze-dried plasma in cattle to appreciate whole experimental effects

G. Masoero[1], G. Bergoglio[1], A. Terzano[1], F. Abeni[1], D. Pavino[2], M.C. Abete[2]. [1]Istituto Sperimentale Zootecnia, Via Pianezza 115, 1015-Torino, Italy, [2]Istituto Zooprofilattico Sperimentale Torino, Via Bologna 148,* 10154-Torino, Italy

Samples of Piemontese cattle plasma (N=327) stored at -20°C since 9-44 months were thawed then freeze-dried in vials. The FT-NIR transreflected spectra were recorded by a P.E. Quantum One (1000-2500nm, 3000 points, reduced to 748) then calibrated to clinical measurements or experimental effects. The effect of storage duration was strongly perceived by FT-NIR (R^2=0.79, SECV=4 months). The whole effects of nutritional treatments received by 130 cows during late gestation in 5 experiments were appreciated with R^2 = 0.12, 0.32, 0.41, 0.41, 0.32 respectively. The calving facility and parity appeared weakly linked (R^2= 0.19 and 0.34). The clinical parameters were only moderately fitted (R^2calibration; ±SECV): PackedCellVolume (0.36;±0.02) estrone sulphate (0.26;±3.4), creatinine (0.34;±0.40), insulin (0.45;±4.4), glucose (0.41;±5.3). FT-NIR of dried plasma appear cheap tool, which can synthesise a whole information about comparative experimental effects by capitalising direct or indirect relationships with conventional laboratory analyses and apparently with denaturative oxidative effects. Study of ethiology of differences will be encouraged if a result is pre-announced or the aimed "substantial equivalence" theory could be affirmed without laboratory tenacity.

 Poster CMNS1.31

The influence of genotype, feeding system and milk yield on the activity of aminopeptidase in whole cow's milk and somatic cells separated from the milk

J. Krzyzewski, A. Józwik, A. Sliwa-Józwik, N. Strzalkowska, A Kotataj Institute of Genetics and Animal Breeding Polish Academy of Sciences, Jastrzebiec, 05-552 Wólka Kosowska, Poland*

The aim of this study was to estimate the influence of genotype (races), feeding system an milk yield on the aminopeptidase activity in the whole cow's milk and in somatic cells, which were separated from the whole milk. It is known that lysosomal system takes part in answers on homeostatic changes in cell. Changes on the activity these enzymes are coefficients of homeostatic disturbances and of sickness - processes.
The experiment was carried out on 40 cows, divided into two groups (20 cows in each): 1 - Polish Red (native race) - the everage milk yield about 4200 kg per lactation
2 - HF - the evarage milk yield about 8500 kg per lactation
In the whole milk and in somatic cells, basing on substrates from SIGMA-ALDRICH Co., the activities of alanyl aminopeptidase (AlaAP, E.C. 3.4.11.2), leucyl aminopeptidase (LeuAP, E.C. 3.4.11.1), arginyl aminopeptidase (ArgAP, EC. 3.4.11.6) were estimated. The activity of AlaAP, LeuAP and ArgAP were determined according to the method of McDonald and Barret (1986). The activity of the enzymes was expressed as nMol/mg of protein/hour. The activity of examined aminopeptidases were significantly higher in HF cows whole milk and somatic cell in compare to Polish Red cows.

Poster CMNS1.32

Effects of different forage system and herd management on milk yield and quality of Girgentana goats

A. Di Grigoli[1], L. Stringi[2], D. Giambalvo[2], G. De Vita[2], A. Bonanno[1], G. Russo[1], M. Alabiso[1]. [1]Dipartimento S.En.Fi.Mi.Zo., sezione Produzioni Animali. [2]Dipartimento ACEP, Università di Palermo, Viale delle Scienze, 90128 Palermo, Italy.

The aim of the present study, carried out in the Sicilian inland, was of evaluating the productivity of different dairy goat management systems: extensive (EXT), based on grazing on improved pasture mainly (60% of surface, 8 goats/ha); semi-intensive (SIN), based on grazing on grown forage species (80% of surface, 12 goats/ha); intensive (INT), involving continuous housing, zero-grazing, stored forage and supplementary feed. The research lasted from March to August 2001 and involved 44 Girgentana milking goats (12, 18 and 14 goats for EXT, SIN and INT groups, respectively). All groups received supplementary feed during the trial. Surveys and analysis of available and selected forage at pasture and milk and cheese were executed. Milk yield of EXT goats was higher than SIN and INT groups (1165 vs 1075 and 1042 g/head/d, $P \leq 0.05$). Milk of INT group was lower in fat ($P \leq 0.01$). The EXT milk had lower somatic cells ($P \leq 0.01$) and higher content in protein ($P \leq 0.05$) and casein ($P \leq 0.05$), responsible of better clotting parameters and slight increase in cheese yield. At the end of the experiment, the INT goats showed higher body weight and BCS ($P \leq 0.01$) than the other groups. These results demonstrate a better productive response of extensively managed goats.

FT-NIR spectroscopy of freeze-dried plasma in poultry to appreciate experimental effects linked to ROM status

G. Masoero[1], Dal Bosco[2], C. Castellin [2], C. Mugnai[2], G. Bergoglio[1], D. Pavino[3], M.C. Abete[3]. [1]Istituto Sperimentale Zootecnia, Via Pianezza 115, 10151-Torino, Italy, [2]Dipartimento di Scienze Zootecniche, Facoltà di Agraria, Borgo XX Giugno, 74-06100, Perugia, Italy, [3]Istituto Zooprofilattico Sperimentale Torino, Via Bologna 148,* 10154-Torino, Italy

Plasma samples collected in two experiments with organic hens (N=25) and broilers (N=22), stored at -80°C since trhee months were thawed then analysed for ROM test produced by DIACRON®s.r.l.(Italy). One ml freeze-dried was transreflected by FT-NIR P.E. Quantum One. The 3000 points were reduced to 748 and chemometrised by Stepwise Regression. FT-NIR enhanced strong capability to separate kind of animal (laying-hens *vs* broilers, R^2c=0.953) and treatments in laying-hens (cage *vs* bioplus, R^2c=0.806), with the involved genetic-type on trial (R^2c=0.950) or in broilers (bio_mouvement *vs* bio_resting, R^2c=0.746). Equivalent figures by ROM analyses were lowered: 0.429; 0.513; 0.247 and 0.546. In general ROMs appeared apparently well estimated by FT-NIR (R^2c= 0.779). This is due because of strong between-groups differences and because of a hypothetic ethiological relationship on the within-group basis. Our expectation can be optimistic by the fact that all the FT-NIR spectra examined in these experiment appeared to be quite homogeneous. Extension of this simple, immediate and synthetic method to researches about oxidative status of the animals can be recommended.

Poster CMNS1.34

Metabolic and oxidative stress response to abrupt dietary starch variation in dairy cows

B. Stefanon[1], E. Binda[2], G. Casirani[2], A. Summer[3], L. Marinelli[4] and G. Gabai[4], [1]Dipartimento Scienze Produzione Animale, via delle Scienze 208, 33100 Udine, Italy, [2]Dipartimento Patologia Animale Igiene e Sanità Pubblica, 20133 Milano, Italy, [3]Dipartimento Produzioni Animali, Biotecnologie Veterinarie Sicurezza degli Alimenti, 43100 Parma, Italy, [4]Dipartimento Scienze Sperimentali Veterinarie, 35020 Legnaro Padova, Italy.*

Ten mid-lactating Friesian heifers were randomly assigned to two groups. Both groups were fed a basal TMR until 167 DIM (24% starch DM). From 170 DIM afterwards, a group of animals continued to receive the same ration, while the other group was allotted to the experimental diets, which consisted in a 7 days dietary starch decrease (21% DM) after 7 days of starch increase (27% DM). Blood samples were collected at DIM 167, 171, 172, 173, 178, 179 and 180 and analysed for metabolic, endocrine, oxidative and immune parameters. Somatic cell count and protein fractions in milk were also measured. The increase of starch in diet affected plasma b-OHB and free fatty acids and reduced malondialdehyde and glutathione peroxidase activity, whilst starch deprivation caused an opposite response. Cortisol and GH concentrations in plasma, lisozyme and NAGase activities in plasma and milk and nitrogen fractions and somatic cell count in milk did not response to the variable availability of glucose. Therefore, the short-term dietary-mediated modification of circulating metabolic parameters and oxidative stress markers were not related to a cognitive stress.

 Poster CMNS1.35

Somatotropin and fat administration to lactating dairy buffalo: effects on milk production and plasma leptin

F. Rosi, L. Pinotti[1], Istituto di Zootecnia Generale, Facoltà di Agraria, [1]Dept. VSA, Facoltà di Medicina Veterinaria, Università degli Studi di Milano, I-20133 Milan Italy.*

The aims of this study were to determine the effects of somatotropin (bST) and dietary Fat administration on milk production, plasma leptin, and selected plasma lipid parameters in dairy buffalo. Forty lactating Italian river dairy buffalo in mid to late lactation were randomly divided into 4 groups: Control, Fat (0.3 kg/d of rumen-protected fat), bST (320 mg/3wk of slow release bST for 4 cycles) and bST+Fat. Milk production was measured weekly. Blood samples were collected weekly at 14.00h and plasma analyzed for leptin, NEFA and triglyceride. Somatotropin administration increased (P<.01) milk yield (6.76, 7.55, 9.03, and 8.99 kg/d in control, Fat, bST and bST+Fat respectively), whereas milk composition was unaffected by treatments. Although plasma NEFA was unaffected by treatments, mean plasma leptin (2.33, 2.81, 2.28, 3.32 µg/l; P<.01) and triglyceride (309, 370, 321, 351mmol/l; P<.05) were increased by Fat supplementation. Results herein presented confirmed a galactopoetic effect of bST in lactating dairy buffalo. On the other hand increased plasma leptin observed in fat supplemented buffalo probably confirm that, like in other mammals, plasma leptin is related to dietary fat composition and to the nutritional status of the animal.

Poster CMNS1.36

Homocysteine plasma levels and lymphocyte proliferation in cows during lactation

E. Chiaradia[1], B. Stefanon[2], A. Gaiti[1], S. Sgorlon[2], S. Testoni[3] and L. Avellini[1], [1]Dipartimento di Tecnologie e Biotecnologie delle Produzioni Animali, Università di Perugia, 06126 Perugia, Italy, [2]Dipartimento di Scienze della Produzione Animale, Università di Udine, 33100 Udine, Italy, [3]Dipartimento di Scienze Sperimentali Veterinarie, Università di Padova, 35020 Legnaro, Italy.*

Fertility reduction in dairy cow depends on several factors, which include high milk productivity, unbalanced diet, environmental factors, endocrine and metabolic conditions and stress-related diseases. In previous observations in the horse, we described that a submaximal exercise stress may induce a reduction of lymphocyte proliferation that could be related to a simultaneous increase of plasma homocysteine. Since the lowering of the immune response is particularly recognized during lactation, we decided to verify whether the lactation period can induce a variation of the cysteine and homocysteine plasma levels as well as a modification of the proliferative capacity of bovine peripheral lymphocytes. Blood samples were collected at 37, 80 and 150 days of lactation from 5 Friesian heifers. Our results indicate that the lactation period may determine a significant change of the thiols plasma levels as well as a variation of lymphocyte proliferation. Further investigation on the role of homocysteine, as possible mediator of the worsening of immunitary function during the transition period, is needed.

 Poster CMNS1.37

The effects of parity and SCC on plasmin and plasminogen content in goat milk

G. Battacone, A. Nudda, G. Pulina, G. Enne, Dipartimento di Scienze Zootecniche, Università di Sassari, Via Enrico De Nicola 9, 07100 Sassari, Italy.

Plasmin (PL), and its inactive zymogen plasminogen (PG), is the most significant protease in milk. It is quite heat stable and affects adversily dairy products. The objective of this work was to investigate about effects of parity and SCC on PL and PG content in goat milk. Forty crossbred goats (Alpine x Saanen x Sarda) at different parity (10 of 2nd, 10 of 3rd, 10 of 4-5th and 10>5th), were used to provide milk samples in 2-mo study. Measurements included milk yield, milk components, milk protein fractions, SCC, PL and PG concentrations. Samples were grouped into 3 classes according to SCC levels: low (L) <$0.5*10^6$; medium (M) = $0.5*10^6$-$1*10^6$ and high (H) >$1*10^6$ SCC/ml. PL content tended to increase as SCC rose (3.58, 4.78, 4.96 µg/ml in L, M and H SCC classes respectively; P = 0.10) whereas PG concentration did not vary (14.52, 13.24 and 13.43 µg/ml in L, M and H SCC classes respectively). This suggests that PL increase can be due to its higher passage from blood to milk rather than to an activation of its zymogen in mammary gland. Parity influenced PL content (5.42, 3.69, 5.66, 2.99 µg/ml in 2nd, 3rd , 4-5th and >5th parity; P<0.01) even if a definite trend was not observed: this trend was not explained by interaction between parity and SCC. This work was supported by the National Strategic Project DIETOLAT (MiPAF).

Poster CMNS1.38

Evaluation of the effect of mycotoxins on primary cell proliferation and the protective role of retinol

E. Fusi[1], R. Rebucci[1], A. Baldi[1], K. Sejrsen[2] and S. Purup[2], [1]Department of Veterinary Sciences and Technology for Food Safety, Via Celoria 10, 20133 Milano, Italy, [2]Institute of Animal Nutrition and Physiology, Danish Institute of Agricultural Sciences, Research Centre Foulum, P.O. Box 50, DK-8830 Tjele, Denmark.

The aim of this study was to evaluate the cytotoxic effects of Ochratoxin A (OTA) and Aflatoxin M_1 (AFM_1), involved in human and animal diseases on primary cells derived from target organs as mammary gland and the possible protective role of retinol. The cell viability and proliferation of bovine primary mammary epithelial cells, isolated from pre-puberal heifers incubated for 24 h with increasing concentrations of mycotoxins in serum free medium were determined.

OTA treatment affected the cell proliferation in a concentration dependent manner. Clumps were pre treated (3 h) with retinol (0.1 ng/ml), which significantly (P<0.05) counteracted the OTA cytotoxicity at the mycotoxin concentration of 10 µg/ml. From this result it could be suggested that retinol modulated OTA damage, which take place scavenging reactive oxy-radicals and thereby reducing lipid peroxidation. In vitro exposure for 24 h of clumps to different concentrations of AFM_1 showed a detrimental effect on cellular viability and proliferation. No significant protective effect of retinol was observed.

To conclude our results showed that OTA was more sensitive to retinol activities than AFM_1, probably due their different mechanism of damage.

 Poster CMNS1.39

Housing system and welfare of buffalo cows

C. Tripaldi[1], F. Napolitano[2], M.C. Scatà[1], F. Grasso[3], G. De Rosa[3], E. Pasqui[1], C. Roncoroni [1] and and A. Bordi[3], [1]ISZ, Monterotondo (Roma), Italy, [2]DISPA, Università della Basilicata, Potenza, Italy, [3]DISCIZIA, Università di Napoli "Federico II", Portici (Naples), Italy.

Twenty-eight buffalo cows were used to evaluate the effect of housing system on a range of behavioural and physiological variables from February to July. Fourteen cows were group-housed in a loose open-sided barn with a concrete floor and 10 m^2/head as space allowance (Group IS). Fourteen others were group-housed in a similar barn but they could also benefit of an outdoor yard with 500 m^2/head as space allowance, spontaneous vegetation and free access to potholes for wallowing (Group TS). Six behavioural recordings were performed using instantaneous scan sampling. Data were expressed as proportion of subjects observed in each behavioural category. Phytoemagglutinin (PHA) and ovalbumin were used to assess cellular and humoral immune responses, respectively. Cortisol concentration was evaluated prior to and after exogenous ACTH injection. The metabolic status of the animals and milk production were also monitored. Immune responses, metabolite concentrations and milk production were not affected by treatment. The provision of an housing system close to natural conditions was able to improve the welfare of buffalo cows as indicated by the expression of some species-specific natural behaviours (i.e. grazing and wallowing) and the reduction of idling ($P<0.001$). Such conditions also determined a lower cortisol response ($P<0.01$) as possible consequence of the higher degree of initiative allowed to TS cows.

Poster CMNS1.40

Effect of genotype α-S1 casein on the yield,chemical composition and technological parameters of goats milk

N . Strzalkowska, J. Krzyzewski, A. Józwik, E. Bagnicka, Z. Ryniewicz, Institute of Genetics and Animal Breeding, Polish Academy of Sciences, Jastrzebiec, 05-552 Wólka Kosowska, Poland.*

The work aimed at analysing the relations between a simultaneus occurence of specific polymorphic forms α-S1 casein and milk yield, its physicochemical compositions and technological parameters.

The investigations were conducted over three concecutive years on 40 (in each year) Polish White Improved goats, divided into two groups:

1- with „strong" (A,B) and 2-with „intermediate" (E) α-S1 casein alleles.The diets were balanced according to INRA system. Once a month, the daily milk yield and SCC, as well as total protein, casein, fat, lactose and total solids were determined. Also the physicochemical properties of the milk were examined- pH, SH as well the quality of casein curd in a fermentation and rennet-fermentation test. The goat' s milk with „strong" variants of casein α-S1 was characterised by a higher concentration of total protein (2,97 vs.2,81%), casein (2,58 vs.2,52%), fat (3,59 vs.3,49%) and lactose (4,77 vs.4,70%). The milk of this goats contained a higher concentration of tatal solids (11,95 vs.11,67%) and has higher SH. The animals with „strong" α-S1 casein alleles produced milk characterised by better quality of casein curd.

 Poster CMNS1.41

Assessing meat quality in Sarda breed and Limousine x Sarda crossbred heifers

A. Gaddini[1], M. Iacurto[1], P. Brandano[2], S. Rassu[2], M. Contò[1], [1]Animal Production Research Institute - Via Salaria, 31- 00016 Monterotondo (Roma), Italy, [2]University of Sassari - Department of Zootechnical Sciences - via E. De Nicola,1 - 07100 Sassari, Italy*

In our work we analyzed quality traits of steaks from heifers of Sarda breed, a typical italian cattle (7 animals), and crossbred Limousine x Sarda (7 animals), all born and fattened with hay and concentrates in Sardinia.
Sample joint dissection was made to calculate the percentage of muscle *Longissimus dorsi* (LD), bone and fat (intramuscular and subcutaneous) on the total weight of the joint. We'll be measuring collagen amount in the joint.
The joints, were thawed for 24 hours at 4°C, then we measured pH, CIELAB colour, shear force on cores (diameter 1/2 inches) of raw and cooked meat, with Warner-Bratzler on Instron, cooking losses after reaching internal temperature of 75°C.
We found a good performance in crossbred heifers about the percentage of LD (35,14%) while Sarda heifers had an higher overall percentage of meat (52,87%).
Cooking losses were low, better for the crossbred heifers (23,63%) than Sarda ones (28,08%).
Shear force measurement on raw meat gave low values for Sarda (2,92 kg), but also for crossbreds (3,50 kg), while on cooked meat, the trend was opposite (4,37 kg for crossbred and 5,94 kg for Sarda), being anyway widely acceptable.

Poster CMNS1.42

Effect of rearing system and homeopathy on milk production of Merino derived ewes

C. Pacelli, A. Braghieri, F. Napolitano, M. Verdone, F. Surianello and A. Girolami, Dipartimento di Scienze delle Produzioni Animali, Università degli Studi della Basilicata, Via N. Sauro 85, 85100 Potenza

The effect of rearing system (extensive vs intensive) and homeopathic therapy on sheep welfare and milk production was investigated on 40 multiparous Merino derived ewes. Twenty animals were housed in an indoor-bedded pen, whereas twenty ewes were allowed to graze on pasture for 9 hours/d. Penned and grazing animals were fed an equivalent diet in terms of dry matter intake, crude protein percentage and energy concentration. In each group, 10 animals were subjected to unicistic homeopathic treatments, while 10 ewes were kept as a control and treated with conventional medicine when necessary. The extensive rearing system had a marked positive effect on in vivo cellular immune response (delayed-type hypersensivity to PHA, $P<0.001$). Grazing animals produced more milk than penned ones (1048.00±75.61 vs 853.04 ±67.78 kg, $P<0.05$), with increased content of milk fat (7.69±0.15 vs 7.25±0.14 %, $P<0.05$). The homeopathic treatments did not affect the immune response and milk production, although they avoided the use of allopathic therapies with no detrimental effects on animal health. Therefore, homeopathy proved to be more economic and safer (no risk of residuals in the products) than conventional medicine. In addition, extensive sheep farming was able to maximise welfare and improve milk production as indicated by the recent EU Regulation on organic farming.

A real-time computer vision system for the quantification of poultry behaviour in furnished cages

T. Leroy[1], J. Ceunen[1], E. Struelens[2], A. Janssen[3], F. Tuyttens[2], K. De Baere[3], J. Zoons[3], B. Sonck[2], E. Vranken[1] and D. Berckmans[1], [1]Laboratory for Agricultural Buildings Research, Catholic University of Leuven, Leuven, Belgium, [2]Agricultural Research Centre, Merelbeke, Belgium, [3]Provincial Centre for Applied Poultry Research, Geel, Belgium

The general purpose of this study is to develop an on-line image-processing technique to quantify the behaviour of laying hens as opposed to the current human visual observation. The contour of the laying hen in each camera image will be extracted using a model-based segmentation method. The parameters from this model are stored as a description of the hen's posture in that image. As a next step, the parameters of the posture as a function of time are approximated by a model within a certain time window. The parameters from this model can then be used to classify the hen's behaviour as e.g. egg laying, wing stretching, pecking.
A first implementation of the system was tested on an image sequence of 640 frames containing 3 different types of behaviour (standing, sitting, pecking). The set of parameters for each image was then plotted, showing 3 clear clusters corresponding to each behaviour class. The objective of further research will be the automatic classification of the feature vector clusters into the different classes of behaviour, and the extension of the classification to up to fifteen different types of behaviour (eating, drinking, walking, egg laying, wing stretching, etc...).

Theatre M2.1

Animal identification, traceability and disease prevention

D. Chaisemartin, Organisation mondiale de la santé animale (OIE), 12, rue de Prony, 75017 Paris, France

The traceability of cattle, sheep, goats and pigs and of their movements is an essential element to the management of the sanitary follow-up of animals, epidemiological surveillance and monitoring, and for the food safety of products issued from these animals.
The traceability is the capacity to find the history, the use or the localization of an entity, with registered identifications.
This concept is more efficient than the identification of animals. It requires that the identification of animals is taken into account from the birth of animals, that this identification is maintained at any time, that all animals' movements are taken into account and that an analysis of the possible failings of the system of animals' traceability are made since the birth of the animals to the animals' products.
This concept of traceability is taken into account by the international organizations working within the framework of the sanitary negotiations (OIE in the field of the living animal and products from the slaughter and the first transformation, Codex Alimentarius for the transformed products and the rest of the food chain), and for the entire production chain of animal foodstuffs, from stable to table, in particular to foster dialogue with all levels of the sector and to avoid conflicts of interest between consumers and producers.

 Theatre M2.2

Results from the IDEA project in view of a future EU legislation

M. Cuypers[1], C. Korn[1], U. Meloni[1], A. Poucet[1], O. Ribo[2], [1]European Commission, Joint Research Centre, Ispra (Va) Italy, [2]Consultant in livestock identification

Since several years, laboratories have been developing technical devices (transponders and readers) and pilot projects have been launched for testing the feasibility and performances of electronic identification, applied to livestock.

In 1998, the EC decided to launch a large scale project, called IDEA, with one million animals, for the identification of bovines, buffalo, sheep and goats. Different identification techniques (ear-tags, ruminal bolus, and injectable transponders) have been used. The IDEA project, which lasted for four years, was performed in six different countries of the EU, involving more than 5000 holdings, and 60 slaughterhouses and a variety of breeds and breeding conditions.

The project was completed in December 2002 and the final report was made available in April 2003.

Based on the positive results obtained, the technical features related to electronic identification have been introduced in the new EC draft legislation for the identification of sheep and goats.

The legislation, presently under discussion by EU Member States, is expected to be introduced for implementation in the near future.

The paper provides the detailed results of the large scale IDEA project, the conclusions drawn and the elements, which have been introduced in the legislation.

Theatre M2.3

Identification and registration with electronic identification in The Netherlands

P.H. Hogewerf, A.H. Ipema and A.C.Smits, IMAG, P.O. Box 43, 6700 AA Wageningen, The Netherlands.*

The Netherlands has decided to allow ear transponders for animal identification and registration (I&R) because: application of ear transponders can be done at a very young age, the transponders do not imply any food safety risks and many farmers have experience with applying and using visual ear tags. Boluses and injectables will be allowed in specific cases.

Before an authority can accept an I&R transponder it has to be evaluated for fraud control, permanency, visual and electronic readability, losses and inflammation rate of the ears per animal species. Considerations around the tests procedures will be presented. As well as developments that have to take place before an I&R system on the basis of transponders can be completely successful applied. These developments have to be focused on equipment and routines for reading individual transponders from groups of animals (during transport), methods for selecting and or marking non recognized animals and re-tagging routines for animals that have a non readable or missing transponder.

The farm process control might face the following conflicting situations: 1) if neck belt transponders will be used for process control next to ear transponders for I&R, 2) if the I&R transponders are used for I&R and process control and 3) farms that already use ear transponders and use readers that are not fully compatible with the I&R transponders. Aspects around these problems will be explained.

Comparison of ear-tag and injectable transponders for the identification and traceability of pigs from birth to slaughter

G. Caja[1], M. Hernández-Jover[1], C. Conill[1,2], D. Garín[1], J. Ghirardi[1], X. Alabern[2] and B. Farriol[3], [1]Departament de Ciència Animal i dels Aliments, Universitat Autònoma de Barcelona, 08193 Bellaterra; [2]Tracex Trazabilidad en Alimentación S.L., 08228 Terrassa; [3]Gesimpex Comercial S.L., 08037 Barcelona, Spain.

A total of 557 piglets (1-2 wk of age) were tagged by using conventional (C) and electronic ear tags (E1 and E2), and injectable transponders of different sizes: 12mm (D12, S12), 23mm (T23), 31mm (T31) and 34mm (S34). Two body positions were compared: subcutaneously in auricle base and intraperitoneally. Performance were recorded during fattening and throughout slaughtering. On farm losses were lower (P<0.01) for C (1.1%) than electronic ear tags (E1, 8.8%; E2, 44.9%). Failures were lower (P<0.001) for E1 (5.5%) than E2 (55.1%).The C and E1 ear tags had similar transport losses (1.2%). Farm losses in auricle base increased (P<0.05) with size (D12, 17.1%; S12, 19.4%; T23, 29.8%; T31, 46.3%; S34, 72.5%). Only one loss (0.4%) was recorded for intraperitoneal position. Slaughtering losses did not differ for C (11.3%) and E1 (6.4%), but a 12.8% more of E1 failed. Injection site affected losses and breakages at slaughtering (auricle base, 6.3%; intraperitoneal, 0%). As conclusion, traceability varied between ear tags (C, 86.7%; E1, 68.1%; and, E2, 0%), auricle base (D13, 75%; S12, 70.7%; T23, 70.2%; T31, 51.2%; and, S34, 17.5%) and intraperitoneal (D12, 100%; S12, 98%, T23, 100%; T31, 100%; and S34, 100%). The intraperitoneal injection with 23 to 34 mm is proposed as a tool for the traceability of pigs.

Theatre M2.5

Development of monitoring system for surveillance of animal welfare during animal transport

G. Gebresenbet, SLU, Box 7032, 750 07 Uppsala, Sweden

Animal transport and handling activities from farms to abattoirs or to farms are increasing within European countries and these activities may compromise animal welfare and reduce the quality of meat. Both welfare and meat quality are the main concern of consumers and meat industries.

Currently, it is a societal demand to acquire a reliable system that could measure the environmental conditions in the vehicle and communicates with control stations.

In line with the above objectives, instrumentation system of different categories has been developed to study air quality, vibration, animal responses in terms of physiological and behavioural alteration during handling and transport from farms to abattoirs.

After identifying relevant parameters, a control system (both soft and hardware) has been developed to continuously measure the following parameters and transfer them using GSM to the control station: (a) the climatic conditions, i.e., temperature, relative humidity, and level of gases in the loading compartment, (b) vehicle performance (particularly vibration), (c) driving routes and performances, (d) animal identification, and (e) animal behaviour when subjected to uncomfortable conditions during transport.

30 cattle transporters have been followed to test the system, and it found that functions satisfactory. The combination of electronic identification and GPS technology allows traceability of individual animals on line during transit, which is important in view of sanitary surveillance and risk assessment.

Theatre M2.6

A framework for animal traceability

Eildert Groeneveld[1], Ralf Fischer[1] and Ulf Müller[2], [1]Institute for Animal Science, Federal Agricultural Research Center, Höltystr. 1, D-31535 Neustadt, Germany, [2] Saxon State Institute for Agriculture, Am Park 3, D-04886 Köllitsch, Germany

In the wake of the BSE crisis traceability has become a major issue in animal production. As a consequence the EU requires the setup of computer systems which allow tracing of animal movements, currently for all cattle but in the future also for other species. The Adaptable Platform Independent Information System (APIIS) developed for the management of individual records in animal production provides a strategy and software framework for following up on animal movements. This is covered by the inbuilt feature to allow for different identifications for one animal, their renumbering and relocation. Technically, this is done by establishing data channels which connect external identifications with unique internal sequences. Furthermore, animal identifications can be reused, still resulting in unique internal identification. As a result, any external animal identification system can be used for animal tracing, without having to introduce globally unique lifetime numbers, thereby making implementation of traceability much easier. Based on an Open Source Relational Database the APIIS program code is freely available under the GNU Public License, thereby allowing the creation of national animal movement databases without licensing costs.

Theatre M2.7

A simulation model for analysis of disease spreading

S. Karsten and J. Krieter, Institute of Animal Breeding and Husbandry, Christian-Albrechts-University, 24098 Kiel, Germany*

Contagious viral diseases like classical swine fever (CSF) have been posed a threat for animal production for a long time. Computer simulation represents a possibility to investigate risk factors and to evaluate epidemiological and economical consequences of control measures.
In this project a stochastic and spatial simulation model has been developed in order to simulate the spread of CSF between farms. Due to spatial as well as on-farm level heterogeneities in pig production the model allows for importing individual farm data. Results show that by disregarding the contact structure between farms the mean size of the epidemic may be overestimated (1178 vs. 7 infected herds). Besides animal, indirect and local contacts artificial insemination (AI) is regarded as a route of transmission. The outcomes indicate that if an AI-centre is infected in the beginning of an epidemic nearly all farms will be infected in the end. Several control measures can be compared relative to their effectiveness in controlling the disease. In addition, contact farms can be traced with variable efficiency. In preliminary calculations tracing of all animal contacts 3 and 4 days after detection of an infected multiplier is assumed with following culling, respectively. The mean period between infection and detection is not shortened (21.2 vs. 21.6 days) but 107 herds are infected instead of 194. Without contact tracing 532 of 2986 farms would be infected on average.

Poster M2.8

Ear tag transponders studied in sheep and goats

J.J. Heeres[1] and P.H. Hogerwerf[2], [1]Research Institute for Animal Husbandry, P.O. Box 2176 , 8203 AD Lelystad, [2]IMAG P.O. Box 43, 6700 AA Wageningen, The Netherlands.

To improve the present Identification and Registration system for sheep and goats in the Netherlands, early 2002 an experiment has started to investigate the functional value of ear tags with transponders. Finally technical specifications applicable to this type of ear tag will be formulated. The experiment exists of three successive steps (1) laboratory test, (2) pilot test with a restricted number of animals and (3) large scale test on sheep and goat farms and slaughterhouses. The tests focus on (a) minimizing loss of ear tags, (b) minimizing irritation; ear tagging must be as animal friendly as possible, (c) readability with electronic reader and visual and (d) fraud proof. First results show that 1/3 of the ear tags offered by companies, passed the laboratory and pilot test after minor modifications. In the pilot test (duration four weeks) it is shown that none of the tested ear tags scored 'animal friendly'. There are concerns about the healing of the wound. Depending on the ear tag, four weeks after tagging 3 tot 38 % of the animals scored healed wounds, whereas 10 to 50 % of the animals scored severe infections. Special attention must be paid to ear tagging of adult sheep. The shell-shaped ear can be susceptible to grazes. Results of the large scale test will be available early 2004.

Poster M2.9

Electronic identification of pigs: injectable transponders in abdominal cavity

F. Chiesa[1], E. Marchi[2], M. Zecchini[1], S. Barbieri[1] and N. Ferri[2], [1] Istituto di Zootecnica, Facoltà di Medicina Veterinaria, Via G. Celoria 10, 20133 Milano, Italy, [2] Istituto Zooprofilattico Sperimentale dell'Abruzzo e del Molise "G. Caporale", Campo Boario, 64100 Teramo, Italy.*

Electronic identification and monitoring of farm animals assure the traceability in the food chain and respect the food safety policy.

A total number of 527 weaned pigs were tested on two commercial farms: 242 in Farm 1 and 285 in Farm 2. Animals were identified by an ear tag in farrowing pen (average age of 18 days in Farm 1 and 16 days in Farm 2) and the ear tag number was linked with the transponder identification code at the injection by a programmable reader. Piglets at an average age of 25 days in Farm 1 and 30 days in Farm 2 were injected in abdominal cavity intraperitoneally, by an injection pistol. 148 passive bio-glass encapsulated HDX 23mm and 379 HDX 32mm transponders were randomly used. Readings of identification device were performed by portable ISO transceivers before injection, after injection, the day after and one week after the injection.

Readings weren't available in five pigs 7 days after application. Within one week from injection, 10 pigs died; autopsy results showed the cause of death was attributed to transponder's injection for two animals. Subsequent readings will be performed by stationary reading unit at fixed time.

Poster M2.10

Automatic readings in electronically identified cattle: first experience in four slaughterhouses

N. Ferri,E. Marchi and C. Di Francesco, Istituto Zooprofilattico Sperimentale dell'Abruzzo e del Molise "G. Caporale", via Campo Boario 64100, Teramo, Italy*

The implementation of an automatic reading system at the slaughterhouse is discussed. 88000 cattle head were identified by electronic ear tag. 47994 passed through four slaughterhouses, equipped with readers, antennas, connection cable, computers, software, data processing, remote data export, reader's network management. Results obtained shows 36727 (76,70 %) valid readings, 11267 not valid readings. According to a specific codification for not valid readings, results were: 8 (0,02%) code 01 (tag not read); 8 (0,02%) code 02 (tag lost); 974 (2,03%) code 03 (tag broken); 6776 (14,15%) code 04 (reader not functioning); 3389 (7,08%) code 10 (reading not performed). The results obtained shows that the system needs to be improved. Slaughterhouse represents a harsh environment for electronic equipment. Humidity, water, dust, steam, electromagnetic pollution, can easily lower the efficiency of the system. Several readers can influence each others, when operating in a restricted area; connecting several reader to a single PC is not always simple. The long distance between readers and antennas can enhance the interference in readings. Cable needs to be protected from damages. Antennas must be adjusted in order to fit the width of corridors. Computer must guarantee a full automation of reading operation, periodical data saving, continuous monitoring of readers operation through automatic enquiry, data downloading and monitoring of the software and system's functionality.

Poster M2.11

Electronic identification in buffaloes breeding

N. Ferri,E. Marchi and T.Di Mattia, Istituto Zooprofilattico Sperimentale dell'Abruzzo e del Molise "G.Caporale", via Campo Boario 64100, Teramo, Italy*

The IDEA project (Identification Electronique des Animaux), has foreseen the use of a tag for buffalo's identification. Buffaloes identification, due to the particular anatomic conformation and living habits of the animals, is particularly difficult. Electronic identification seems to be able to solve these management problems and guarantee a unique and inalterable identification of the animals.Buffaloes. A total number of 1611 buffaloes at different ages (from two days to twenty years) has been identified using a ceramic ruminal bolus 66x15 mm, 50 gr. weight (Innoceramics-Castelli, Italy), provided with a transponder HDX type (TIRIS Texas Instruments)-, glass encapsulated, 32x3,8 mm. A bolus gun administered the ruminal bolus. Control readings performed for 18 months, shows positive results in 98,77% of identified animals. No injuries to the animals have been reported. Data recorded shows that the time required for buffaloes tagging varies from a farm to the other, according to the facilities available to restrain the animals. It goes from 12 adult animals/hours, in farms were no restraining tools were available, to 60-70 adult animals/hours, in well-equipped farms. Electronic identification in buffaloes resulted to be highly compatible with a full automation in the milking procedures; results obtained in two farms equipped with automatic reading systems in the parlor, showed good results in the management of the animals electronic identification has been done in four farms in the province of Caserta (Italy).

Poster M2.12

Electronic identification and molecular markers for improving the traceability of livestock and meat

G. Caja[1], M. Hernández-Jover[1], A. Sánchez[1], A. Poucet[2], C. Korn[2], J. Capote[3], J.F. Vilaseca[4], G. Wendl[5], R. Webber[6], N. Ferri[7], M.A. Toro[8], C. Meghen[9], and I. Gut[10]. [1]Universitat Autònoma Barcelona, Spain; [2]Joint Research Centre-EC, Ispra, Italy; [3]Instituto Canario Investigaciondes Agrarias, Spain; [4]Gesimpex Com., Spain; [5]Technical University of Munich, Germany; [6]Shearwell Data, United Kingdom; [7]Istituto Zooprofilattico Sperimentale dell'Abruzzo-Molise, Italy; [8]Instituto Nacional Investigaciones Agrarias, Spain; [9]IdentiGen, Ireland; [10]Centre National Genotypage, France.

Traceability is a sensitive point for consumers. Despite this, methods for tracing meat are poorly developed. A double system based on electronic identification (EID) and DNA profiling for tracing animals and meat, has been developed in a EU FAIR 5th project (QLK1-CT2001-02229). The EID provides a tagging and real time tracing-back methodology for use until slaughtering, and DNA profile is used to audit the tracing-back of animals, carcasses and meat in the whole chain. Limiting factors of the use of bolus (ruminants) and injectable (pig) transponders in practice and the transfer of data from animals to carcasses and meat are studied. A selection of DNA markers is used and different biopsying and sampling methods tested. Finally, the project implements and evaluate the double system for tracing 7500 cattle, 2000 sheep and 9000 pigs from farm to consumer, including data base management and cost-benefit analysis. The project makes up a loose cluster with two other FAIR projects on food traceability and integrates the previous research on EID of livestock in the EU.

Poster M2.13

Electronic boluses features and retention law in the reticulorumen of cattle

J. Ghirardi, G. Caja, D. Garín, and M. Hernández-Jover , Universitat Autònoma de Barcelona, Spain.

A total of 782 beef calves were used to evaluate different electronic identification boluses. Milk fed calves were bolused at 2-5 wk of age, fed with milk (1 month) concentrate and straw and slaughtered at 380-480 kg. Size of the reticulo-omasal orifice was measured in 70 males and 42 females. Bolus consisted of two series of ceramic capsules containing a glass encapsulated half duplex transponder (31.8×3.8 mm). Series #1 (n=544) consisted of six prototypes with same dimensions (68×21 mm) but different specific gravity (2.39, 2.9, 2.79, 2.95, 3.12 and 3.36); and series #2 (n=238) of different commercial boluses varying in dimensions and specific gravity (39×15, 3.08; 51×15, 3.00; 64×16, 3.63; 68×17, 3.60; 62×19, 3.60; and, 66×20, 3.11). Bolus retention was checked at mo 1, 5 and 7, and at slaughter by using a handheld transceiver. Retention rate until slaughter varied quadratically (R^2=0.96) with a plateau according to bolus weight for the two serials: #1 (89.5 to 100%) and #2 (76.2 to 100%). Minimum weight and specific gravity to reach the 98% retention rate established by ICAR were estimated to be 65 g and up to 3.00 for cattle. Reticulo-omasal orifice differed in males vs. females (32.5 vs 29.9 mmØ) and was greater than diameter of retained boluses. As a conclusion, bolus features need to be optimized in order to achieve their maximum retention in cattle.

Poster M2.14

First results of a comparative trial of different rumen boluses in the electronic identification of US dairy sheep

G. Caja[1], D. L. Thomas[2], M. Rovai[1], and Y. M. Berger[2]. [1]Grup de Recerca en Remugants, Universitat Autònoma de Barcelona, 08193 Bellaterra, Spain, [2]Department of Animal Sciences, University of Wisconsin-Madison, Madison, WI 53706, USA.

A total of 368 dairy sheep at the Spooner Agricultural Research Station were used to study the effectiveness of three types of electronic rumen boluses for identification and milk recording. All sheep carried at least one ear tag. The boluses consisted of ISO radio frequency transponders of different technology encased in capsules of different construction: B1 (full duplex; 20_74 mm, 70 g, white plastic cover), B2 (half duplex; 21×68 mm, 79 g, white ceramic cover), and B3 (half duplex; 12×42 mm, 16 g, brown ceramic cover). Boluses were given orally to sheep on the same day. Bolus readability was checked immediately before and after administration, and at 1, 9, 32, 72, 102 and 154 d, using handheld transceivers. Animals ranged in weight from 33 to 117 kg, and there were no injuries or deaths from bolus administration. Application and reading times averaged 65 and 19 s, respectively. Five months after administration, bolus readability varied by bolus type (B1, 41.5%; B2, 100%; and B3, 97.5%; $P < 0.001$). Ear tag losses were 2.7%. The B1 and B3 boluses were insufficiently readable for ICAR requirements of 98% readability, but the B2 was very effective in identification and milk recording of sheep.

Poster M2.15

Livestock identification in Ukraine

R. Kravciv[1], V. Kvachov[1], D.Yanovich[2], [1]Lviv State Academy for Veterinary Medicine, Pekarska str. 50, Lviv, [2]Lviv Region State Depertment for Veterinary Medicine, 79024 Promyslova str. 9, Lviv, Ukraine*

Livestock identification in Ukraine includes a number of actions such as ears tagging with unique and invariable identification code, issue of cattle passports and veterinary cards and filing the information about animals and their displacement to the database of livestock Register. Livestock Register is the automatic electronic net, which is responsible for gathering, accumulation and processing data about identified livestock during the whole life period. Information about separate animals displacement and their owners and veterinary and sanitary state of their economies are noted in the Register.

With the aim to conduct animal identification in Ukraine state enterprise “Animal Identification and Registration Agency” was established. At this time an experimental introduction of livestock identification is realized in Kiev, Lviv, Dnipropetrovsk, Odessa, Vinnica, Sumi, Cherkassi and Hmelnisk regions. First stage of identification is accented on breeding farms. Next stage is planned to be conducted in private sector. Work on animals identification in regions is conducted by agents, those authorized by Animal Identification Agency.

 Poster M2.16

Farm certification: the next phase in the Identification & Registration of cattle

P.J.B. Galesloot[*1], H.B. Jansen[1], A.L.W. van Gee[2] and R.W. de Koning[2], [1]NRS B.V., P.O. Box 454, 6800 AL Arnhem, the Netherlands, [2]Animal Health Service, P.O. Box 9, 7400 AA Deventer, the Netherlands.*

The Identification and Registration (I&R) systems are implemented in the past ten years in the EU countries with the main objective of tracing all animal movements from birth to slaughter. This traceability of animals is a prerequisite for disease eradication and control. The Dutch I&R system has been expanded by the Animal Health Service (AHS) with a Certification Operating System (COS). This system is used to manage automatically the monitoring and certification programs for diseases like Brucellosis, Bovine Leucosis, IBR and BVD. COS is fed by systems like the national I&R system, the commercially available IRIS system and the Laboratory Information Management System. COS improves the quality and efficiency of decision making by considering all key factors. It facilitates the selection of animals for sampling, the mailing of instructions for sampling to veterinarians and farmers, the recording and interpretation of the laboratory results and the determination of the health status of farms. Another important function of COS is the automatic planning of farm visits by veterinarians within the framework of the Milk Quality Assurance Program (KKM) for dairy producers. In conclusion: COS is an application that manages the process of farm certification, the corner stone of farming in the coming years.

Theatre M3.1

Bioaerosols in farm animal houses

J. Hartung, Institute of Animal Hygiene, Animal Welfare and Behaviour of Farm Animals, Bünteweg 17P, D-30559 Hannover

The air in farm animal houses contains considerable amounts of so-called bioaerosols which are composed of viable and nonviable particles which may carry gases and which remain suspended in the air for longer periods because of their minute dimensions of between 10^{-4} and approximately 10^{2} µm. The bioaerosols give cause for concern: (1) microbial pathogens may cause directly infectious and allergic diseases in humans and farm animals. (2) they entail complaints of nearby residents about possible respiratory health effects. The concentration of airborne microorganisms in livestock buildings are between some 100 and several 1000 per liter. Staphylococcae, streptococcae, colilike bacteria, fungi, moulds and yeasts are regularly found. The 24 h average concentrations of dust in animal barns vary considerably. In poultry houses the highest inhalable resp. respirable dust concentrations (up to 10 mg/m^3 resp. 1.2 mg/m^3) were found, followed by pig houses (5.5 mg/m^3 resp. 0.46 mg/m^3) and cattle barns (1.22 mg/m^3 resp. 0.17 mg/m^3). Endotoxins in airborne dust can range from 0.6 ng/m^3 (cattle respirable dust) to 860 ng/m^3 (laying hens, inhalable dust). Presently discussed occupational health threshold at the workplace is around 5 ng/m^3 (50 EU/m^3). The emission rates for respirable dust are from piggeries about 60 mg/h, from poultry houses nearly 300 mg/h and from cattle barns at 20 mg/h, related to 500 kg liveweight of the animals. The reduction of indoor pollution to improve health of animal and man and the establishment of safe distances to neighbouring residential areas are essential for the future development of sustainable animal farming in Europe.

 Theatre M3.2

Dust in different housing systems for growing-finishing pigs

A.J.A. Aarnink[1], N. Stockhofe[2] and M.J.M. Wagemans[1], [1]Institute of Agricultural and Environmental Engineering (IMAG), P.O. Box 43, 6700 AA Wageningen; [2]AnimalSciences Group, P.O. Box 65, 8200 AB Lelystad, The Netherlands.*

The objective of this project was to determine dust concentrations and sources of dust in different housing systems for growing-finishing pigs. Three housing systems were studied: 1. common housing (in The Netherlands) without straw; 2. common housing with use of little 'activity' straw; 3. housing with a thick layer of straw bedding and an outside yard.
Inhalable and respirable dust and endotoxine concentrations were measured at different locations at different moments during the fattening period. By elementary analysis of collected airborne dust and dust generated in the lab from different dust sources (feces, feed, skin dust, straw) the contribution of each source to dust production was determined. In the slaughterhouse the lungs of the pigs were checked for pneumonic lesions.
The results showed higher concentrations of inhalable dust ($p<0.05$) and endotoxine ($p<0.05$) for the housing with straw bedding, while respirable dust was lower in the beginning and higher at the end of the fattening period in the straw housing ($p<0.05$). The straw bedding significantly contributed to airborne dust at the end of the fattening period. The lung study showed a higher number of pigs with a mild focal pleuritis in the straw bedding house than in the common housing systems.

Theatre M3.3

Air quality in pig facilities in relation with physiological stages

N. Guingand, Institut Technique du Porc, BP 35104, 35651 Le Rheu cedex, France

One of the missions of the Technical Institute for Pig is to study different aspects of pig breeding in relation with air quality inside the building. In this paper, data collected since several years have been analysed in order to compare air quality in relation with physiological stages and season. In each building, different parameters concerning physical aspects of air quality (ambient temperature, outside temperature and ventilation rate per animal) and environmental aspects as dust concentration, ammoniac concentration in the ambience and in the exhaust air and odour emission were measured. Buildings involved in this paper are considering representing of buildings existing in major French pig facilities. Great differences were observed between physiological stalges. Although dust concentrations were higher in post-weaning rooms, the highest concentrations of ammonia and odour were measured in fattening rooms. Season appears to have a great effect on dust, ammonia and odour whatever physiological stages considered. Relation between ammonia and odour was described showing the absence of correlation between those both parameters whatever season and physiological stages. At the end of this paper, dust and ammonia concentrations in the ambient were analysed in relation with labour conditions of pig farmers.

Occurence of fungi and yeasts in pig facilities in dependence on stable equipment and feeding technique

R. Böhm, University of Hohenheim, Institute of Environmental nd Animal Hygiene, Garbenstraße 30, D-70953 Stuttgart

In one pig facilities with liquid and solid feeding airsamples during feeding time and during rest period were taken in several functional areas using 3 different airsamplers (PGP-system, Andersen-airsampler, Respicon).
In the samples the cultivatable mesophilic and thermophilic fungi and yeasts were examined and the total fungi count was determined using the CAMNEA-technique.
The measured cultivatable fungi and yeast concentrations in the pig facility were low. The total fungi count was more than 10^3 to 10^6 times higher than the cultivatable counts.
No noteworthy differences in the results of investigations were seen between the different feeding techniques nor between feeding time and rest period.

Theatre M3.5

Isolation and identification of cocci in the air of animal houses

J. Schulz, Institute of Animal Hygiene, Animal Welfare and Behaviour of Farm Animals, Bünteweg 17P, D-30559 Hannover

Airborne micro organisms present in poultry livestock houses are rich in variety and quantity. The two most prominent genera that have been recovered from the air are staphylococcus and streptococcus. Currently, the quantity and associated health risks on humans and animals from the pathogen cocci is relatively unknown.
Therefore, this work focussed on developing an analytical procedure to separate stapyhylococci within animal house air, and to identify the species by biochemical and molecular biological methods.
After air sampling staphylococci were separated from other genera by a culturing step. Simple biochemical tests followed to identify the genus and further biochemical tests along with an ITS-PCR were used to detect the species. This method has proved to be useful for rapid identification of airborne staphylococci species.
The first results taken from a poultry livestock building showed that different staphylococcus species could be isolated and identified within 36-48 hours. The sampling method provides the means to quantify the species per cubic meter of air.
Similarly this method can also be applied to investigate airborne streptococcus species.
The potential exists for this application to characterise the germ spectra of animal house air and in more detail providing a better assessment of the health risks for humans and animals that are exposed to airborne bacteria.

Theatre M3.6

Techniques for reduction of ammonia release in a cowshed with tied dairy cattle

G. Gustafsson[1], K-H. Jeppsson[1], J. Hultgren[2], J. Sannö[2], [1]Department of Agricultural Biosystems and Technology, P.O. Box 86, S- 230 53 Alnarp, Sweden, [2]Department of Animal Environment and Health, P.O. Box 234, S- 532 23 Skara, Sweden.*

The influence of different techniques to reduce the ammonia emission from a cowshed with 42 tied dairy cows has been investigated. The following changes of the building design were made; slurry instead of semi solid manure handling; improved gutters with a 3% slope towards a urine drainage channel equipped with an auger; cooling of manure by water pipes in the gutters; manure gas ventilation from the urine channels and manure culvert; and cleaning of the exhaust air by a biofilter of woodchips and straw prepared with a bacteria culture. The release of ammonia from the building was measured continuously before and after steps were taken to reduce the emission by using an infrared spectrophotometer in outlet air and outlet impellers. Before changing the building design the average ammonia emission was 24 g/cow and day, indoor ammonia concentration was 8 ppm. After the changes had been made the ammonia release through the exhaust air before the biofilter was reduced with 20 % to 18 g/cow and day. Average indoor ammonia concentration was 3 ppm. In most cases, it was not possible to detect ammonia in the air after the biofilter, implying that the total emission from the facility was negligible.

Theatre M3.7

Comparing and evaluating suitable tracer gas methods to estimate ventilation rates in naturally ventilated broiler livestock houses

L.C. Formosa, Institute of Animal Hygiene, Animal Welfare and Behaviour of Farm Animals, Bünteweg 17P, D-30559 Hannover

Increasing concern over bio-aerosol and greenhouse gas emissions from livestock farming enterprises into local and global environments has lead to the need to quantify these emissions. Currently the majority of livestock housing systems throughout the world are Louisiana or naturally ventilated design, whereby the ventilation rate is dependent on the weather. In these types of livestock houses, ventilation rate measurements are difficult to perform and subject to many errors. The best options available for quantifying ventilation rates include tracer gas techniques adopting natural and/or artificial tracer gases and/or mass balance models. This paper looks at the principles of these methods and compares their advantages and disadvantages using a broiler barn as an example. The use of natural tracer gas methods (CO_2) requires detailed knowledge on heat and respiratory carbon dioxide balances, regarding the production of CO_2 from animals and subtracting for interfering sources. On the other hand the more expensive release of artificial tracer gases requires knowledge of the internal airflows, which windows and chimneys act as inlets and/or outlets and under what weather conditions. Therefore, knowledge of air circulation patterns and the position of samplers are crucial. Due to different architectural designs and the random nature of such measurements, the best method for one livestock building may not be for another, therefore the technique should be selected with regards to the requirements of the investigation and design of the livestock house.

 Poster M3.8

Microenviromental parameters and air quality in a swine housing

M. Guarino, A. Costa, G. Agnelli and P. Navarotto Dipartimento di Scienze e Tecnologie Veterinarie per la Sicurezza Alimentare, Università degli Studi di Milano - Via Celoria, 10 -20133 Milano - Italia*

Swine welfare and human health, in modern intensive swine breeding, depends mostly on indoor air quality. The interaction among the environmental parameters, type of floor, ventilation system, and growth performance of pigs were studied in a trial conducted from the 17th July to 13th November 2002 in a swine finishing building in Northern Italy. The building was subdivided in three rooms varying in floor type, ventilation system. The floor in the three rooms, was partially slatted, or totally slatted or continuous. A score was assigned to estimate the amount of manure lying on the floor. In all rooms, ammonia concentrations were generally higher than the 7 ppm except for the totally slatted floor room, but lower than the 25 ppm value indicated by ACGIH (1993). Ammonia concentration and relative humidity were significantly lower in the totally slatted floor room. Ammonia level is inversely related to temperature, in agreement with studies lead by Aarninck (1992) and by Gustaffson (2002). Relative humidity seems positively related to ammonia levels. The floor ventilation system, when compared to the ceiling system, seems to affect positively indoor air quality. It can be concluded that floor ventilation system and the totally slatted floor can concur to improve air quality and growth performance in a swine housing.

Theatre M4.1

Teaching animal bioethics in Europe: present situation and prospects

M. Marie[1], S. Edwards [2], E. von Borell [3], G. Gandini [4], [1]Sciences Animales, ENSAIA-INPL, B.P. 172, 54505 Vandœuvre lès Nancy, France, [2]Department of Agriculture, University of Newcastle, King George VI Building, Newcastle upon Tyne NE1 7RU, United Kingdom, [3]Institute of Animal Breeding and Husbandry, Martin-Luther-University Halle-Wittenberg, Adam-Kuckhoff-Str. 35, 06108 Halle, Germany, [4]Dipartimento di Scienze e Tecnologie Veterinarie per la Sicurezza Alimentare, Facoltà di Medicina Veterinaria, Università degli Studi di Milano, Via Celoria 10, 20133 Milano, Italia.*

A survey has been conducted in 17 European countries, in 106 agricultural or veterinary higher education institutions delivering courses in animal bioethics. Information regarding the nature of the curriculum, number and background of the teachers, pedagogic methods, topics covered (nature and time dedicated) has been collected for 199 courses. The wide disparity in the structures for delivering training, the different approaches and histories of teaching in this domain are presented. For now, teaching is biased towards ethical issues relating to the human-animal interaction and animal welfare, and much less attention is paid to other issues. The paucity of PhD or post-graduate courses, and so the few opportunities for young scientists to become specialised in animal ethics is evident. Difficulties, assets and strategies for developing curricula in this field are analysed. An on-line searchable and continuously updating database has been implemented. Contacts and collaborations between teachers, information and virtual or physical mobility of students are expected outcomes (see: http://www.ensaia.inpl-nancy.fr/bioethics).

Theatre M4.2

Improved rabbit housing management for female growth and reproduction

G. Masoero, G. Bergoglio, R. Chicco.* Istituto Sperimentale Zootecnia, Via Pianezza 115, 10151-Torino, Italy.

A complex experiment with four housing systems for growing rabbit females (N=168, of which 36 slaughtered at 120d), and successively reproduced (N=110), in a standard flat-deck or in a improved two-floor cage housing system was carried on. The growth in the pre-reproductive phase was similar in small, medium and in large collective (3 females), but increased in large single cages (+22%). Hind-leg bones weight was reduced by 10% in small cages, while muscle/bone ratio appeared reduced in large collective cages. Low availabilty of space in growth period was negative for reproductive fitness till to 1st kindling (20% discarded vs 6%; P=0.087) and produced the lowest litter size. The colony rearing for young females strongly affected productivity as total weaned weight (-14%). In the two-floor cages fertility was reduced (-15%), incidence of abortion increased (17 vs 10%; P< 0.05) and the litter size decreased about 5%. The weight of the kit at 19d appeared reduced by 4%, because significant reduction of feed intake of the family (-6.5%), but at weaning no difference was found. Management solutions adopted for females in pre-reproductive growth period and increased housing volume of the cage, conceived for rabbit does welfare can significantly affect, in negative sense, reproductive performance.

Theatre M4.3

Productivity of free-nursing rabbit does and their litters submitted to a split 48-hour separation

A. Bonanno, F. Mazza, A. Di Grigoli, M. Alabiso, Dipartimento S.En.Fi.Mi.Zo., sezione Produzioni animali, Università di Palermo, Viale delle Scienze, 90128 Palermo, Italy.*

In order to prevent weight loss in litters subjected to doe-litter separation (DLS), whilst maintaining its beneficial effects on fertility, the standard DLS, lasting 48 h before artificial insemination (AI), was split into two periods of 24 h by a controlled suckling.

Initially, 105 does of different parity were divided into three groups. During the free-nursing the does were treated as follows: standard DLS (ST), the nest-box was closed for 48 h from day 9 to 11, before AI; split DLS (SP), the nest-box was closed for 24 h and, after suckling, for other 24 h, before AI; control (C), does had free access to the nest-box.

Fertility improved similarly (P≤0.05) in ST (60.9 %) and SP (59.4 %) does, compared to C does (44.1 %), especially in does of parity 1 (+20.8 and +19.4 %) and 2-3 (+25.8 and +18.5 %; P≤0.05). ST and SP does showed lower rabbit losses from day 14 to 35 (P≤0.001) and higher litter sizes at weaning (P≤0.05) than C does. The ST reduced growth from day 9 to 14 (P≤0.001) and the weaning weight of rabbits (732, 777, 780 g for ST, SP and C, respectively; P≤0.01). Productivity improved by 35.4 % and 44.2% with ST and SP respectively.

Illumination or guiding light during night hours in the resting area of AM-barns

Gunnar Pettersson and Hans Wiktorsson, Department of Animal Nutrition and Management, Swedish University of Agricultural Sciences, S-75007 UPPSALA 7, Sweden

It is a common practice to have full illumination day and night in AM-barns. It is however questioned whether cows prefer/need guiding light/darkness during night hours. The aim was to investigate if dairy cows actively choose light or dark area for resting during night hours. The study was conducted in an AMS research barn with 4 rows of cubicles. The resting area was divided into 2 identical section, but the passages remained unaffected. One half of the resting area had full lighting (app. 200 lux), while the other had guiding light (5 - 7 lux) from 23:00h to 05:00h. After 3 weeks the lighting in the two sections was reversed. Manual identification of every cow in the resting area was performed every 12:th minute during 48 consecutive hours in each experimental period.

The results of the studies did not reveal obvious preference for a special side because of the illumination. The conclusions of the study are: 1) no difference between full lighting or guided light could be seen on herd level; 2) number of milkings were not affected; 3) cows did not change their resting periods; 4) individual preference of full lighting or guided light could be observed, but was not due to ranking order.

Theatre M4.5

Husbandry systems from the animal's point of view: Pigs

K.H. de Greef[2], W.G.P. Schouten[1], C.M. Groenestein[1], R.G. ten Hoope[1] and M. de Jong[3], Wageningen-UR ([1]Wageningen and [2]Lelystad) and [3]Dutch Society For the Protection of Animals, The Hague, The Netherlands

In a multi-disciplinary research group, the biological needs of animals were chosen as a basis for the design of a husbandry system. Rationale for this is the view that satisfying the needs of animals is a minimum standard for acceptance. Knowledge of the natural behaviour of the animals is highly important in formulating the behavioural needs of animals but not all natural behaviour is necessary in husbandry systems e.g. anti predator behaviour, sexual behaviour in most slaughter animals. Therefore needs are defined from the motivation of the animals (what do animals want) rather than from the natural behaviour of the animals (what the animals are able to). A total of 59 requirements for a stable for fattening pigs were formulated. The basic assumption for including the requirements was: do we wrong the animals in not accepting a given requirement. Definition of requirements for adequate health (absence of discomfort due to disease) is less clear than for the other needs. Lack of unequivocal definitions and absence of animal motivation aspects are major factors in this. The required space for fattening pigs decreased with increasing group size. Beyond a group size of 50 pigs this decrease became marginal. For a group of 50 fattening pigs the amount space was about 2m^2/pig. Outdoor access could not be supported being essential to the animals. This is one of the key factors in which an animal-oriented design deviates from public ideal views.

Rearing piglets with a sensor controlled mash feeder: performance, eating behaviour and animal health compared with the conventional tube feeder

E.F. Hessel[1], K. Cordes[1] and H. Van den Weghe[2], [1]Institute for Agricultural Engineering, Georg-August-University of Göttingen, Gutenbergstr. 33, 37075 Göttingen, Germany, [2]Research Centre for Animal Production and Technology, Georg-August-University of Göttingen, Driverstr. 22, 49377 Vechta, Germany.*

The sensor feeding system for weaned piglets shall reach a smooth transition from the sows' milk by ration out mash in time intervals. Thus weaning problems are supposed to be reduced.
In this investigation the influence of a sensor controlled mash feeder versus a tube feeder on performance, behaviour and animal health was determined. Therefore in one compartment with two pens piglets were housed in groups (25 animals). In one group piglets were fed with the sensor feeder the first 14 days of rearing, in following three weeks they were fed with the tube feeder. In the second group piglets were fed with the tube feeder during the whole weaning period. This trial was repeated three times.
After 14 days of rearing piglets fed with the sensor feeder showed significantly higher weight gains. After five weeks of rearing this advantage was still detectable, especially with piglets weighing less than 5.0 kg by the time of stalling in. Also, in this group significantly more concerns around the feeder and a significant higher number of head injuries were detected after two weeks of rearing. Furthermore, significantly more piglets attempted to get some food but failed because of occupied feeding places.

Theatre M4.7

Health status of finishing pigs in different environments

J. Krieter[1], R. Badertscher[2], R. Schnider[2], K.-H. Tölle[1]. [1]Institute of Animal Breeding and Husbandry, Christian-Albrechts-University, 24098 Kiel, Germany, [2]Swiss Federal Research Station for Agriculture Economics and Engineering, 8356 Tänikon, Switzerland*

The aim of the study was to investigate the health status of finishing pigs in different environments. Pigs (n=11,163) were checked twice in 92 farms (slatted floor, n=36; concrete floor with straw bedding and outdoor area) by one person (at the beginning and the end of the fattening period in summer or winter). Animal health was described by skin lesions, lameness, sneeze, cough and tail biting. Housing and management conditions were registered by an detailed questionnaire. After merging health information with the questionnaire the data were analysed using generalized linear models In addition to the random farm effect different housing and management factors (fixed) were included in the model depending on the trait considered.
Housing affected skin lesions (p=.002), lameness (p<.0001) and tail biting (p<.0001). The risk (odds ratio (OR)) of skin lesions was lower at concrete floor (OR=.40) compared to slatted floor (OR=1.00); restricted straw increased OR (2.35) in contrast to the deep litter system. Lameness enhanced with concrete floor and outdoor area (OR=3.03), restricted straw use showed higher OR. Tail biting was positively affected by straw (OR=.22). In addition season (winter/summer) and different management factors (e.g. all in/all out, purchase, cleanliness, antibiotics) and the random farm effect had a great impact on the animal health status at farm level.

Use of a test day model in an extension education and outreach program for a dairy farming community using an on-line system

G. Azzaro[1], S. Ventura[1], J. Carvalheira[2], M. Caccamo[1], G. Licitra[1,4], E. Raffrenato[1,3,] and R.W. Blake[3]. [1]CoRFiLaC, Regione Siciliana, s.p. 25 km 5, 97100 Ragusa, Italy. [2]Instituto de Ciências Biomédicas Abel Salazar and Centro de Investigação em Biodiversidade e Recursos Genéticos, Universidade do Porto, Rua Padre Armando Quintas-Crasto, 4485-661 Vairão, Portugal. [3]Department of Animal Science, Cornell University, USA. [4]D.A.C.P.A., Università di Catania, Italy.*

Dairy extension programs in southeastern Sicily have been restructured to meet the needs for specialization by potentially highly productive managers. An integrated information system was developed to evaluate the effects of management changes and to inform farmers about the results. This system uses an autoregressive test-day animal model to estimate the genetic (co)variance components and parameters. The edited data were 214,650 (15,161), 44,768 (3,049) and 8,669 (660) records of yields (cows) of milk, fat and protein in first three lactations of Friesian, Brown Swiss and Modicana breeds. Parameter solutions were applied using the model to routinely update monthly estimates of management factors affecting herd performance for the 12 months prior to the current test day. Management response curves for milk and components revealed within-year variation in average daily yields and seasonal effects of quality, availability and cost of feed, thus facilitating evaluation of the feeding and management program. Using the internet, producers and technicians can now query and interact with the integrated system, obtaining monthly updates, which are intended to better inform decision making.

Poster M4.9

Environmental control in an intensive rabbit rearing

P.A. Martino[1], F. Luzi[2], M. Verga[2], [1]Dipartimento di Patologia Animale, Igiene e Sanità Pubblica Veterinaria, [2]Istituto di Zootecnica, Via Celoria 10, 20133 Milano, Italy*

The environmental conditions play a pivotal role in maintaining the health and the welfare of the animals in intensive breeding. This is also valid in rabbit, a species particularly sensitive to environmental changes and to pathogenic microorganisms (e.g., bacteria, fungi). Aim of this work is the evaluation of the number and kind of bacteria and fungi to which rabbits, breeded in sheds with natural ventilation, are exposed. In detail, for fungi, we have evaluated not only the typical environmental ones but also the dermatophytes (*Microsporum* and *Trichophyton*). Data was collected during summer and autumn (July - October) in doe's sheds, in nests and in fattening sheds. We have used, for all the environments, "opened plates" containing *Tryptic Soy Agar, Sabouraud Agar* and *Dermasel Agar* (Oxoid).
Escherichia coli, *Staphylococcus* spp. and *Micrococcus* spp. was the most frequently isolated bacteria, with a bacterial charge, on average, more than 50 UFC/plate. Among fungi, *Aspergillus*, *Penicillium* and *Alternaria* was the most spread; this result confirms their "omnipresence" and the unavoidable exposure of the animals. It's important to underline the isolation of a high number of dermatophytes such as *Microsporum canis*, *Microsporum gipseum* and *Trichophyton mentagrophytes* with charge extremely variable (10-50 UFC/plate). This result have a great importance for animal welfare but, above all, for human health because these microorganisms have a zoonosic potential.

Poster M4.10

Effect of the environmental enrichment and group size on performance and carcass traits in rabbits

F.M.G. Luzi[1], V. Ferrante[1], E. Heinzl[1], D. Zucca[1], M. Verga[1], M. Bianchi[2], C. Cavani[2] and M. Petracci[2], [1]Istituto di Zootecnica Veterinaria, Università di Milano, via Celoria, 10, 20133 Milano, Italy, [2] Dip. di Scienze degli Alimenti, Università di Bologna, Via S. Giacomo 9, 40126 Bologna, Italy.*

Aim of this research was to test the effect of environmental enrichment (presence of a peace of wood inside the cage) and group size on performance and carcass traits of fattening rabbits. This trial was carried out in a commercial facility, situated in the North of Italy (Lombardia region). Animals were housed in cages (2, 3 and 4 animals per cage) at the same density. Animals were weighted at 35, 55, 75 days. There were no significant differences in any selected productive parameters (alive weight and daily weight gain) among treatment groups. Animals were slaughtered at 75d of age under commercial conditions. A total of 102 carcasses were used to establish loin and hind cut yields as well as perirenal and scapular fat deposits. *L. lumborum* muscles were analysed for colour, pH, drip and cooking loss, moisture and LF-NMR parameters. There were no significant differences in any selected carcass traits among treatment groups. Rabbits held with environmental enrichment exhibited meat with significantly higher moisture (76.0 vs. 75.7%, $P<0.05$) and lower redness (a*, 2.65 vs. 3.22, $P<0.05$) in respect with those kept under standard conditions, whereas group size did not influenced any selected meat quality parameters.

Poster M4.11

The effect of creep boxes with covered openings on the growth and behaviour of piglets

V. Juskiene, R. Juska, Lithuanian Institute of Animal Science, R. Zebenkos 12, LT-5125 Baisogala, Radviliskis distr., Lithuania.

A study was conducted to determine the effect of creep boxes with covered openings on the growth of suckling piglets, their behaviour and morphological-biochemical profile of blood. The experiments were carried out on 233 piglets of the Lithuanian aboriginal breed. The piglets were allotted to 2 groups. Pigs in the control group were heated with 250W lamps from birth to weaning, while the lying areas of pigs in the experimental group were equipped with creep boxes of 1 m^2 area and having 0.26 m openings covered with curtains made of synthetic fabrics. The experiments indicated that the temperature in the creep boxes was on the average by 13.1°C higher, but CO_2 concentration was also by 3-5 times higher than that in the pig-house. At weaning the experimental piglets weighed on the average by 300 g less than the control piglets. The analysis of blood indicated no significant differences between the groups except for the alkaline reserve, which at 50 days of piglets age was by 18% lower in the experimental group. Behaviour studies indicated lower agility of the piglets in the experimental group. In conclusion, our study indicated that if creep boxes are used for equipping the lying areas of suckling pigs, it is advisable not to cover the opening of the box at all or to keep it covered only for the first two weeks.

Effects of gender on the resistance to *Ascaridia galli* infections in poultry

M. Gauly, T. Homann and G. Erhardt. Department of Animal Breeding and Genetics, Justus Liebig University of Giessen, Ludwigstr. 21 B, D-35390 Giessen, Germany*

55 male and 75 female chickens were each experimentally infected with 250 Ascaridia galli eggs at the first day of live to estimate sex differences of parasite resistance. All animals were slaughtered 6 weeks *post infection,* faecal egg counts (FEC) determined, guts removed and the adult worms collected. Worm establishment rates were not significant different between the sexes. However mean FEC of male chicks (411 ± 355) and worm burden (2.69 ± 2.24) were in tendency higher ($p > 0.05$) compared with female animals (334 ± 361; 2.26 ± 2.21), which confirms studies in other species. FECs were significantly ($p < 0.01$) positive correlated with worm burden ($r = 0.43$). Size and weight of female worms were significantly ($p < 0.01$) negative correlated with bird weights at 6 weeks of age ($r = -0.30$; $r = -0.53$). Significantly ($p < 0.01$) negative correlations were estimated for total worm burden and the size and weight of female worms ($r = -0.21$, $r = -0.34$). Fertility per female worm was significantly ($p < 0.01$) positive correlated with the worms weight ($r = 0.25$).

Poster M4.13

Relationship between broiler performance and hygiene variables

S. Gürler[1] and M.N. Orman[2], [1-2]Ankara University, Faculty of Veterinary Medicine, Department of Biyostatistics, 06110 Diskapi Ankara, Turkey.*

The objective of this research was to determine the effects of some hygiene variables on performance of commercial broilers. Investigation data coming from 1430 commercial broiler flocks kept on 298 broiler production units were collected in sixteen moths of time from April 1999 to October 2000. European Efficiency Factor (dependent variable) was used as a quantitative measure of the flock performance. Thirty seven hygiene variables (independent variables) with two responses were defined. The stepwise regressions were performed using of a software program. An index for hygiene variables associated with EEF was developed at the end of analysis. In the final regression model, the following hygiene variables were found to be significantly ($P<0,01$) associated with broiler performance: epidemic diseases, dead-bird management, structure of the house, presence of different age groups or other poultry in the farm, distance to the nearest poultry house, removal of litter in the end of rearing period, disinfection of the footwear at the entrance of broiler house, age of broiler house, flock size, type of ventilation system, and heating system. The R^2 ($P<0,01$) showed that the model could explain 49% of the differences in flock performance. As the result of this investigation it can be stated that efficiency of broiler flocks can be improved by means of improving the hygiene variables related with house, equipment, management and bio-security.

Poster M4.14

The effect of rearing season and region on performance of commercial broilers in Turkey

S. Gürler and M.N. Orman, Ankara Univ, Veterinary Medicine 06110 Diskapi Ankara, Turkey.*

The aim of this study was to determine the effects of rearing season and region on performance of commercial broilers. Investigation data from 1430 commercial broiler flocks were kept on 298 broiler production units. Livability (L), feed conversion ratio (FCR), live weight (LW) and European Efficiency Factor (EEF) were used as a quantitative measure of the flock performance. The effect of the season and region on the FCR, LW and EEF was determined by two ways analyses of variance. Despite very similar genetic backgrounds, statistically significant differences between flock performances were found. The mean EEF figures for different rearing seasons, winter, spring, summer and autumn, were 194,1; 196,3; 185,1 and 202,6 respectively ($P<0,01$). For the different geographical regions, Mudurnu, Bolu, Dörtdivan, Sakarya, Ankara and Eskisehir, mean EEF figures were 181,4; 218,3; 208,5; 217,7; 224,7 and 216,3 respectively ($P<0,01$). While FCR figures for winter, spring, summer and autumn were not significant statisticaly, those for regions were found to be significant. The mean LW(g) figures for winter, spring, summer and autumn were 1767,1; 1777,2; 1717,5 and 1805,4 respectively ($P<0,01$). The mortality rates (%) for the seasons were 10,21; 10,34; 11,33 and 9,18 respectively ($P<0,01$). In conclusion, the least production figures were obtained from the flocks raised in the summer and it was determined that rearing season and region have a significant effect on performance characteristics.

Poster M4.15

Influence of egg weight on ostrich (*Struthio camelus*) chick growth in Northern Italy

I. Zoccarato[1], L. Gasco[1], K. Guo[1], G. Picco[1], G. Masoero[2], [1]Dipartimento di Scienze Zootecniche, Università di Torino, Via Leonardo da Vinci 44, 10095 Grugliasco (Torino), [2]Istituto Sperimentale per la Zootecnia (ISZ), via Pianezza 115,10151 Torino, Italy.*

From 1997 to 2001 ostrich chick growth from hatching to 56 days of age were recorded. Ostriches were kept in sex ratio (M:F) of 1:1. In all 610 eggs were weighed at laying and twice during incubation while 409 chicks were weighed at hatching, 7, 14, 28 and 56 days of age.
Laying season could range from February/March to October but in practice the induction to stop laying was carried out in August. The total number of eggs laid per female ranged from 21 to 52. The fertility was around 70%. The overall hatchability was higher than 60%, while the hatchability of fertile eggs was higher than 90%. During 5 years the egg mass increased constantly, the weight ranged from 1220 to 1427 g. The percentages of weight losses during incubation were around 9.9% and were not affected by years of laying and egg weight. Egg weight changed in different months and years and showed a positive linear relationship (R^2=0.84) with the chick hatching weight. The effect of egg weight on chick weight decreased as chicks grew and became insignificant at 56 days of age. The average weight of chick was around 800 g and 11000 g respectively at hatching and 56 days.

Poster M4.16

A comparison of different kind of bedding materials for dairy free stalls

P. Rossi, A. Gastaldo, M. Borciani, C.R.P.A. spa, C.so Garibaldi, 42, 42100 Reggio Emilia, Italy*

A trial was carried out in an experimental free-stall barn comparing 3 different kind of bedding: straw (ST), sawdust (SW) and sand (SA). The survey on time spent by the cows resting and in activity has been carried out with the aid of a closed circuit video camera with time-lapse recorder; cubicles were observed in summer and winter conditions. The time spent lying down in cubicle was, on average, 15 h/cow/day in cubicles with ST and SW and 12 h/cow/day in cubicles with SA. The average number of daily rest frequencies was 8÷9 and the duration of rests was 90÷100 min. Higher frequencies of rests were observed in ST (+ 44 %) in SW (+69 %), compared with SA. In cubicles with SA the average duration of resting periods was higher than in cubicles with ST and SW. On daily basis the results show two principal resting periods. The longer period starts at 20 and finish at 6; the shorter period stars at 9 and finish at 16. Higher attendance had been noticed in cubicles with ST and SW, during the first hours of each daily resting period, while cows were able to choose among different bedding. In conclusion cows showed higher preference for ST and SW, because they tend to rest in cubicles with sand only when they have no other chances.

Poster M4.17

Preferences of dairy cows for different kind of cubicle flooring

M. Intini[1], L. Calamari[2], G. Lombardi[1] and L. Stefanini[1], [1]Azienda Sperimentale "V. Tadini", 29027 Podenzano, Piacenza, Italy, [2]Istituto di Zootecnica, Facoltà di Agraria, Via Emilia Parmense, 84, 29100 Piacenza, Italy.*

A trial was carried out on 60 lactating dairy cows in an experimental free-stall barn comparing 4 different bedding surfaces: straw, rubber mat, mattress and sand. In a first period (26 days) cows were allowed to choose between 15 cubicles of each bedding material. Rest area was filmed to record the total duration of lying down and the duration and frequency of lying bouts. In a second period, lasted 50 days, the cows were subdivided in 4 groups, each one was raised in a pen with one kind of cubicle flooring. Checks on metabolic conditions, milk yield and milk characteristics were performed. The time spent lying down in cubicle was 631 minutes/cow/day, mainly on sand (41.5%) and straw (28.2%) respect to mat (15.3%) and mattress (14.9%). Higher number of bouts was observed on sand and straw and cows laid down longer in each bout on these bedding surfaces (62.1' and 54.5'/bout on sand and straw respectively) respect to mattress and mat (39' and 38.6' respectively). During the trial milk yield decreased more in mattress and less in sand. These results, together to the lower values of plasma total protein and higher of albumin and calcium in sand respect to mattress, seem to indicate better comfort conditions for sand and straw.

Poster M4.18

Computerised image analysis application for the linear morphological evaluation of dairy cows

G. Bianconi and P. Negretti, Dipartimento di Produzioni Animali, Università della Tuscia, Viterbo, Italy.*

Modern technologies for computerised image analysis allow to carry out morphological measurements on live animals with no need for a direct contact. The experiments by which the general criteria of the methodology were established, have been performed on Holstein Friesian dairy cows. Results obtained after comparison of measurements were determined by biometric traditional instruments (ippometro) and the computerised method; they gave very small differences (0-3 %) for all selected parameters such as Height Withers (H.WI.), Rump Height (RU.H.), and Thorax Height (TH.H.). Such a result was also obtained after comparing the average differences of parameters measured with ippometro (H.WI. 142.3 ± 5.0; RU.H. 144.4 ± 5.4 ; TH.H. 80.20 ± 4.6), and that measured with the opto-informatic system (H.WI. 142.7 ± 5.1; RU.H. 144.7 ± 5.4; TH.H. 81.10 ± 4.9); furthermore such differences were no significant. These values, previously obtained with other species and zootechnical animals, have supported the quality and the reliability of the developed methodology. The high standard achieved with opto-informatic systems allows nowadays to evaluate experimentally the morphologically linear analysis. The greatest result was to compare the official (at naked eye) analyses, altered by subjective factors, with the real biological analyses, that are not possible to get anymore in the farming business with the traditional tools of zootechnical biometry.

Poster M4.19

Role of acid-base disturbances in perinatal mortality of calves

O. Szenci, Szent István University, Faculty of Veterinary Science, H-2225 Üllö, Dóra major, Hungary

The profitability of cattle breeding is greatly influenced by the rate of calves born alive and reared to adulthood. In spite of the speedy development of animal breeding, perinatal mortality is still very high (4 to 7%) and constitutes approximately a half of the total calf losses. Perinatal mortality (stillbirth) is interpreted as the death of mature calf foetuses during calving or in the first 24 h of postnatal life.

Direct and indirect asphyxia was suggested as the causes of death because in 73 to 75% of the calves died in the perinatal period no pathological changes were detected. In a recent study, occurrence of asphyxia in calves dying perinatally was 58.3%. Since, due to disturbances occurring during parturition in the uteroplacental circulation as a result of the rupture of fetal membranes and uterine contractions, all fetuses develop a more or less severe hypoxia and a consequent acidosis. The duration of survivable asphyxia always depends on the reserves of glycogen in the heart muscle. The surviving period for calves with induced anoxia changes between 4 to 6 or 8 minutes. Four of 6 fetuses subjected to 4 minutes of anoxia survived whereas all others died when the umbilical cord was clamped for 6 or 8 minutes. The degree of asphyxia can be evaluated by measuring the acid-base parameters in the blood. The present paper is focused on the acid-base disturbances during and after parturition and their effect on the rate of perinatal mortality in the cow.

Poster M4.20

Indirect determination of weight in Mediterranean Buffaloes by the opto-informatic methodology

P. Negretti1, G. Bianconi[1]*, *S. Bartocci[2], S. Terramoccia[2] and M. Verna[2] , [1]Dipartimento di Produzioni Animali, Università della Tuscia, Viterbo, Italy, [2]Istituto Sperimentale di Zootecnia, Monterotondo, Roma, Italy.*

The research activity was carried out on a sample of 104 Mediterranean Buffaloes during lactation, and it was focused on the indirect determination of live weight by opto-informatic techniques. Such methods have already allowed to get, for other interestingly zootechnical species, precise measures throughout photographic analyses and computerised evaluation. The measured parameter for the weight evaluation was the Side Surface (S.S.) that can be determined by the computerised system. The Back Surface (B.S.) parameter was also evaluated in order to find out a possible correlation between the morphological analysis and the fattening state of the animal.
Results showed a high correlation between the S.S. parameter and the real weight ($r = 0.97$; $P < 0.01$), thus allowing to obtain with 50 individuals randomly sampled a regression equation with good statistically significance ($P<0.01$); this equation was later evaluated with the remaining 54 animals. The difference among real weight averages (763.56 ± 98.72) and indirect weight averages obtained with the opto-informatic system (764.95 ± 96.66) was not significant. A good correlation was also found between the S.S. parameter and the fattening state, as measured by 5 evaluators, equal to $r = 0.88$ ($P<0.01$).

Poster M4.21

Weights of carcasses of stags, hinds and fawns of the Red Deer (*Cervus elaphus* L.) from North-Eastern Poland

W. Szczepanski and P. Janiszewski, University of Warmia and Mazury in Olsztyn, Faculty of Animal Bioengineering, Oczapowskiego 5/140A, 10-719 Olsztyn, Poland

The experimental material were 1 320 larder carcasses of red deer shot in north-eastern Poland (near the city of Olsztyn - 20°30'E; 53°47'N). The data were collected during 15 hunting seasons, from the season 1986/1987 to 2000/2001. They included the weights of larder carcasses of 293 stags, 643 does and 384 fawns. The aim of the studies was to analyzed the average larder carcass weight in particular groups in one hunting season within one hunting ground, i.e. under comparable natural conditions, and to determine changes in the weights of carcasses of stags, does and one-year-old fawns in successive months of a given hunting season.
The average larder carcass weight in the group of stags (without the head), hinds and fawns was 114.5 kg, 76.6 kg and 43.5 kg respectively. It was found that the hunting season affected the larder carcass weight of males. The differences in this trait between particular years were ca. 30 kg. In the case of stags the carcass weight depends on their physiological condition and the month in which they were shot. The heaviest stags are those shot in September and October, whereas the lightest - in January and February. The hunting season and the month in which they were shot have a slight effect on the weights of carcasses of hinds and fawns.

Poster M4.22

Comparison of reproduction performance of chinchillas held in rooms with or without access of natural light

Lidia Felska[1], Marian Brzozowski[2]. [1]Department Ruminant Animal Science, Laboratory of Fur Animals, Agricultural University of Szczecin, ul. Doktora Judyma 12, 71-460 Szczecin, Poland. [2]Division of Fur and Pet Animals, Warsaw Agricultural University, ul. Ciszewskiego 8, 02-786 Warszawa, Poland.*

The aim of the study was to compare reproduction performance of chinchillas kept in rooms with or without access of natural light. The study was carried out in two chinchilla farms; farm A, with glow-discharge tubes as the only light source, with 12-hour light regime, and farm B, with the same lamps, but also with windows. From 1 November until end March, the lamps in farm B were on between 6.00 and 16.00 hours, i.e. light day lasted about 10 hours. Then, the lamps remained off and the chinchillas were under natural light only, which meant quite ample diel light intensity fluctuations. Mean litter size, mean number of the weaned per litter, and death rate of cubs during nursing were investigated. No significant differences were found in the number of born and weaned cubs per litter between the farms A and B. Keeping in artificial light only results in higher both litter size and weaned number, respectively 2.20 and 1.93 chinchillas (farm A), compared with the farm B, respectively 2.07 and 1.78 chinchillas. This may be a result of more even and better illumination of cages with artificial light. A generally higher death rate of young chinchillas was at farm B.

The project was financed by State Committee for Scientific Research, grant no. KBN-3PO6Z 02623

Poster M4.23

Analysis of hip dysplasia in the Italian dog population

E. Sturaro[1], P. Piccinini[2], G. Bittante[1], P. Carnier[1], L. Gallo[1]. [1]Dept. of Animal Science, University of Padova. [2]Centre for the screening of skeletal diseases (Celemasche), Ferrara, Italy.*

This study aimed to investigate frequency of hip scores (FCI method) and risk factors for hip dysplasia (HD) in 6 dog breeds in Italy. Screening data for hip dysplasia of 27278 x-rayed dogs of 6 breeds (German Shepard, Boxer, Labrador, Golden Retriever, Terranova, and Rottweiler) were analysed. Frequency of dogs showing “A” and “B” hip scores was high for all breeds and the frequency of “C”,”D” and “E” scores ranged from 4.2 to 32.8%. Analysis of risk factors was performed considering dogs with “A” and “B” scores as “not affected” and dogs scored “C”, “D” or “E” as “affected” by HD. Logistic regression was used. For most breeds, females were more at risk of hip dysplasia than males. Age of animals at x-ray assay was not a significant risk factor for most breeds. Recent years of birth showed a decreasing risk of HD, and dogs born in spring and winter were more at risk than dogs born in summer or fall. A limited experience of the x-raying veterinarian was often a risk factor for hip dysplasia. A joint analysis of screening results of all breeds indicated that Rottweiler was the least at risk breed for HD. However, selection of dogs for official screening performed by the breeders might have caused biased results.

Poster M4.24

WebCase: Design, delivery and support of web-based agricultural case studies for use in teaching and training across Europe

P.J. Cain[1], G. Brunori[2], J. Fischer[3], S. Heath[4], L.S. Jensen[5] and K. Kajari[6], [1]University of Newcastle upon Tyne, UK, [2]University of Pisa, Italy, [3]University of Tuebingen, Germany, [4]University of Aberdeen, UK, [5]KVL, Denmark, [6]Szent Istvan University, Budapest, Hungary.*

WebCase is an EU Socrates Minerva Programme project which is piloting agricultural case studies for use in on-line learning. It has produced 6 case studies representing animal production systems, agronomy, agribusiness and rural development situations in UK, Italy, Denmark and Hungary. The case descriptions are complimented with appropriate student projects and uploaded to the web using a simple common template. A suite of cases has been mounted in a Managed Learning Environment with communication tools for both teachers and learners. The cases are written in English with local language glossaries.

The case studies and associated projects have been piloted in the class room across Europe, delivered both locally and internationally. A simple Guide has been produced to provide teachers with straight-forward advice on writing, uploading, delivering and supporting web-based case studies. Information on the project and its outcomes is available from:
www.webcase-online.info

Poster M4.25

Micronucleus test application in evaluation of environmental genotoxicity in pigs

I. Sutiaková[1], L. Hetényi[2], J. Buleca Jr.[1], P. Reichel[1], M. Húska[1], V. Sutiak[1], L. Bajan[1], [1]University of Veterinary Medicine, Komenského 73, 041 81 Kosice, Slovakia, [2]Research Institute of Animal Production, Hlohovská 2, 949 92 Nitra, Slovakia

Pigs as a species are very susceptible to impaired life conditions. The micronucleus test enables to state chromosomal damage caused by genotoxic substances in the environment in which the organism is living. The bioclimatic indices in the environment of the piggery under examination were proved to be appropriate. The regime in the stables depended on the temperature dynamics of the outer environment, so it was strongly season dependent. The micronuclei were identified according to the criteria of Countryman and Heddle (1976).The frequency of micronuclei were determined for each animal. The frequency of micronuclei in boars reached 9,3 ± 2,49 per 1000 binucleated cells whereas in sows prior to and after delivery 6,98 ± 4,75 and 6,82 ± 2,66 micronuclei were stated per 1000 binucleated cells, respectively. Irrespective of sex the frequency of micronuclei in pigs reached 7,7 ± 3,45 per 1000 binucleated cells whereas in sows at different stages of the reproductive cycle 6,9 + 3,7 micronuclei were counted per 1000 binucleated cells. Biomarkers should serve as early indicators of health risks.

Poster M4.26

Sexual performance of Awassi, Awassi x Charollais and Awassi x Romanov yearling rams exposed to Awassi x Romanov females

R.T. Kridli[1], M. Momani Shaker[2], A.Y. Abdullah[1] and I. Sada[2], [1]Department of Animal Production, Faculty of Agriculture, Jordan University of Science and Technology, Irbid 22110, Jordan, [2]Institute of Tropical and Subtropical Agriculture, Czech University of Agriculture, Prague, Czech Republic*

This study was designed to compare sexual performance of Awassi (A, n=7) with F1 Awassi x Charollais (AC, n=7) and F1 Awassi x Romanov (AR, n=8) yearling rams. Sexual performance was recorded on three occasions, each 2 days apart. During each occasion, rams were individually exposed to two estrous Awassi x Romanov ewes (short tail) for 15 min during which sexual behavior was monitored. Bouts of leg kicking were greater in A and AR than in AC rams. Frequency of anogenital sniffing and mounting was similar in all genotypes. Ejaculation rate was greater in AR and AC ($P < 0.05$) when compared with A rams. Mating efficiency (mounts/ejaculation) was greater ($P < 0.05$) in AC than A rams with no differences among AC and AR rams. Day of testing influenced mounting frequency ($P < 0.01$), ejaculation rate ($P < 0.001$) and mating efficiency ($P < 0.05$). Time to next activity following ejaculation was similar among genotypes. Latency to next ejaculation, however, was shorter ($P < 0.001$) in AR than AC and A rams. Results indicate that crossbred AR and AC rams had an overall better sexual performance than A rams.

Poster M4.27

Effect of different protein/energy ratios on growth performance of Nile Tilapia (*Oreochromis Niloticus*) fish

S.M. Hashish[1], F Hafez[2], O Hussiny[3] and A El-waly[1], [1]NRC,Dokki, Cairo,Egypt, [2]Central Lab. for Aquacultural Res Abbassa,Egypt, [3]Faculty of Agric.,Cairo Uni.

Tilapia fingerlings were transferred with special care after weighing and distributed into sixteen experimental ponds to represent 16 nutritional treatments(3 replicates for each nutritional treament).Tilapia were stocked in pond using the optimum stocking rate of tilapia (2 fish/m^2)(16 fingerlings per each pen).Two metabolizable energy levels (3000 and 3500 Kcal/Kg diet) and two protein levels (30 and 35%) were used to prepare four protein/energy ratios (CP/E ratio,mg/Kcal/Kg diet) (100 ,110 ,90 and 100).Four replacements were done between dietary soybean meal protein and fish meal protein (30% : 60% ; 50% : 50% ; 50% : 40% ; 60% : 30%) in each diet in a 4 x4 factorial design ,the experimental period lasted 98 days. Significant improvement of tilapia body weight gain ,specific growth rate and feed conversion ratio were achieved when dietary P/E increased while decreasing dietary P/E ratio reduced feed consumption and increased condition factor. The highest values were obtained for fish fed diets containing 60 %: 30 %fish meal protein : soybean protein.

Theatre M5.1

Assessment of the impact of locomotion on animal welfare

J.H.M. Metz[1] and M.B.M. Bracke[2], [1]Wageningen University, Farm Technology Group, P.O. Box 43, 6700 AA Wageningen, the Netherlands, [2]Institute for Animal Science and Health, Edelhertweg 15, P.O. Box 65, Lelystad, the Netherlands.

Locomotion is an important element of the animal's activity. It may take various states as regards gait and speed. Moreover, it supports all main behavioural functions in that. locomotion enables the animal to act properly, in space and time, serving its different needs. For this reason impaired locomotion is an important threat to survival in free living animals, and probably perceived as such in all animals, including the domesticated species.

The impact on welfare in farm animals should be considered in relation to this multifunctional nature of locomotion. But then the question arises as to how to assess the impact of impaired locomotion in proportion to other conditions affecting the animal?

We will propose to follow the decision support model for integrated welfare assessment developed by Bracke et al. (J.Anim. Sci, 80 (2002), 1819-1834). Fundamentally, welfare is assessed from the state of the biological needs of the animal. This welfare definition provides transparency and allows scientific verification.. A list of biological needs has been worked out for sows, but analogous lists are easily made for other species. The model allows a systematic weighting of the consequences of impaired locomotion in the various biological functions such as foraging behaviour, body care and safety. The model allows not only an assessment of impairment due to lameness, but also of the consequences of restraint or inconvenient floors.

Theatre M5.2

Foot lesions and lameness in dairy cows feet - what are the real risks for locomotor disorders?

L.E. Green, Ecology and Epidemiology Group, Department of Biological Sciences, University of Warwick, Coventry CV4 7AL, UK.

There are now many studies into locomotion disorders of dairy cattle. Some studies have used presence of lesions and others occurrence of lameness as an indicator for locomotion disorders. From these papers current factors considered to be important in cattle lameness include previous locomotor disorder, transition housing and feeding of heifers and dry cows, floor surface, diet, floor hygiene, parity and milk production, walking surfaces.

This paper will discuss the relative merits of using foot lesions versus lameness as measures for locomotor disorders and the confidence that we can have in currently identified risk factors from these studies.

Theatre M5.3

Locomotor disorders in pigs - genetical and environmental factors

Bente Jørgensen, Danish Institute of Agricultural Sciences, Research Centre Foulum, P.O. Box 50, DK-8830 Tjele, Denmark.

In Denmark as well as in other countries with intensive pig production, leg problems constitute a large welfare problem both in the slaughter pig production and in the sow population. By leg problems is meant clinical leg problems and locomotion disturbances as well as the joint diseases osteochondrosis and osteoarthritis, and claw disorders. In sows, leg weakness is a main cause of lameness which ultimately leads to culling, and 29% of dead sows examined post mortem in Denmark were found to have been euthanized due to leg weakness. Other studies found that between 10 and 25% of the sows are culled due to locomotory problems making it the second most important cause of culling among sows. There is a negative genetic correlation between leg weakness and meat content, which is an important selection goal in many countries. The possibility exists of reducing the incidence of leg problems genetically since moderate heritabilities of about 0.3 have been found for several of the causes of leg problems, including osteochondrosis. Many different environmental factors may be contributing to or provoking the outbreak and development of the problems. Among these, adverse effects have been found of especially a high feeding intensity, porcine growth hormone administration, limited possibility of exercise either as a result of small pens or high density, and inappropriate floor type. This presentation reviews the results from studies carried out at the Danish Institute of Agricultural Sciences.

Theatre M5.4

Prevalence of Osteochondrosis in offspring from 15 Norwegian Landrace sires

*E. Grindflek[*1,2], B. Ytrehus[3], J. Teige[3], E. Stubsjøen[1], S.Ekman[4], T. Grøndalen[5], [1]NORSVIN, N-2341 Hamar, Norway, [2]Agricultural University of Norway, Dept.Animal Science, N-1432Ås, [3]Norwegian School Vet.Sci., Div.Pathology, N-0033Oslo, [4]Swedish Un. Agricultural Sciences, Dept.Pathology, S-75007Uppsala, [5]KOORIMP, N-0513Oslo*

Leg weakness is a major economical and welfare problem in swine production, and the main cause of this clinical syndrome in Norway is articular osteochondrosis (OC). The aim of this study was to determine the difference in incidence of OC in Norwegian Landrace sires, by evaluating 1645 offspring from 15 boars. All animals were raised under similar conditions in one herd. The average slaughterweight was 82 kilogram. For OC evaluation the distal femur and humerus were sawed in 3 mm thick slabs, cut coronally and perpendicular to the length direction of the bone. The presence and extent of macroscopic OC lesions was evaluated by visual analogue scale (0-5) in seven locations. Results show that the prevalence of OC is highest in the trochlea of humerus with 45% of the individuals scoring higher than 0, and the medial condyle of femur follows with prevalence of 40%. This frequency is lower than earlier observed in Norwegian Landrace. For all elbow locations the effect of sire was highly significant ($P<0.001$), and significance ($P<0.05$) was also found for most of knee locations. All this traits, except from capitulum of humerus, were also significant ($P<0.001$) for sex differences (castrates showing more OC). Growth rate did not show any significant effect on OC.

Inter-rater agreement between different evaluaters using a broiler gait scoring system

C. Berg[1], G.S. Sanotra[2], A. Butterworth[3] and S. Kestin[3], [1]Department of Animal Environment and Health, SLU University, POB 234, SE-532 23 Skara, Sweden, [2]Department of Animal Science and Animal Health, KVL University, Grønnegårdsvej 8, DK-1870 Frederiksberg C, Denmark, [3]Department of Clinical Veterinary Science, Univeristy of Bristol, Langford, Bristol BS40 5DU UK.*

The Bristol gait scoring method for visual assessment of lameness in broilers has been used by a number of different researchers in several countries to estimate the prevalence of leg weakness in experimental studies and on commercial farms. The gait scoring scale ranges from 0 (perfect) to 5 (unable to walk), from which a mean can be calculated. The method was used in a recent Swedish survey, where a number of risk factors for lameness in commercially grown broilers were analyzed. It was also used in a recent survey organized by the British broiler industry. Our study was made as a comparison of gait scoring results by the rater in the Swedish survey (A) and two raters from the Bristol research group (B and C), and again as a comparison between rater A and two raters from the British industry study (D and E). At each occasion 2 groups of 50 birds were scored, each being scored by all three raters. The results showed a very good agreement between raters A (mean value 1.7), B (1.9) and C (1.8) at the first comparison. At the second comparison, there was a good agreement between raters D (mean value 0.6) and E (0.5), but their results were significantly different from rater A's (1.4). From this we conclude that raters D and E used a different - milder - standard compared to the others, resulting in a different interpretation.

Theatre M5.6

The effect of digital disorders and flooring system on locomotion score

J.G.C.J. Somers[1,2,], J.H.M. Metz[1], W.G.P. Schouten[1], E.N. Noordhuizen-Stassen[2] and K. Frankena[3], [1]Institute of Agricultural and Environmental Engineering (IMAG), P.O. Box 43, 6700 AA Wageningen, The Netherlands, [2]Faculty of Veterinary Medicine, Utrecht University, P.O. Box 80.151, 3508 TD, Utrecht, The Netherlands, [3]Wageningen Institute of Animal Sciences, Wageningen University, P.O. Box 338, 6700 AH, Wageningen, The Netherlands.*

Lameness in dairy cows is a serious welfare problem. Ninety % of the locomotory disorders result from claw diseases. So far no clear association has been demonstrated between locomotor disorders and (subclinical) claw diseases. One of the objectives of our running study was to investigate the development over time of the most frequently occurring digital disorders, i.e. interdigital dermatitis together with its symptom heel erosion (IDHE) and digital dermatitis (DD), by regularly inspectations of the hooves of individual cows. Subsequently, the effect of a certain claw disease on a cow's locomotion pattern was evaluated. In addition to claw disease, the effect of flooring system on the locomotor process was taken into account. The cows were housed either in cubicle houses with a slatted floor, solid concrete floor, grooved slotted floor, or in a straw yard. Hind hooves of 240 dairy cows coming from 12 commercial farms were inspected at monthly intervals throughout one year. The severity of IDHE (6-point scale) and DD (5-point scale) was recorded, as well as the presence of any other claw disorder. After each hoof inspection, the locomotion of a cow was recorded with a digital camera. The easiness of movement will be assessed according to the locomotion score developed by Manson and Leaver.

Theatre M5.7

Locomotion of lame and healthy cows on different floors

E. Telezhenko[1], C. Bergsten[1, 2]. [1]Swedish University of Agricultural Sciences, Department of Animal Environment and Health, P.O.Box 234, SE-532 23 Skara, Sweden, [2]Swedish Dairy Association, P.O.Box 234, SE-532 23 Skara, Sweden.*

Trackway measurements (space measurements between footprints) were used for gait analysis in lame and healthy cows. Lameness was scored subjectively with a scale from 0 to 2 (normal, mild lameness and severe lameness). Cow trackways were assessed on solid and slatted concrete floors with and without KEN rubber mats (Gummiwerk Kraiburg, Germany). A pressed sand surface was used in the study as a reference for the objective judgment about deviations from normal locomotion. Severely lame cows were characterised by the biggest step asymmetry (length difference between consecutive steps), shorter stride and step length and smaller step angle than mildly lame and normal animals. Cows with mild lameness did not differ significantly from non-lame cows in stride and step lengths but had a larger positive overlap (distance between the imprints of front and hind hoofs of the same side) and a shorter diagonal support. Lame cows decreased the step angle both on solid and slatted concrete floors, while non-lame cows decreased their step angle only on concrete slats. Mildly lame cows increased the asymmetry on the both types of slatted floor. Cows with severe lameness decreased the step asymmetry on the floors with rubber covering, in contrast to concrete; although the smallest asymmetry they had on the sand surface.

Theatre M5.8

The biomechanical effect of claw trimming

P.P.J. van der Tol, J.H.M. Metz, E.N. Noordhuizen-Stassen, W. Back, C.R. Braam and W.A. Weijs, PO Box 80157, NL-3508 TD, Dept of Veterinary Anatomy, Faculty of Veterinary medicine, Utrecht University.

Increased use of artificial housing in dairy cattle husbandry led to higher prevalence of claw disorders. Claw disorders affect cattle behavior and reduce animal welfare. The body weight of the cow is applied to the four feet and distributed over the contact area of the claws, resulting in pressures at the soles. It is easy to assume that high pressures could result in horn-fractures and haematoma. To prevent claw disorders, trimming is often applied as a management routine.

The force and pressure distribution under ten Holstein-Friesian hind feet were measured before and after trimming (according the Dutch method) while standing on a Footscan® pressure plate, firmly embedded on a Kistler® force plate at 250 measurements/second, to test the biomechanical effect of trimming.

The vertical loading of the hind limb was exerted for 30 % at the medial and 70 % at the lateral claw. Although after trimming the hind feet remained heavily unbalanced, it decreased the pressures exerted to the weight-bearing parts of the feet, since the total contact area was increased. It was concluded that the risk of unbalanced feet was less, compared to the risk of high pressures at the sole. Therefore, trimming needs to prevent overloading of the horn, particularly at the softer parts of the sole at the lateral hind claw.

Sole ulcer and lameness at claw trimming associated with reproductive performance, udder health, and culling in Swedish dairy cattle

J. Hultgren, T. Manske and C. Bergsten, Department of Animal Environment and Health, Swedish University of Agricultural Sciences, P.O.Box 234, SE-532 23 Skara, Sweden*

In an observational study of 2,963 dairy cows in 102 Swedish herds, effects of sole ulcer and lameness found at routine claw trimming during the first 6 mo of lactation were investigated. Outcome traits were indices of reproductive performance, udder health, milk production, and culling in the same lactation. The data analysis was performed by mixed multivariable linear, logistic and Poisson regression modelling at the cow level, accounting for herd clustering and using the MIXED procedure or GLIMMIX macro in SAS statistical software. Significant associations were found between sole ulcer and first-service conception rate in the first study year (OR 0.59), calving interval (2% longer), treatment for anoestrus (OR 1.61), 305-d milk yield (479 kg ECM higher), and 60-180-d milk yield (136-308 kg ECM higher in cows calving between February and October). There was also a significant association between lameness and culling (OR 1.81). The results provide evidence of a negative effect of sole ulcer on reproductive performance, and of lameness on longevity. The positive association between sole ulcer and milk yield is probably due to high-producing cows being more prone to develop the disease. Finally, the study shows the importance of recording the presence of foot lesions and not only lameness in hoof-health research.

Poster M5.10

Study of "arthrogryposis" in Piedmont cattle breed by microsatellite analysis

A. Galli[1], G. Bongioni[1], M. Bona[2], M. Zanotti[3], M. Longeri[3], [1]Istituto Sperimentale Italiano "Lazzaro Spallanzani", Località La Quercia 26027 Rivolta d'Adda, Cremona, Italy, A.N.A.Bo.Ra.Pi, *Strada Trinita' 32/a, 12061 Carru',Cuneo, Italy, [3]Istituto di Zootecnica, via Celoria 10, 20133, Universita' degli Studi, Milano, Italy.*

"Arthrogryposis" is a congenital malformation characterised by curvature of limbs and multiple articular rigidity. In Brown Swiss and Holstein Friesian cattle congenital contractures have been classified as spinal muscular atrophy (SMA). In Italy, since 1980, National Association of Piedmont Cattle (A.N.A.Bo.Ra.Pi) recorded 7912 out of 438638 new-born calves as arthrogryposis affected (1,8%). The higher frequency in males (3.3%), the evidence of similar genetic forms in other cattle breeds, the absence of toxic-infectious agents or distocia and the presence of the disorder in related animals justify a study by genetic approach. Survival motor neuron (SMN) gene is responsible for several arthrogryposis forms in man. Four microsatellite loci, closely mapping to the SMN locus, have been chosen and have been amplified on 69 Piedmont cattle owing to 8 familiar groups showing 25% of affected animals. Linkage analysis recorded a Lod Score of 1,33. Our data suggest the presence in the chosen chromosomal region of a gene affecting the character and encourage more detailed studies. That will help to eradicate a quite high incidence defect, which determines economic losses in terms of management, reduction of productive life of the animal and loss in carcass weight at slaughter in one of the most valuable autochthonous Italian breed.

 Theatre Ph1.1

Mechanism of action and immune-modulatory actions of conjugated linoleic acid

S. Banni[1] and C. Corino[2], [1]Department of Experimental Biology, Experimental Pathology Section, University of Cagliari, 09042 Monserrato, Cagliari, Italy, [2]Department of Veterinary Sciences and Technologies for Food Safety, University of Milan, 20133 Milan, Italy.

Conjugated linoleic acid (CLA) is a naturally occurring fatty acid that is produced by a bio-hydrogenation process in the rumen, and thus is present in dairy products and ruminant meat. In this case the predominant isomer formed is 9cis, 11trans. However, CLA includes 28 positional and geometrical isomers, of which only 9cis, 11trans and 10trans, 12cis have thus far been proven to possess biological activities which include anti-obesity, antiatherogenic and anticarcinogenic activities, demonstrated in a wide range of animal models. Both of these CLA isomers have been shown to undergo elongation and desaturation processes similar to those that occur with linoleic acid, maintaining the conjugated diene structure. There are evidences supporting the hypothesis that CLA metabolism may interfere with eicosanoid formation, thus also influencing immune functions. As a matter of fact, CLA had a favorable influence on immune competence in nursery and weaned piglets. Recent study reported that immunoglobulin G concentration was higher in colostrum of CLA-fed sows than in colostrum of control sows and that serum IgG and lysozime concentrations were increased in CLA-fed sows. A dietary treatment of periparturient sow enhances passive immunity of piglets with positive effects on growth.

Theatre Ph1.2

Effect of milk peptides on the immune system with emphasis on gastro-intestinal immune response

I. Politis, Department of Animal Science, Agicultural University of Athens, 11855 Athens, Greece

The importance of milk in the nutrition of all mammals has been recognized from time immemorial. The proteolytic breakdown of milk proteins generates a number of peptides endowed with biological including immunomodulatory properties. All milk proteins are destined to be broken down during the digestive process. Milk proteins are also subjected to inadvertent proteolysis during milk storage or deliberate proteolysis by lactic acid bacteria during yoghurt manufacturing and cheese ripening. Recent research indicated that the hexapeptide Pro-Gly-Pro-Ile-Pro-Asn and the tripeptide Leu-Leu-Tyr corresponding to residues 63-68 and 191-193 of the bovine beta-casein respectively modulated the function and the activity of porcine monocytes/macrophages. In vitro experiments revealed that both peptides significantly suppress chemotactic activity, membrane-bound urokinase-plasminogen activator and the production of major histocompatability class II antigens by porcine macrophages obtained from the newly weaned piglet. The immune system of the newly weaned piglet has not reached its full maturity. In contrast, both peptides had no effect on the function or activity of macrophages obtained from mature animals. The down-regulation in several functional properties of porcine macrophages caused by two milk-born peptides could be related to development of immunocompetence and prevention of undesirable immune responses to dietary proteins. Research on the significance of milk-born peptides on gastrointestinal immunology is at its infancy and the role of these peptides must be evaluated in vivo.

 Theatre Ph1.3

Leptin in bovine plasma, colostrum and milk during the first month of lactation

L. Pinotti, F.Rosi, Dept. VSA, Facoltà di Medicina Veterinaria; Istituto di Zootecnia Generale, Facoltà di Agraria. Università degli Studi di Milano, I-20133 Milan Italy.*

The objective of this study was to determine leptin content in bovine colostrum and mature milk during the first month of lactation, and their possible relation with plasma leptin. Five multiparous Holstein dairy cows homogenous for parity and meam production in the previous lactation were used. Colostrum and milk yield and composition were measured on day 0, 10, 20, and 30 of lactation. Blood samples were collected on day 0, 10, and 20 post-calving. Plasma, skim colostrum and skim milk were analysed for leptin content using a commercial multi-species leptin RIA kit. Leptin concentration was 56% lower in mature milk than in colostrum (13.90 vs. 6.14 μg/l; $P<.01$), while no significant differences were observed during the first month of lactation (5.88, 6.16, 6.38 μg/l on day 10, 20 and 30, respectively). Leptin daily secretion in mature milk was 21% lower than in colostrum (220.0 μg/d vs. 173.2 μg/d; $P<.01$). Plasma leptin at calving was 2.64 μg/l, decreasing by 18% during post-partum (2.17 μg/l; $P<.05$). Although, both plasma and milk leptin concentrations showed a similar decreasing time trend during the first month of lactation, colostrum and milk showed a higher leptin level than plasma, suggesting that transfer of leptin from the blood accounts only partially for its milk content.

Theatre Ph1.4

Bovine milk: nutritional and non-nutritional components and their importance for the newborn calf

J.W. Blum, Division of Nutriton and Physiology, Institute of Genetics, Nutrition and Housing, University of Berne, Bremgartenstrasse 109a, CH-3012 Berne, Switzerland

The adaptation of bovine neonates is critical and characterized by high morbidity and mortality rates since the GH -IGF axis is not fully functioning and nutrition is changing from parenteral to enteral supply. Colostrum contains nutrients, immoglobulins (Ig) and bioactive substances and its ingestion is essential to stimulate growth of the small intestine and enhance absorptive capacity, partly associated with reduced apoptosis. mRNA of members of the GH-IGF-axis are present along the entire gastro-intestinal tract (GIT) in a way which is site-specific, changes in the perinatal period and is influenced by postnatal feeding, being stimulated by colostral bioactive factors. Feeding of IGF-I alone does not influence GIT development, but an extract derived from colostrum selectively stimulates small intestinal epithelial proliferation and villus size. There are marked differences in proliferation and apoptotic rates and in the number and of B- und T-lymphocytes dependent on whether or not colostrum is fed. The status of glucose, plasma amino acids and the glutamine/glutamate ratio, non-esterified fatty acids, triglycerides, phospholipids, essential fatty acids, β-carotene, retinol and α-tocopherol depends on whether or not colostrum is fed early postnatally. The timing and amount of colostrum intake also influences the endocrine status, such as of gastrin, glucose-dependent insulinotropic hormone, insulin, glucagon, IGF-I, IGF binding proteins, and cortisol. In conclusion, C intake not only influences GIT development, the status of passive immunity and thus the timepoint needed to start active immune responses, but also markedly changes metabolism, endocrine systems and nutritional status.

Theatre Ph1.5

Variation in nutritive constituents, hormones and insulin like growth factor-1 of bovine colostrum in response to time after calving

Y.M. Hafez and S.M. Salem, Animal Production Department , Faculty of Agriculture, Cairo University, Giza, Egypt.

A total of 300 colostrum samples represent the first three successive milking (100 sample/ milking) were analyzed to study changes in their constitution associated with time after calving (6 hrs intervals). First milking colostrum contains the highest (g/dl) dry matter (22.5), protein (17.4), fat (3.4) and solids not fat (19.1) and the lowest lactose (1.6). Furthermore, it contains the highest alpha-lactalbumin (1.43 mg/ml), citrate (98.7 mg/dl) and colostrometer reading 98 mg Ig/ml. Colostral insulin, prolactin and IGF-1 were the highest in the first milking colostrum, 40.2, 92.8 and 1132 ng/ml, respectively. Time after calving significantly affects colostral dry matter ($P<0.001$), protein (P0.001), SNF($P<0.001$), colostrometer reading ($P<0.001$), insulin ($P<0.01$), prolactin ($P<0.05$) and IGF-1 ($P<0.001$). Colostrometer reading , insulin, prolactin and IGF-1 of the second milking colostrum samples were higher than that of the third milking colostrum samples by 114, 39, 27 and 32 %, respectively. Colostrometer reading had a positive gross correlation with dry matter (0.66), SNF (0.77), citrate (0.52), protein (0.51), insulin (0.72) and IGF-1 (0.79). In conclusion, First milking colostrum are the best to fed and save. Also, specific gravity of colostrum in terms of colostrometer reading is a good measure for colostrum quality and its adequacy for feeding the new born calf.

Theatre Ph1.6

Enrichment of goat's colostrum and milk in n-3 long-chain polyunsaturated fatty acids by maternal dietary fish oil

D. Cattaneo[1], G. Savoini[1], A. Agazzi[1], V. Bronzo[2], P. Moroni[2] and V. Dell'Orto[1]. Università degli Studi di Milano [1]Dipartimento di Scienze e Tecnologie Veterinarie per la Sicurezza Alimentare, Via Trentacoste 2, 20134 Milano,Italy. [2]Dipartimento di Patologia Animale, Igiene e Sanità Pubblica Veterinaria, Via Celoria 10, 20133 Milano,Italy.

Long-chain n-3 polyunsaturated fatty acids (PUFAs), particularly docosahexaenoic acid (DHA, C22:6 n-3), have been shown to play specific functional roles during perinatal growth and development of mammals. During pregnancy and foetal development, maternal requirements for DHA increase and DHA status of the neonate and the mother may be sub-optimal if maternal intake is insufficient. The study examined whether dietary fish oil during pregnancy and lactation would increase the proportion of n-3 PUFAs in colostrum and milk of dairy goats. From three weeks before kidding throughout 42 days of lactation, 14 Saanen dairy goats were fed either a control diet or a diet containing 1.20% fish oil. Fatty acid profiles of colostral and mature milk were altered by the dietary treatment: proportions of C18:0 and C18:2 were reduced, while occurrence of C16:1 and long-chain (≥C20) n-3 PUFAs, mainly EPA (C20:5 n-3) and DHA were enhanced. Apparent transfer efficiency from fish oil to mature milk was 14% for EPA and 7% for DHA. Thus, a greater occurrence of n-3 PUFAs in goat's colostrum and milk can be obtained through maternal dietary fish oil during pregnancy and lactation.

 Theatre Ph1.7

Periparturient changes in the constituents of blood and mammary gland secretions of Friesian cows

Y.M. Hafez[*1], *S.A. Ibrahim*[1], *B. Rabie Zenate*[2], *and Alyate A. Hassanein*[2], [1]*Animal Production Department, Faculty of Agricultture, Cairo University, Egypt,* [2]*Animal Producttion Research Insitute, Egypt.*

A total of 16 pregnant multiparous Friesian cows used to study changes in blood and mammary secretions constituents around parturition (-7 through +7 days). Plasma cortisol increased gradually, being the highest at parturition (9.13 ng/ml) and declined thereafter. Meanwhile, plasma progesterone decreased sharply and reached the minimum at parturition (0.62 ng/ml) then slightly increased. Plasma IgG decreased gradually being 952.5 mg/dl at parturition. Both total protein (TP) and ttotal lipid (TL) in plasma showed the same trend in which they declined gradually till parturition (7.4 g/dl and 9.1 g/l, respectively). Activity of GPT was the lowest at parturition (18 U/ml) even greater values were obtained following parturitionrather than that before. While, activity of GOT was the highest at parturition (45 U/ml). Stored mammary secretions during prepartum period had higher Somatic cell count (SCC), it declined at parturition ($3674.2x10^3$/ml) and sharply declined thereafter (814.2×10^3/ml at + 7 days). Highest values of total solids, protein and solids not fat in mammary gland secretions were obtained at -7 days and decreased gradually thereafter to be the minimum at + 7 days postpartum which indicate the changes from colostrum to transitional milk. Fat content in mammary secretions was the highest during the period of colostrogenesis whereas lactose showed a reversed trend.

Theatre Ph1.8

Thyroid hormone levels are correlated with the tocopherol and retinol transport in the milk

M.S. Spagnuolo[1*], *L. Cigliano*[1], *F. Sarubbi*[2], *F. Polimeno*[2], *L. Ferrara*[2], *P. Abrescia*[1], [1]*Dipartimento di Fisiologia Generale ed Ambientale - Università di Napoli Federico II, via Mezzocannone 8, 80134 Napoli, Italia,* [2]*ISPAAM, CNR, via Argine 1085, 80147 Napoli, Italia.*

Thyroid hormones stimulate oxygen consumption and heat production, inducing the synthesis of reactive oxygen species, which in turn trigger several pathologies including mastitis, and infectious diseases in the newborn calf. The retinol and tocopherol seasonal levels were measured by HPLC in the milk of buffalo cows (winter: 1.60 and 1.20 ?g/ml respectively; summer: 0.71 and 0.76 respectively). In the plasma, seasonal changes for the levels of both antioxidants were not found. The retinol levels in the milk were positively correlated with the plasma levels of T_3 ($P<0.05$), thus suggesting hormone-dependent retinol accumulation. This hypothesis was supported by the finding of increased levels of retinol in the milk (29 or 65%) of cows injected with T_3 (2.2 or 4.0 µg/Kg respectively). The cytosol fraction, extracted from alveolar epithelial cells of mammary glands was incubated with ^{3}H- retinol and, after gel filtration chromatography, one radioactive protein fraction ($M_r = 30000$) was detected. The amount of labelled proteins was 126% higher in winter ($T_3 = 1.53$ ng/ml) than in summer ($T_3 = 0.84$ ng/ml).

We suggest that, in winter, both liposoluble antioxidants are more efficiently transported through the blood-mammary barrier, and that T_3 might enhance the retinol uptake by the mammary gland.

Poster Ph1.9

Leptin distribution in goat milk fractions

F. Rosi, L. Pinotti[1], A. Campagnoli[1], D. Magistrelli, Istituto di Zootecnia Generale, Facoltà di Agraria. [1]Dept. VSA, Facoltà di Medicina Veterinaria. Università degli Studi di Milano, I-20133 Milan Italy.*

The aims of this study were to determine the effects of morning vs. evening milking time on blood and milk leptin. Six lactating (120±12 DIM) Saanen goats were randomly selected for this experiment. On two subsequent milkings, blood and milk samples were collected and milk yield and composition measured. On plasma and whole sonicated milk and skim milk, leptin content were analyzed. Mean morning milk yield, fat, and protein were respectively, 1.36 kg/d, 3.84 %, 3.58 %, whereas on evening milking the same variable measured were 1.11 kg/d, 3.97 % and 3.57 %. Morning and evening whole sonicated milk leptin content and total secretion did not show significant differences (17.91 vs. 23.77 µg/l, and 24.33 vs. 24.32 µg/milking, respectively), but a wide range of variability was observed. Skim milk leptin was higher ($P<.05$) in morning milk than evening one (5.43 vs. 4.53 µg/l), without significant correlation to plasma leptin at correspondent sampling time (4.05 vs. 3.90 µg/l). Three main conclusions can be drawn: 1) no correlation was observed between milk and plasma leptin; 2) skim milk showed a higher leptin level than plasma, suggesting a possible mammary secretion; 3) of total leptin measured in milk, 57% was associated to fat fraction, remarking that milk sampling and handling procedures must be as accurate as possible.

Poster Ph1.10

Role of polyamines on bovine primary cell proliferation

E. Fusi[1], F. Cheli[1], R. Rebucci[1], K. Sejrsen[2] and S. Purup[2], [1]Department of Veterinary Sciences and Technology for Food Safety, Via Celoria 10, 20133 Milano, Italy, [2]Institute of Animal Nutrition and Physiology, Danish Institute of Agricultural Sciences, Research Centre Foulum, P.O. Box 50, DK-8830 Tjele, Denmark.

Colostrum and first milk contains the highest level of nutrients, growth factors, immunoglobulins and polyamines. It is generally accepted that milk composition reflects the requirement of a newborn mammal. The highest secretion rate of polyamines in the mammary gland at the beginning of the lactation coincides with the highest demands of a newborn calf for these compounds, especially in the development of the gastrointestinal tract. Intracellular polyamines homeostasis is regulated by a complex feedback mechanisms, controlling polyamines biosynthesis, degradation and equally important, uptake from the extracellular space.
The aim of the study was to evaluate the role of polyamines in a primary culture model of bovine Mammary Epithelial Organoids (MEO) grown three dimensionally within rat collagen. Increasing concentrations of putrescine, spermine, and spermidine were added to cell cultures and the cell proliferation was determined by tritiated thymidine incorporation. During the 48 hour of putrescine treatment MEO underwent to a proliferation. Spermidine has significantly ($P<0.01$) affected the MEO proliferation. At low concentrations, spermine confirmed significantly ($P<0.01$) its stimulating activity, but at higher concentrations was cytotoxic. Analysis of mammary epithelial cells in vitro supported the role of polyamines in the induction of proliferative-cytotoxic effects in dose-response manner.

Poster Ph1.11

Cloning and expression in *Pichia pastoris* yeast of full length porcine lactoferrin cDNA

C. Pecorini[1], P. Martino[1], S. Reggi[2], L. Sangalli[1], A. Baldi[1], C. Fogher[3], [1]Faculty of Veterinary Medicine, University of Milan, via Celoria 10, 20133 Milano, [2]Plantechno, via Staffolo 60, 26040, Vicomoscano (CR), [3]U.C.S.C., via Emilia Parmense 84, 29100, Piacenza, Italy.*

Lactoferrin is a polyfunctional glycoprotein that has many biological activities, including nonimmune disease protection, immunoregulation, antiinflammation, prebiotic support of intestinal microflora and growth promotion. Lactoferrin in milk is likely to be of particular importance to neonatal mammals that are born in an immature immune and digestive state of development, such as piglets. We report the production of recombinant porcine lactoferrin (rpLF) in methylotrophic yeast *Pichia pastoris*. The full length cDNA of pLF was obtained by reverse reaction from total RNA of sow's mammary gland. The cDNA was cloned in the expression vector pPIC9, downstream the α-factor, that drives the production of the recombinant protein in the growth medium and under the control of alcohol oxidase 1 promoter, that allows the expression of lactoferrin in the presence of methanol as inducer. SDS-PAGE and Western techniques showed the presence of a band of about 80 KDa, corresponding to rpLF, indicating a *Pichia pastoris*-porcine similar pattern of glycosylation. Current studies are evaluating the biological activity of the protein against bacterial strains isolated from piglets with diarrhoea. The production of rpLF by *Pichia pastoris* can provide an effective tool to support the piglets health during weaning period.

Poster Ph1.12

Identification of minor proteins of goat colostrum and milk by two dimensional eletrophoresis and maldi tof spectrometry

P. Roncada[1-3], F. Carta[2], and G.F. Greppi[3], [1]LEA Laboratory of Applied Epigenomic, Institute L. Spallanzani, Lodi, Italy, Dip. of Biology, Genetic and Biochemistry University of Turin [3]Department of Veterinary Clinical Science, University of Milan

The post genomic era has brought exciting and challenging prospects for proteomics. With the availability of many completed genomes, we now have the opportunity to study protein expression levels, structure modifications and interactions in complex systems, which lead to a comprehensive understanding of their biological functions. 2D-PAGE offers parallel analysis of hundreds to thousands of proteins and post translational modifications that can be readily detected and analysed, with help of mass spectrometry. Our work is to analysed, understanding behaviour of goat milk proteins, because goat milk can be a valid alternative of vaccine milk in allergies. The colostrum samples were obtained 12-24 hours after parturition and mature milk at 3 months postpartum from 10 Orobica goats. We have identified in milk and colostrum some key proteins, and we have traced typical constellations of goat milk. Differences were observed when we analyzed samples of colostrum and mature milk. Protein identification was carried out by MALDI-TOF and mass fingerprinting database searching was carried out using ProFound. Furthermore we identified several minor proteins including FABP, clusterin, fructose-bisphoshate aldolase A, as well as several fragments of milk protein. This technique will be an effective approach to identify and characterize new and interesting proteins.

Theatre Ph2.1

The role of IGFBP-5 in mammary gland development

G.J. Allan and D.J. Flint, Hannah Research Institute, Ayr, KA6 5HL, Scotland, UK.*

Mammary gland development involves a phase of proliferation during pregnancy, a period of cellular differentiation during lactation followed ultimately, at the end of lactation, by a rapid and co-ordinated programme of cell death during involution. We demonstrated that this cell death occurred via apoptosis, which is normally suppressed by an important survival factor for the mammary gland, insulin-like growth factor-I (IGF-I). However, during involution, mammary epithelial cells produce copious amounts of an IGF-binding protein (IGFBP-5) which we proposed to act as a mechanism to sequester IGF-I and thereby initiate the cell death programme. In order to test the hypothesis that IGFBP-5 can induce apoptosis, we generated transgenic mice expressing IGFBP-5 on a mammary-specific promoter to target its expression to the mammary gland. These animals showed impaired mammary development, impaired milk synthesis and elevated concentrations of caspase-3, a pro-apoptotic molecule, and of plasmin, a marker of extracellular matrix (ECM) degradation. Thus, these studies clearly implicate IGFBP-5 as a pro-apoptotic molecule with potential therapeutic value. In addition to promoting cell death through activation of caspases, our preliminary experiments would indicate that IGFBP-5 is also able to inhibit the actions of plasminogen-activator inhibitor-1 (PAI-1), thereby promoting ECM degradation. As a consequence, we would propose that IGFBP-5 may play a central role in co-ordinating both cell death and ECM remodelling. Experimental evidence will be presented in this talk which supports this hypothesis.

Theatre Ph2.2

The role of the GH/IGF-I axis in muscle tissue development and its significance for the performance of meat animals

Niels Oksbjerg, Pia M. Nissen, Margrethe Therkildsen, and Mogens Vestergaard. Danish Institute of Agricultural Sciences, Research Centre Foulum, DK-8830 Tjele, Denmark.

This presentation describes the basic events in prenatal muscle development and postnatal muscle growth and how these events are controlled by various regulatory factors including IGFs and growth factors. The prenatal events or myogenesis (muscle fibre formation) encompass the rate of proliferation, the rate and extent of fusion, and the differentiation of three myoblast populations. The three populations of myoblasts give rise to a primary- and a secondary fibre population, and a satellite cell population, respectively. Muscle fibre formation is terminated late in gestation and the number of muscle fibres is a determinant of the postnatal growth rate. Furthermore, the postnatal events contributing to postnatal muscle growth comprise satellite cell proliferation and protein turnover; the latter being the difference between the rate of protein synthesis and the rate of protein degradation. Factors to be dealt with of importance for muscle development and postnatal growth comprises transcription factors, growth factors (endocrine vs. para/autocrine), the nervous system, proteolytic enzymes, and external factors like maternal nutrition, feeding strategies, and selection for increased performance.

Theatre Ph2.3

Regulation of lipogenesis by growth hormone and insulin in isolated porcine adipocytes in culture: involvement of SREBP-1?

I. Louveau and F. Gondret, INRA, Unité Mixte de Recherches sur le Veau et le Porc, 35590 Saint Gilles, France.*

The ability of growth hormone (GH) to decrease fatness and insulin-regulated events such as lipogenic enzyme activities, is well known in pigs. Nevertheless, the precise mechanism underlying these actions has not been elucidated yet. Expression of the transcription factor sterol regulatory element binding protein (SREBP)-1 has been reported as a key mediator of insulin action in rat hepatocytes and adipose cell lines. The present study aimed to determine whether the regulation of lipogenesis by GH and/or insulin in porcine adipocytes also involved SREBP-1. Isolated adipocytes, obtained from perirenal or subcutaneous (s.c.) adipose tissue samples of female pigs (51 ± 0.4 kg ; n=15), were cultured in serum-free medium in the absence or presence of these hormones for up to 4 days. Glucose incorporation and fatty acid synthase (FAS) activity were increased by insulin in a dose-dependent manner in adipocytes of both sites. The increase was maximal at 1.7 and 17 nM in s.c. and perirenal adipocytes respectively, indicating inter-depot differences in the regulation of lipogenesis by insulin. These insulin-stimulated events were decreased by pGH (1 nM). No change in SREBP-1 mRNA level was observed in response to GH and/or insulin. Taken together, these data indicate that the regulation of lipogenesis by insulin and GH appears to not involve change in SREBP-1 expression in porcine adipocytes.

Theatre Ph2.4

Effects of maternal nutrition on serum growth factors in the sow and foetuses, and on serum-induced proliferation and differentiation of primary myoblasts

P.M. Nissen, M. Vestergaard and N. Oksbjerg, Danish Institute of Agricultural Sciences, P.O.Box 50, 8830 Tjele, Denmark.*

The objective of this study was to examine the effect of increased maternal nutrition on changes in serum growth factors of the sow and foetuses. Furthermore, the effect of foetal sera on *in vitro* proliferation and differentiation of porcine primary myoblasts was examined. Pregnant sows were either fed restrictively (2 kg/d) until day 50 or 70 (C) of gestation or fed restrictively until day 25 and then *ad libitum* until day 50 or 70 (A) (2×2 factorial design). Sows were slaughtered at day 50 or 70, respectively. Serum from sows and pools of cord-blood serum from each litter were analysed for insulin, IGF-I and -II and IGFBPs. IGF-I ($P<0.01$), IGFBP-3 ($P=0.08$) and IGFBP-4 ($P=0.07$) were higher in A compared with C sows, and IGFBP-1 was higher ($P=0.06$) and IGFBP-2 lower ($P=0.10$) in serum from day 70 compared with day 50 sows. There was no effect of feeding level on growth factor concentrations in foetal serum and on serum-induced proliferation and differentiation of myoblasts. IGFBP-1, -2, and -3 were all higher ($P<0.05$) and serum-induced proliferation and differentiation were lower on day 70 than day 50. In conclusion, no effects of maternal nutrition were found on serum growth factor concentrations in the foetuses or on serum-induced proliferation and differentiation of primary myoblasts.

Theatre Ph2.5

Treatment with somatotropin during early gestation affects maternal metabolic and hormonal status and offspring growth in swine - summary of a comprehensive study

C. Rehfeldt, G. Kuhn, K.Ender, Research Institute for the Biology of Farm Animals, Wilhelm-Stahl-Allee 2, D-18196 Dummerstorf, Germany*

To investigate the effects of elevated circulating concentrations of maternal somatotropin during early gestation, crossbred gilts received daily i.m. injections of either 6 mg of recombinant porcine somatotropin (pST) or of a placebo (control) from day 10 to 27 of gestation (EXP1) or with gradual withdrawal from d 28 to 37 (EXP2). A series of changes was found with regard to maternal circulating hormones and growth factors as for example increases in IGF-I and decreases in thyroxine and progesterone concentrations. Nutrient availability was elevated in terms of glucose and free fatty acids. Changes in placental regulatory proteins of the ST-IGF axis were found, and placental and fetal growth was stimulated by pST. Skeletal muscle development was markedly influenced as seen by increases in muscle fibre number, in the expression of *Myf5* and *MyoD* transcripts, in creatine phosphokinase activity, DNA and protein concentrations. Treatment with pST from d 10 to d 37 of gestation (EXP2) had only minimal effects on postnatal growth and carcass and meat quality. Nevertheless, an increased balance between littermates in muscle growth was apparent. In conclusion, elevated ST concentrations during early gestation cause considerable endocrine and metabolic changes and is capable to alter fetal and postnatal growth.

Theatre Ph2.6

Effect of the donor's age on bovine oocyte maturation and early embryonic development in vitro

T.I. Kuzmina[1] , H. Torner[2], H. Alm[2] and W. Kanitz[2], Research Institute for Farm Animal Genetics and Breeding, St.Petersburg-Pushkin, 19625 Russia, [2]Research Institute for Biology of Farm Animals,18196 Dummerstorf, Germany

The objective of the present study was to compare the developmental potential of bovine oocytes depending on animal's age and culture system (S). We used cumulus-oocyte complexes (COC) from the cows (5-6 lactation)-exp.1, heifers (1,5-2 years)-exp.2 and calves (1-2-month-old)-exp-3. Three systems were used for culture of COC: S1-TCM 199 (Sigma) with 10% fetal calf serum (Gibco); S2-TCM 199 with 10% eostrus serum; S3-TCM 199 with 5% proteins of follicular fluid (PFF - molecular weight more than 65 kDa). PFF were precipitated by ammonium sulphate (T.Kuzmina et al., 1993). A total of 1369 COC were cultured. There was no difference in the rate of oocytes maturation, in percentages of oocytes with chromosomes degeneration, in proportion of fertilized oocytes depending on culture system and age's group. Development rates for calf and cow oocytes did not differ significantly in similar culture systems. The proportion of late morulae and blastocyst stage in exp.3 was significantly higher following oocyte's maturation in TCM 199 and eostrus serum (22,6% - Exp.3-S2, P<0.05) or in TCM 199 with 5% PFF (28,6%-Exp.2-S3, P<0.01), than in TCM with 10% fetal calf serum (13,6%). These results indicate the possibility of using donor's oocytes from calves (1-2-month -old) in the reproduction biotechnology for reducing the generation interval in breeding schemes.

Theatre Ph2.7

Influence of breed and diet on leptin state in cattle

C. Pirotte, F. Wergifosse, J.L. Bister, R. Paquay. Department of Animal Physiology, The University of Namur, 5000 Namur, Belgium*

The aim of the study is to determine the relation between leptin state (plasmatic concentration, mRNA, receptors) and intramuscular fat content in beef cattle. Three cattle breeds (*Angus*, *Limousine* and *Belgian Blue*), differing in their ability to deposit fat within muscle tissue, and two diets (barley and beet pulps) were compared. Six groups (3 breeds x 2 diets) of six steers were fed *ad libitum* and slaughtered after 120 to 150 days. Blood, muscle and subcutaneous adipose tissue samples were taken.

Plasma leptin concentration was determined by RIA. Amount of leptin mRNA and leptin receptor gene expression were analysed by RT-PCR in comparison with a house keeping gene, β-actin. At slaughtering, content of plasma leptin was 2.60±1.91, 2.52±1.35 and 2.15±1.10 ng/ml respectively for *Angus, Limousine* and *Belgian Blue*, but differences were no significant. Ratio of leptin to β-actin mRNA was respectively 1.23±0.29, 0.90±0.23 and 0.39±0.15 for *Angus, Limousine* and *Belgian Blue* and was significantly different ($P \leq 0.05$) between *Belgian Blue* and the two others breeds.

Plasma leptin concentration and mRNA leptin expression were positively correlated ($r=0.99$) between the three breeds. There was no influence due to the diet on plasma leptin concentration and mRNA expression whatever the breed may be. These data show clearly the effect of the breed on leptin state in cattle.

Theatre Ph2.8

The variation of leptin plasma concentration in growing buffaloes

F. Polimeno[1], M.S. Spagnuolo[2], F. Sarubbi[1], L. Cigliano[2], L.Ferrara[1] and P. Abrescia[2], [1]ISPAAM-CNR Via Argine 1085, 80147 Naples, Italy, [2]Dipartimento di Fisiologia Generale ed Ambientale - Università di Napoli Federico II, via Mezzocannone 8, 80134 Naples, Italy.

Leptin, a hormone mainly secreted by adipose tissue, is involved in the regulation of food intake, energy expenditure and whole-body energy balance. The aim of this study was to evaluate whether leptin concentration changes in growing buffaloes. The correlation between plasma leptin level and some haematic parameters as well as between leptin level and some growing indices was also analysed. Plasma level of glucagone, insulin, glucose, NEFA and 3-hydroxybutyrate were measured. Liveweight, rump area, compactness index, bodily index, tronco-thoracic index and average daily gain were chosen as somatic parameters. Blood samples were collected at 30 days intervals for ten months from 20 young growing buffaloes, starting from animals 130 days old. We found that plasma leptin level increased with weight gain. In particular, plasma leptin level decreased between the 7th and 9th month of age, anddramatically increased between the 10th and the 12th month of age. Plasma insulin and somatic parameters were positively correlated with leptin level while glucose and NEFA were negatively correlated with leptin plasma level. These results suggest that leptin might play a central role in the regulation of glycaemia and fat mobilization during growth in buffaloes.

Poster Ph2.9

Granulosa cell-mediated actions of prolactin and somatotropin on bovine cumulus cells in vitro

I. Yu. Lebedeva[1], T.I. Kuzmina[1], T.V. Kibardina[1], F. Schneider[2], H. Alm[2] and H. Torner[2], [1]Research Institute for Farm Animal Genetics and Breeding, St.Petersburg, 196625 Russia, [2]Research Institute for the Biology of Farm Animals, 18196 Dummerstorf, Germany*

The aim of the present study was to examine whether some actions of prolactin (PRL) and somatotropin (ST) on bovine cumulus cells (CC) are mediated by granulosa cells (GC). Bovine GC from follicles of 2-5 mm in diameter were cultured for 48 h in TCM 199 containing 10 % fetal calf serum in the absence (control) or presence of bovine PRL (50 ng/ml) or bovine ST (10 ng/ml). Estradiol and progesterone concentrations were measured in GC-conditioned media by RIA. Cumulus-oocyte complexes (COC) isolated from follicles of 2-6 mm in diameter were cultured for 24 h in the conditioned media. The rate of CC with normal chromatin and that of CC at prophase stage were determined after culture. Neither PRL nor ST affected steroidogenic activity of GC. The addition of ST to GC culture resulted in a rise in the rate of CC with normal chromatin during the subsequent culture of COC ($p<0.01$). The similar effect of PRL was less significant. Moreover, proliferative activity of CC cultured in the medium conditioned by PRL-treated GC was considerably higher than in control ($p<0.05$). The data indicate that PRL and ST actions on CC can be mediated by GC without the change in steroidogenic activity of these latter.

Poster Ph2.10

Analysis of plasma IGF-I hormone level and its correlation with live weight and age in Holstein-Friesian heifers

M. Horvai-Szabo, Szent István University, Godollo, Hungary.

The aim of this study was to evaluate the changes and relation of live weight and IGF-I plasma concentration during the rearing period in HF heifers. Number of animals was 85 kept in similar housing and feeding conditions. Blood samples were collected monthly at the same hour of the day and weight of the calves were scaled simultaneously up to the 14th month of age. Plasma IGF-I c.c. was measured by RIA procedure. Data were analysed by SPSS 10.0 version and Post Hoc Test programs. Results of this work allow to clonclude that change of IGF-I c.c. and live weight show similar trend. Rearing phase of calves shows three peaks: 1th at birth, 2nd closed to sexual maturity, 3rd closed to first service. IGF-I profile can be taken as similar for all individual and animals can be categorised into groups with low or high hormone c.c. There is only negative correlation (r=-0,24) between IGF-I levels at birth and at 4 months of age. Bull have special effect on IGF-I c.c. at birth, at 5th, 13th and 14th months of age ($P<0.1$). On contrary to previous findings IGF-I level and weight of calves correlated negatively ($r=-0.31$, $P<0.05$) in the whole population, while within progeny groups positive and negativ correlation may occur, too. Negativ correlation prove the compensation ability of animals in growth rate. IN comparison with the overall mean of IGF-I c.c., the subpopulation below average has lower live weight, too and with high IGF-I level a higher love weight is bound.

 Poster Ph2.11

Plasma concentrations of IGF-1 and thyroid hormones in pre-weaning Angus-Nellore crossbred calves supplemented with recombinant bovine somatotropin (rbst)

R.C. Cervieri[1], M.D.B. Arrigoni[1], H.N. Oliveira[1], A.C. Silveira[1], L.A.L. Chardulo[2], C.L. Martins[1], [1]Faculdade de Medicina Veterinária e Zootecnia (FMVZ)-UNESP, Rubiao Júnior, P.O. Box 560, Botucatu, Sao Paulo, Brazil, [2]Instituto de Biociencias (IB)-UNESP, Departamento de Química e Bioquímica, Rubiao Júnior, Botucatu, Sao Paulo, Brazil.*

The objective of this study was to determine the recombinant bovine somatotropin (rbST) effect on plasma IGF-1 and thyroid hormone (T3 and T4) concentrations. We used thirty-six 1/2 Angus-Nellore crossbred bull calves, with 63 ± 17 days old and weighting 76,8 ± 14,7 kg, creep-fed, grazing *Brachiaria decunbens,* supplemented or not with rbST until the weaning (217 days). Eighteen calves received 0,10mg/kg/day of rbST (Boostin®) and eighteen control calves received saline solution, both every 14 days. Supplemental creep feed was supplied free access to all caves to compensate for an increased protein and energy requirement in calves given rbST. The blood collection was made by jugular venipuncture every 28 days throughout the 140-day period. The rbST-treated calves had higher plasma IGF-1 (213,60 vs 159,28 ng/ml, $P<0,05$) and T4 (8,59 vs 7,43 µg/dL, $P<0,05$) concentrations than control calves. However, plasma concentrations of T3 were not affected by rbST. Recombinant bovine somatotropin administration altered the hormonal status in pre-weaning creep-fed bull calves, mainly plasma IGF-1, which is closely involved with growth metabolism.

Theatre NPPh3.1

Effects of nutrient intake during pregnancy on fetal and placental growth and vascular development

D.A. Redmer[1], J.M. Wallace[2] and L.P. Reynolds[1], [1]Department of Animal and Range Sciences, North Dakota State University, Fargo, North Dakota, USA, [2]Rowett Research Institute, Bucksburn, Aberdeen, United Kingdom.*

Remarkable diversity of size and health of offspring exists after normal pregnancies. Pregnancies complicated by factors such as under or over nutrition will substantially affect birth weight and health of the neonate. Numerous studies have led to the conclusion that this diversity is essentially determined by the intrauterine environment. The placenta is the organ through which respiratory gases, nutrients, and wastes are exchanged between the maternal and fetal systems. Thus, transplacental exchange provides for all the metabolic demands of fetal growth. Transplacental exchange is dependent upon uterine and umbilical blood flow, and blood flow rates are in turn, dependent in large part upon vascularity of the placenta. Therefore, factors that influence placental vascular development have a dramatic impact on fetal growth and development, and thereby on fetal and neonatal mortality and morbidity. Recent work from our laboratories has focused on effect of nutrient intake during pregnancy on placental growth and vascular development and subsequent fetal growth. Both nutrient restriction and overnourishment of the dam during pregnancy suppress placental cell proliferation and vascularity. Furthermore, placental expression of angiogenic factors and their receptors, factors that are known to affect vascular growth, are perturbed by level of nutrition. Studies in this area will lead to improved methods to manage nutritionally-compromised pregnancies.

 Theatre NPPh3.2

Effects of increased porcine maternal nutrition on postnatal growth and meat quality of offspring

P.M. Nissen and N. Oksbjerg, Danish Institute of Agricultural Sciences, P.O.Box 50, 8830 Tjele, Denmark.*

The objective of this study was to examine the effect of increased maternal feed intake during early to mid gestation, on postnatal growth and meat quality (pH_{24}, colour, drip loss and pigmentation) of the offspring in pigs. Pregnant sows were either fed restrictively (2 kg/d) throughout gestation (C) or fed ad libitum from d 25-50 (A_{25-50}) or d 25-70 (A_{25-70}) and as C in the remaining periods. Offspring were slaughtered litter wise at an average age of 158 ± 10 days. Only the lightest, middle and heaviest weight pig by slaughter weight of each sex within litter was used for analysis. The weight of Semitendinosus and the muscle deposition rate was lower in A_{25-50} pigs compared to C (P = 0.019 and P = 0.038, respectively). Also the average daily gain and muscle mass was numerically lower for A_{25-50} pigs. Interactions between treatment and pig weight was found for muscle mass (P = 0.024) and muscle deposition rate (P = 0.003). The lightest A_{25-50} pig had lower muscle mass and muscle deposition rate than the lightest C pig. We found no effect of treatment on meat quality traits in the offspring. Thus, no beneficial effects on performance of offspring following increased maternal feed intake were observed.

Theatre NPPh3.3

Influence of pig birth weight on postnatal growth, muscle characteristics and meat quality traits at commercial slaughter weight

F. Gondret[1,], L. Lefaucheur[1], I. Louveau[1], B. Lebret[1] and X. Pichodo[2], [1]INRA, UMR Veau et Porc, 35590 Saint-Gilles, [2]EDE-Chambre d'Agriculture de Bretagne, 29100 Quimper, France.*

High prolificacy of sows in French breeding led to an increased within-litter variation in piglet birth weights. This study aimed to determine whether light *versus* heavy weight at birth could influence postnatal growth, biochemical and histological muscle characteristics, and in fine, meat quality traits at slaughter. A total of 19 piglets (10 females and 9 barrows) were allocated within litters to either light (LBW, n = 9) or heavy (HBW, n = 10) birth-weight groups. Light birth weight significantly impaired average daily gain (ADG) during lactation (P = 0.02) and post-weaning period (P < 0.001), whereas ADG was similar in the two groups during the growing-finishing period. At a constant weight at slaughter (102 kg ± 0.6 kg), LBW were 12 days older than HBW littermates. Back fat depth, muscle mass, and muscle biochemical composition did not differ between groups. On the opposite, the total number of myofibers was reduced (-13% in *semitendinosus* and -20% in *rhomboïdeus*, P < 0.10) whereas myofiber mean size was increased (+14% in *semitendinosus*, +20% in *longissimus* and *rhomboideus*, P < 0.05) in muscles from LBW compared to those from HBW pigs. Ultimate pH in the loin meat was not affected by birth weight.

Theatre NPPh3.4

Body composition and organ development in neonatal piglets

I. Wigren[1], M. Neil[1], J. E. Lindberg[1], and S. Stern[2], [1]Department of Animal Nutrition and Management, [2]Department of Animal Breeding and Genetics, Swedish University of Agricultural Sciences, Funbo-Lövsta, 755 97 Uppsala, Sweden.*

Neonatal piglet mortality rate remains a dilemma in modern pig production. Most deaths occur within the first 3 days after birth. A large difference among littermates in birth weight and growth rate affects mortality. Genetic selection against piglet mortality may not automatically increase birth weight, but could have an effect on body composition and development. The purpose of this study was to examine body composition and the proportional organ weights of a typical newborn piglet and compare with the extremes in the same litter at one day of age. Data were collected from litters of 12 multiparous Swedish Yorkshire sows. Immediately after birth a representative piglet was sacrificed. At 24 hours of age the lightest and the heaviest piglet in the same litter were also killed. Piglets were weighed and selected organs were dissected and weighed. The carcasses (including head) were analysed for ash, moisture, crude protein and fat content. Crude protein content was lower in the newborn than in light or heavy piglets ($p<0.001$), and lower in light than in heavy piglets ($p<0.05$) Fat content was lower in the newborn, than in the heaviest piglet ($p<0.01$). Proportional liver weight was reduced in lightweight piglets, compared with heavy piglets. Additional data is to be analysed within this project.

Theatre NPPh3.5

Dry period management strategies

R.J. Collier[1], E L. Annen[1] and M.A. McGuire[2], [1]University of Arizona, Tucson, AZ and [2]University of Idaho, Moscow, ID

A 40-60 d dry period is a routine management practice in the dairy industry. When dry periods are shorter than 40 d, subsequent milk yield is reduced by 5 to 15%, whilst absent dry period results in production losses of 20 to 40%. This study evaluated milk production after shortened or omitted dry periods in high producing cows treated with bovine somatotropin (bST). The study utilized 3 herds and four treatment groups with five multiparous and five primiparous cows from each farm in each group. Treatments included: 1) 60 d dry period, label bST (control; label=bST started at 57-70 DIM, end 2 wk before dry-off), 2) 30 d dry period, label bST, 3) continuous milking, label bST and 4) continuous milking with continuous bST. Average milk yield was reduced ($P<0.05$) during the first 17 weeks postpartum for treatments 2, 3 and 4, compared with controls (42.9, 37.5, 39.9, vs. 45.0 kg/d, n=95). However, the treatment-induced reduction in milk yield occurred in primiparous cows (40.1, 32.2, 34.6, vs. 43.1 kg/d; $P<0.01$), as milk for multiparous cows was not affected by treatment (45.6, 42.0, 45.5 vs. 47.3 kg/d; $P>0.8$). We hypothesize that a shortened or omitted dry period may alter mammary growth in primiparous animals and may have minimal production effects in multiparous cows treated with bST. We are currently evaluating whether increasing the number of milkings in early lactation reverses the negative effects of no dry period in primiparous cows.

Theatre NPPh3.6

The effects of milk feeding with different amounts in different periods on growth performance of Friesian Female calves in 0-12 month age period

Ö. Sekerden[1] and M. Sahin[2], [1]Mustafa Kemal Univ., Fac. of Agric., Dept. of Anim. Sci., P.O.Box 31034, Antakya, Turkey, [2]Directorate of Agriculture of Hatay State Farm, Hatay, Turkey.

In this research it was aimed to determine effects of different amounts of milk feeding in different periods on growth performance of Friesian female calves in 0-12 months of age period. The material of the research was formed by 62 Friesian female calves. The calves born in the unit were allocated into 3 milk feeding group as follows; 1st, 2nd and 3rd groups were fed with milk 2, 2.5 and 3 months respectively and total amount of milk fed were 212 kg whole milk +49 kg diluted milk, 226 kg whole milk+105 kg diluted milk, 226 kg whole milk+140 kg diluted milk for 1st, 2nd and 3rd groups respectively.Various body measurements (height at withers, body length, chest girth, chest depth, chest width and shin girth) and live weight (in first 6 month age) of the trial animals were determined in 0-12 month age period with 3 month intervals. Effects of lactation order, birth season and milk feeding group on the characteristics were investigated by using Least Squared Analysis Method. Standardization was applied on the characteristics for the effects which were found statistically significant.
It was concluded that milk feeding with different amounts in different periods did not have statistically significant effect on body size and weights obtained in 6 and 12 month ages.

Theatre NPPh3.7

Influence of changing feeding intensities during the weaning period on the growth performance of goat kids

C. Kijora, K. J. Peters and A. Müller Institute of Animal Sciences, Humboldt-University Berlin, Philippstr. 13, Building 9; 10115 Berlin, Germany*

The utilisation of compensatory growth during suckling and in mature animals is not fully clarified. The aim of the experiment was to investigate how different and changing feeding levels effect the performance and body composition of goat kids. It was also tested whether a lower milk consumption is compensated by a higher concentrate intake. A total of 64 goat kids were divided into 4 feeding groups. A first suckling period (7-weeks) was followed by two feeding periods over 4 weeks each (Exp. 1) and 7 weeks (Exp. 2),resp.. Control animals were exposed to a high (HHH; 2.4 x maintenance) or a low (1.4 x maintenance, LLL) feeding level over all three periods. Two experimental groups were subjected to changing feeding levels (HLH, LLH). As expected the performance difference between the control groups was highly significant. Feed restriction even for one period was not compensated during subsequent realimentation, irrespective of length of the feeding period. However, the restricted groups show a higher live weight gain during realimentation than the energy intake explains. No differences were observed between feeding groups in the body nutrient composition but significant differences in organ weight. The milk restriction leads to a higher intake of concentrates, which did not fully compensate the reduced milk nutrients. A milk restriction of 60% during suckling is possible, when the intake of quality feed (energy and protein) in the first or second post weaning period is guaranteed.

Effect of dietary undegradable intake protein in postpartum reproductive performance of Awassi ewes

S. Haddad R. Kridli and D. Alwaadi, Department of Animal Production, Jordan University of Science and Technology, P.O. Box 3030, Irbid 22110, Jordan*

To evaluate the effect of feeding high level of undegradable intake protein (UIP) on the return to estrus during the early postpartum (PP) period, thirty multiparous Awassi ewes were fed three experimental diets for 62 days. Diets were isonitrogenous, isocaloric, and were formulated to contain 17 (CON), 25 (MSBM), and 33 % (HSBM) of the dietary CP as UIP. Ewes were housed in individual pens for 5 weeks. Animals were then removed and combined into 3 separate groups (CON, MSBM, and HSBM). One fertile, harnessed ram was allowed with each group for 34 days. The UIP intake and metabolizable energy intake were higher ($P < 0.05$) for ewes fed HSBM diet compared with ewes fed MSBM and CON diets. Ewes fed HSBM gained more ($P < 0.05$) weight compared with ewes fed MSBM and CON diets. Ewes fed the HSBM had higher ($P < 0.01$) pregnancy rate compared with ewes fed MSBM and CON diets. Pregnancy rate of ewes fed HSBM diet was 100% (10/10), compared with 70% (7/10) and 40% (4/10) for ewes fed MSBM and CON diets, respectively. Lambing rate was greater ($P < 0.05$) for ewes fed HSBM (9/10) diet compared with ewes fed MSBM (5/10) and CON (4/10) diets. These results indicate that Awassi ewes receiving adequate nutrition and adequate UIP are capable of returning to estrus within one month postpartum and are able to lamb every 6 months.

Poster NPPh3.9

Nitrogen balances in relation to carcass composition changes of Boer Goat bucks fed winter veld hay and supplemented

A.M. Almeida[1], L.M Schwalbach[2], H.O. de Waal[2], J.P. Greyling[2] and L.A. Cardoso[1], [1]Centro de Veterinária e Zootecnia, Faculdade de Medicina Veterinária, Rua Prof. Cid dos Santos 1300-477 Lisboa, Portugal, [2]Faculty of Natural and agricultural Sciences, Department of Animal Science, University of the Free State, PO Box 339, Bloemfontein 9300, South Africa*

Fifteen Boer goat bucks (6 - 8 months old, 28 kg), were allocated to two groups. WH group (n=8) received a chopped diet consisting of a *Themeda trianda* grass hay from a natural pasture (veld) and WH+S group (n=7) received a chopped diet of the same hay, supplemented with maize, molasses and urea. Animals were housed individually for 30 days. Food Intake was recorded daily and Faeces and urine were collected once a week in order to determine nitrogen balances (NB). At the end of the experimental period, animals were slaughtered and carcass chemical characteristics determined. WH animals lost 20 % of their initial body weight, while WH+S increased only 10 %. Since WH+S animals had a very small increase in body weight it was considered that carcass chemical composition was stable throughout the assay in this group. Carcass composition changes were hence determined. Significant differences were recorded between the two groups at the last collection date (NB of -1.47g in WH and 3.12g in 3.12). Regarding carcass changes WH+S group had an increase in Dry matter, water, protein, fat and energy contents (approximately 105 % for all characteristics in comparison with the initial date). WH animals lost 82 % of their Dry Matter 86 % of the water and protein contents, 75 % fat content and 70 % of crude energy content.

Poster NPPh3.10

Effect of royal jelly on reproductive responses of Awassi ewes synchronized using CIDR-G with or without PMSG

M.Q. Husein S.G. Haddad and H.A. Ghozlan, Department of Animal Production, Jordan University of Science and Technology, P.O.Box 3030, Irbid 22110, Jordan*

The objective was to evaluate the effect of royal jelly (RJ) treatment on reproductive responses of ewes synchronized using CIDR-G with or without PMSG. Forty 3-6-yr-old Awassi ewes were allocated into four groups namely, RJ-PMSG, PMSG, RJ and control. All ewes were synchronized to estrus using CIDR-G for 12 days. During this period half of the ewes (RJ-treated) received a total of 4.8 g RJ given i.m. in 12 equal doses of 400 mg/ewe/day. At the time of CIDR-G removal (0 h, 0 day), half of the ewes in RJ and non-RJ groups received an injection of 500 IU PMSG. Blood samples were collected from day -12 until day 0 and thereafter until day 20 for progesterone analyses. Four intact rams were turned in with ewes from 0h for 4 days. The incidence and duration of estrus were not influenced by either RJ or PMSG treatments and averaged 82% and 20.6±0.8 h, respectively. Intervals from 0h to onset of estrus were shorter ($P<0.01$) in PMSG-RJ-, PMSG- and RJ-treated than control ewes. Royal jelly treatment resulted in a greater rate of decline and lower ($P<0.02$) progesterone concentrations between days -10 and 0. Neither RJ nor PMSG affected pregnancy (36%) and lambing (33%) rates. In conclusion, RJ and PMSG treatments were equally effective in occurrence and duration of estrus. Both treatments induced estrus in >80% of the ewes and resulted in shorter intervals to onset of estrus.

Poster NPPh3.11

Molecular tests and pig productivity

T.A. Dementyeva, L.V. Lazareva, A.V. Dementyev, G.V. Korotkova, Novosibirsk State Agrarian University, 630039 Novosibirsk, Russia.

The experiment was done in the experimental training farm "Tulinskoye" under Novosibirsk State Agrarian University and in the pig breeding complex "Chistogorsky" Kemerovo region. The activity of alanine-aminotransferase was examined in mitochondrions and supernatant of skeletal muscles, liver and heart of the pig breeds: Large White(LW), Kemerovskaya(K), Landras(L) and their three - way crosses. The study in the alanine - aminotransferase activity in the mitochondrial fraction of cardiac muscle revealed its activating in the crosses of all the groups. The most expressed increase of the fermentative activity (by 21.78%, $p<0.001$ as compared to the control) was determined in the pigs whose fathers were Landras boars, sows were KxLW crosses. The crosses produced with the use of Landras boars and the Kemerovo sows of KxLW and LWxL were characterized by the higher alanine-aminotransferase activity for the control values in the skeletal muscle metochondrions. The highest level of amino-transferase activity in the liver mitochondrions was marked in the crosses whose fathers were the Landras and Large White boars, the sows were KxLW and KxL crosses. The results of the experiment can drive us to the conclusion that the metabolic processes of three breed crosses run more intensively than those of pure breed animals that testifies to their higher precocity and viability.

Poster NPPh3.12

Formation of MLLT in slaughter pigs in relation to age

M. Sprysl, R. Stupka, Czech University of Agriculture, Department of Pig and Poultry Science, Prague, Kamycka, 165 21, Czech Republic

The test included 144 currently used final hybrids of the (DxPN)x(LWxL) genotype of balanced sex. The increasing age of the animals and consequently also their weight is accompanied by an increase of the MLLT area, width, height and the height of fat above MLLT. Until 134 days of age and live weight of approx. 70kg and starting from 162 days of age and the average weight of approx. 96kg the increase of the MLLT area is low. In the period between 134th day and 162nd day of age a significant increase of the MLLT area was registered.
During the testing period the MLLT area increased by 1471mm2 , i.e. 55,2%. The width increased by 13,8% and the height by 29,2%. The comparison of the area of the A section (between 2nd and 3rd last but one rib) and B (between 4th and 5th lumbar vertebra) of the loin in the course of the growth showed in point B lower values in the MLLT area and width and on the contrary higher values in the depth. The assessment of the height of the fat in point B proved that it reaches during the growth lower values as compared to point A with more significant differences registered starting from the live weight of 75kg.

Poster NPPh3.13

Nutrient digestibility in weanling pigs fed starter diets with three dry wheys

T.C.R. Souza[1] and G.L. Mariscal[2], [1]Universidad Autónoma de Querétaro, Av. 16 de Septiembre 63, 76000, Querétaro - Qro, México. [2]CENID Fisiología - INIFAP, 76280 Querétaro - Qro, México.*

One experiment was conducted with 12 male crossbred weanling pigs (6.8 ± 0.9 kg; 17 ± 0.5 days of age) canullated at terminal ileum to determine the effect of dry whey type on nutrient digestibility and pH of gastric and small intestinal digesta. Three diets were formulated with sorghum, soybean meal, soy protein concentrate, spray dried porcine plasma and acid dry whey (ADW), sweet dry whey (SDW) or neutralized dry whey (NDW). Total tract (TTAD) and ileal (IAD) apparent digestibilities were measured on the same piglets in three periods. For TTAD: 27th - 28th, 34th - 35th and 41st - 42nd day of age. IAD was measured at 28th - 29th, 35th - 36th, and 42nd - 43rd day of age. IAD of DM (69.8, 71.0, 68%), CP (71.1, 71.0, 67.1%) and energy (67.9, 69.2, 67.4%) were not different ($P > .05$) among diets. Dry matter TTAD was higher ($P < .05$) in piglets fed ADW (83.2^{a}, 81.0^{b}, 81.4^{b} % for ADW, SDW and NDW, respectively). There were not period or period x diet interaction effect on digestibilities determination. There were not whey type effect in gastric pH. Intestinal pH was lower in piglets fed ADW (5.9^{b}, 6.5^{a}, 6.1^{ab} for ADW, SDW and NDW, respectively).

Poster NPPh3.14

The study of the influence of lysine and threonine in diet on quantity and composition of sow milk

J. Bojcuková, F. Krátky, Research Institute of Animal Production, Prague, workplace 51741 Kostelec nad Orlicí, Czech Republic.

The aim of the experiment was to study the influence of various levels of lysine and threonine in complete feed mixtures for the lactating sows on milk production and quality. There were 30 sows of the breed Large White in the trial (3 groups- I.,II.,III.). The content of lysine in diets was 10,90 g/kg; 15,19 g/kg and 8,46 g/kg for the individual groups, threonine content was 6,75 g/kg; 9,85 g/kg; 5,22 g/kg. We examined the influence on litter weight at the age of 0, 7, 14, 21 days and milk composition on the 3rd day post partum and further at weekly intervals until the weaning. The highest average litter weight was at the age of 14 days at group II. 49,88±8,67 kg, on the 21st day as well at group II. 65,88±9,83 kg. Lysine content in milk was the highest at first samples (the 3rd day post partum) and at group II., namely 11,92±2,62 g/16gN, the same tendency was at threonine - group II. 5,93±1,08 g/16gN.

The results suggest that the increase of lysine and threonine in the feeding ration of the suckling sows influences quantity protein and amino-acids in milk, especially at the beginning of the lactation. Protein and amino acids in milk further influence litter weight on the 21st day of life.

Poster NPPh3.15

The influence of some complete feed with different energy concentrations on the productive performance in the "Robro" Romanian Broiler

Minodora Tudorache, I. Van, M. Nicolae, Elena Popescu Miclosanu, I. Custura, University of Agronomical Sciences and Veterinary Medicine Bucharest, Faculty of Animal Sciences, 59 Marasti Blvd., 1 sector, Romania*

On five hen broiler groups, each of them having 500 chicken, and bred on permanent litter, in three phases (starter - 0-3 weeks; grower - 4-5 weeks, and finisher - the sixth week), differentiated upon the energy level from the complete feed (+ 5, + 10, - 5, - 10% comparison to the control), but keeping all the other nutritive parameters at a constant level, the feed consumption, daily weight gain, and gain composition were analysed.

The energy level into those three diets at the control group was 12.56, 13.07, respectively 13.13 MJ/kg.

The duration of the experiment was 42 days, and the feeding was ad libitum. The increasing in energy concentration have had as effect a decreasing of feed consumption up to 11.2%, and its decreasing determined a larger consumption up to 8.7%. Increasing the energy parameter leaded to a better gain, by up to 4.7% comparison to control, but the difference being non-significant ($P > 0.05\%$), while its decreasing determined a significant decreasing in gain ($P < 0.05\%$). The ratio between protein and lipids retained per kg net weight, at the end of experiment, decreases up to 0.828 when the energy level increases, and it increases up to 1.017 when the energy level decreases.

Poster NPPh3.16

Preliminary studies on an effect of captopril on the activity of angiotensin converting enzyme (ACE) in the blood of newborn calves

M. Ozgo, W.F. Skrzypczak, A. Dratwa. Department of Animal Physiology, Agricultural University, Doktora Judyma 6, 71-466 Szczecin, Poland.*

The experiment was carried out on 9 Black-&-White calves. Blood was taken from the external jugular vein from 1 to 7 days of life. Every day, after the first blood sampling, the calves were p.o. administered with 0.3 mg/kg b.w. of captopril (Sigma). Next, the blood was collected in 0.5, 1, 2, 4, and 6 hours after the captopril administration. The concentration of angiotensin convertase in blood plasma was determined spectrophotometrically (using FAPGG-furylacryloylphenyl-alanine, Sigma Diagnostics). Preliminary results display high ACE activity during the calves' first days. Before captopril administration, it varies within a relatively wide range, from 70 to 290 μ/l, which means, on one hand, that individual differences occur and, on the other hand, ACE activity decreases with the age of the calves. After the blocker had been applied, an increase in the enzyme blood concentration was observed, especially in 1-2 hours after its administration. It was also observed that an increase in ACE concentration is the higher, the lower its concentration before captopril administration is. The results of this study will be comparable with the results of parallel analyses of captopril concentration in blood, renin-angiotensin-aldosterone system activity analysis, and atrial natriuretic peptide concentration in serum.

The study was financed by Committee for scinetific Research (grant No. 3 P06D 028 22)

Poster NPPh3.17

Atrial natriuretic peptide (ANP) concentration in the blood of newborn calves

W.F. Skrzypczak, A. Dratwa, M. Ozgo. Department of Animal Physiology, Agricultural University, Doktora Judyma 6, 71-466 Szczecin, Poland.*

The experiment was carried out on 10 Black-&-White calves. Blood was taken daily from the external jugular vein on the 1, 2, 3, 4, 5, 6 and 7 days of postnatal life, always at the same time of day (8.00-9.00 a.m.). The concentration of atrial natriuretic peptide in blood serum was assayed immunoradiometrically (immunoradiometric assay kit - SHIONORIA, CIS Bio International, France). ANP concentration in plasma blood was steady, ranging from 5.73 to 16.44 pmol/l. On the first day of life, the concentration of the hormone was the lowest (5.73 pmol/l). A statistically significant increase in ANP concentration was observed on the 2nd day of life (9.39 pmol/l). In the subsequent days, further growth in the hormone level was recorded, which reached its maximum, 16.44 pmol/l, on the 6th day of age. It should be stressed that a wide range of individual variability was observed in the concentration of ANP in the blood of the calves, particularly during the first two days of their life. The results of our studies will correspond with the results of renin-angiotensin-aldosterone system activity analysis, which is being carried on simultaneously, as well as with the results of complex, clearance studies on renal function.

The study was financed by Committee for Scientific Research (grant No. 3 P06D 028 22)

Poster NPPh3.18

Comparative fattening potential and carcass characteristics in Simmental and Brown Swiss beef crossbred calves

A. Fayyaz and M.A. Jabbar, Livestock Production Research Institute, Bahadurnagar, Okara, Pakistan.

Twenty (20) crossbred calves (Simmental and Brown Swiss crossbred with local non-descript cows) were included in this study. Four groups representing the genotypes of either sex were formulated. They were given fattening ration ad-libitum containing 13.7% CP and 70% TDN along with 5 kg of green fodder, daily on individual feeding basis for a period of 120 days. Average feed intake in male and female Simmental crossbred calves was 8.56 and 8.59 kg while similar values for male and female Brown Swiss was 7.22 and 6.68 kg, respectively. The average daily weight gain over this period was 1210, 1340, 920 and 950 gms in respective groups. The FCR values were 7.14, 7.36, 7.88 and 7.02 percent for these groups. The carcass percentage was slightly higher in female (57.9 vs 58.9) in Simmental crossbreds as well as in Brown Swiss crossbred calves (56.9 vs 57.9). The meat bone ratio was 62:38, 61:39, 62:38 and 62:38 in Simmental and Brown Swiss crossbred calves. Statistically the difference for all these parameters was non-significant among the groups.

Poster NPPh3.19

The nutritive effect of rumen protected methionine on haematological values and some metabolic parameters in growing beef cattle

Lina Bacar-Huskic[2],B. Liker[1], V. Rupic[1], N. Vranesic[2], M. Knezevic[1], B. Stuburic[2], J. Leto[1].[1]Agricultural University, Svetosimunska 25, Zagreb, Croatia, [2]Pliva d.d., Development of Vet. and Agric., Ulica grada Vukovara 45, Zagreb, Croatia.*

The nutritive effect of rumen protected methionine on haematological value (RBC, haemoglobin, haematocrit, WBC, lymphocites, monocites, neutrophils, eosinophils, basophils) and on some metabolic parameters in blood plasma (total protein, albumine, triacylglycerols, cholesterol, glucose, urea, creatinine, ALT, AST, GGT, and AP) was investigated.

Twenty two beef cattle, devided in two groups equial in number: one control (C) and one, experimental group (E) were included in trial and were fed hay, silage and 500 g fodder mix (35% CP). Added to the fodder mix, the group E received 10 g rumen protected methionine per animal. Blood samples were colleced et 1st, 34th, 68th and 102nd day of trial.

Total blood leukocyte ($P<0,05$) of C group was increased on 68th day. The values of glucose were significantly higher ($P<0,05$) on 68. and 34. day in the control group and the value of urea was significantly lower ($P<0,05$) on 34. day. Methionine supplementation affected slightly antistressfully.

Poster NPPh3.20

Factors affecting longevity in maternal Duroc swine lines

J. Tarrés[1], J. Tibau[2], J. Piedrafita[1], E. Fabrega[2], J.Reixach[2], [1]Departament de Ciència Animal i dels Aliments , UAB 08193 Bellaterra, Spain, [2]Institut de Recerca i Tecnologia Agroalimentàries, 17121 Monells, Spain, [3]Selecció Batallé , Riudarenes 17421 Spain*

Longevity of sows is affected by genetic background, environmental influences and management practices. The most important reasons for culling are reproductive (fertility and productivity) and locomotor problems. Preparation of pre-farrowing gilts is a key stage for future productivity of any swine herd. If feeding and management are not all appropriate, the true reproductive potential will not be likely expressed, leading to an early culling of sow. The goal of this study was to evaluate the influence on longevity of several non-genetic pre-mating factors, like average daily gain (ADG) and back fat thickness (BF). Data from 567 duroc sows were analysed. The influence of the factors was assessed by means of survival analysis (Proportional Hazard Model) using the program 'The Survival Kit v3.12'. A higher ADG from the end of the growth period until mating increased culling rate. The optimal BF at first parturition was found to range from 17 to 19 mm, whereas at the end of the growth period this optimal BF was higher than 16 mm. Culling rate was reduced when body weight was close to 140 kg at first mating. Therefore, it is suggested that an appropriate pre-mating management, mainly associated with the nutrition level, can help to decrease culling rate of the future sow.

Poster NPPh3.21

The influence of feeding technique on performance and economy in fattening pigs

T. Neuzil[1], J. Cítek[1], T. Cervenka[1], A. Kodes[2], [1]Czech University of Agriculture Prague, Department of Pig and Poultry Science, 165 21 Prague, Czech Republic, [2]Czech University of Agriculture Prague, Department of Nutrition and Feeding of Husbandry Animals, 165 21 Prague, Czech Republic.

70 hybrid pigs of the (LW_SxBL) x (LWxL) genotype were divided into three groups and the impacts of feeding technique and quality of feed mixture on fattening capacity, slaughter value, and their production economy were compared. The first group of pigs was ad-libitum fed with the mixture richest in nutrients. The second and the third groups were subject to semi ad-libitum feeding at a higher/lower nutrient level.

The maximal genotype production efficiency manifested itself in the ad-libitum fed group when that group (1) clearly reached the highest growth intensity in comparison with other groups (827 vs. 768 ($P \leq 0.05$) or 730 g/day ($P \leq 0.01$)) with demonstratively higher ($P \leq 0.01$) daily feed intake (2.47 vs. 2.29 kg). The impact of feeding technique and quality of feed mixture on the meatiness of individual groups was not proven. In terms of economic analyses, the semi ad-libitum feeding technique based on leaner feed mixtures seems to be the most convenient technique.

Poster NPPh3.22

Certain biochemical parameters in crossbred pigs during growth

Dilip Kumar Garikipati[1] and P.E. Prasad[2], [1]Washington State University, [2]A.N.G.R.Agricutural University*

Biochemical changes taking place during different stages of growth have been attributed to the changes in the activities of certain enzymes and biochemical constituents which have clinical importance in assessment of their growth, health, nutritional status, diagnosis and prognosis of metabolic disorders. The present research has been under taken to study the enzymes-AST, ALT, ALP, LDH and certain biochemical constituents like glucose, total proteins, albumin, globulin and urea concentrations of blood in crossbred pigs during growth. The level of AST, ALT, ALP, and LDH enzymes in serum decreased significantly ($p<0.01$) as the age of piglets increased from 60 days to 120 days. However, the AST and ALP level at 90 days age are not significantly different from 120 days age. The level of glucose at 90 and 120 days was significantly lower compared to 60 days age. The total serum protein and albumin concentrations significantly ($p>0.01$) increased as the age of the piglets increased. The serum urea concentration of the growing piglets did not differ significantly as age advanced.

Poster NPPh3.23

Manipulation of rumen fermentation, microbial population and blood metabolites of Holstein neonatal calves using Yeast Culture as a microbial additive

B. Saremi, A.A. Naserian, Animal Science Department of Ferdowsi University of Mashhad, Khorasan, Iran*

Eighteen female Holstein neonatal calves were randomly placed on treatments and fed colostrums at 10% of birth weight and milked until 45 days old. All calves were fed calf starter (NRC 2001) containing high quality alfalfa (15%) from seven days of age and weaned at 45 days. Calf starter was offered until 90 days old and the yeast was added at 0, 0.5 and 1% to the calf starter, which was, used daily. Rumen (pH, N-NH3, Microbial population (MP)) and blood samples (Total protein (TP), Glucose (GLS), (BUN)) were taken from 0 to 90 days in regular periods. In day 90, feed and feces samples obtained to determine, nutrient digestibility. The design was completely randomized. Means were compared with Duncan test. Data showed that Yeast culture could not significantly alter protein, NDF, ADF and Ash digestibility, also have no effect on MP, pH, N-NH3 of the rumen. It couldn't affect TP and GLS in blood plasma. But BUN, OM and DM digestibility were significantly different ($P=0.05$). Results showed that addition of yeast culture to calves starter could improve DM and OM digestibility and also reduced BUN. We suggested that better weight gain and reduced DMI (Data not shown) could be result of better digestibility and the less losses of ammonia in the rumen.

Poster NPPh3.24

Neonatal proteinuria in kids

D. Drzezdzon, W.F. Skrzypczak. Department of Animal Physiology, Agricultural University, Str. Doktora Judyma 6, 71-466 Szczecin, Poland.*

The aim of this study was to evaluate adaptational capability of kid kidneys during the first month of postnatal life, in the scope of glomerular-tubular barrier against plasma proteins. The analyses were carried out using clearance methods in the first month of postnatal life. On each day, analyses were done in 12-hour intervals (at 7.00 a.m. and 7. p.m.). In the blood (collected from external jugular vein) and urine samples, the concentration of endogenous creatinine (for determination of GFR) was measured spectrophotometrically, while total protein concentration was established with Lowry's method. Electrophoretic separation of the blood and urine proteins was done in 12.5% polyacrylamide gel with an addition of SDS, according to Laemmli's method. In the morning, the average daily total protein excretion rate ranged between 0.324 and 0.181 g/24h/kg b.w. and was lower than in the evening, which indicates a transient proteinuria. Total protein clearance decreased during the first 10-12 days of life (which was accompanied by growing tubular reabsorption), and grew significantly again after this period (accompanied by decreasing tubular reabsorption). At the same time, total protein concentration in blood serum was found to decrease. The electrophoretic image of urine proteins of the examined kids revealed fractions of their molecular weight ranging from 151 to 11,8 kD.

The study was financed by Committee for Scientific Research (grant No. 3 P06D 034 24)

Theatre Ph4.1

Mammary cell proliferation, apoptosis and enzymatic activity during lactation

Martin T. Sørensen and Kristen Sejrsen, Danish Institute of Agricultural Sciences, Foulum Research Centre, DK-8830 Tjele

Milk yield of the dairy cow follows the lactation curve. We have investigated the cellular background for this pattern. During the lactation and reproduction cycle we collected seven mammary gland biopsies from each of ten cows, two times during the dry period (48 and 16 days before calving) and five times during lactation (14, 42, 88, 172 and 347 days after calving). The samples were analysed for cell proliferation and apoptosis and for three enzymes central for milk synthesis, i.e., fatty acid synthetase (FAS), Acetyl CoA-carboxylase (ACC) and galactosyl transferase (GT).

Cell proliferation of alveolar cells (staining for Ki67) was much higher during the dry period than during lactation, i.e., approximately 10-fold higher in the early dry period and 18-fold higher in the late dry period. Cell proliferation had its nadir 12 weeks after calving. Apoptosis was low, i.e., 0.1-0.4 % of alveolar cells, except during very early lactation where appoximately 0.8 % of alveolar cells were apoptotic. The activity of all three enzymes were low during the dry period and high during lactation. The highest level of enzyme activity was not reached at the very early stage of lactation but rather 6 (FAS and ACC) or 12 (GT) weeks after calving. GT was the only of the three enzymes that had a drop in activity at late lactation.

We conclude that mammary cell proliferation is substantial during late pregnancy but otherwise low. The activity of enzymes central for milk synthesis is low during the dry period but generally high throughout lactation.

Theatre Ph4.2

Existence of different shapes of lactation curves in Italian Water Buffalo

N.P.P. Macciotta[1], A. Carretta[2], G. Catillo[2], A. Cappio-Borlino[1]. [1]Dipartimento di Scienze Zootecniche, Università di Sassari, Italia, [2]Istituto Sperimentale per la Zootecnia, Monterotondo (Roma,) Italia.*

In order to evalue the influence of main environmental factors on the lactation curve shape for milk yield in Buffalo, the Wood incomplete gamma function $y=at^b e^{(ct)}$ was fitted to 938 lactations of Italian buffalo cows. Within the group of individual curve showing the best fit (adjusted r-square>0.75), the existence of two families of lactation curves, one with the typical form and the other characterised by the absence of the lactation peak, has been evidenced. The two groups were separated according to the values of the ratio *b/c* and showed different averages of all the parameters. Parameters were then analysed with a linear model that included the fixed effects of age at calving, season of calving, herd and pregnancy status. The analysis was carried out both for the whole data set and separately for each of the two shapes of curve. Results were quite different in the two groups, even if they could be explained by considering the two shapes, whereas the analysis carried out in the whole data set resulted in meaningless estimates of parameter averages. As an example, the time at which the peak is attained was around 30 days, whereas it should be at around 60. These results suggest a great attention in using average lactation curves for prediction and management purposes but also fitting of indivual curves for genetic evaluations requires a particular care.

Theatre Ph4.3

Responses of long-term administration of bovine growth hormone (BST) on the lactating performance of Egyptian dairy buffaloes

F.I.S Helal, Animal Production Department, National Research Centre, Dokki, Great Cairo, Egypt.

Twenty-five Egyptian lactating buffaloes (first to fifth lactation) were used to evaluate the efficacy of a prolonged administration of bovine Somatotropin hormone (BST). All buffaloes were fed ad-libitum a complete mixed diet and milked twice daily. Tested animals were (15 lactating buffaloes) receiving 500 mg. Somatotropin hormone at 14 - days intervals starting at 60 (+ or - 7) days postpartum and continuing for 20 weeks. The other group (10 lactating buffaloes) was used as a control group.

Treatment with somatotropin increased milk yield with at least 35% (Kg./d) in all animals under test (primiparous and multparous buffaloes). Milk constituents of lactose and minerals were not affected, but fat and protein were greater (5%) in milk compared with the control one.

Over the treatment period (140 days) Somatotropin - treated animals increased voluntary feed intake to a sufficient extent so that the treated group recorded better body weight gains than control.

Results demonstrate that bovine Somatotropin administration for prolonged period is effective in improving milk yield and composition of Egyptian lactating buffaloes.

Theatre Ph4.4

Electrical conductivity in milk-validation of different conductivity parameters for detection of mastitis

E. Norberg[1], I.R. Korsgaard[1], N.C Friggens[2], and P. Løvendahl[1]. Danish Institute of Agricultural Sciences (DIAS), [1]Dept. of Animal Breeding and Genetics, [2]Dept.of of Animal Health and Welfare, P.O. Box 50, DK-8830 Tjele, Denmark.*

Electrical conductivity (EC) in milk has during the last decades been introduced as an indicator trait for mastitis. Traditionally, EC level during milking has been used as the parameter for detection of mastitis. However, infected quarters may also show large variation in EC measurements within a milking. In this study, parameters reflecting level and variation of EC during milking were compared for detection of mastitis. The experiment was performed at Ammitsbøl Skovgaard, Denmark. 549 lactations were included in the study, and 1353 cases of clinical and 778 cases of subclinical mastitis were recorded. The EC level, the variance, and inter quarter ratios for both parameters were calculated for every milking. All parameters increased significantly when a quarter was infected. A simple detection model based on threshold values and a discriminant analysis were executed to validate the parameters. Performance of the models was expressed as sensitivity and specificity. The inter quarter ratio for the level showed highest sensitivity and specificity. About 80% of the clinical and 45% of the subclinical cases were detected when specificity was 75%. The parameters reflecting the variance did not perform as good as the parameters reflecting the level. However, a combination of these two parameters improved the detection of mastitis.

Theatre Ph4.5

The influence of feeding intensity on growth curves of body traits in Holstein heifers: A twin study

U. Mueller[1], J. Hoessler[2], L. Panicke[3], L. Hasselmann[1], S. Betzin[1], R. Staufenbiel[2], [1]Humboldt University of Berlin, Dep. of Basic Science of Husbandry, Philippstr. 13, G-10115 Berlin, [2]Free University Berlin, Clinic of Cattle and Pigs, [3]Research Institute for the Biology of Farm Animals, Dummerstorf*

In the field of animal production the term "growth" means the ability of individuals to gain live weight and to increase skeleton measurements. To describe the growth mathematically it is probably insufficient to use a standard curve for all traits, in all spezies, and in all environments.
The aim of our investigation was to analyze the effect of feeding intensity on the growth curves for three body traits (body weight, withers height, back fat thickness). Data from 15 female twin pairs of the HF-breed were used. Each animal was measured repeatedly in the time from birth to an age of 23 months. Each twin belonged to a separate feeding group and was raised equally with the exception of feeding.
The results of both groups indicate that the development of body weight was nearly linear, whereas the developments of back fat thickness and withers height follow an exponent and a power function, respectively. The linear development of body weight is probably the result of many different growth processes. Maybe feeding intensity does influence only the the growth rate of some traits but not the kind of mathematical function of the growth.

Theatre Ph4.6

Patterns of follicular waves and corpus luteum development throughout the abnormal estrous cycles of Egyptian buffaloes

A.H. Barkawi, Y. Hafez, Amal K. El-Asheeri, S.A. Ibrahim, and N.G. Othman, Animal Production Department, Faculty of Agriculture, Cairo University, Giza, Egypt.*

Buffaloes are reported to have irregular ovarian activity during the summer season. Poor estrous behavior, irregular ovarian activity and sustained anestrous are the common reproductive phenomena observed during the hot season. Throughout the hot months (May to September), 9 cyclic buffaloes were investigated to monitor the type(s) of ovarian activity (follicular and corpus luteum development). Both ovaries were daily examined using the ultrasound technique. Blood sampling every 3 days were proceeded to assay the progesterone concentration in peripheral blood plasma in relation to corpus luteum development.

Forty-four abnormal estrous cycles were detected during the experimental period. The detected types include; short and long cycles. Clinical examination and progesterone concentration indicated that long cycles were attributed to one of delayed ovulations, anestrous incidence, persistency of corpus luteum or incidence of cystic follicles. In each type, follicular growth pattern, corpus luteum growth features and concentration of progesterone were obviously differed. Each type is discussed individually at the present study.

Theatre Ph4.7

Measurment of faecal progesterone metabolites by using of EIA as an aid for pregnancy diagnosis in buffalo-heifers

K.A. El-Battawy, Animal Reproduction and A.I Dept., National Research Centre, Tahrir Street, Dokki, Egypt.

The objective of this study was to find out whether the concentrations of progesterone metabolites in faeces would reflect the concentrations of progesterone in blood and consequently be used as a non invasive method monitoring of the reproductive status in buffalo-heifers.

In this investigation, five heifers were randomly selected from a group of cycling buffalo-heifers after being rectally palpated twice at an 11 day interval. The estrous cycles of those heifers were synchronized with prostaglandin F2 alpha where all heifers came in heat then they were allowed to be mated with fertile bull.

Blood samples were collected twice weekly from each animal starting from the day of synchronized estrus and for a period of six weeks for assessment of progesterone in the blood. On the other hand, faecal samples were collected at the same time as the blood samples to measure faecal progesterone metabolites (20-oxo-pregnanes).

In conclusion, faecal 20-oxo-pregnanes concentrations during the experimental period is clearly correlated with the concentrations of progesterone in the blood and could be used as a valuable non invasive technique for pregnancy diagnosis in buffalo-heifers.

Feeding rabbits on diet contaminated with lindane, zinc and their combination. 2- effect on hematological and biochemical parameters

A.A.A. Hassan[1], M.H.M. Yacout[1], H.Z. Ibrahem[2], M.I. Yousef[2], [1]Animal Production Reseach Institute, Ministry of Agriculture, Dokki, Giza, Egypt, [2]Department of Environmental Studies, Institute of Graduate Studies and Research, University of Alexandria, P. O. Box 832, Alexandria 21526, Egypt.*

The objective of the present study was to assess the potential effects of two chemical contaminants, lindane (HCH), zinc chloride ($ZnCl_2$) and interactive of them on growth performance of rabbits. Twenty-four male New Zealand White growing rabbits aged one month were randomly divided into 4 equal groups, on body weight basis, each treatment consists of 6 individual rabbits.Lindane and the combination of lindane and zinc treatment caused a significant decline ($P<0.05$) in hemoglobin (Hb) concentration, total erythrocyte counts (TEC) and packed cell volume (PCV), but total leucocyte counts (TLC), blood glucose and cholesterol were significantly increased compared to the control animals. While, treatment with zinc alone did not cause any effect on the above parameters. Lindane and its combination with zinc treatment caused a significant decreased ($P<0.05$) in serum total protein, albumin and albumin/globulin ratio. However, they caused a significant increase ($P<0.05$) in urea, creatinine, plasma aspartate aminotransferase (AST), alanine aminotransferase (ALT), alkaline phosphatase (AlP) and lactic dehydrogenase (LDH). But acid phosphatase (AcP) and plasma acetylcholinesterase (AChE) caused a significant decrease ($P<0.05$) during treatment with lindane and their combination. The activities of liver AST, ALT, AlP and LDH were significantly ($P<0.05$) decreased during treatment with lindane, zinc and their combination, but AcP was decreased. The activities of liver Mg^{++}-ATPase, testes Na^+, K^+-ATPase were significantly ($P<0.05$) decreased during treatment with lindane, zinc and their combination, while brain total ATPase, brain Mg^{++} and Na^+, K^+-ATPase were decreased.

Poster Ph4.9

Effect of semen extender type on rabbit semen metabolism under different storage temperatures

W. Kishk[1], K. Suvegova[2] and J. Rafay[2], [1]Suez Canal University, Faculty of Agriculture, Animal Production Dept., Ismailia, Egypt, [2]Research Institute of Animal Production, 94992 Nitra, Hlohovska 2, Slovakia

Three extenders were used in this experiment. These extenders were commercial diluent (com.), Sodium citrate-Egg yolk (S.C-EY) and Sodium citrate free of Egg-yolk (S.C). The storage period for extended semen was 2, 4 and 24 hrs. at 0, 5, 15 and 25 ºC. Three parameters were carried out after 0, 2 and 24 hrs. These parameters were, sperm motility (SM%), methylene blue reduction-time (MBR-T) and smears for sperm morphology. The results showed that, overall means of (SM%) for three semen extenders at different storage periods and different storage temperatures were 65.1 ±6.1, 56.2 ±7.6 and 53.2 ±8.4 for (com.), (S.C-EY) and (S.C) extenders, respectively. (SM%) differed significantly between initial diluted semen and other storage periods but did not differ significantly between 2 and 4 hrs storage period. While (SM%) differed significantly between 2, 4 and 24 hrs storage period. Methylene blue reduction-time (mbr-t) was 10.1 ±2.12, 14.5 ±2.68, 26.3 ±2.33 and 32.8 ±2.59 for initial, 2, 4 and 24 hrs storage period for extended semen, respectively. Fertility rate was recorded for Com., S.C-EY and S.C extender was 75, 70 and 53% in the same order and differed significantly between Com., S.C-EY and S.C extender.

Poster Ph4.10

An attempt at metabolic typing of juveniles using GTT in association with dairy performance

E. Szücs[1], H. Febel[2], M. Mézes[1], G. Holló[3], Gy. Huszenicza[1], J. Seenger[1], T.A. Tran[1], Cs. Ábrahám[1], A. Gáspárdy[1], and I. Györkös[2]. [1]Szent István University, Gödöllö-Budapest, [2]Research Institute for Animal Breeding and Nutrition, Herceghalom, [3]Kaposvár University, Kaposvár, Hungary*

Glucose Tolerance Test (GTT) has proved to be useful in assessing endocrine-controlled metabolic processes. The mobilisation cattle type is characterised by high milk yield, while the opposite is true for deposition one. Early typing may have concern for the breeder and efficiency. Holstein calves (N=19) weighing 100kg were administered 0.2g glucose i. v. per kg $BW^{0.75}$ at 70 days of age (*Lovendahl, 1997*). Serial blood samples were taken at 0, 0.5, 1, 2, 3, 4 and 5 h and analysed for cortisol, glucose insulin and FFA. The response was evaluated by the area under the curve. Based on insulin animals were assigned into high (HR) or low (LR) response groups. Between HR and LR animals no statistical difference was found in 305 day milk yields, means were 8072±1503 vs. 7713±971kg (P>0.05), resp. Bivariate coefficients of correlation reveal negative, and mostly loose relationship between response to GTT for cortisol, insulin, or FFA and ADWG during growth (P>0.05). Negative correlation of glucose to milk, butterfat and protein yield, and protein percentage (r=-0.45, -0,67, -0.65 or -0.65; P<0.10 and P<0.01), insulin to butterfat percentage (r = -0.43, P<0.10), or FFA to butterfat yield (r=-0.44, P<0.10) were calculated.

Poster Ph4.11

The influence of high frequency ultrasound on some indices of mineral and water-salt metabolism

O.I. Sebezhko, O.S. Korotkevich, Institute of Veterinary Genetics and Selection of Novosibirsk State Agrarian University, 160 Dobrolubov Str., 630039 Novosibirsk, Russia

1.5 month Precocious Meat piglets were taken to examine the influence of high frequency ultrasound (0.88MHz) with low therapeutic intensities 0.2-0.4 Wt/cm^2 on blood serum mineral composition and content of electrolytes under the piglets' lung meidian biologically active points (BAPs) exposure to the ultrasound. It was established that the content of calcium was below the physiological norm in all the piglets. In the experimental group after the ultrasound therapy the level of calcium increased by 24% (P<0.001) from 1.20 to 1.58 mmol/l. Moreover, the level of inorganic phosphorus and the calcium/phosphorus ratio did not change. These indices can characterize the activization of parathyroid glands function due to the ultrasound effect on vegetative nerve system. The content of sodium, potassium and chlorides is one of the most stable constants of an organism. In all the examined piglets both in the experiment and control groups the content of chlorides, sodium and potassium was within the physiological norm: 86.19 - 91.92 mmol/l; 143.11 - 143.77 mmol/l and 4.77 -4.78 mmol/l, respectively. Under the ultrasound affect there were no true changes in the content of the studied electrolytes. Thus, the ultrasound produces biomodel effect on animal organism, stimulating metabolism, and its function has low level and doesn't change the constants which are within the physiological norms.

Poster Ph4.12

Effect of under-feeding on reproduction and plasma metabolites in the ewe: impact of FGA treatment

N. Debus, F. Blanc and F. Bocquier, UMR "Elevage des Ruminants en Régions Chaudes", 2 pl. Viala, 34060 Montpellier Cedex 1, France.*

Oestrus synchronization is often used in studies on the effects of nutrition on ewes' reproduction. As in goat, we suspected that FGA treatment may alter blood metabolites response to under-feeding. We tested; first if FGA induces an effect on plasma NEFA in ewes, second how under-feeding alters their reproduction. Control (n=10) and under-fed (n=10) ewes have been studied during four successive sexual cycles either FGA-induced (C1 and C3) or not (C2 and C4).
FGA treatment limited the food restriction-induced NEFA increase in ewes. Long-term food restriction (C4) decreased the number of ewes in oestrus (67% vs 100%), delayed the beginning of oestrus (15.8±0.2 d vs 14.6±0.15 d) and reduced the oestrus duration (1.2±0.35 h vs 2.9±0.3 h). Although food restriction did not alter the ovulatory activity, maximal progesterone concentrations were higher and the time of the progesterone fall was delayed in under-fed ewes compared to well-fed ewes.
In conclusion, we observed for the first time in ewes that FGA treatment blocked NEFA response to under-feeding and that food restriction altered oestrous behaviour without change in ovulatory activity. In order to avoid the side-effect of oestrus synchronisation on food restriction-induced NEFA signals, we recommend studying the effects of feeding level on reproduction during the natural cycle following a synchronised cycle.

Theatre GPh4.1

Steps towards an imprinting map of the porcine genome

G. Jensen[1], N. Reinsch[2], M. Schwerin[2], E. Kalm[1], [1]Institut für Tierzucht und Tierhaltung, Christian-Albrechts Universität, D-24098 Kiel, [2]Forschungsinstitut für die Biologie landwirtschaftlicher Nutztiere, D-18196 Dummerstorf, Germany*

Genomic imprinting effects in pigs have been mapped in several whole genome scans on F_2 line-cross experiments. The recognition of imprinting effects at a QTL requires a higher marker density and/or a higher marker polymorphism compared to the detection of a mendelian QTL. This condition is however difficult to achieve over the whole genome. On the other hand it is well known that imprinted genes occur in clusters, highly conserved across species. Therefore,we propose a targeted increase of the marker density and/or marker information content in and around these imprinting clusters in order to produce a map of phenotypic effects of these clusters on important traits in pigs. A comparison of porcine ESTs with mouse and human sequence data was performed in order to develop primers, which were subsequently used to screen a PAC-library for clones containing stretches of pig DNA from imprinted genes. The function of these genes is mainly in muscle and tissue development. These clones were analysed for the presence of new microsatellites and SNPs. Roughly one dozen of new markers have been identified so far and are currently checked for their PCR-conditions, exact map position, and polymorphism. An overview of the targeted search for markers, the results of this search, and the use of these markers in mapping experiments is given.

Expressed Sequence Tags derived from prenatal development of skeletal muscle in pigs: A source of functional candidate genes for pork quality

E. Muráni, M. Muràniová, S. Ponsuksili, K. Schellander and K. Wimmers. Institute of Animal Breeding Science, University of Bonn, Endenicher Allee 15, 53115, Bonn, Germany.*

One factor known to influence meat quality is the myofibre type composition. Contractile and metabolic properties of myofibres and their number and proportion are to a large extent predetermined during prenatal development. We study prenatal gene expression at seven key stages of myogenesis in Duroc and Pietrain pigs known to be significantly different in muscularity and meat quality. Therefore RNA was isolated from day 14 embryo pools, 21 day whole embryos and from longissimus dorsi muscle at days 35, 49, 63, 77 and 91 of gestation. RNA pools were set up from either 5 embryo pools or 10 individuals per stage per breed (7×2 = 14 pools). Expression profiles were derived by differential display using 70 combinations of anchored and arbitrary primers. A total of 122 fragments differentially expressed between both breeds were identified of which 23 were sequenced. Additionally, 251 fragments with stage specific expression patterns were identified and 16 of these EST were sequenced. These preliminary results already revealed a number of EST that represent functional candidate genes for pork quality.
This work is part of an EU-funded project (PorDictor - QLK5-2000-01363). We acknowledge the contribution of BHZP, LRS and IPG.

Theatre GPh4.3

Identification of quantitative trait loci affecting carcass composition in beef cattle

H.E. Rushdi[1], J. Canón[2] and S. Dunner[2], [1]Faculty of Agriculture, Cairo University, 12511 Giza, Egypt, [2]Laboratorio de Genética, Facultad de Veterinaria, Universidad Complutense de Madrid, 28040 Madrid, Spain.*

A search for quantitative trait loci (QTL) affecting hot carcass weight (HCW) and conformation (CNF) traits was performed in the Asturiana de los Valles breed by using the half-sibs design. A total of 228 sons belonging to 6 families were genotyped with 6 and 2 microsatellite markers on chromosome 3 and 10, respectively. The chromosomal regions involved in this study were chosen based on the comparative mapping strategy to segments of porcine chromosomes 4 and 7 in which some QTLs affecting performance and carcass traits have been previously detected. Each marker was tested for effects on HCW and CNF by using regression, Wilcoxon rank-sum test (RS) and maximum likelihood. The empirical values of statistical significance thresholds were determined from interval mapping of 10,000 random permutations of the experimental data. The individual family analysis revealed the presence of three QTLs segregating with significant effects in two families. In family 1, a QTL for HCW was detected on chromosome 10 by regression ($P < 0,041$) and by using RS ($P < 0,034$). Moreover, a significant marker effect on CNF was also found on chromosome 10 by RS ($P < 0,036$). In the family 6, a siginificant QTL for HCW was identified by regression ($P < 0,023$) on chromosome 3. Although there are some published reports about QTLs affecting meat production traits in the bovine species, the QTLs detected in this study have not been previously described.

 Theatre GPh4.4

Preparation and validation of a bovine muscle cDNA library to identify genes which determine beef sensory traits

K. Sudre[1], G. Rolland[2], C. Leroux[1], A. Listrat[1], I. Cassar-Malek[1], B. Meunier[1], P. Martin[2], and J.F. Hocquette[1], INRA, [1]Theix and [2]Jouy-en-Josas Research Centers, France

A bovine muscle cDNA library has been designed and constructed to identify genes which determine muscular characteristics and hence beef sensory traits. This work is part of an INRA programme devoted to the analysis of farm animal genomes (AGENAE). Messenger RNAs (mRNA) were extracted from oxidative and glycolytic muscles of bovine foetuses or animals, of different ages, sexes and breeds. After retrotranscription and directional cloning of cDNA in pUC18, 1595 clones were sequenced. Sequence quality was checked and uninformative parts (low quality regions, repetitions, vector, linkers, contamination, etc) were masked using bioinformatic tools. The 1062 valid sequences were clustered and annoted using the SWISSPROT public library. The cDNA library redundancy was 48.3%. The results were gathered on a private website (http://sigena.jouy.inra.fr). Amongst the 549 contigs, 415 cDNA were amplified, printed on glass slides and nylon filters, then hybridised with total RNA labelled by fluorescence and with mRNA labelled with ^{33}P[dCTP], respectively. RNA prepared from two muscle types of two Charolais lines divergently selected on their muscle growth potential were hybridised independently. About 30 to 60% of hybridisation signals could be exploited with both approaches. Although data analysis is still in progress, it is clear that this library may be used for transcriptome studies on bovine muscles.

Theatre GPh4.5

Exploring the synergy between *in vitro* embryo production and sexed semen technologies

R.D. Wilson, K.A. Weigel, P.M. Fricke, M.L. Leibfried-Rutledge, D.L. Matthews, and V.R. Schutzkus. Department of Dairy Science, University of Wisconsin, Madison, USA.*

Our objective was to develop a system for producing extra replacement heifers on commercial dairy farms using sexed semen and *in vitro* embryo production. Genetically superior cull cows were used as donors, and ovaries were collected at the time of slaughter. Oocytes were aspirated, fertilized 20-24 hours later, and matured to the morula or blastocyst stage before transfer into recipient cows and heifers on these farms. Thus far, 165 embryos have been produced from 42 donor cows using sexed semen from three Holstein sires. An average of 3.9 transferable embryos (including 1.7 grade one and 1.5 grade two). Individual farms have averaged from 1.5 to 6.7 embryos per donor. Recipients that have shown standing estrus have a pregnancy rate of 0.19, while those resulting from an estrus synchronization program have a pregnancy rate of 0.11. Recipients that were synchronized to ovulate a day later (than for traditional embryo transfer) have a pregnancy rate of 0.30, as compared with a pregnancy rate of 0.03 for "conventionally" synchronized animals. These results, although preliminary, suggest that low cost *in vitro* embryo production may have promise as a system for utilizing sexed semen in dairy cattle breeding programs.

Theatre GPh4.6

IGF-1 Plasma levels and GH polymorphism as an indicator of the productive potencial in beef cattle

L.G.G. Silveira[1], L. Suguisawa[1], C.L.Martins[2], L.C.A. Regitano[3], M.M. Alencar[3], A.C. Silveira[4] and H. N. Oliveira[4], [1]Graduate Students-UNESP/Botucatu, [2]Pos-doctor-UNESP/Botucatu, [3]Researchers-Embrapa-CPPSE, [4]Professor-Department of Breeding and Animal Nutrition Universidade Estadual Paulista, C.P. 560, 18618-000, Botucatu/SP, Brazil.*

The IGF-1 plasma concentrations were related to the polymorphism of the GH gene as a productive potential of beef cattle to use it as an auxiliary trait to the meat production selection. Blood samples of 210 Canchim male calves, with known sires, seven to ten months old, were taken to determine the IGF-1 plasma concentrations and for DNA extraction. The DNA amplification was made by PCR and the identification of the ALU-I and DDE-I restriction enzymes was analysed by SSCP and by RFLP method. Data were analyzed by Qui-square test to verify the genotypes distribution. The genotypes effect on the predicted animal genetic values was analysed for each polymorphic site. Using the least square means and the observed allelic frequencies, estimates of the medium genic substitutions effects were made, only for the polymorphic sites with significant effects. The results indicated that the polymorphism found in GH gene can be important to the selection of growth traits and, in the herd studied, the haplotype that contains the restriction sites for the two enzymes lead to higher weaning weights. The plasma IGF-1 concentration were not significantly affected by the GH genotype but showed an association with the animal's growth characteristics.

Poster GPh4.7

New polymorphism in the bovine STAT5A gene and its association with meat production traits in beef cattle

K. Flisikowski, J. Oprzadek, E. Dymnicki, A. Oprzadek L. Zwierzchowski, Institute of Genetics and Animal Breeding, Polish Academy of Sciences, Jastrzebiec, 05-552 Wólka Kosowska, Poland.*

STAT5 are transcription factors that mediate signals from prolactin and growth hormone. Therefore, STAT5A gene is a candidate marker for quantitative traits in farm animals. In this study the new nucleotide sequence polymorphism was found in the coding region of the bovine STAT5A gene - substitution C/T at position 6853 within the exon 7. As this mutation creates new AvaI/DdeI restriction site it could be easily detected by PCR-RFLP analysis. The RFLP-AvaI polymorphism was studied in different cattle breeds. The overall frequency of alleles C and T were 0.82 and 0.18, respectively. The genotype TT was found Polish Red and Bialogrzbietka only. For the first time an association was reported between STAT5A gene polymorphism and production traits in the cattle. Beef cattle with CC variant of the gene were superior over CT animals in the live body weight at 9 and 15 months, weight gain, and carcass traits, but consumed less feed and used less feed for maintenance and meat production.

Poster GPh4.8

Mapping of Quantitative Trait Loci (QTL) for Growth and meat quality in Korean native pigs

I.S. Choi[1], T.H. Kim[2], S.S. Lee[3], H.K. Lee[3], K.J. Jeon[3], J.Y. Han[1] and Y.I. Park[1], [1]School of Agricultural Biotechnology, Seoul National University, Suwon 441-744, Korea, [2]National Livestock Research Institute, Rural Development Administration, Suwon 441-744, Korea, [3]Department of Genomic Engineering, Genomic Informatics Center, Hankyong National University, Ansung 456-749, Korea.

Molecular genetic markers were genotyped used to detect chromosomal regions which contain economically important traits such as growth and meat quality traits in pigs.Three generation resource population was constructed from a cross between the Korean native boars and Landrace sows. A total of 193 F_2 animals from intercross of F_1 were produced. Phenotypic data on 13 traits, birth weight, body weight at 3, 5, 12, 30 weeks of age, live empty weight, backfat thickness, muscle pH, meat color, drip loss, cooking loss, and shear force were collected for F_2 animals. Animals including grandparents (F_0), parents (F_1), offspring (F_2) were genotyped for 194 microsatellite markers covering from chromosome 1 to 18. Least squares regression interval mapping was used for quantitative trait loci (QTL) identification. Significance thresholds were determined by permutation test. Fifteen QTL were detected at 5% chromosome-wide significance level for growth traits on chromosome 1, 5, 7, 13, 14, and 16, and for meat quality traits on chromosome 5, 6, 7, 10, 11, 15, and 18. Two QTLs out of these were significant at the 1% Chromosome-wide level for meat color on chromosome 7, and for muscle pH on chromosome 11.

Poster GPh4.9

Detection of imprinted Quantitative Trait Loci for growth and meat quality in porcine chromosome 2, 6 and 7

H.K. Lee[1], S.S. Lee[1], T.H. Kim[2], G.J. Jeon[1] and I.J. Jung[2], [1]Department of Genomic Engineering, Genomic Informatics Center, Hankyong National University, Ansung 456-749, Korea, [2]National Livestock Research Institute, Rural Development Administration, Suwon 441-744, Korea.

As an experimental reference population, crosses between Korean native pig and Landraces were established, and information on growth and meat quality was recorded. Animals were genotyped for 24 microsatellite markers covering chromosome 2, 6, and 7 for partial-genome scan to identify chromosomal regions that have effects on growth and meat quality. The QTL effects were estimated using interval mapping by the regression method under the line cross models with a test for imprinting effects. For test of presence of quantitative trait loci (QTL), chromosome-wide and single position significance thresholds were estimated by permutation test and normal significance threshold for the imprinting test were derived. For tests against the Mendelian model, additive and dominance coefficients were permuted within individuals. Thresholds (5% chromosome-wide) against the no-QTL model for the analyzed trait were ranged from 4.53 to 4.99 for the Mendelian model and from 4.08 to 4.81 for the imprinting model, respectively. Partial-genome scan revealed significa nt evidence for 7 QTL affecting meat quality (one QTL was imprinted), and 4 QTL affecting growth (2 QTL were imprinted). This study demonstrated that testing for imprinting should become a standard procedure to unravel the genetic control of multi-factorial traits. The models and tests developed in this study allowed the detection and evaluation of imprinted QTL.

Poster GPh4.10

Detection of mutations in the GDF8 (Growth differentiation factor 8) gene: comparison of Denaturing HPLC (DHPLC) with other conventional techniques

C. Marchitelli, A. Crisà, M.C. Savarese, L. Buggiotti, A. Nardone and A.Valentini, Dipartimento di Produzioni animali, Università degli studi della Tuscia, Viterbo, Italy*

In several beef breeds double muscling can be attributed to mutations at the myostatin locus, that exhibits a large number of variants. While in some populations the alleles are fixed, in others they are still in segregation and there is an objective interest for a selection assisted by genotyping- in order to vary the frequency of double muscled subjects. However, genotyping the various mutations at myostatin gene may involve several tests, some of them rather difficult, especially for single nucleotide polymorphisms (SNP) for which there are no restriction enzymes available.
Here, we report the analysis of different polymorphisms of GDF8 gene in several cattle breed using Denaturing High Performance Liquid Chromatography (DHPLC). This method is a fully automated system for separation, quantification of double-stranded nucleic acid fragments and for mutation detection (SNP, insertion and deletion) in unpurified PCR products.
Pair of primers were designed to generate different PCR product of myostatin gene (promoter, first, second and third exon) and were analysed by Wave System (Transgenomic, Inc, San Jose, CA) at different denaturing temperature. The results were cross-checked by sequencing.
DHPLC has proven to be a simple, accurate, rapid technique for the typing of GDF8 locus, easily detecting all the mutations within the amplified DNA fragments.

Theatre Ph6.1

Metabolic properties of bovine muscles: regulation by genetic and nutritional factors

J.F. Hocquette[1], J.F. Cabaraux[2], C. Jurie[1], I. Dufrasne[2], and L. Istasse[2], [1]INRA, Herbivore Research Unit, Theix, France and [2]Nutrition Unit, Veterinary Faculty, Liege University, Belgium*

Among other factors, muscle metabolic properties influence beef sensory traits by playing a role in intramuscular fat deposition and also tenderness (Hocquette et al., 1998, 2001). The general objective of this work was thus to assess to what extent muscle metabolic indicators are regulated by genetic and nutritional factors. A total of 36 young bulls were equally divided according to three breeds (Aberdeen Angus, Belgian Blue, Limousin) and according two diets (barley-rich diet and sugar beet pulp based diet). They were slaughtered at 14-15 months of age. Activities of five metabolic enzymes in three muscles (*rectus abdominis* [RA], *semitendinosus* [ST] and *longissimus thoracis* [LT]) were determined. Only significant differences at 5% are indicated. Generally, LT had the highest activities and ST the lowest. Based on two mitochondrial enzymes (citrate synthase, cytochrome-*c* oxydase [COX]) and on one glycolytic enzyme (lactate dehydrogenase [LDH]), muscles from Belgian Blue were less oxidative (about -30%) and those from Angus less glycolytic (-20%), but differences were more evident in ST and LT than in RA. COX activity was higher with beet pulp in RA only (+19%), and LDH activity was higher with barley in ST only (+5%). In conclusion, muscle metabolic type was more affected by genetic than by nutritional factors, and this metabolic regulation is clearly muscle-specific.

Theatre Ph6.2

Modelling muscle characteristics of beef cattle according to different animal types and muscles: Influence of age and energy supply on fibre type, area and enzymatic activities

T. Hoch, M. Bécart, C. Jurie, J. Agabriel, D. Micol, R. Jailler and B. Picard, Institut National de la Recherche Agronomique (INRA), Centre de Clermont-Theix, 63122 Saint-Genès-Champanelle, France

Muscle fibre characteristics (fibre type, area and metabolic properties) of beef cattle are linked with meat quality, and especially tenderness. These characteristics vary between breeds, sexes and muscles. The evolution of muscle characteristics depends on the age of the animal and on the feeding level. However, the effect of these factors appears to be complex. In order to synthesize such a multifactorial phenomenon, a modelling approach has been chosen. A compartmental model has been developed, that take into account major fibre types (I, IIA and IIB). The fibre types evolved through conversion processes, depending on the age of the animal and its physiological age. The physiological age is estimated by the ratio "live weight of the animals / live weight at maturity" and reflects the influence of the growth type on fibre characteristics. Independantly from fibre type simulation, fibre area and enzymatic activities, associated with each fibre type, are included in the model. Different parameter sets are considered to account for various animal types and muscles. Apart from the elaboration of the model, simulations realized with this model allow to set up a hierarchy between the different factors involved in beef muscle characteristics.

Theatre Ph6.3

***In vitro* muscle protein degradation is dependent on the feeding strategy in pigs**

M. Therkildsen and N. Oksbjerg, Danish Institute of Agricultural Sciences, P.O. Box 50, DK-8830 Tjele, Denmark.

Several pieces of evidences indicate that the rate of muscle protein degradation (MPD) *in vivo* is related to the tenderization of meat *post-mortem*. This has prompted us to study MPD following different feeding strategies with the aim to develop alternative strategies with the purpose to improve meat tenderness of pork. Nine litters of eight pigs (4 female and 4 castrated male pigs) were fed either ad lib (AA), restrictively (RR), or restrictively from d 28 to either d 80 ($R_{28\text{-}80}A$) or d 90 ($R_{28\text{-}90}A$) followed by ad lib feeding until slaughter at d 140. Within 10 minutes *post-mortem* muscle strips (80 mg) were prepared from the medial red part of *M. semitendinosus* and used to study tyrosine (total MPD) and 3-methylhistidine (3-MH, myofibril MPD) release to the incubation medium. μ-Calpain was determined by zymography on *M. longissimus* samples taken immediately after slaughter. Tyrosine release ($P<0.03$) and μ-calpain ($P<0.01$) were lowest in RR pigs and highest in $R_{28\text{-}80}A$ pigs. The release of 3-MH was not significantly affected by feeding strategy. The data indicate that MPD vary among feeding strategies, and especially that compensatory growth prior to slaughter ($R_{28\text{-}80}A$ pigs) stimulates MPD, which in turn may cause variations in the tenderization of meat.

Poster Ph6.4

Influence of cadmium on quality of meat

L.I. Lisunova, V.S. Tokarev, A.V. Lisunova, Novosibirsk State Agrarian University, 160 Dobrolubov Str., 630039, Novosibirsk, Russia.

High parameters of reproduction, energy of growth, payment of forage by production favourably distinguishes poultry farming from other branches of animal industries. Research on studying influence of ions of cadmium on aminoacids structure of meat of a bird was carried out. Chickens - broilers in the age of 20 day together with fodder received sulfate of cadmium in concentration of its ions of 2 mg on 1 kg of fodder. Experience proceeded within 30 days. For the analysis muscular fabrics were taken. It is established, that inclusion in fodder of cadmium concentration lizin in meat decreases on 3,8 % ($P < 0,01$) and leichin - on 2,7 % ($P < 0,05$), but treonin the contents is increased by 20,5 % ($P < 0,001$) and metionin on 7,1 % ($P < 0,05$) in comparison with control group. On triptofan and oksiprolin between skilled and control groups of distinctions it is not revealed.
Correlation is applied to an estimation of quality of meat in it of aminoacids - triptofan and oksiprolin. The relation triptofan/oksiprolin is higher, the high-grade fibers and the above biological value of meat more contains. In our research the relation triptofan to oksiprolin was the following: in control group 6,71, in skilled group - 6,62. These data testify that addition in a diet of cadmium promotes deterioration of meat.

Poster Ph6.5

Utilisation of nitrogen and energy at meat type of pigs

A. Kodes, B. Hucko, Z. Mudrík, L. Kacerovská, Dpt. of Animal Nutrition, Czech University of Agriculture in Prague, 165 21 Prague 6, Suchdol, Kamycká 129, Czech Republic

There were organised three series of classic balancing experiments on 6 four bred hybrids of the meat type. The followings were carried out under generally accepted usances in the 14th, 17th and 22nd week of age of pigs, which corresponds to an average life weight of 40.37 kg, 65.17 kg and 91.08 kg at growth intensity represented as daily gain in the balancing periods 880 g, 980 g and 910 g. And feed conversion corresponding the value of 2.06 kg, 2.56 kg and 3.08 kg.
The coefficients of true digestibility NL (80,84 - 76,82 - 76,15) were in the all cases of the balances about 2 - 4% higher than the coefficients of apparent digestibility (78,03 - 73,77 - 72,06).
Average values of the digestibility of energy of feed mixtures oscillated around the value of 84% (84,40 - 83,03 - 83,77).
The hypothesis of the necessity of a repeated assessment of exactness of the prediction MEp in mixtures for pigs of the meat type and the validity of the equation of the calculation of the need of MEp for growing fattening pigs.
The study was financed by Committee for Scientific Research (grant MSM 412100003).

Poster Ph6.6

Evaluation of the formation of the lean meat of the belly meat part in relation to sex of pigs

R. Stupka, M. Sprysl, Czech University of Agriculture, Department of Pig and Poultry Science, Prague, Kamycka, 165 21, Czech Republic

The tests included 194 final pig hybrids of the genotypes currently used in the Czech Republic in a balanced sex. Evaluation was focussed on the formation of the lean meat of the belly in relation to sex. The belly in total and the EU belly reached in barrows the weight of 7,85kg and 4,35kg, respectively, and in gilts 7,66kg and 4,12kg, respectively. In barrows the belly accounted with practically identical weight of the carcass for a higher share, i.e. 9,96% as compared to 9,56% in gilts. In terms of percentage the gilts had a statistically significantly higher share of lean meat in the EU belly, namely by 3,32% as compared to barrows. All measurements showed a higher total area of the belly in barrows in comparison with gilts. The comparison of the percentage share of the meat area and the total area in the individual points of measuring revealed that gilts reached a statistically evidently higher value as compared to barrows. It has been proved that from section 1 (behind the last rib), 2 (between 10th and 11th ribs) as far as section 3 (between 7th and 8th rib) there is a higher deposition of fat in barrows.

Poster Ph6.7

Effect of slaughter weight, genotype and sex on pig carcass value in hybrid pigs

J. Citek, M. Sprysl, R. Stupka, T. Neuzil and M. Pour. Czech University of Agriculture Prague, Department of Pig and Poultry Science, 165 21 Prague 6-Suchdol, Czech Republic.

The problems of the effect of slaughter weight, genotype and sex on carcass value in the pure breed in CR is continuously examined. However, the influence of these factors in the hybrid pigs is not objectively known yet. The study was conducted on 199 hybrid pigs of eight different genotypes in the test station. For determination of carcass value the classic dissection has been made.

On the basis of obtained results it can be stated that sows in comparison with barrows have larger area of MLLT, lower fat of bisector section, higher percentage of lean meat stock, higher percentage of main meat parts (MMP) and lower weight of fat. The quality of selected characteristics of slaughter efficiency varied significantly with different hybrid combinations. From the viewpoint of the selected slaughter value characteristics, it was hybrid combination CMPx(LWxL) that proved unsuitable in relation to other combinations, while combinations OLWx(LWxL), (OLWxBL)x(LWxL) and Seghers proved suitable. The increased carcass weight would go hand in hand with worse meat stock quality from the viewpoint of the selected slaughter efficiency characteristics. Regarding the meat stock weight range under examination, the highest increase was demonstrated in the weight of fat. Lower increase was demonstrated in MMP free of fat layer.

Poster Ph6.8

Effects of early castration of Charolais steers on animal performances, carcass quality, muscular characteristics, and sensory traits

D. Micol, M.P. Oury, B. Picard. URH, Institut National de la Recherche Agronomique (INRA), Centre de Clermont-Theix, 63122 Saint-Genès-Champanelle, France.

Management practices of beef cattle have a significant effect on meat sensory attributes. Castration was tested in the young age as a way to control meat quality.

Two groups of Charolais steers, castrated early (3 month old) or late (9 month old) were compared. Both groups were fed with grass at the INRA experimental farm (63, France), and slaughtered at 26 months of age, at the same weight and the same body score. Two muscles, Rectus Abdominis and Triceps Brachii, with different androgen sensibility, were analyzed. Animals performance (growth, daily gain, food efficiency, fat score), slaughtering ones (live weight, carcass weight, fat content, carcass composition), muscular composition (type and growth of fibres, enzyme activities, total and soluble collagen, lipids, proteases) and meat quality (sensory panel) were studied.

Ages at the castration achieve the same result on animal performances, slaughter, muscular characteristics and sensory assessments. The small difference that exists, concerns daily gain during the finishing period, carcass weight and proteases content. These results are favorable to early castrated animals.

Early castration can be recommended as a rearing practice, giving the same results on growth, muscle characteristics and meat quality with a low stress for the animals in the young age.

Poster Ph6.9

Morphological characterization of *semitendinosus* muscle fibers in pre-weaning Angus-Nellore calves supplemented with recombinant bovine somatotropin (rbst)

R.C. Cervieri[1], M.D.B. Arrigoni[1], H.N. Oliveira[1], A.C. Silveira[1], L.A.L. Chardulo[2], C.L. Martins[1], [1]Faculdade de Medicina Veterinária e Zootecnia (FMVZ)-UNESP, Rubiao Júnior, P.O. Box 560, Botucatu, Sao Paulo, Brazil, [2]Instituto de Biociencias (IB)-UNESP, Departamento de Química e Bioquímica, Rubiao Júnior, Botucatu, Sao Paulo, Brazil.*

The objective of this study was to determine the recombinant bovine somatotropin (rbST) effect on type, frequency and diameter of *semitendinosus* muscle fibers. We used thirty-six 1/2 Angus-Nellore crossbred bull calves, with 63 ± 17 days old and weighting 76,8 ± 14,7 kg, creep-fed, grazing *Brachiaria decunbens,* supplemented or not with rbST until the weaning (217 days). Eighteen calves received 0,10mg/kg/day of rbST (Boostin®) and eighteen control calves received saline solution each 14 days. Two muscle samples were taken from nine animals per treatment at 150 days (biopsy), and at 217 days old, when five animals per treatment were slaughtered. The rbST-treated calves had larger fast-twitch-glycolytic (FG) fibers than control calves at 150 (47,42 vs 41,11 mm, $P<0,05$) and at 217 days old (56,32 vs 45,66 mm, $P<0,10$). No differences between fast-twitch-oxidative-glycolytic (FOG) and slow-twitch-oxidative (SO) diameters and FG, FOG and SO frequencies were observed at 150 and 217 days. The somatotropin administration lead to a greater hypertrophy of the white fast-twitch-glycolytic muscle fibers in creep-fed bull calves, but did not affect the percentage distribution of the three fiber types.

Theatre CM3.1

Physiological and pathological adaptations that may lead to increased susceptibility to periparturient metabolic diseases

J.K. Drackley, 260 Animal Sciences Laboratory, University of Illinois, Urbana, IL 61801 USA.*

Tremendous metabolic and physiological adaptations occur in dairy cows during the transition from late gestation to early lactation, likely contributing to the high incidence of infectious diseases and metabolic disorders during this time. Imbalances between demand for calcium and magnesium for milk production and their supply from diet and bone may lead to hypocalcemia or hypomagnesemia and associated problems. Dietary supply of glucose precursors is less than needed to furnish glucose for milk synthesis. Rates of skeletal muscle protein breakdown are increased, and hepatic capacity for glucose synthesis from alanine is increased, during the first 14 d postpartum. Deficiencies of metabolizable protein may compromise the immune system. Lipolysis in adipose tissue increases in response to negative energy balance. Increased nonesterified fatty acid (NEFA) uptake, coupled with increased esterification capacity in liver, may lead to hepatic lipid infiltration. Lipid accumulation may predispose the liver to decreased function or increased oxidative damage. Deficiencies of glucose and high rates of NEFA mobilization may increase hepatic ketogenesis. High blood concentrations of NEFA and ketone bodies in blood may inhibit function of the immune system. Prepartum nutrition may modulate the capacity for long-chain fatty acid oxidation in liver. Because these adaptations normally are exquisitely coordinated, management or environmental factors that impinge on feed intake or activate the immune system may be components of increased peripartal disease.

Theatre CM3.2

Interaction between energy metabolism, oxidative status and immune response in periparturient dairy cow

B. Ronchi, U. Bernabucci, N. Lacetera and A. Nardone. Dipartimento di Produzioni Animali, Università della Tuscia, Italia*

In the periparturient period dairy cow experiences a set of physiological and nutritional changes which are critical to health, productive and reproductive efficiency. In particular during that period oxidative stress occurs with increase of reactive forms of oxygen and reduction of antioxidant defenses. The oxidative stress of transition cows is related with increased metabolic processes and with metabolic disorders. Periparturient cows with higher body condition, more pronounced body condition losses and higher plasma nonesterified fatty acids and beta-hydroxybutyrate show higher reactive oxygen metabolites and lipoperoxydes, and lower levels of antioxidants. Oxidative stress may lead on the other hand to alteration of metabolic pathways, with further consequences on cow health and productivity. Both impairment of energy metabolism and of prooxidant-antioxidant balance result associated with reduced immuneresponsiveness of periparturient cow and with increased susceptibility to infectious diseases during lactation. The real beneficial effects from supplementation with nutrients involved in antioxidant defense is on discussion.

Lipomobilisation syndrome and metabolic disorder in dairy cows in peripartal period

P. Reichel[1], J. Szarek[2], J. Buleca Jr.[1], M. Húska[1], E. Pilipcinec[1], A. Bugarsky[1], P. Zachar[1], [1]University of Veterinary Medicine, Komenského 73, 041 81 Kosice, Slovakia, [2]Agricultural University of Cracow, Al. Mickiewicza 21, 31 103 Cracow, Poland

Disturbances and failures in dairy cows nutrition result to alimentary dysfunction of rumen and lead to metabolic production diseases. The most critical period, from the view of nutrition and energy demand, is period of early lactation, in which negative energetic bilance uprise. Longterm discrepancy between nutritives intake and their demand interfere with interior and metabolism can results in development of lipomobilisation syndrome (Roberts et al., 1981). Clinical manifestation of the syndrome in peripartal period involve increased lipid reserves loss, weight reduction, digestive and metabolic disorders, hepatal steatosis and following complication. Results of rumen content analysis signify decreased volume of volatile fatty acids in the group of dry cows and calved cows with percentual increase of acetic acid content at the expense of propionic acid, which is according to feed with sufficient amount of dry matter and gross fiber and insufficient energy coverage. Insufficient energy and protein coverage organism compensates by increased lipolysis and proteolysis, which induces higher hepatal endurance and vitamin and macroelements metabolism disorders.

Theatre CM3.4

Inflammatory conditions in peri-parturient cows and anti-inflammatory treatments

E. Trevisi, F. Librandi, G. Bertoni. Istituto di Zootecnica, Facoltà di Agraria, U.C.S.C., 29100, Piacenza, Italy*

The release of pro-inflammatory cytokines is particularly dangerous around calving; in fact they increase body reserve mobilization, reduce DM intake and increase disease susceptibility, causing an impairment of health, milk and fertility levels. Several factors are responsible of cytokine release (i.e. diseases, trauma, endotoxins, stress etc.). With the aim to attenuate the redundancy of cytokine effects at calving, treatments with anti-inflammatory drugs were used. Immediately after calving, 61cows received lysine acetylsalicylate (LAS) or meloxicam (ME) or placebo (CTR). Milk yield and composition, disease occurrence, BCS, fertility and blood samples (metabolic profile) were continuously monitored. LAS (but not ME) have increased milk yield and reduced somatic cell count (both $P<0.05$). Fertility was ameliorated with both LAS and ME (i.e. 46% of cow pregnant after 1st insemination vs 18% in CTR). Nevertheless, LAS have shown a higher incidence of early lactation metritis (25% vs 15% of CTR), although the rate of total gynaecological disorders was not modified. About metabolic profile, LAS (but not ME) have shown a reduction of inflammation indices (i.e. ceruloplasmin) and an increase of proteins usually synthesized by liver, suggesting a better hepatic function. At calving time many causes of cytokine release can occur and the inhibition of their effects, besides a reduction of these causes, seems very useful to improve health status and therefore milk yield, fertility and welfare of dairy cows.

Theatre CM3.5

Dairy production and metabolic traits of Friesian cows in continuous lactation

A. Bortolozzo[1], G. Gabai[2], R. Mantovani[1], L. Marinelli[2], L. Bailoni[1], G. Bittante[1], [1]Dept. of Animal Science and [2]Dept. of Veterinary Basic Science, Agripolis, 35020 Legnaro (PD), Italy*

Continuous lactation is supposed to be a means to reduce milk yield and body energy mobilisation after calving, thus limiting the metabolic challenges of the high yielding dairy cow. Milk yield, milk quality and metabolic traits of two groups of Friesian cows balanced for milk yield, days in milk and parity, were evaluated. The first group of cows (CTR; n=5) was traditionally conducted (a dry period of 55 d and a calving interval of 13 months) while the second one (CON; n=6) undergone to continuous lactation (dry period suppression). Daily milk yield from 74 d before the calving date to 103 d after was recorded. Milk and blood samples were collected at fixed dates during the trial. Animals received a complete mixed diet and an individual concentrate supplementation by electronic feeder according to their nutritional requirements. During the trial the cows were weighed and body condition was scored (BCS). The CTR group produced +1.28 kg/d of milk compared to CON group throughout the trial. After calving and up to the lactation peak, milk yield of CON cows was lower than CTR group. No differences between groups were observed on milk quality, except for protein content, higher in the CTR group at calving (13.8 vs. 11.1%), due to higher immunoglobulins content in the colostrum. Among different metabolic traits, NEFA content, as expected, was higher for the CTR group in the post-calving period (0.52 vs. 0.35 meq/l), indicating a higher energy mobilisation, confirmed also by a slightly lower BCS.

Theatre CM3.6

Hepatic expression of ApoB$_{100}$ is downregulated, and ApoE and microsomal triglycerides transfer protein are up-regulated in periparturient dairy cows

U. Bernabucci[1], B. Ronchi[1], L. Basiricò[1], D. Pirazzi[1], F. Rueca[2], N. Lacetera[1] and A. Nardone[1].*
[1]DiPA, Università della Tuscia, Italia, [2]Sez.Med.Vet.Int., Università di Perugia, Italia

Limitation of VLDL secretion in dairy cows in the early postpartum is strongly related with metabolic disorders. Presently it is not known which role plays ApoB$_{100}$, ApoE and microsomal triglyceride transfer protein (MTP) in that VLDL limitation. To our knowledge, no studies have simultaneously measured ApoB$_{100}$, ApoE and microsomal triglyceride transfer protein (MTP) mRNA in periparturient dairy cows. Therefore, a trial was conducted to assess liver gene expression of these proteins in transition dairy cows. Eight multiparous Holstein cows were monitored during the transition period. To evaluate metabolic and nutritional status body condition score was registered and plasma indexes of energy metabolism were determined from -35 to 35 from calving. Liver biopsies were performed on d -35, 3, and 35 relative to day of calving and gene expression of ApoB$_{100}$, ApoE and MTP were determined on liver tissue. Body condition and plasma glucose decreased ($P<0.01$), and plasma NEFA and BHBA increased ($P<0.01$) after calving. Compared with values of day -35, on day 3 after calving the ApoB$_{100}$ mRNA synthesis was lower ($P<0.05$), whereas MTP and ApoE mRNA synthesis were higher ($P<0.05$). Negative ($r = -0.55$, $P<0.05$) correlation between plasma NEFA concentration and ApoB$_{100}$ mRNA abundance was observed at 3 days postpartum. Our results suggest that the limitation of VLDL secretion occurring in dairy cows after calving might be associated with down-regulation of ApoB$_{100}$ expression.

Theatre CM3.7

The effects of milk fraction, milk interval, and udder health on acetone in milk in relation to its use for monitoring ketosis in dairy cows

N.I. Nielsen, N.C. Friggens and K.L. Ingvartsen. Department of Animal Health and Welfare, Danish Institute of Agricultural Sciences, P.O. Box 50, 8830 Tjele, Denmark*

Ketone bodies in blood, milk and urine have been used to characterise ketotic dairy cows. Acetone is a ketone body that is advantageous to measure in milk because milk is easy to collect and technical equipment with high capacity has been developed to measure acetone in milk. Therefore, it is of interest to evaluate the use of milk acetone to monitor dairy cows for ketosis and to identify possible factors affecting the concentration of acetone in relation to milk sampling. We conducted an experiment where acetone in milk was measured daily in 67 cows from calving and throughout their lactation. These individual profiles clearly indicated the potential of using daily measurements of acetone for early identification of clinical ketosis. Furthermore, 10 cows were used to examine the effects of milk fraction, milk interval and udder health on the concentration of acetone in milk. These cows had either 1 or 2 mastitic quarters and 2 or 3 healthy quarters and were milked with both 6 and 12-hour intervals. Milk samples were collected from each quarter every 45 seconds throughout milking. The results of this study indicated that the time of sampling during milking, the interval with which the cow is milked and the health status of a quarter had only minor effects on the concentration of acetone in milk. It is concluded that milk acetone has the potential to provide a simple, non-invasive, indicator of ketosis.

On-line metabolic profiling for nutritional management of dairy cows

L.L. Masson[1], T.T. Mottram[1] and P.C. Garnsworthy[2], [1]Silsoe Research Institute, Wrest Park, Silsoe, Bedfordshire, MK45 4HS, U.K., [2]University of Nottingham, Sutton Bonington Campus, Loughborough, Leicestershire, LE12 5RD, U.K.*

On-line monitoring of milk composition with biosensors may be useful for nutritional management of dairy cows. Acetone, urea, fat and citrate are constituents in milk that could possibly be used to monitor metabolic and nutritional status. For daily monitoring, several sources of variation (between and within cows throughout lactation) need to be determined and quantified for accurate data interpretation. Several experimental protocols were used to investigate sources of variation within cows and to determine whether dietary adjustment could be detected through changes in milk composition. These studies involved 54 cows and 1500 milk samples. Significant variation was found between and within days for several parameters, which would make interpretation of daily measurements difficult. Mean citrate concentrations (± standard error) changed significantly with stage of lactation ($P<0.001$), being 10.89 ±0.24mM, 9.76 ±0.14mM and 10.26 ±0.15mM in early, mid and late lactation cows respectively. Changing the starch to fibre ratio in the diet had no effect on milk acetone, but significantly affected urea, fat and protein when dietary changes were extreme ($P<0.001$). Further research on a larger scale is needed to determine whether this system of nutritional management will be feasible.

Poster CM3.9

Correlation between liver TAG and glycogen content and plasma concentration of NEFA and glucose in early lactating dairy cows

J.B. Andersen and K.L. Ingvartsen, Department of Animal Health and Welfare, Danish Institute of Agricultural Sciences, P.O. Box 50, 8830 Tjele, Denmark

The objective was to examine the correlation between liver TAG (triacylglycerol) and glycogen content and plasma NEFA and glucose concentration in early lactating dairy cows. The cows were fed two different energy density diets (High vs Low) and were milked 2 or 3 times daily in a 2 x 2 factorial design. Forty multiparous Danish-Holstein dairy cows were used in the first 8 weeks after calving. Liver biopsies were taken in weeks 2 and 7 from calving and blood was sampled every week in the experiment. Liver TAG content was 48% lower for cows fed diet H compared with diet L, but liver glycogen was not affected by treatment. Overall there was no effect of milking frequency on liver parameters. Plasma concentration of glucose was increased (3.19 vs. 3.43 mmol/l) for cows fed diet H compared with diet L, but decreased (3.42 vs. 3.20 mmol/l) for cows milked 3 times vs. 2 times daily. There was no effect of treatments on concentration of NEFA in plasma. The correlation between plasma concentration of NEFA and liver TAG content was not obvious and differed between week 2 and 7 after calving. Plasma concentration of glucose and liver glycogen content were significantly correlated in early lactation ($R^2 > 0.12$).

Poster CM3.10

Morphological studies on digestive tract of high productive cows with ketosis

A. Jemeljanovs[1], M. Pilmane[2] and I.Zitare[1], [1]Research Centre "Sigra" of the Latvia University of Agriculture, Instituta Street 1, Sigulda LV-2150, Latvia, [2]Institute of Anatomy and Anthropology of the Riga Stradins University, Dzirciema Street 16, Riga LV 1007, Latvia

Ketosis is one of the most spread metabolic diseases of high productive cows in Latvia and often is related to structural changes of animal digestive tract. Thus, the aim of this work was histochemical and immunohistochemical investigation morphofunctional changes in different levels of cows with ketosis. We examined tissues of 42 animals; 8 of them possessed laboratory affirmed diagnosis.
Results showed the main changes in cows' forestomach and abomasum, and small intestine: atrophy in the ruminal villi, the regional inflammation and parakeratosis. Relatively similar changes were seen in small intestine mucosa. However, abnormal fusing of villi and detaching of epithelium often took place.
Inflammation was mainly expressed in large intestine mucosa. Submucosa of all intestinum was filled with conglomerates of secondary nodules. The neuropeptides-containing innervation was fragmentary, week and mainly decreased in tissue of cows with ketosis.
In conclusion, our studies discovered serious morphofunctional changes, including the immunoreactive innervation decrease in forestomach, abomasum and small intestine of digestive tract in cows with acute ketosis, suggesting about reduced morphofunctional activity in these parts of gastrointestinal system.

Poster CM3.11

Metabolism disorders in barren high yielding dairy cows: vitamin A, calcium and phosphorus metabolism

I.A. Porfiriev, E.M. Boldyreva, Russian University of People's Friendship, Miklukho-Maklaia, 8, building 2, 117198, Moscow, Russia.*

The purpose of the research was to study metabolism in barren high yielding dairy cows, especially of vitamin A, calcium and phosphorus. In 1970-2000 years a complex gynecological examination of barren cows of holmogorsk, switz, simmental, sychev, black-and-white, jersey, Dutch and other breeds at 29 livestock complexes on 91 Russian farms was conducted. Different diseases of ovaries and uterus were revealed. Clinical examination, morphological and biochemical examinations of blood, milk and urine showed subclinical chronic disorder of carbohydrate, lipid, protein, iodine metabolism, acidosis, liver malfunction, alterations in blood morphology, cardiovascular, endocrine, respiratory and nervous systems. Detailed examination of vitamin A, phosphorus and calcium metabolism was done. Carotene and vitamin A concentration in blood serum samples was 2-7 times less than normal indices. Their concentration was 3 and 1.85 times more in summer in comparison with that in winter respectively. The level of calcium in the blood was 20% and of phosphorus - 61.1% less than normal indices respectively. As a result of improvement of cattle keeping conditions, increase in feed production, changes in the technology of feed storage, ratio balancing of nutrients and sugar-protein proportion the metabolism and reproductive function became normal. The number of calves per cow increased by 20-30%, milk productivity increased by 20-250% and loss of newborn calves decreased by 15-40%.

Poster CM3.12

Vitamin E dietary supplementation and oxidative stress in the dairy cow

A. Formigoni[1], P. Pezzi[2], D. Calderone[3] and G. Biagi[2], 1Dipartimento di Scienze Veterinarie ed Agroalimentari, Università di Teramo,P.zza Aldo Moro, 64100 Teramo, Italy, [2] Sezione di Zootecnia, Nutrizione ed Alimenti, DIMORFIPA, Università di Bologna, via Tolara di Sopra 50, 40064 Ozzano Emilia, Italy, [3]Consorzio del Prosciutto di Parma, Via Marco dell'Arpa, 8/b, 43100 Parma, Italy.

Thirty days before calving, 40 Italian Friesian cows were divided in two homogenous groups. Animals received a basal diet (hay + 10 kg of a total mixed ration for lactating dairy cows; control group) added or not with vitamin E (dl-alpha-tocopheryl-acetate; 13 g/head/d; treated group) until calving. After calving, vitamin E supplementation was suspended and all animals received a common diet for lactating dairy cows for 4 more weeks. Blood samples were collected weekly. Body Condition Score (BCS) was evaluated weekly. Milk yield, milk fat and protein content and somatic cell count were recorded. Haemoglobin and ROMs plasma concentration and plasmatic glutatione peroxidase (GSH-Px) activity were not influenced by treatment. Plasma vitamin E levels were significantly higher in treated animals until 18 days after calving ($P < 0.05$). Vitamin E supplementation did not influence BCS, milk yield and milk quality. In conclusion, it seems that vitamin E supplementation does not influence the oxidative status of the transition cow. However, throughout the study, multiparous cows showed higher GSH-Px and ROMs plasma values than primiparous animals ($P < 0.05$). This result deserves further investigation.

Poster CM3.13

Effect of silymarin on oxidative status in periparturient dairy cows

M. Balestrieri[1], D. Tedesco[2], S. Galletti[2], [1]ISPAAM, CNR, Via Argine 1085, 80147, Napoli, Italy, [2]Department of Veterinary Science and Technologies for Food Safety, Via Celoria 10, 20133 Milano, Italy.*

The periparturient and early lactation periods are critical for the health of dairy cows. Oxidative stress may be involved in etiologies of certain disorders of transient cows. Plasma concentrations of retinol and a-tocopherol can be considered as markers of oxidative status. The aim of this study was to test the effects of silymarin, a natural acknowledged antioxidant and hepatoprotective substance, on transient dairy cows oxidative status. Twenty dairy cows in the dry period were chosen from a commercial dairy herd. Animals were divided into two groups according to health condition, parity (≥2), and previous milk production. From day 10 before calving to 15 days after calving, 10 cows received 10 g/d of silymarin as a water suspension by oral drench. Blood samples were taken at d-7, 0, 7, 21 from calving and at birth in newborn calves. Plasma concentrations of retinol and a-tocopherol were evaluated by HPLC. There was no distinct trend in the change of plasma retinol and α-tocopherol due to silymarin treatment. Plasma retinol and α-tocopherol concentrations increased from parturition (0.76 and 2.74 micro g/mL, respectively) to early lactation (1.14 and 4.20 micro g/mL). Plasma retinol and α-tocopherol concentrations in mothers and calves were not correlated.

It is concluded that antioxidant status in periparturient dairy cows was not improved by feeding silymarin.

Poster CM3.14

Metabolic traits and the metabolic status by heifers in the glucose tolerance test

L. Panicke[1]; U. Müller[2], H. Behn[3], R. Staufenbiel[3], A. Oprzadek[4], [1]Research Institute for the Biology of Farm Animals, Dummerstorf, Germany, [2]Humboldt University Berlin, Inst. of Farm Animals, Philippstr. 13, Berlin, Germany, [3]Free University Berlin, Animal Clinic, Koenigstrasse 65, Berlin, Germany, [4]Institute of Genetics and Animal Breeding, Jastrzebiec, Poland*

The possible applications of the glucose tolerance test (GTT) as an index of the quantification of the metabolic capability of cows is reported. The aim was to determine the influence of the systematic factors like age and feeding by 15 one-egg twins heifers. The common contemplation of genetic and physiological aspects seems to be very important. The measurement of the glucose reaction during an induced metabolism burden in the glucose tolerance test (GTT) offers a possibility of the quantitation of the metabolic capability of cows (Burkert 1998, Panicke et al., 2001 and 2002). 15 one-egg twins induced by embryo splitting and embryo transfer were analysed. These animals were fed intensively energy-rich, and extensively, energy-poor. Intravenous glucose tolerance tests in the age of 6 weeks, 6, 12, and 17 months were executed regularly. The glucose half-life (GHWZ) decreased with the age and the body weight in the examined period. The biggest difference was proved at the age of 12 months. Exactly at this time, according to our own results (Panicke et al. 2001 and 2002) the highest relationships of r = 0.4 - 0.5 to the daughter's performance was estimated.

Poster CM3.15

The cows and calves blood plasma free amino acids changes in different physiological stages

A. Jemeljanovs, J. Miculis and I. Zitare, Research Centre "Sigra" of the Latvia University of Agriculture, Instituta Street 1, Sigulda LV-2150, Latvia

Quantitative content of free amino acids in blood plasma indicates metabolism processes in animals organism depending on reproductive cycle and other physiological states of organism.
To determine dynamics of free amino acids concentration in blood plasma of Latvian Brown Breed cows and calves, clinically healthy group of cows of 3-5 lactations was selected 10 days before calving. Animals were analogues according to different physiological indices. Samples of cows blood were taken 15 minutes, 2 hours, 5-7 days, 4 and 6 months after calving and of calves blood - before first time feeding and in 5-7 days age. The free amino acids of blood plasma were analysed by amino acids analyser. The obtained results showed that in calves blood plasma free amino acids spectrum the highest level had arginine, glycine, alanine, glytamic acid, leucine. After 5-7 days of calving the significant changes of amino acids content were observed, level of lysine increased from 0.68 up to 1.15, histidine from 0.46 up to 0.68, asparagine acid from 0.69 up to 0.96, threonine from 0.43 up to 0.69, proline from 0.59 up to 0.70, cystine from 0.44 up to 0.84, valine from 0.63 up to 1.34, thyrosine from 0.45 up to 0.58 mg%. The level of free amino acids of cows blood plasma decreased promptly after calving and significantly increased 5-7 days after calving. The sum of cows blood plasma free amino acids had non significant changes during lactation but had a tendency to increase at the end of lactation.

Poster CM3.16

Sources of variation of dry period length in Italian Holstein cows

F. Cesarini, C. Romani, B. Contiero, P. Carnier, M. Cassandro and L. Gallo, Department of Animal Science, University of Padova, Agripolis, 35020 Legnaro (PD), Italy*

The magnitude and the effects of several sources of variation of dry period length (DPL) were investigated using field data recorded in 101 herds located in northern Italy throughout 4 years of study. Dry period length (69 ± 33 d), available for over 11000 lactations of Italian Holstein cows, was analyzed according to a model accounting for the effects of herd, year and season of dry-off and data of previous lactation such as calving season, parity, lactation length, cumulated milk yield at 100 DIM, occurrence of mastits and lameness, daily milk yield near dry-off and several interactions. R^2 of the model was 21% and most effects were highly significant ($P<0.01$). Herd effect alone explained over 11% of dry days variation, and LS means for dry days in different herds ranged bewteen 48 and 118 d. DPL increased at increasing parity number and was highest for previous lactation shorter than 280 d. Milk yield potential after 100 DIM of lactation slightly affected dry-days, but DPL significantly decreased at increasing daily milk yield near dry-off. The occurrence of mastitis or lameness during previous lactation did not affect DPL. Similarly, DPL was not affected by BCS at previous calving, but tended to increase at increasing condition score near dry-off.

Poster CM3.17

Effect of dry period length on milk yield, body condition score, somatic cell counts and health disorders in subsequent lactation in Italian Holstein cows

M. Cassandro, P. Carnier, B. Contiero, G. Bittante and L. Gallo, Department of Animal Science, University of Padova, Agripolis, 35020 Legnaro, Padova.*

Effects of dry period length (DPL) on milk yield, body condition score (BCS), somatic cell count and health disorders in subsequent lactation were studied using 76399 test-day records from 7299 Italian Holstein cows reared in 115 herds of northern Italy from 1998 to 2001. Dry period length (DPL) was grouped in 4 classes: DPL1 (1-35 d); DPL2 (36-55 d); DPL3 (56-80 d) and DPL4 (81-220 d). Milk yield, BCS and log-transformed SCC (SCS) were analyzed according to a mixed linear model accounting for herd-test day, parity, DPL, days in milk and animal effects. DPL affected milk yield of subsequent lactation, and DPL1 cows evidenced a reduction of milk yield at peak, of milk in 305 d and an increase in persistency with respect to other DPL classes. DPL did not affect change of BCS and SCS in the subsequent lactation. A logistic regression analysis was used for estimating the effect of DPL on the risk of contracting mastitis, lameness, retained placenta and mammary edema. Several models considering single or multiple health disorders were applied. DPL did not appear associated with the risk of health disorders occurrence, but some other factors (herds, parity, exposition time and cow breeding values) were important as predisposing factors.

Poster CM3.18

The effect of condition of heifers before preparation on milk yield in the first lactation

E. Báder[1], I. Györkös[2], A. Muzsek[1], P. Báder[1], J. Szili[3], Ms. A. Kovács[1], Z. Gergácz[1], Ms. Kertészné Györffy E.[1], [1]University of West Hungary, Faculty of Agriculture, Vár, 2, 9200 Mosonmagyaróvár, Hungary, [2]Research Institute for Animal Breeding and Nutrition, Gesztenyés srt. 1, 2053 Herceghalom, Hungary, [3]Aranymezo Ltd. 7671 Bicsérd, Hungary*

The influence of pre-calving condition of heifers on first lactation was studied. Condition scoring was carried out at the beginning of preparation. The experiment involved 554 Holstein-Friesian cows. Evaluation of condition was made on a 5-score-scale.
Pre-calving condition of heifers before preparation has a considerable effect on the first lactation. Cows with 2.0-2.5 condition scores produced 8943 kg milk in the first lactation. 2.6-2.9 and 3.0-3.2 condition scores is connected with 9092-9087 kg milk yield. Milk production was the highest (9287 kg) in the group of cows with optimal condition (3.3-3.4 scores) and this production level is approached (9195 kg) by heifers with 3.5 condition scores. Heifers with reasonable condition (3.6-4.0 scores) could also produce high milk yield (8977 kg). There was a considerable decrease in milk yield (8002 kg) in the group of animals which start the preparation period with over-condition. The above results confirmed the importance of condition scoring in heifers.

Theatre C4.1

Relationships between lactation stage with milk yield amount and constituent heritabilities of milk constituents

Ö. Sekerden, Mustafa Kemal Univ., Fac. of Agric., Dept. of Anim. Sci., Antakya, Turkey

This study was carried out to investigate the relationships between lactation stage with milk yield and constituents and estimation of heritabilities of milk constituents on 371 Black Pied cows. At control days of the farm, daily milk yields were determined and milk samples were taken from each cow in 30±15, 90±15, 150±15 and 210±15 days of lactations at morning milkings in order to determine fat, protein, total dry matter(TDM) and solids non fat (SNF) rates.
By using standardized (for claving season and year and lactation order effects) data, heritabilities of milk constitutients were calculated. Results of analysis belong to 4 seperate stages were evaluated all together in investigation of relationship between 305-day milk yield and lactation stages. Following results were obtained; Fat and SNF percentages in first two stages, protein percentage in first 3 stages; TDM percentage in every stage (except 2nd stage) resemble to each other; Relationships are not significant between 305-day milk yield with fat and protein rates in the 1st lactation stage; Relationships between 305-day milk yield with lactation fat, protein, SNF and TDM rate means are not significant. Heritabilities for fat, protein, SNF and TDM percentages were estimated as 0.379±0.176, 0.248 ±0.149, 0.303 ±0.160 and 0.180 ± 0.134, respectively.

Theatre C4.2

Some productive characteristics of F_1, B_1 and F_1xB_1 crossbreds from Simmental x SAR crossbreeding

M.N. Orman[1] O. Ertugrul[2], I.S. Gürcan[1], O. Alpan[2], [1]Ankara University, Faculty of Veterinary Medicine, Biostatistics Department 06110, Diskapi, Ankara, Turkey, [2]Ankara University, Faculty of Veterinary Medicine, Genetic Department 06110, Diskapi, Ankara, Turkey.*

South Anatolian Red (SAR) cattle breed is well adapted to the arid, hot and harsh conditions of the region and has the highest milk yield among the local breeds of Turkey.
The aim of this research project was to determine the main productive characteristics, such as viability, reproduction and milk production of F_1, B_1 and F_1xB_1 crossbred genotype groups from Simmental x SAR crossbreeding.
ANOVA was used for three group comparisons and t test was used for two group comparisons. In cases of insufficient or small group sizes Kruskall-Wallis and Mann-Whitney U test were used where appropriate.
There was no birth difficulties in all the crossbred groups. Viability rates for bull calves were 100% in B_1, and 97.3% in F_1xB_1 crossbred groups, while 92.3% in B_1 and 94.6% in F_1xB_1 groups for the heifer calves. The high surviving abilities of the groups indicate the success for the crossbreeding program. The average milk yields of F_1 and B_1 genotype groups were similar to those of SAR. However, there were big variations in the genotype groups for milk production indicating that selection for milk yield would be highly promising. It may be stated that the crossbreeding program would be beneficial for viability and milk production.

Theatre C4.3

Modeling daily somatic cell score and milk yield

G.J. Jeon[1], P. Madsen[2] J. Jensen[2], E. Norberg[2], and P. Lovendahl[2], [1]Dept. of Genomic Engineering, Genomic Informatics Center, Hankyong National University, Ansung City, Kyonggi-Do, Korea, [2]Dept. of Animal Breeding and Genetics, Danish Institute of Agricultural Sciences, P.O. Box 50, DK-8830 Tjele, Denmark*

Daily milk yield (**DMY**) and somatic cell score (**SCS**) were analyzed using random regression models. The data consisted of daily recordings from 268 primiparous cows. Univariate REML analyses were conducted to determine the order of fit needed for both additive genetic and permanent environmental effects for **DMY** and **SCS**. Based on likelihood ratio tests, the sufficient orders of fit were 3 and 3 for **DMY** and 0 and 3 for **SCS** for genetic and permanent environmental effects, respectively. Despite that, estimates of heritabilities for **SCS** from random regression models with higher order of fit were in better agreement with estimates obtained from analysis when lactation stages were defined in 30 days periods.
The problems in finding the "best" model for **SCS** could be related to the nature of **SCS**. Elevated levels of **SCS** are associated with mastitis and the distribution of **SCS** may not be equal for healthy and infected cows. Therefore, **SCS** can be regarded as a mixture trait. In this study, a mixture model using a Bayesian approach via the Gibbs sampler was used to estimate parameters for **SCS**. Genetic and permanent environmental effects and heterogeneous residual variance for the two classes of the mixture were accounted for.

Theatre C4.4

Mature equivalent adjustments for yields of Italian buffalo population

M. Fioretti and R. Aleandri, Associazione Italiana Allevatori, Via Nomentana 134, 00162 Roma, Italy.*

Buffalo breeding in Italy is of major importance, with 33.928 controlled cows in 286 farms in 2001. Controlled buffaloes are continuously increasing in Italy. from Buffalo milk has a high fat content (up to 15%) and is used for the production of mozzarella, a typical Italian cheese well known world-wide. Performance recording activity allows a genetic evaluation by BLUP-AM; the evaluated traits are 270-days yields for mozzarella, milk, fat, protein and fat and protein percentage. Selection aim is to increase mozzarella cheese production. A study has been performed to determine, for milk, fat, protein and mozzarella yield, a set of coefficient to calculate, from a 270-days reference production, an Equivalent Mature Buffalo (EMB) yield, that is, an estimated yield supposing the animal be the Mature Buffalo cow, the reference lactating female. Solutions from a BLUP-AM were used to determine the above mentioned coefficients. The EMB yield will be useful for both management decisions for the farmer, allowing to compare in the same farm animals with different physiological conditions and age, and genetic evaluation purpose.

Theatre C4.5

Comparison of rearing systems at low environmental impact: the beef cattle of central Italy

M. Iacurto, A. Gaddini, S. Gigli, M. Mormile, F. Vincenti, Animal Production Research Institute - Via Salaria, 31, 00016 Monterotondo (Roma), Italy*

We analyzed *in vita* and slaughtering performances of Chianina bulls reared in different conditions: slatted floor (SF, 10 animals), feed-lot (FL, 14 animals) and pasture (PA, 9 animals). The FL fed according to PGI mark “Vitellone Bianco dell’Appennino Centrale”. The PA had a summer integration with maize grains (1 kg/100 kg BW).

The animals, all born in pasture, were taken back from rangeland and weaned at 6 months of age, then started the trial at 10 months and were slaughtered at commercial maturity; the PA had an higher live weight (+7,8 p.p. (percent point) compared to SF), and an older age at slaughter.

All the groups had good conformation score (U- to U), but we found a significant difference in fatness score (SF:2; FL:2-; PA:1+); these values are confirmed by a percentage of intramuscular (-3,36 p.p.) and subcutaneous (-1,84 p.p.) fat.

PA had an higher percentage of lean meat (+3,9 p.p.) and bone (1,14 p.p.), in comparison to SF. The PA compared to SF showed lower dressing percentage (-3,00 p.p.) and net dressing percentage (-2,27 p.p.) and an higher difference between fore and hind quarters weights (22,17 kg vs 20,85 kg), as typical of animals raised at pasture, due to an higher and different physical activity.

Theatre C4.6

Influence of rearing system on slaughtering performances and carcass of Piemontese young bulls

C. Lazzaroni, D. Biagini. Department of Animal Science, University of Turin, Via Leonardo da Vinci 44, 10095 Grugliasco, Italy.*

To verify the effect of different rearing systems on slaughtering performances of Piemontese young bulls, a trial was carried out to evaluate the influence of the local traditional rearing systems in tied stall compared with the EU free range system in group pen. The animals, 15 in tied stall (TS) and 15 in pens (GP; 4.8 m^2/head), were raised in the same environmental conditions and following the same feeding system. The rearing period was 285 days, from about 7 month of age and 230 kg l.w., until the same commercial fattening degree (about 16 month of age). At slaughter, live weight, so as head, shanks, skin, guts, and offal, until carcass and sides weights were recorded. After cooling (1 d) carcass sides were weighted, evaluated and measured. At slaughtering the GP animals were heavier than the ST (579 *vs*. 539 kg; $P<0.05$), but no significant differences were founded in slaughtering data. Again, after cooling GP sides were heavier than TS ones (196 vs. 183 kg; $P<0.05$), with a wide chest depth (42 *vs*. 39 cm; $P<0.05$) and a thin leg (max width 31.13 *vs*. 31.60 cm; $P<0.01$), probably due to different movements of animals, while no differences were found in conformation and fatness. The group pen rearing system, besides to assure the minimum standards for the calves' welfare provided by the European regulation, allows so to obtain slaughtering performances and carcasses comparable to the old rearing system in tied stall.

Theatre C4.7

Beef production from New Zealand, European/American and Belgian Blue x Holstein-Friesian male cattle

M.G. Keane, Teagasc, Grange Research Centre, Dunsany, Co. Meath, Ireland.

The objective was to evaluate the male progeny of New Zealand (NZ) and European/American (EU) Holstein-Friesians, and Belgian Blue x Holstein-Friesians (BB) for beef production. NZ were imported as embryos and implanted into heifers. EU were the progeny of high genetic merit Irish cows and European/North American-bred bulls. BB were the progeny of Belgian Blue bulls and Holstein-Friesian cows. A total of 96 spring-born animals (32 per genotype) were used in a 3 genotypes (NZ, EU and BB) x 2 production systems (bulls and steers) x 2 slaughter weights (550 and 630 kg) factorial experiment. For NZ, EU and BB, respectively, mean carcass weights per day were 425, 459 and 528 (s.e.d. 3.8) g and mean kill-out proportions were 496, 508 and 554 (s.e.d. 2.8) g/kg. Carcass conformation score, carcass fat score, fat depth and *m. longissimus* area did not differ between NZ and EU, but BB had higher values for carcass conformation and *m. longissimus* area and lower values for the fatness indicators. Compared with NZ, EU had more muscle and bone and less fat in the ribs joint, while BB had more muscle and less fat and bone than the dairy strains. Bulls had higher carcass weights and a higher proportion of muscle than steers. Delaying slaughter increased slaughter and carcass weights but there was no significant effect on composition. It is concluded that EU were slightly superior to NZ for beef production and BB were considerably superior to both dairy strains.

Theatre C4.8

Real-time ultrasound measurements in fattening bulls from three different breeds

A. Delobel[1], J.F. Cabaraux[1], J.L. Hornick[1], L. Istasse[1] and I. Dufrasne[2], [1]Nutrition Unit, [2]Experimental Station, Animal Production Department, Veterinary Medicine Faculty, Liège University, Belgium.*

Real-time ultrasound data - area and depth of *longissimus thoracis (LT),* back fat thickness and echogenicity of muscle - were obtained on 21, 20 and 14 growing fattening bulls respectively from the Belgian Blue double muscle breed (BB), the charolais breed (CH) and the limousin breed (LI). The animals have been offered a concentrate fattening diet.
The area of the LT was 111.1, 110.3 and 105.3 cm^2 ($P=0.38$) in the BB, CH and LI bulls respectively. The corresponding data for depth of LT were 82.6, 83.7 and 80.8 mm ($P=0.38$). By contrast, breed significantly affected ($P<0.001$) the back fat thickness at 2.50, 3.26 and 2.81 cm. There were no effects ($P<0.44$) of the breed on the echogenicity, a measure of intra-muscular fat, at 15.5, 16.6 and 17.7% respectively. Correlation coefficients were calculated between ultrasound data and different parameters from slaughter characteristics. The relationships(r) were significant ($P<0.01$ or 0.05) between depth or area in the LT and final live weight (0.43 and 0.46); carcass weight (0.43 and 0.51) muscle weight (0.42 and 0.55) and bones weight (0.35 and 0.39). The correlation coefficients were also significant between back fat thickness and killing-out percentage (-0.38), muscle weight (-0.25) and adipose tissue weight (+0.52). By contrast, the echogenicity was significantly correlated only with the killing-out percentage (-0.37).

Theatre C4.9

Proteomic analysis applied to bovine muscle hypertrophy

J. Bouley, C. Chambon[1], G. Renand[2], J.F. Hocquette, B. Picard, INRA, U.R.H., [1]S.R.V., 63122 Saint-Genès Champanelle, [2]S.G.Q.A., 78 352 Jouy-en-Josas, France*

Different studies have clearly shown that a high bovine muscle development from monogenic (double-muscled genotype, DM) or polygenic origin (divergent lineages) is accompanied by particular characteristics. They act in favour of improvement of meat tenderness but against improvement of flavour. The aim of this study was to develop a proteome analysis permitting the simultaneous study of hundreds of proteins to identify markers related to both muscle hypertrophy and tenderness.
Two-dimensional electrophoresis, covering a pH range of 4-7, were applied to *Semitendinosus* (ST, mixed fast glycolytic).With a colloïdal Coomassie blue procedure more than 500 proteins spots were detected with a high reproducibility. These data indicate the feasibility of the method for differential display analysis and for the construction of a reference map of bovine skeletal muscle which is in progress.
An analysis was conducted on ST of bovine with high or low muscle growth : Belgian Blue bulls homozygote DM, heterozygote DM, homozygote non DM and charolais bulls lineages with high or low muscle growth. Less than 10 % of the revealed proteins were altered between low and high muscled animals. Some of them had an intermediate expression in heterozygote DM. For example, contractile proteins which were altered include troponin T slow and fast isoforms, Myosin binding protein H isoforms. These proteins variably expressed in our different models could be markers for muscle hypertrophy.

Poster C4.10

Milk recording methods: effects on phenotypic variation of lactation records

R. Aleandri and A. Tondo, Associazione Italiana Allevatori, via Nomentana 134, 00162 Roma Italy.*

The accuracy of different recording methods have been compared on dairy production records. The effect of different methods has been evaluated both on lactation calculation and test day. Lactation calculation: a set of milk production data from lactometers have been used to evaluate the accuracy of different Milk Recording Methods on lactation calculation at different stages (100, 240, 305 days). Test day: an experimental dataset have been used to simulate different Daily Recording Methods and the accuracy of the estimates of 24 hour milk, fat and protein (Test Day) with different methods has been compared.
The spread of new technologies (lactometers and robots) will move dairy production recording towards the use of automatic recording systems which have great accuracy.

Poster C4.11

Change and genetic aspects of body condition score (BCS) in Italian Brown cattle

R. Dal Zotto[1], M. Cassandro[2], C. Valorz[1], P. Zischg[1], L. Gallo[2], P. Carnier[2] and G. Bittante[2], [2]Department of Animal Science, University of Padova, Agripolis, 35020, Legnaro, Padova, Italy, [1]Consortium Superbrown of Bolzano and Trento, Via Lavisotto, 125, 38100, Trento, Italy.*

Body condition score (BCS) at approximately four-week intervals were taken during over 2 years (from 2001 to 2002) on 1,323 Italian Brown cattle reared in 50 farms. The aims of this study were to investigate the pattern of changes during lactation of BCS and to estimate heritability value of BCS and its genetic correlations with daily milk yield, using a test-day model. A total of 10,460 records of BCS were available for statistical analysis. Only cows with at least two records were analyzed and repeated observations per cows were considered repeated measurements of the same trait. Data were analyzed using ANOVA according to a time-dependent model based on days in milk. R_ accounted for 72% of total variation of test-day BCS. The pattern of change in BCS appeared closely related to stage of lactation. Body reserves decreased from calving until first 3 months of lactation and were restored in mid and late lactation. Variance and covariance components and related parameters were estimated using a REML bi-trait procedure (unequal design) for BCS and milk yield. Heritability estimates for BCS and daily milk yield were 0.31 and 0.19, respectively. Condition score was negatively correlated (-0.32) with daily milk yield.

Poster C4.12

Pre-calving condition in heifers and during the first four lactations

I. Györkös[1], E. Báder[2], A. Muzsek[2], J. Szili[3], P. Báder[2], Ms. A. Kovács[2], Z. Gergácz[2], Ms. Kertészné Györffy E.[2], [1]Research Insitute for Animal Breeding and Nutrition, Gesztenyés str.1, 2053 Herceghalom, Hungary, [2]University of West Hungary, Faculty of Agriculture, Vár 2, 9200 Mosonmagyaróvár, Hungary, [3]Aranymezo Ltd. 7671 Bicsérd, Hungary*

The experiment involved 1317 Holstein-Friesian heifers or cows. Evaluation of condition was made on a 5-score-scale.
On the basis of results the following conclusions can be made. 20% of the heifers had less than 3 condition scores just before calving. According to the bibliography, limits of condition scores at calving were 3-4, the optimal score was 3.5 75% of the heifers belongs to this category. Only 0.9% received high condition scores (4-5) indicating plus condition. Number of the cows with poor and plus condition increased at the end of the first lactation. 69.9% of cows had acceptable or desirable condition. Rate of cows with poor condition was quite similar, (16.4-18.6-17.6%) at the end of the 2nd, 3rd and 4th lactation. Rate of obese cows (9.7-12.1-9.8%) increased in the subsequent lactations compared to the first lactation. Rate of the cows with good condition just before calving was around 70%. The rate of the optimal condition (score 3.5) among heifers and cows during the first 3 lactations was around 10.7-14.8%, but in the 4th lactation was reduced to 5.9-9.8%.

Poster C4.13

Index of height at withers at take in breeding in Holstein-Friesian heifers

E. Báder[1], I. Györkös[2], J. Bartyik[3], P. Báder[1], Z. Gergácz[1] and Ms. A. Kovács[1], [1]University of West Hungary, Faculty of Agriculture, Vár 2, 9200 Mosonmagyaróvár, Hungary, [2]Research Institute for Animal Breeding and Nutrition, Gesztenyés str.1, 2053 Herceghalom, Hungary,*
3Enyingi Agrár Company, Farm Kiscséripuszta, 8130 Enying, Hungary

For observing the development of heifers the wither height index is more exact than the body condition scoring. The body weight, height of withers and the index were at 14 months of age: 376 kg, 121 cm, 3.11, at the age of 16 months: 404 kg, 126 cm, 3.21, at the age of 18 months 458 kg, 132 cm, 3.47 respectively. At the age of 14 months the 65% of animals belonged to the suggested weight category, at 16 months of age of heifers that rate was 56%, at the age of 18 months it was 68%.
At the age of 14 months the 64% of the individuals had an ideal wither height, at 16 months of age it was 80%, and at the age of 18 months was 90%.
The ideal wither height index was calculated for 41.3% of the population at 14 months of age with slight surplus condition. Wither height indices of 43% of animals at 16 months of age were ideal. This ratio became better at 18 month of age, while 55.2% of heifers had ideal index, 25.6% had low and 19.2% had high index.

Poster C4.14

The relationships between 305-day milk yield with live weight, udder and some body measurements at black pied heifers

Ö. Sekerden and Y.Z. Güzey, Mustafa Kemal Univ.,Fac. of Agric., Dept. of Anim. Sci., Antakya-Turkey

In this research, it was aimed to investigate relationships between 305 day milk yield with various udder measurements(Height of rear udder, udder length, rear udder depth, distances of front and rear teats to ground, width of rear udder, distances of front, rear and side teats to each other, lenghts of front and rear teats, diameters of front and rear teats), live weight, body measurements (Height at withers, body length, chest depth, chest girth, shin girth, abdomen girth) in various stages of pregnancy and 1st lactation period (150, 210 and 265 days of pregnancy; 7., 21., 35., 49., 90., 150., 210. and 270 days of lactation) of Black Pied heifers.
The material of the research was consisted of various data of 20 Black Pied heifers. Daily milk yield, live weight, udder and body measurements of trial animals were determined mentioned times.
The correlation coefficients between 305-day milk yield with each investigated characteristic were calculated at each pregnancy and lactation stages investigated and results obtained were interpreted.

Poster C4.15

Age correction factors for milk yield of Holstein Friesian cattle in Turkey

*H. Atil[1] and A.S. Khattab[*2]. [1] University of Ege, Faculty of Agriculture, Department of Animal Science, Izmir, Turkey, [2]University of Tanta, Faculty of Agriculture, Animal production Department, Tanta, Egypt*

A total of 2257 normal first lactation records of Holstein Friesian cattle kept at five herds in west Turkey during the period from 1971 to 1987 were used. The influence of herds , season and year of calving and age at first calving (AFC) on 305 day milk yield (305 d MY) was investigated. A least squares analysis of variance of the data showed significant effects of herds, season and year of calving on 305 d MY ($P < 0.01$) . Estimates of partial linear and quadratic regression coefficients of 305 d MY on AFC were significant and being 30. 19 + 5.48 kg/mo, and - 1.15 + 0.32 kg/mo ^{2} , respectively. A set of multiplicative age correction factors was derived for each season of calving and for all season by fitting a polynomial of second degree of production on age at first calving.

Poster C4.16

Relationships between functional traits, longevity and milk performance of Estonian Red cows

E. Orgmets and O. Saveli. Estonian Agricultural University, Institute of Animal Science, Kreutzwaldi 1, 51014 Tartu; Estonia*

The body conformation, age at 1st calving, productive lifetime, longevity, milk productivity and culling reasons of the culled Estonian Red dairy cows in last decade were analyzed. Total of 20,054 cows were studied. It was found that the average age of the Estonian Red cows was 83 months, the age at first calving 31 months, and the productive lifetime 52 months or four lactations. From economic aspect it is considered too short. The main reasons for culling were udder diseases (26.0%), sterility (23.1%), low milk productivity (13.1%), gynaecological diseases (6.8%), and feet diseases (6.0%). The percentage of other reasons was lower. As for the analysis of longevity and type traits, most of the linear traits of the cows with longer stayability are closer to the ideal, compared with those of the earlier culled cows. A stronger correlation was observed between longevity, rump width, feet and udder traits (r= 0.15...0.17). The productive lifetime and stayability were also positively correlated with body region scores and the final score of exterior. The cows with higher scores of general impression, udder, stronger feet and legs lasted longer (r= 0.13...0.23). The latter had a higher total score of exterior as well (r= 0.26). A lifetime milk production was more strongly correlated with body depth, rump width and udder traits (r= 0.15...0.22). The cows with stronger body conformation had significantly higher type score, milk production and longer stayability.

Poster C4.17

Factors affecting fat and milk solids non fat yields of Black Pied Cows and estimation of heritabilities of the yields

Ö. Sekerden, Univ. of Mustafa Kemal, Fac. of Agric., Dept. of Anim. Sci., Antakya, Turkey.

This research was aimed to investigate the factors affecting of milk, fat, total dry matter (TDM), solids non fat (SNF) yields of lactation. The material was formed by data belong to 348 Black Pied cows. Daily milk yields determined and fat, TDM and SNF rates were analysed in milk samples taken from each trial animal in the morning milkings at 30±15, 90±15, 150±15 and 210±15 days of their lactation,. By using averages of the data for each cow, lactation yields of fat, protein, TDM and SNF were calculated.

Variance analysis were applied on the investigated characteristics for environmental factors. Standardization was applied for the effects found significant statistically. Heritabilities of yields of fat, protein, SNF and TDM were estimated.

Variance analysis were repeated as considering firstly, calving season and calving year, secondly calving year and lactation order. Standardization was applied on the characteristics again two times seperately according to results of both of variance analysis groups. Means of fat, protein, TDM and SNF yields were determined according to lactation orders and calving seasons. Heritabilities for fat, protein, SNF and TDM yields as 0.244±0.148, 0.072±0.100, 0.136±0.124, 0.136±0.124 were estimated respectively.

Poster C4.18

Factors associated with milk urea concentrations in Korean Holstein cow

K.J. Han[1], D.H. Lee[2] and S. Islam[2], [1]Dairy Cattle Improvement Center, NACF, 201-64 Wondang-Dong, Kyonggi-Do, Korea, [2]Hankyong National University, Seokjeong-Dong, Ansung, Kyonggi-Do, Korea

Generalized linear model was used to investigate the relationships between milk urea nitrogen (MUN) concentrations and milk productuion and somatic cell scores (SCS) in Korean dairy herds. More than one million test-day data on milk yield, fat%, protein%, solids-not-fat%, somatic cell scores, and MUN were collected from dairy herds by national dairy herd improvement program (Korean DHI) from 1999 to 2002. The MUN estimates were increased from first parity (16.8-17.0 mg/dl at 75-90 DIM) to later parities (17.4-17.6 mg/dl at 75-90 DIM) and onward in the stage of lactation and same estimates were found in parturition year and season. In the milking performances, MUN influenced milk production within a certain range (<10-27> mg/dl). At concentration of <10 mg/dl for MUN, milk production was lowest (25-26 kg); at 21-24 mg/dl for MUN, milk production was highest (29-30 kg). SCS(s) were high (3.45-3.50) at concentration of <10 mg/dl for MUN and showed a gradual decrease following by the gradual increase of MUN level up to 24-27mg/dl and SCS(s) was little higher (3.25-3.5) at 27< mg/dl. These results indicate that the more increase of parity, the more increase of MUN and the more increase of milk production.

Poster C4.19

Comparison of bulk somatic cells counts after changes in management style and intra-mammary infection control program

G. Pisoni[1], A. Casula[1], V. Bronzo[1], G. Gnemmi[1], F.M.G. Luzi[2], P. Moroni[1]. [1]Dipart. Di Patologia Animale, Igiene e Sanità Pubblica Veterinaria, [2]Istituto di Zootecnica, via G. Celoria, 10, 20133 Milano, Italia.*

The study describes the results of a program of management improvement in 26 farms with high somatic cells count (SCC) in bulk milk (BM). During the period 1999-2002 we examined monthly BM samples for SCC and total bacterial count. Farms were divided in three groups according to the most prevalent microrganisms isolated in the intramammary infections (IMI): contagious pathogens (*Streptococcus agalactiae, Staphylococcus aureus*), coagulase-negative staphylococci (CNS) and environmental pathogens (*Streptococcus spp., E. coli*). In 1999, mean BMSCC was 493 x 10^3cell/ml. The application of an improving management program has been successful in the reduction of mean BMSCC and the incidence of IMI. The total decrease of SCC among all farms was approximately 102 x 10^3cells/ml. Reduction of SCC was more evident in those farms with high prevalence of IMI due to CNS and environmental pathogen: decrease of mean SCC was of 141 x 10^3/ml and of 171 x 10^3/ml respectively. The effect of management was not so evident on mean SCC in farms with contagious micro-organism infection, reduction of mean SCC was only of 50 x 10^3/ml. Intervention strategies need to be implemented for contagious IMI: strict segregation of cattle with IMI, intensified culling of cattle with multiple-quarter IMI and the use of long-acting intramammary dry therapy.

 Poster C4.20

The factors affecting somatic cell count in milk

H. Kiiman, O. Saveli, T. Kaart. Institute of Animal Science, Estonian Agricultural University, Kreutzwaldi 1, Tartu 51014, Estonia

The somatic cell count (SCC) is commonly used as measure of udder health as well as milk quality. High SCC is almost always result of mastitis infection. Mastitis remains a major source of economic loss to dairy cattle farmers, mainly through the veterinary treatments, increased cost of replacement and reduced milk yield. Somatic cell count becomes very essential as a genetic tool for reducing mastitis in addition to management initiatives. In Estonia there are several problems with somatic cell count.

The objective of this study was to estimate the factors affecting somatic cell count in milk. The experimental dairy farms were chosen from agricultural enterprises applying different milking and cow-keeping technologies. Data about ten-month milk yield, fat and protein content and SCC were collected. Cows' sire, enterprise, birth-year, lactation, calving month, milking equipment and milking operator were fixed in data-base. Monitoring of working operations of the milkers were performed. SAS- program were used for data processing. Procedure REML was used to estimate dispersion components and heritabilities. From these data analysis observed that the milking operator had an essential effect on the milk SCC ($P<0.001$), as well as agricultural enterprise and lactation number ($P<0.01$). The milking equipment was not essential to milk SCC.

Poster C4.21

Investigations on somatic cell count in milk

G.G. Karlikova[1] and A.Z. Kaneev[2], [1]All-Russian Research Institute of Animal Husbandry, Dubrovitsy 142132 Moskovskaya Oblast, Russia, [2]NP 'Mosplem', Susczhevskaya ul. 27, Moscow, 103030 Russia*

Studies on somatic cell count (SCC) in milk of Ayrshire; Russian Black-Pied and Kholmogor cows determined monthly by Fossomatic milk analyser were conducted for one-year period.

Cows were classified as healthy if SCC was below 250 000 cells per ml milk, risk group (SCC >250 000 and <500 000), probability of udder inflammation high (SCC >500 000 and <900 000), probability very high (SCC >900 000 and <1 500 000) and mastitis (SCC is over 1 500 000 cells). Distribution of SCC classes did not depended from month of the year. Frequencies of SCC classes were influenced by management (barn and group of dairymaid). In a herd Black-Pied cows per cent of healthy cows was in range 42 to 57% in various barn groups, in Kholmogor herd 39 to 83% and Ayrshire herd 28 to 71% ($P<0.05$).

A statistically significant difference between farms breeding three breeds of cattle in respect of SCC distribution with lower per cent of healthy group in Black-Pied breed (46%), than in Ayrshire and Kholmogor breeds (64 and 54% respectively, $P<0.05$) was found. Accordingly classes of cows with SCC >500 000 - <900 000 and SCC >900 000 - <1 500 000 cells was smaller in Ayrshire herd than in other two breeds. There were no significant differences between farms in respect of mastitis incidence.

Poster C4.22

Udder morphological investigations by ultrasound in a Hungarian Simmental population

B. Húth[1], R.D. Fahr[2], F. Rosner[2] and I. Hollo[1]. [1]University of Kaposvar, Faculty of Animal Science, H-7401 Kaposvar, P.O. Box 16, [2]Martin-Luther University, Institute of Animal Production, D-06108 Halle, Adam-Kuckhoff 35.*

As it's known the state of the udder's health is one of the most important factor in realising the genetically determined qualitative milk production. The mastitis is a polifactorial sickness, in the same time the milking ability and udder conformation is one of the most important factors.
The examinations were to follow the change of the teat canal closing muscle barrier by the effect of milking and the correlation between the anatomical structure of the teat and parameters of the milking ability. The udder morphology was observed by ultrasound at 72 Hungarian Simmental cows.
The milking ability was examined by milk quantity measuring instruments *(Lacto Corder)*. The udder morphology was examined by *Hitachi Oculus 9100 type ultrasound*. Examining the udders by ultrasound, it can stated that the length of the teat canal and the surface of the closing muscle grows according to mechanical effects of the milking and later on and as a result of the regeneration it declines. Parallel to the tendency of increasing the length of the teat canal the average and the maximal milking speed shows a decrease. Finally higher somatic cell number at the longer teat canal was experienced.

Poster C4.23

Milk performance of automatic milked cows and conventional milked cows

N. Wirtz[1], K. Oechtering[1], E. Tholen[1] and W. Trappmann[1], [1]Institute of Animal Breeding Science, University of Bonn, Endenicher Allee 15, 53115 Bonn, Germany*

Between May 1999 and September 2001 a comparison of an automatic milking (AM) system with a conventional milking parlour was perfomed in an experimental herd of 104 HF-cows in North Rhine-Westfalia (Germany). 52 cows were milked automatically by a one box milking robot, 52 comparable cows were milked conventionally by a 14 places rotation milking parlour in the same barn. All cows were fed with a mixed ratio of grass silage, maize silage and concentrates (covering around 25 kg energy corrected milk yield) and concentrates depending on milk yield.
Due to technical problems in the first nine months the AM-cows were not able to pick up their own milking rhythm. In this period the milk yield of the automatic milked cows was significantly lower. However, after solving the problems and reaching a milking frequency of 2.75 per day the milk yield did not increase as expected. During the whole experiment the cows in the AM-system realized only 91 % of the 305-day-milk yield of the conventionally milked cows (7.747 vs. 8.479 kg). A significant decrease of the milk fat content in the AM-group was observed (3.98 % vs.4.17 %). No differences were found in the milk protein content (3.32 vs. 3.35 %).
Our results indicate that in comparable environmental conditions, cows in AM-systems don't necessarily realize a higher milk yield than cows in conventional milking parlours.

Poster C4.24

Effect of the AMS on milk quality in a farm of the Parmesan cheese area

Luca Bertolini, Paolo Liberati, Gian Battista Castagnetti, Giovanni Ferri, Università di Bologna DIPROVAL Via F.lli rosselli, 107 42100 Reggio Emilia Italy

Quality parameters of milk milked by means of an automatic milking system (AMS) were compared to those milked in a conventional milking parlour based on two milkings per day in a farm located in *Parmigiano Reggiano* production area.
Data were collected for one year between January 2002-January 2003. The parameters were: Total plate count (TPC), bulk somatic cells (BMSCC), freezing point (FP) and lipase, protease activity , protein %, fat %, Lactose %, Urea g/L, pH tritrable acidity, and Freezing point (FP).
Introduction of an AMS in a traditional area like *Parmigiano-Reggiano* production zone, from a technical point of view, seem to improve some milk quality aspects like the BMSCC and the gross chemical components. Overall AMS milk show: an increase in the residues of lipase and proteasis activity that are correlated with a significant increase in the psytrophic bacteria count; an evident reduction of somatic cells was also seen in comparison with conventional milking parlour; a lesser increase of TPC in the summer time; FP decrease along all the evaluation period.
Problems related to the legal implications of the introduction of the AMS in the *Parmigiano-Reggiano* typical zone were finally taken in account.

Poster C4.25

Factors affecting somatic cell count in buffalo milk

B. Moioli, F. Napolitano, G. Catillo and C. Tripaldi, Istituto Sperimentale per la Zootecnia, via Salaria 31, 00016 Monterotondo, Italy

This papers aims to estimate the effects of year and season, age at calving, stage of lactation and herd on somatic cell count (SCC) in buffalo and the effect of SCC on milk yield and composition. For this purpose, 9,807 observations of test-day SCC of 1,785 calvings (1996 to 2002) of 757 buffaloes were used. Average SCC was 181,000 (S.E. 343,000) and was significantly affected by the considered environmental effects. The highest SCC levels were found in the year 2002, in the months of May, August and December, in the older buffaloes and at end lactation. On the contrary, lowest SCC levels were found in the years 1998-1999, in April and October, in the youngest buffaloes and at mid-lactation (4th to 7th month). The effects of the age of the cow and lactation stage showed the same trend as in dairy cows. Herd effect was highly significant.
Milk yield, fat and protein percentage were negatively affected by SCC; an increase by 100,000 in SCC produced a decrease of 0.85 kg in the daily milk yield; a decrease of 0.028 in fat percentage and of 0.043 in protein percentage.
Because of the lower average values of SCC in buffalo milk, the physiological threshold used as an indicator of pathological status for this livestock is likely to be different from that of the dairy cow.

Poster C4.26

Mastitis of cows and the use of homeopathic preparations for the treatment

E.M. Boldyreva, Russian University of People's Friendship, 26 Bakinskikh comissarov, 7-6-28, 119571, Moscow, Russia.

Mastitis is one of the most spread diseases of dairy cows. This disease leads to the decrease in production and milk quality and causes considerable damage to livestock farming. Preparations used for treatment are not always effective and harmless for animals and for people consuming milk.

In the research conducted different methods of treatment of cows with serous and catarrhal mastitis were studied. Mastitis was caused mainly by improper milking machine work and had traumatic etiology. Two experiments were conducted. In control groups of both experiments antibacterial preparations were administered. In experimental groups different homeopathic remedies with antibacterial preparations of control groups were used. Homeopathic preparations had not been used in Russia for the treatment of mastitis before. An average duration of illness in experimental groups of the 1st and 2nd experiment was 2.4 and 1.9 days less than that in control ones correspondingly. In control groups the period of illness was prolonged and 27.3-31.7% of cows recovered only after the 10th day of illness (up to 3-4 weeks) while in experimental groups all the animals had been cured to the 10th day. The treatment in experimental groups was more economical than in control groups. Homeopathic preparations are harmless, do not cause side effects. Milk after the treatment with homeopathic remedies may be used without restrictions that makes their administration preferable.

Poster C4.27

Prediction of the breeding value of dairy heifers using equations based on animal factors and blood physiological traits

A. Oprzadek, J. Oprzadek, Z. Reklewski, E. Dymnicki, Institute of Genetics and Animal Breeding, Jastrzebiec, 05-552 Wólka Kosowska, Poland.*

Feed intake, growth rate and levels of the blood physiological indicators: thyroxine, triiodothyronine, insulin, alanine aminotransferase, aspartate aminotransferase, alkaline phosphatase, urea, glucose, creatinine and cholesterol were measured from 109 Friesian growing heifers (7-8 months of age). Blood samples were collected: 1) on day 1, after they had been fed in the morning; 2) on day 4, after 36 h fasting; 3) on day 46, after 6 weeks when feed intake was measured and heifers were fed concentrates and hay *ad libitum*; 4) after 36 h fasting on day 48. Multiple regression analyses were employed to construct prediction equations that were restricted to a maximum of four traits. These equations showed much greater prediction value of blood physiological indicators than feed intake and growth rate traits. The reliability (R^2) of equations was higher where blood indicator levels were measured after fasting and ranged from 0.36 to 0.48. The best results were obtained for the index constructed for prediction of milk yield ($R^2 = 0.48$; P £ 0.001). The equation contains the following elements: triiodothyronine, alkaline phosphatase, alanine aminotransferase and daily gain.

Poster C4.28

Cholesterol content in the blood serum of Black and White breed cows with different share of Holstein - Friesian genes

A. Tomaszewski, A. Zachwieja, M. Bohdanowicz-Zazula, Institute of Animals Breeding, Department of Cattle Breeding and Milk Production, Agricultural University of Wroclaw, Chelmonskego str. 38D, 51-630 Wroclaw, Poland.

138 cows of Black and White breed were taken into consideration. Cows were divided into five groups depending on different share of genes of Holstein - Friesian breed: I - pure black and white lowland breed, II - below 50%, III - more than 50% to 75%, IV - from 75,1% to 93,8%, V - over 93,8%. Moreover, cows were combined into groups according to age and stage of lactation. Blood samples were collected from common carotid vein. After centrifugation in obtaining blood serum total cholesterol and HDL and LDL were indicated by the enzymatic method. To the measurement automat EXPRESS PLUS (BAYER) was performed. It was found that the lowest level of total cholesterol and its fractions was in blood serum of Black and White cows (group I), adequately: 172.35, 95,30 (HDL) and 73,10 mg/dl (LDL). Along with extension share of genes of Holstein-Friesian breed there was observed systematic increase of cholesterol content. In blood serum from cows with over 93,8% share of genes of Holstein - Friesian breed the content of total cholesterol was higher more than 36%, HDL over 23% and LDL more than 56%. Differences between I and IV and V were significant ($p \leq 0.05$). The results show clear influence of cow's genotype on cholesterol content in cow's blood serum. Similar results were obtained in cow's milk.

Poster C4.29

Prolonged calving interval and reduced supplementation in an organic dairy herd

J. Sehested and A. Danfær, Danish Institute of Agricultural Sciences, P.O. Box 50, DK-8830 Tjele, Denmark.*

The proportion of organic feed in the total ration for dairy cows has to reach 100% in 2005, and there is a demand for 60% roughage in the total ration. This puts pressure to the market for supplementary feeds, and gives basis for an increasing proportion of roughage in the feeding ration and thereby a decreasing intake of energy. Long calving interval could be a strategy for adapting organic dairy production to a high proportion of roughage in the diet and a high degree of self-supply or local supply of feeds. A two times two factorial design including reproduction strategy (12 or 18 month calving interval) and feeding strategy (balanced standard supplementation of concentrate feed or no supplementation) were applied to a dairy herd of 60 Danish Holstein cows at the organic research station Rugballegaard from mid 2000. The experiment will run untill mid 2004. The main feed has been grass clover herbage as grazing or silage. Respons parameters were animal performance and health, milk production and quality, efficiency of production and persistency of lactation. Milk production was affected by feeding strategy as expected. Preliminary data indicates interaction between feeding strategy and reproduction strategy on persistency of lactation. Number of services per gestation and frequency of clinical treatments were not affected by treatment. Calving intervals were equal at the two feeding strategies.

Poster C4.30

Calving interval in a spring calving suckler herd

M.J. Drennan, Teagasc, Grange Research Centre, Dunsany, Co. Meath, Ireland.

In the period 1987 to 1999, 978 spring calving suckler cows in the Grange herd were bred using artificial insemination or natural mating. Mean calving date was March 15, mean turnout date to pasture was April 19, breeding commenced in early May and weaning (and housing) was in November. Adult cows were offered grass silage only in winter while first calvers (2-years of age) were also offered 1.5 kg daily of concentrates post-calving until grazing commenced. All cows were offered a mineral/vitamin supplement in winter. Mean pregnancy rate was 94% with a mean calving interval (CI) of 367 days. CI was affected ($P<0.001$) by previous calving date but there was no effect of either cow age or previous calving difficulty. CI values for cows calving before March 6, from March 6 to April 1 or after April 1 in the breeding season were 382 (se 1.8), 366 (se 1.8) and 347 (se 2.8) days respectively. Corresponding winter liveweight losses were 83 (se 3.4), 59 (se 3.4) and 41 (se 5.3) kg and summer weight gains were 100 (se 3.6), 84 (se 3.7) and 75 (se 5.7) kg. Body condition scores followed a similar trend. From post-calving to mid June first calvers had lower liveweight (1 v 28 kg) and lower body condition score (0 v 0.37 units on scale 1 to 5) gains than cows in lactations 2 to 7. First calvers lost 0.66 units of a body condition score over the year while the older cows gained condition. Thus, first calvers require higher winter feeding levels than older cows.

Poster C4.31

Indirect effects of the mating sire on cows' milk production

G. Freyer[1], U. Kadow[2], J. Wolf[3] and L. Panicke[1], [1]Research Institute for the Biology of Farm Animals, D-18196 Dummerstorf; [2]Informa Software Consult, Liese-Meitner-Ring 7, D-18059 Rostock, [3]D-18196 Petschow*

The amount of cows' individual milk production is affected by several internal (mainly genetic) and external (environmental) factors. Dividing both types seems to be obvious, in general. The indirect effects of the father of the embryo on mates' milk production seem to be a combination of genetic and environmental factors influencing cows' performance. A further orientating analysis was carried out, using two independent data sets of mother-daughter pairs from the German Black Pied cattle, containing about 13000 (sample 1) and 8800 (sample 2) pairs. Developing and using a computer program, based on the methodological approach by van Vleck (1980), we estimated direct (father) and indirect (mating) effects of the sires on cows' milk production. These direct and indirect effects were negatively correlated for the milk traits. The variance components of indirect effects on milk production were in average about 5 %, varying from 2 to 10 %. The heritability estimates were nearly half as high as for the direct effects. We present results from the subsequent lactations. The highest indirect effects were obtained in third lactations for sample 1, and in second lactations for sample 2. The genetic and physiological backgrounds of the indirect effects in linkage with the direct effects are worth to be further investigated.

Poster C4.32

Estimation of genetic and phenotypic parameters of milk yield and fertility traits in a dairy cattle population after a rapid progress in milk yield

G. Seeland and C. Henze, Institut of Animal Science, Agricultural and Horticultural Faculty of the Humboldt-University, Invalidenstr. 42, 10155 Berlin, Germany.

The purpose of the study was to estimate genetic parameters for milk production and fertility traits as well as their genetic and phenotypic correlations. The study included data on about 75 000 first and 40 000 second parity cows of German Friesian. The model included the fixed effects of herd and calving season and the random effect of the sire. The variance and covariance components are estimated by using REML.
The estimated coefficients of heritability for milk, fat and protein yield were in comparison to previous estimates relative high (0,314-0,409). In contrast to that, heritabilities of fat and protein content were very low and amounted to 0,474 and 0,353 in the first and to 0,420 and 0,317 in the second lactation. As expected, heritabilities of fertility traits were very low, ranging from 0,009 to 0,127, depending on traits. Genetic correlation between milk, fat and protein yield on the one hand in fertility traits on the other were high and unfavourable, reflecting an antagonism. The estimated environmentals correlations coefficients are negligible. This may be one cause of the fact that the phenotypic correlation always less strong than the genetic onces. The genetic regression coefficients between milk yield and fertility traits are small and weak the antagonism.

Poster C4.33

Study on some reproduction indicators in Frizian cows breed in Southern Romania

Vidu Livia, Gheorghe Georgescu, Ion Calin, Elena Nistor - University of Agricultural Sciences and Veterinary Medicine Bucharest, Departament Cattle Husbandry*

In Romania, the Frizian ranks second in the breed structure, i.e. 35%. This breed is grown for milk production and was certified in 1987.
The present paper aims at pointing out several reproduction indices: age at first calving, calving interval and mammary repose.
Research was carried out on lot of 557 milk cows grown on farms located in Southern Romania.
The studied population had different precociousness according to the genetic potential and growing conditions. The calving interval was influenced both by the age vof the cows and the farms (481,58 days).
The mammary repose recorded an average of 63,06 days, with a very high variability.
The present study points out that the Frizian breed grown in Southern Romania records average values similar to the active population, and also to the Holstein Frizian populations grown all over Europe.

Poster C4.34

Survival probabilities of calving interval and gestation length the young and the mature cows in Simmental x South Anatolian Red Crossbred

I.S. Gurcan[1] and M.N. Orman[1], Ankara University Faculty of Veterinary Medicine,Department of Biometrics,06110 Diskapi, Ankara, Turkey.

Survival analysis can be described as a collection of statistical procedures for data analysis in which the outcome variable of interest is time until an event occurs.
Survival analysis, a statistical method developed for research in medicine, can be used in analyzing longevity data and combines information on dead (uncensored) and alive (censored) individuals, enables proper statistical treatment of censored records and account for nonlinear characteristics of longevity data. Survival analysis has been appliying to animal breeding since the beginning of the 1980.
Many methods have been proposed for estimating the survival function S(t). the Kaplan-Meier method is a commonly used method in survival analysis. Cox's regression is another method for analyzing data. Cox proportional hazard model is preferred to other method since, generally, it gives the relationship between the covariates and the dependent variable, survival time when a collection of censored data is considered.
The purpose of this study is to compare survival probabilities of calving interval and gestation length the young and the mature cows in Simmental x South Anatolian Red crossbred.

Poster C4.35

Causes of increasing calf losses in dairy farms in Schleswig-Holstein

K.-H. Tölle, G. Springer, J. Krieter , Institut of Animal Breeding and Husbandry, Christian-Albrechts-University, 24098 Kiel, Germany*

The aim of this study was to investigate causes of the continuously increasing calf losses in dairy farms.
In a first part 7,100 annual reports from 2,039 farms were analyzed. In herds with Black Holsteins stillbirth rate and calf losses in rearing were higher than in herds with Red-Pied cows (+0.9% and +2.0%, resp.). Farms with tie-stall barns had about 1% lower stillborn calves than farms with cubicle houses. With increasing level of herd milk yield calf losses in rearing decreased up to 3%. Herd size had no significant influence on calf losses.
In a second investigation data from 879 calving Black Holsteins (weight, body condition score, hipbone and ischium width) and newborn calves (weight, head circumference) were recorded on 11 farms with cubicle houses. Heifers and multiparous cows with weights lower than 600kg had a significant higher risk of stillbirth (14.9% and 14.6%, resp.) compared with heavier cows (10.4% and 7.2%, resp.). The stillbirth rate increased (4.5% to 20.8%) if cows needed assistance at birth. Cows with a hipbone width lower than 53cm required nearly the double frequency of assistance at birth in comparison with cows with wider pelvics. Calves with a birth weight above 50kg and light calves lower than 41kg had a higher stillbirth risk. If the head circumference of calfs exceeded 51cm the stillbirth rate increased (8.5% to 14.8%).

Poster C4.36

Production of bovine embryoes by ICSI

R. Puglisi, M. Mokrani and A. Galli, Istituto Sperimentale Italiano "Lazzaro Spallanzani", Località La Quercia, 26027 Rivolta d'Adda, Cremona, Italy

ICSI procedure can be succesfully utilized for the production of viable human, mice and horse embryoes. In bovines, the same technique cannot be employed with encouraging results because of the different ovocyte physiology and the particular compact structure of the sperm DNA. The aim of our study was to optimize an ovocyte activation protocol after ICSI for the production of bovine embryoes. The tail scoring method to improve the decondensation of the sperm into male pronucleus was also tested.

In our first experiment, groups of matured ovocytes were fixed after activation with calcium-ionophore (50μM, 5min) leading to 45% of female pronuclear formation that increased to 96% when calcium-ionophore were followed by cycloheximide treatment (10μg/ml for 3,5hrs).

In the second experiment a total number of 205 matured ovocytes have been injected with motile-immobilized sperms after a vigorous aspiration of the ovocyte cytoplasm. These, were then activated by calcium-ionophore (10μM, 5min) and cycloheximide. The presunted zygotes were cultured for 8 days and 32 developed to the blastocyst stage (16%). A control group of 66 non injected ovocytes were activated parthenogenetically with the same modality and only one blastocyst were formed. In conclusion this method of activation togheter with the tail scoring method can be used for the production of bovine embryoes with a very low incidence of parthenogenesis that with others protocols is still very high.

Poster C4.37

The impact of dairy cow fertility on methane emissions

P.C. Garnsworthy, University of Nottingham, School of Biosciences, Sutton Bonington Campus, Loughborough, LE12 5RD, UK

Dairy cows account for 20% of methane emissions worldwide. The aim of this study was to model the influence of fertility on methane production. Improved fertility increases annual milk yield, feed intake and methane emissions per cow. However, reduced cow and replacement numbers, and lower forage proportions, reduce methane. A model was constructed to calculate the combined effects of these factors. Heat detection (HD) and conception rate (CR) were used in a decision tree to calculate pregnancy probabilities for a Markov chain that determined calving intervals, herd structure and replacement rate. Nutrient intakes were used to calculate methane emissions. Fertility scenarios were L) low - HD 50%; CR 38%, G) good - HD 55%; CR 47% and H) high - HD 70%; CR 65%.

For a milk quota of 1 Ml, under scenario L, herd methane emissions decreased from 54 to 20 t/yr as milk yield increased from 4000 to 9000 l/cow/yr.

With the same quota, at 6000 l/cow/yr, methane emissions were 35, 31 and 29 t/yr for scenarios L, G and H; at 9000 l/cow/yr they were 20, 16 and 14 t/yr. Without milk quotas, a 100-cow herd produced 21, 20 and 19 t methane/yr under scenarios L, G and H.

These results suggest that moving from low to high fertility status can reduce herd methane emissions by up to 25%.

Poster C4.38

Factors affecting labour efficiency of milking

B. O'Brien[1], K. O'Donovan[1, 2], J. Kinsella[2], D. Ruane[2] and D. Gleeson[1], [1]Teagasc, Moorepark Research Centre, Fermoy, Co. Cork, Ireland, [2]Department of Agribusiness, Extension and Rural Development, University College Dublin, Ireland.*

A high labour demand associated with milking may influence limitation of herd size in future. The objective of this study was to investigate structural and procedural limitations to efficient milking.
Labour demand was measured on 141 dairy farms on 3 or 5 days/month between February, 2000 and January, 2001. Time spent at milking was investigated for a subset of farms, which comprised 75 spring-calved herds (quota range 136 x10^3 to 591 x10^3 litres), during the month of June. Milking facilities and practices were also studied on these farms. Mean times were calculated using SAS and Microsoft ACCESS packages.
Average time taken for milking (cluster-on/off) and average time taken per milking row for the 33 % most and least efficient herd groups were 1.7 and 2.7 h per day, and 7.1 and 11.1 min, respectively. Proportionally 0.08 and 0.68 of herds in the most and least efficient groups, respectively, had a cow:unit ratio greater than 7. Cows entering the parlour through narrow doorways and herds having exit gates operated from any point in the milking pit were observed on 0.28 and 0.56 of herds and on 0.68 and 0.30 of herds in the most and least efficient groups, respectively. In addition, milking efficiency was improved when the milker did not leave the pit during milking.

Poster C4.39

A profile of the working year on Irish dairy farms

B. O'Brien[1], K. O'Donovan[1, 2], J. Kinsella[2], D. Ruane[2] and D. Gleeson[1], [1]Teagasc, Moorepark Research Centre, Fermoy, Co. Cork, Ireland, [2]Department of Agribusiness, Extension and Rural Development, University College Dublin, Ireland.*

The objective of this study was to quantify and characterise the labour consumed by the dairy system and to establish the influence of production scale and seasonality on labour demand.
The study incorporated 141 dairy farms ranging in milk quota size from 136 x10^3 to 1,455 x10^3 litres. The time associated with carrying out 29 separate farm tasks was measured on these farms between February 2000 and January 2001. Data was recorded using timesheets (98 farms) and electronic data loggers (43 farms) for consecutive 3- and 5-day periods, respectively, once every month. Data from 94 spring-calved herds was analysed using SAS and Microsoft ACCESS.
The average daily labour input per farm over a 12-month period was 10.1 h. Of this, 9.1 h was directly associated with dairying. Average daily labour demand peaked in March at 12.4 h, due mainly to the milking process, calving and calf care and office including management. The lowest labour input per day occurred in December at 7.3 h. The labour input over the 12-month period was significantly affected by both month ($P<0.001$) and milk produced ($P<0.001$).
In conclusion, the results indicate where new technology and labour supply need to be directed in order to maximise labour efficiency on dairy farms in the future.

Poster C4.40

Comparison of colostrum and milk components of different aged Charolais cows in a Hungarian herd

R. Zándoki[1], J. Csapó[2], Zs. Csapó Kiss[2], I. Tábori[1], G. Holló[2] and J. Tözsér[1], [1]Szent István University, H-2103 Gödöllö, [2]University of Kaposvár H-7400*

Milk and colostrum production is a very important factor in calf rearing ability of cows. Authors' aim was to investigate if there are any differences between colostrum and milk components (%) of younger (<5 years, n=5) and elder (>5 years, n=10) Charolais cows in the first week after calving. Cows were hand-milked right after calving, and also, 24, 48, 72 hours and 7 days after calving. Right after calving there was a difference only in non proteinic nitrogen content, to the advantage of elder cows (+0,06%; p<0,05). Milk of cows younger than 5 years was richer in crude protein (+1,33%; p<0,05), true protein (+1,49%; p<0,05), whey protein (+2,33%; p<0,005) and true whey protein (+2,11%; p<0,005) on the first day after calving. While differences observed in crude- and true protein disappeared on the 2nd or 3rd day after calving, there were decreasing, although significant differences (p<0,05) between the two groups of cows in crude- and true whey protein rate throughout the whole week. In the case of casein content, values for younger cows became larger after 48 hours (+0,36%; p<0,05), and the difference increased until the 7th day (+0,41-46%; p<0,058).

Poster C4.41

The yield and composition of beef cows' milk and the results of calf rearing

Z. Litwinczuk[1] and J. Król[2], [1]Department of Cattle Breeding, [2]Department of Evaluation and Use of Animal Raw Materials, Agricultural University of Lublin, Akademicka 13, 20-950 Lublin, Poland

An analysis has been performed of the yield and composition of milk from cows of three beef breeds - Limousine, Hereford and Simmental. Simmental cows had the highest milk yield, while the Hereford cows - the lowest. The milk from Hereford and Limousine cows was characterized by a significantly lower content of dry matter and fat as compared to the milk of Simmental cows, but had a similar lecel of lactose. The highest concentration of protein was recorded for the milk from Limousine and the lowest - from Hereford cows. A directly proportional relation was observed between the milk yield of the dams and the live body weight of their progeny at the day 210 of live.

Poster C4.42

Research on growth, food conversion and qualitative parameters of meat production in Frizian breed

Ion Calin, Gheorghe Georgescu, Vidu Livia- University of Agricultural Sciences and Veterinary Medicine Bucharest, Departament Cattle Husbandry*

Nowadays, Romania has a total meat consumption of 63,5 kg per capita per annum, out of which 21% is bull meat (13,3 kg per capita per annum). The most important meat quantity results from intensive fattening.

The present experiment was carried out on 15 young bulls belonging to the Frizian breed a local mixed breed. Research was performed in two stages, as follows: the pre-experimental (three months) and experimental stage (about nine months).

The animals were fed on manually administered rations, differentiated according to season; the forage was weighted daily,

At the beginning of the experimental stage proper, the weight of the young bulls was 138 kg, while at the end (14 months of age) it was 466,6 kg.

Generally, the daily average growth increase achieved by the 15 bulls varied according to age, from 1,250 kg (5 months) to 1,520 kg (10 months) and 1,029 kg (14 months), with an average specific consumption of 5,72 feed unit/kg of body weight increase and 510,57 digestible gross-protein/kg of body weight increase.

The quantitative parameters achieved were superior: 508,8 kg weight at slaughter time, 291,33 kg (warm carcass) and a low variability coefficient (9%).

Poster C4.43

Effect of pronifer supplementation on the performance of Holstein Friesian calves

A.A. El-Shahat[1], E.M. Ragheb[2] and A.A. El-Basiony[3], [1]Anim.. Prod. Dept. National Res. Centre, Dokki (12622). Cairo, [2]Anim. Prod. Res. Institute, Dokki and Anim. Prod. Dept. Fac. of Agric. Ain Shams University, Cairo, Egpyt.*

Forty growing Holstein Friesian Calves (22 males and 18 Females) were used to study the effect of probiotic pronifer supplementation on the performance of growing friesian calves. The animals were fed berseem hay *ad. lib.* In addition to concentrate feed mixture (CFM) at the level of 2% of their body weight, either without or with pronifer which was in the rate of 0.1% of CFM. Mean values (±S.E.) of the initial livebody weights of the males and females were (39.27± 0.97) kgs. and (35.33 ±0.59) kgs., respectively. The live body weight (LBW) was individually recorded monthly. The concentrates were monthly adjusted according to LBW changes. The experimental period lasted for about 90 days. The most interesting features of the present results is that the experimental treated animals gained slightly faster than the control ones. The data indicated also that no significant differences were d!etected between the two sexes. The statistical analysis revealed also that the efficiency of utilization expressed as feed conversion, calculated as the amount of livebody weight gain per either dry matter, starch equivalent or digestible crude protein consumed were somewhat higher for calves fed pronifer supplemented ration than those of the control ones. That may be due to the better response of rumen fermentation to the used additive. The results will be discussed on the basis of animal nutrition and cattle production.

Poster C4.44

Variability and heritability of growth traits and body measurements in performance tested dual-purpose bulls

V. Bogdanovic[1], R. Djedovic[1] and M. Petrovic[2], [1]Institute of Animal Sciences, Faculty of Agriculture, University of Belgrade, Nemanjina 6, 11080 Zemun-Belgrade, Serbia, [2]Institute for Animal Husbandry, 11080 Zemun, Serbia.*

Performance test of young bulls represents the first step for genetic improvement of cattle. This procedure is important especially for beef and dual-purpose breeds and for those traits that are measurable in the live animals. Also, in the most case those traits are suitable for direst selection and they have influence on production traits later in the life of animals. Target traits in performance testing of bulls are growth traits and body development traits. These two groups of traits are consisting of various production characteristics. In order to estimate heritabilities of several measured traits, data on 371 Simmental performance tested bulls was used. Analysed traits were body weight, average daily gains, and linear body measurements. Since that structure of data disables implementation of Animal Model procedure, heriatbilities were obtained using restricted maximum likelihood (REML) methodology applied to sire model. Heritability estimates for birth weight, body weight at the start of test, body weight at age of 365 days, pre-test, in-test and lifetime average daily gain were 0.23, 0.25, 0.30, 0.27, 0.39, and, 0.29, respectively. Heritability estimates for linear body measurements were 0.43, 0.30, 0.33 and 0.29 for test-off height at withers, circumference of chest, depth of chest and body length, respectively.

Poster C4.45

Fattening of young bulls: comparison of three breeds and two managements

J.F. Cabaraux[1], J.L. Hornick[1], L. Istasse[1] and I. Dufrasne[2], [1]Nutrition Unit, [2]Experimental Station, Animal Production Department, Veterinary Medicine Faculty, Liege University, Belgium.*

A total of 88 bulls were equally divided according to 3 breeds (Belgian Blue, Limousin and Charolais) and 2 fattening systems (an indoor system or a system with a grazing period followed by an indoor finishing). The experiment was repeated over 2 years. The pasture was managed in order to produce good quality young grass. The concentrate diet for the indoor fattening and the indoor finishing was based on sugar beet pulp and was supplemented with cereals and protein sources of vegetable origin. The overall initial and final live weights were 362.9 and 589.4 kg. The duration of the fattening was significantly longer (219.5 *vs* 139.5 d; $P<0.001$) and the average daily gain was significantly reduced (1.132 *vs* 1.524 kg/d; $P<0.001$) when the bulls were previously grazed. The breed significantly influenced animal performances. The average daily gain was the highest with the Charolais at 1.462 *vs* 1.261 kg/d ($P<0.001$) in the 2 other breeds. It was with the Belgian Blue bulls that the killing-out percentage and the proportion of muscle in the carcass were the highest (64.95 *vs* 61.05 or 59.55% and 75.7 *vs* 71.0 or 69.0%; $P<0.001$ for the Belgian Blue, Limousin and Charolais respectively). By contrast, the ranking was opposite for the proportion of the adipose tissue (11.8, 16.0 and 16.8; $P<0.001$).

Poster C4.46

Carcass value indicators in Hereford bulls according to SEUROP category

V. Nová, D. Vanek, V.Bukac, Czech University of Agriculture, Department of Cattle Breeding and Dairying, Prague, Kamycka, 165 21, Czech Republic

Hereford bulls (34 heads) were used for fattening after being weaned at the age of 210 days. Slaughter bulls were slaughtered in an average slaughter weight of 550 to 590 kg. Evaluation of indicators of the carcass value was carried out during the check slaughters when carcass bodies were cut into the individual butcher pieces. The following indicators were observed within the tests of the carcass value of bulls both in general and according classification into classes due to their meatiness (according to SEUROP): whole-life average daily gain in grams, life weight before slaughter in kg, carcass weight in kg, carcass efficiency of life weight before slaughter in %, percentage of individual meat parts and bones of the carcass body in %, percentage of meat and bones of the carcass body in %, ratio of meat:bones. For the indicators listed below the basic statistical characteristics were calculated by using of SAS program - a linear module. In comparison of indicators of carcass value statistically provable differences were discovered ($P < 0.05$) in weight of JUT between the classes U (298.9 kg) and R (285.5 kg). Statistically provable differences between the classes of U and R were found in the parts of high sirloin, sub-shoulder and neck altogether without a bone ($P < 0.01$) and then in low sirloin, meat of silverside, weight JUT ($P < 0.05$).

Poster C4.47

Effect of breed and sex on tissue composition of the carcass of animals slaughtering 24 months olds

L. Monserrat[1], A. Varela[1], J.A. Carballo[1], L. Sánchez[2], [1]C.I.A.M. Aptdo. 10. 15080. A Coruña (Spain). [2]Facultad de Veterinaria. Aptdo. 280. 27002. Lugo, Spain.*

The effects of breed and sex on tissue composition of the carcass were studied with the aim of produce red meat with the most important breeds in Galicia (Holstein-Friesian -HF- and Rubia Gallega -RG-). 7 & 6 bulls and 8 & 6 steers of RG and HF grazed in a rotational system and were finished indoors with maize silage *ad lib* and concentrate (4 kg/animal/day) for 3 months before slaughtering at 24 months. The data were analysed with ANOVA. The RG bulls had heavier carcass than HF bulls (478 *vs.*. 385 kg, $P<0.001$) and there were not differences between steer carcasses. Carcasses of RG respect HF had higher lean percentage (79.4 *vs.* 74.3%, $P<0.001$ & 74.7 *vs.* 70.1%, $P<0.01$). They also had better distribution of high and low-priced cuts, and lower fat (4.6 *vs.* 6.9%, $P<0.001$ & 7.3 *vs.* 9.9 $P<0.1$) and bone percentages (16.0 *vs.* 18.8% & 18.0 *vs.*20.1%, $P<0.01$). The RG and HF bulls had higher meat percentage and lower fat and bone percentages than RG and HF steers. It would be better to use RG animals when leaner carcasses were required meanwhile HF animals would be more adequate to produce fattened carcasses.

Poster C4.48

Comparison of slaughter parameters in bulls of different ages

P. Polák, L. Hetényi, E.N. Blanco Roa, M. Oravcová, J.Huba, Research Institute for Animal Production, Hlohovská 2, 949 92 Nitra, Slovak Republic.*

The analyses of carcass traits on 148 fattened bulls of the Holstein breed were done. Bulls were slaughtered at the age of 9, 12, 15, 17 and 19 months. Weight before slaughter, weight of carcass, weight of meat and proportion of valuable cuts increased with the increasing age of bulls.
The lowest dressing percentage (45.31 %) was found in bulls at the age of 9 months and the highest (52.72 %) at the age of 17 months. Proportion of meat in carcass was increasing up to the age of 15 months. After its maximum reached in 15 months, proportion of meat in carcass showed tendency to fall down in older animals, mainly due to rising proportion of fat. In comparison, proportion of valuable cuts calculated from total meat showed the highest value (55.64 %) in bulls of 9 months and the lowest value (53.21 %) in bulls of 19 months. Proportion of valuable cuts calculated from weight of carcass tended to be stable (38 %) and independent on the age of bulls. According to results of our experiment we recommend to finish the feeding period of the Holstein bulls within the age of 15 or 17 months as the maximum.

Poster C4.49

Carcass traits and meat quality of Lithuanian Black and White bulls offered different silages

V. Vrotniakiene, J. Jatkauskas and D. Urbsiene. Lithuanian Institute of Animal Science, R. Zebenkos 12,LT-5125 Baisogala, Radviliskio raj., Lithuania*

The aim of research was to assess the growth rate, slaughter value and meat quality of young bulls (n=6 in group and 143 days trial) fed wilted clover-timothy grass silage (dry matter (DM) content of the whole plant at harvest was 308 g kg^{-1}), maize silage (DM content 205 g kg^{-1}/DM) and maize with whole crop barley-oat-wetch mixture (DM content 276 g kg^{-1}/DM). The treatments: Control (grass silage, C), II group (maize silage, M) and III group (maize + 15% whole crop mixture, M+M). Control slaughtering data indicated that carcass and abdominal fat yield in M and M+M groups was by 0.3 ($P>0.4$) and 0.51% ($P>0.2$) higher than that in C group. The chemical composition of ground meat and long dorsal muscle showed no significant differences between the groups. A tendency was determined towards lower content of saturated fatty acids and higher content of unsaturated fatty acids in M and M+M groups. 0.23% ($P<0.025$) increase of polyunsaturated acid 18:2 in the fat of long dorsal muscle was determined in M+M group. In M and M+M groups, the pH-value of the long dorsal muscle were, respectively, by 0.16 ($P<0.01$) and 0.04 ($P>0.1$) unit higher, cooking losses by 1.93 ($P<0.01$) and 2.51% ($P<0.001$) lower, water binding capacity by 3.54 ($P<0.05$) and 1.49% ($P>0.2$) higher and protein value index by 22.9 and 6.81% higher in comparison with the C group.

Poster C4.50

Slaughter results, carcass traits and chemical composition of muscles of Holstein- Friesian bulls at different age

F. Szabó, J.P. Polgár , Cs. Szegleti, Z.E. Farkasné, Z. Lengyel, I. Holló., Veszprem University, Georgikon Faculty of Agriculture, Keszthely, Deák. F. u. 16. 8360 Hungary*

Slaughter results and chemical composition of three muscles of Holstein-Friesian bulls in different age groups (number 1, 2 and 3) 203-, 435- and 537 days of age, respectively, were analysed and compared. Carcass data and results of laboratory analysis of meat samples taken from roll (*muscle longissimus dorsy*) tenderloin (*muscle psoas major*) and eye round (*muscle semitendinosus*) were computed. The laboratory and carcass data analysis (SPSS PC 9.0) were carried out at the Department of Animal Husbandry of Georgikon Faculty of Agricultural Sciences. Dressing out percentage (50.91, 54.57, 57.46%) and lean meat ratio (65.78, 68.50, 70.21%) increased, while the ratio of bone (26.67, 22.25, 20.37% espectively) decreased with the increase of slaughter weight. Differences were significant. Fat percentage at the group 1 was significantly lower than groups 2 and 3 (4.24, 5,05 and 4.92%). Dry matter content of the tree examined muscles were between 24.6% and 28.8%, and protein content varied from 20.9-24.78%. The intramuscular fat content was low, 0.5-2%. The highest protein content was observed at the group number 2 (435 days of age and 371 kg slaugter weight).

Poster C4.51

The quality of meat from the carcasses of young bulls and heifers classified according to the EUROP system

M. Florek[1] and Z. Litwinczuk[2], [1]Department of Evaluation and Use of Animal Raw Materials, [2]Department of Cattle Breeding, Agricultural University of Lublin, Akademicka 13, 20-950 Lublin, Poland

A comparison was made of physico-chemical properties (pH, cooling rate, electrical conductivity, water holding capacity, colour, tenderness and marbling) and the chemical composition of meat obtained from young bulls and heifers classified according to the EUROP system. In all the conformation and fatness classes of carcasses of both bulls and heifers similar and desirable course of glycolisis was observed. An increase in the adiposity of bull or heifer carcasses lead to an increase of the per cent of intramuscular fat. Simultaneously the colour of meat was lighter and marbling more pronounced. A relation was demonstrated between the EUROP classification and the process of chilling carcasses. A lower rate of cooling was observed in the carcass-sides from bulls with higher muscle deposition and in the more more fathy heifer carcass-sides.

Poster C4.52

Estimation of genetic parameters for growth, slaughtering performance and meat quality in cattle

J.J. Frickh[1] and J. Sölkner[2], [1]Agricultural Federal Research Company, [2]Department of Livestock Sciences (University of Natural Resources and Applied Life Sciences Vienna) and the "Federation of Austrian Cattle Breeders"

The aim of this investigation was to estimate population parameters for Simmental bulls. At least approximately 920 data for analysis were available.
Represented are the results of the estimation of genetic parameters (heritabilities, genetic correlations). Estimated were genetic trait relations between characters of meat quality and fattening and slaughtering performance.
A distinct trait antagonism between the characters of meat quality and the characters of fattening and slaughtering performance is shown.
Increasing daily gains are connected with a lower feed conversion and a lower fatty tissue class and higher carcass leanness. There is a positive correlation to the meat quality traits end pH-value, brightness, shear force and fat area, but a negative one to the traits redness and water holding capacity (dripping-, grilling-, cooking loss). There exists no correlation to marbling.
Increasing net gains as well as growing muscularity (carcass leanness) is related with higher pH-values, lower water holding capacity, a reduction of marbling fat, a brighter meat colour and higher shear force values. Also the genetic trait relations within the meat quality traits show that meat quality traits should be included in the genetic evaluation.

Poster C4.53

In vivo performance, carcass and meat quality of young bovine and buffalo bulls

E. Piasentier, M. Spanghero, L. Gracco and R. Valusso, Dipartimento Scienze Produzione Animale, Università di Udine, Via S. Mauro 2, 33010 Pagnacco, Udine, Italy*

The research was performed on four Italian Mediterranean buffalo and four Italian Simmental young bulls, slaughtered at 10 months.
Buffalo grew at a lesser daily rate than bovine (930 vs. 1040 g/d), reaching a comparable live weight (320 kg, on average) in a period 2 weeks longer than cattle. At 10 months, buffalo achieved shorter body and carcass lenght than cattle and presented wider rump and thicker and shorter thigh. Dressing percentage did not differ between species, although buffalo had hide and head relatively heavier than bovine, the hindquarter of which provided a greater proportion of lean, owing to a minor proportion of trimmed fat.
Buffalo meat was redder and tender (WBSF: 46.3 vs. 68.8 N) than beef in both *longissimus thoracis* (LT) and *semitendinosus* (ST) muscles; LT was darker, redder and tender than ST in both species. Buffalo intramuscular fat had higher saturated fatty acid than bovine, owing to a greater concentration of stearic acid (21.54 vs. 14.36%). It was also richer of oleic acid (32.81 vs. 28.76 %) and poorer of palmitic acid (1.57 vs. 2.76 %) as well as of PUFA, while had significantly higher n6-PUFA/n3-PUFA ratio (16.69 vs. 12.29). Consumers rated differently cooked buffalo and bovine meat for flavour, tenderness and overall liking, with higher hedonistic scores for the buffalo product.

Poster C4.54

Organic beef production system: carcass and meat quality

C. Russo and G. Preziuso, Department of Animal Production, University of Pisa, Viale delle Piagge, 2, Pisa, Italy*

The aim was to verify organic system effect on carcass and meat quality of beefs. Twelve carcasses derived from Limousine x Red Pied beef, reared in the San Rossore Park (Tuscany) and slaughtered at 24 months of age, were used. After 24h post-mortem, carcasses were evaluated according to UE classification grid: on right half carcasses several measurements were taken and carcass compacteness was calculated. After 7 days of ageing longissimus thoracis, semitendinosus and triceps brachii muscles were analysed for pH, meat colour, water holding capacity, tenderness, chemical composition, fatty acid and cholesterol content. Results underlined the good quality of meat obtained from organic system in terms of colour, tenderness, water holding capacity and suitability for domestic storage. The meat had a low content of intramuscular fat; atherogenic and thrombogenic indices were rather high, testifying the high saturated fatty-acids content, probably due both to the inadequate finishing period, both to the high slaughtering age. An appropriate finishing period, in respect of the organic guidelines, should anticipate slaughtering age and improve carcass performance, obtaining higher intramuscular fat, and perhaps lower atherogenic and thrombogenic indices. Semitendinosus appeared more agreeable due to its paler and lighter meat, but was less tender and had worst water holding capacity; instead longissimus thoracis and triceps brachii, although slightly darker, gave meat more tender and with better water holding capacity.

Poster C4.55

Investigation about livestock farming systems in the Sibillini National Park area (Umbria - Italy)

L. Morbidini[1], M. Pauselli[1], D. Donnini[2] and R. Torricelli[2], [1]Dipartimento Scienze Zootecniche, Borgo XX Giugno, 74, 06121 Perugia, Italy, [2]Dipartimento Biologia Vegetale e Biotecnologie Ambientali, Borgo XX Giugno, 74, 06121 Perugia, Italy.*

An investigation about structure of 60 cattle and sheep farms in the Sibillini National Park (Umbria - Italy) were performed. The mountain farms (range: 350-1500 m a.s.l.), had a Useful Agricultural Surface from 0 to 390 ha, 33% of which in ownership and 67% in rental (collective pastures). The average age of shepherds was of about 47 years. Sixty-one % of farms practised 6 months of transhumance in the collective spaces, with 50 cattle/farm or 260 sheep/farm. Organic farming systems involved 31% of farms; 13% practised agri-tourism. Forty-one % of farms raised cattle (average 63 heads/farms), 60% of them were dairy herds (kg 4.866 of milk/head). About 84% of farms raised (alone or with other species) sheep (229 sheep/farm); 53% of the herds milked (62 kg of milk/head). Sixteen % of farms raised goats and 5% swine, for self-consumption. Dairy cattle were primarily Holstein, beef one were crossbreds or Chianina or Marchigiana. Most of sheep were crossbreds (on Sopravissana and Comisana basis) or Apennine or Suffolk. Market aspects pointed out the local sale either for the milk/cheese or for the calves/lambs. The results showed the need of qualification by tying local productions to the Sibillini park image, through the use of labels or traceability.

Poster C4.56

Beef quality meat on Piemontese breed: ageing effect on tenderness and myofibrillar degradation

S. Failla, G.M. Cerbini, F. Saltalamacchia, A. Di Giacomo, D. Settineri, Animal Production Research Institute - Via Salaria, 31, 00016 Monterotondo (Roma), Italy*

An effective control and a continuous improvement of the meat products quality are more and more important to assure consumer satisfaction and to increase the product market.
The target of this work is to verify if it is possible to make some consideration about final meat quality through non-destructive analysis, carried out in the first days after slaughter.
The tests have been executed on fifteen animals of Piemontese breed of an average weight at slaughter of 528,8 kg, and analysed parameters were pH, colour through spectrophotometric analysis (as non-destructive index), MFI, drip loss and tenderness. Samples have been drawn at different moments from the slaughter, exactly at 0, 24, 48, 72 hours and at 5 and 8 days.
We found a colour increase, particularly in Soret peak (420 nm) and between 24h and 8d, lightness (L*) values grew from 39,75 to 44,00, while redness (a*) grew from 14,84 to 16,71 and yellowness (b*) from 12,17 to 15,70. The pH decreased immediately from 6.51 ± 0.177 at 0h to 5.56± 0.05 at the 8th day from slaughter. MFI increased gradually until the 8th day.
The analyzed parameters are highly correlated with tenderness on cooked meat at 8d (5,31 kg) and can be used as predictor.

Poster C4.57

Assessment of genetic variation in meat quality and the evaluation of the role of candidate genes in beef characteristics with a view to breeding for improved product quality (GemQual)

J.L. Williams[1], J. Wood[2], P. Ertbjerg[3], S. Dunner[4], C. Sanudo[5], P. Albertí Lasalle[6], A. Valentini[7], S. Gigli[8], H. Leveziel[9], J-F. Hocquette[10], [1]Roslin Institute (Edinburgh), Roslin Midlothian EH25 9PS Scotland., [2]University of Bristol, Langford, Bristol BS18 7DY UK, [3]Royal Veterinary and Agricultural University, Rolighedsvej 30, 1958 Frederiksberg C, Denmark, [4]Facultad de Veterinaria, University of Madrid, Madrid 28040 Spain, [5]Facultad de Veterinaria, University of Zaragoza, Miguel Servet 177, 50.013-Zaragoza Spain, [6]Servicio de Investigación Agroalimentaria, Apartado 727, 50080 Zaragoza. Spain, [7]Universita della Tuscia, via de Lellis, 01100 Viterbo, Italy, [8]Istituto Sperimentale di Zootecnia, Via Salaria 31, Monterotondo, Rome 00016, Italy. [9]INRA-Université de Limoges,123, Avenue Albert Thomas 87060 LIMOGES cedex, [10]INRA-Centre de Clermont-Fd/Theix, Theix, 63122 Saint-Genès-Champanelle, France*

There are undoubtedly genetic factors influencing meat quality, such as fatty acid composition, fat distribution, muscle fibre type, connective tissue properties etc and there is mounting evidence that there is variation in the quality of meat from different cattle breeds, but this has not been rigorously tested. This EC funded project is examining the genetic component of variation in meat quality by carrying out detailed measurements on genetically diverse breeds of cattle reared, as far as possible, under uniform conditions. Candidate genes, which may affect meat quality, have been selected and polymorphisms are being identified within these genes. The association between polymorphisms in the genes and the observed variation in meat quality will then be tested.

Theatre C5.1

Different approaches for giving advice to cattle farmers: the chart of good practices

A.C. Dockès, C. Hedouin, Institut de l'Elevage 149 rue de Bercy 75595 Paris cedex 12

Cattle breeders are permanently making technical and economic decisions about their farms. They use their knowledge, their social representations, discussions in social groups and the practical aspects involved. Advice can help them to make these decisions. Advisory operations can be managed as projects and take into account the diversity of breeders' expectations. A collective approach of advisory operations aims at maintaining the efficiency of the small group advice while applying to the greatest number of breeders. In this paper, we are going to present a Charter of 35 good practices which has been proposed to cattle farmers for 3 years. This charter concerns different aspects of the cattle farms and different questions asked by the consumers: cattle identification, sanitary aspects, food quality and trace back, animal welfare and environment. The Charter is organised at National and Regional levels. 50 000 farmers have signed this Charter, and a pool of 2500 technicians have been trained to advice and accompany them. A recent evaluation of the Charter has been realised, which shows the necessity: to increase the communication around the Charter; to train frequently the technicians; to give farmers some tools to explain their action to the public; to organise specific advice to small farmers. These different aspects will be the main objectives of the next years.

Theatre C5.2

How environmental problems are adressed to farmers - pyramid model, research, knowledge transfer, practices and attitudes

K. de Grip[1], A. Kuipers[2] and P.J .Galama[3] ,[1]Communication and Innovation Studies, [2]Expertisecentre for farm management and knowledge transfer, [3]Institute for Animal Husbandry, Wageningen University &Researchcentre, The Netherlands

In the 1990's the public extension service was privatised. The Ministry of Agriculture continued to support extension activities in areas such as environment and nature management. A pyramid model shows the know-how development and transfer of environmental activities in the dairy sector. From top to bottom we find research farm(s), discovery farms, demo-farms and the large group of "average" farms. As research farm, The Marke was founded in 1990, where management practices were examined to diminish mineral losses. Later, 17 discovery and 175 demo-farms were established to further test and gain on-farm experiences with the various management practices. Besides reports, know-how transfer was performed through field days, farmers meetings and study-groups. Keywords appeared to be clear goals, farmer-to-farmer exchange, objectivity and an open attitude. However, studies indicated that these activities were not enough to reach the "average" farmers sufficiently. A Mineral-management Support Unit was set up in 2002 to stimulate knowledge exchange and to experiment with demand driven extension. 80.000 farmers could request a free voucher worth € 250,- to buy a knowledge product, which were exposed in the 'knowledge shop' on website. Farmers could also join a study group to articulate their need together and buy a 'knowledge product' collectively. Trained farmers coordinated these groups. The Support Unit also developes a quality system by use of client satisfaction studies to contribute to a transparant knowledge market.

 Theatre C5.3

Know-how transfer in animal breeding - the power of integrated cow data bases for farmer´s selection of bulls to improve functional traits in dairy cows

J. Philipsson[1], *Jan-Åke Eriksson*[2] *and Hans Stålhammar*[3], [1]*Dept. of Animal Breeding and Genetics, SLU, Box 7023, SE-750 07 Uppsala, Sweden.* [2]*Swedish Dairy Association, Hållsta, SE-631 84 Eskilstuna,* [3]*Svensk Avel, Örnsro, SE-532 94 Skara, Sweden.*

Animal breeding research is usually based on different types of data, e.g. from laboratory analyses, selection experiments and field records. The latter type plays an important role in linking research with practical animal husbandry and breeding. Information about large animal populations in normal production systems is collected from the routine recording schemes, such as milk- and beef-recording, and artificial insemination services (AI). These data provide two essential roles in context of research and know-how transfer: i) In providing data for analyses, research results will be implemented through improved methods directly applied in the recording schemes, or information that these provide to farmers, e.g. improved estimates of breeding values of bulls and cows. ii) Integrating data from different sources enables more holistic farm and animal analyses, and as regards genetics, to estimate breeding values for a range of production and functional traits. In Sweden this integration of different sources of data and computer systems started already in the sixties and has allowed dairy farmers in the last two decades to select AI bulls according to production, female fertility, calving performance, health and conformation traits, all incorporated into a Total Merit Index.

Theatre C5.4

Extension work in dairy and beef husbandry in Slovenija

*J. Osterc** *and M. Klopcic, Biotechnical Faculty, Zootechnical Department, Groblje 3, 1230 Domzale, Slovenia.*

In CEE countries a trend of decreased milk and beef production has been observed after the year 1990. In Slovenia, milk deliveries increased 30 % in this period, while veal and beef production stayed at the same level as it was in 1990. Milk yield of recorded cows increased from 4,131 kg in 1990 to 5,561 kg in 2002, and the percentage of recorded cows from 33 to 66 % of dairy cows. Both, microbiological and hygienic quality of milk substantially improved. In 1994, only 60 % of purchased milk contained less than 100,000 m.o./ml, and 97 % in 2002. In the same period the percentage of milk with less than 400,000 SCC/ml increased from 75 to 93 %. The improvements are mostly due to the efficient extension work, backed by the Zootechnical Department. Up to the year 1990, the extension work was performed through farm cooperatives, partly financed by the state. After the independence of Slovenia the extension work became part of the Ministry of Agriculture and financed from the state budget. Since 2000, extension work as well as milk recording and animal breeding have been under the responsibility of the Agricultural Chamber. The government finances most of these activities. These changes ensured the continuation of successful extension work. Recently, a change of A4-to alternating (AT) recording is analysed and proposed. Concerning quality, further activities are under way to improve research, educational and extension work.

Theatre C5.5

Factors determining technology adoption by beef producers in the United States

L.L. Berger, University of Illinois, 164 Animal Sciences Lab, Urbana, IL. 61801 USA*

The cattle industry in the USA is divided into three distinct segments, dairy production, beef cow-calf production and beef feedlot production. There are 840,000 cow-calf producers, with 78% of the producers having less than 50 cows. In contrast, there are just over 2000 feedlots that market 87% of all the finished cattle. Economics drives technology adoption, but the magnitude of improvement has to be much greater for cow-calf producers than feedlots. Ease of technology application is also much more important for cow-calf producers. We developed alkaline peroxide treatment of low quality forages with the cow-calf producer in mind. This treatment process could decrease feed cost by increasing the digestibility of crop residues from 50% to 70%, while costing approximately $40 per metric ton. The adoption of this technology has been slow due to low corn prices, and the need for special pumps, scales and mixers which most producers saw as too expensive and complicated. In contrast, we have been working with local feedlots to use ultrasound carcass evaluation as a tool to sort feedlot cattle for niche markets. Despite the fact that the technology cost over $20,000 and the return per head is likely $10-20, an increasing number of feedlots are using this method to sort cattle. Because of the large volume, small improvements per head will justify the adoption of this technology.

Theatre C5.6

Focushed research, information transfer and advising: first evaluation of a new approach undertaken in Emilia-Romagna

A. Magnavacchi[1] and G. Cargioli[2], [1]Centro Ricerche Produzioni Animali CRPA SpA, C.so Garibaldi 42, 42100 Reggio Emilia, Italy, [2]Regione Emilia-Romagna, Direzione Agricoltura, Viale Silvani 6, 40122 Bologna.*

The high quality products made in an environmentally friendly manner has always been the goal for the agricultural policy of the Regione Emilia-Romagna. Parmesan Cheese, Parma Ham, Culatello and a number of other animal products are the testimonials of the success of such a policy. In order to enforce the application of the political guidelines the Regional administration designed a «system for agricultural development» based on private guidance, competition and transparency. The paper illustrates the experience of CRPA SpA, a mixed public/private organization operating in the animal production sector with the role of catching the research need, setting up and managing projects, disseminating the findings of the researches. Figures of structural aspects as well as about the effect of «privatising» the traditionally public system and promoting competition, show that strong improvement in efficiency can be reached. Less clear results can be cited for technology transfer and knowledge exploitation where the lack of tools and methods for impact benchmarking does not allow a definitive evaluation. Success cases and general hypothesis will then be presented as well as some early trial to measure the efficiency of the information flow and the impact of the new approach at the farm and at the sector level.

Theatre C5.7

The impact of the Zimbabwean change process on dairy farming and farmer attitudes

S.M. Makuza[1] and C.B.A. Wollny[2], [1]Department of Animal Science, University of Zimbabwe, P. O. Box MP 167, Mount Pleasant, Harare, Zimbabwe, [2]Institute of Animal Breeding and Genetics, University of Göttingen, Kellnerweg 6, 37077, Göttingen, Germany

Approximately 95% of Zimbabwean milk is produced by the large scale commercial sector and only 5 % is contributed by the small scale farmer. Foreign currency shortage is affecting genetic improvement, which depends on imports of genetic material. In the smallholder sector lack of a national breeding programme resulted in indiscriminate crossbreeding. In 1980 Zimbabwe's Land Reform and Resettlement Programme was implemented. In 2000 it was fast tracked for political reasons with the following effects: reduction of the large scale commercial dairy farm sector, destocking of herds, changing of land use and ownership patterns, or relocating to neighbouring countries. Consequently the number of dairy farmers declined by 43%, the national dairy herd by 63% and milk deliveries by 50% since 1999. Currently there are milk and dairy product shortages. The relationship between commercial dairy farmers and the Government is characterised by a negative, hostile and confrontational interaction and attitude. The drastic impact of the ongoing change process requires development of adequate breeding programmes and policies for the future of the dairy industry. Regardless of the legal status the newly resettled Zimbabwean farmers require adequate economic and technical training to improve their skills, knowledge and understanding of dairy farming.

Theatre C5.8

Diagnosis and design of smallholder dairy recording in Malawi

A.C.M. Msiska[1], M.G.G. Chagunda[2], H. Tchale[3], J.W. Banda[1],and C.B.A. Wollny[4], [1]Department of Animal Science, University of Malawi, , Lilongwe, Malawi, [2]Department of Animal Health and Welfare, Danish Institute of Agricultural Sciences, Foulum, Denmark, [3]Center for Development Research (ZEF), University of Bonn, Bonn, Germany, [4]Institute of Animal Breeding and Genetics, University of Göttingen, Göttingen, Germany*

Adoption of dairy recording schemes remains poor in Malawi. To investigate some of the root causes, a study on farmer perception on record keeping and factors affecting its adoption was conducted. Eighty-six smallholder farmers from six dairy cooperative schemes of Lilongwe were randomly interviewed. A logit regression approach was used to analyze the adoption decision. The results indicated a positive relationship between participation in dairy recording and the individual assigned the recording task ($P<0.01$), milk recording using simple calibrated containers ($P<0.05$) and also herd size ($P<0.05$). A negative relationship was found between recording participation and the following factors: recording using calibrated scales ($P<0.01$), sale of milk at the informal market ($P<0.10$) as opposed to the formal market, and use of natural service ($P<0.10$) as opposed to artificial insemination for breeding. Farmer education level, cattle genotype, and daily milk yield had no significant influence on the adoption of milk recording. Based on the experiences and lessons learnt, a farmer-participatory recording system using simple equipment like calibrated one-litre cups and based on daily recording was designed, successfully tested and adopted.

Theatre C5.9

Use of management practices to differentiate dairy herd environments in Southeastern Sicily

E. Raffrenato[1,2,], P.A. Oltenacu[2], R.W. Blake[2] and G. Licitra[1,3]. [1]CoRFiLaC, Regione Siciliana, s.p. 25 km 5, 97100 Ragusa, Italy, [2]Department of Animal Science, Cornell University,Ithaca, NY, USA, [3]D.A.C.P.A., Università di Catania, Italy*

An outreach program with modest resources must set priorities for maximum impact. The objective of this study was to develop methodology for defining the target population for a program focusing on herd management practices. Information from 254 herds collected in the summer of 2000 using a direct interview questionnaire described 23 nutritional, udder health, milking and reproductive management practices. The 183 Friesian herds in the study averaged 35 lactating cows and 8640 kg/lactation of milk; 71 Brown Swiss herds averaged 25 lactating cows and 6443 kg milk. For Friesian (Brown Swiss) herds 10 (11) practices were significantly associated with milk production and 9 (8) practices were associated with somatic cell score. A clustering procedure (flexible beta method) permitted defining low and high opportunity herd environments based on these practices. The average difference between low and high Friesian (Brown Swiss) environments were 2007 kg (1792 kg) milk and -0.72 unit (-0.41 unit) somatic cell score. The clustering method was an effective way to identify the target population of herds and the management practices for priority attention.

Poster C5.10

Results of a PreSynch OvSynch protocol in nine Ragusa dairy herds

J.D. Ferguson[1,], D.T. Galligan[1], J.W. Brooks[2], G. Azzaro[2], S. Villari[2], S. Ventura[2] and G. Licitra[2,3]. [1]University of Pennsylvania, Kennett Square, PA; [2]CoRFiLaC, s.p. 25 km 5, 97100 Ragusa, Italy; [3]D.A.C.P.A., Università di Catania, Italy.*

Nine Holstein herds (SYNCH) (size:30-140 cows) participated in a breeding protocol with Presynch-Ovsynch-Postsynch. The trial included cows calving between Mar., 2001 to Feb., 2002 (2001). Nine herds (CON, matched on size, production, artificial insemination) served as contemporary controls. Historical herd records were collected for cows calving Mar., 1999 to Feb., 2000 (1999). The Presynch-Ovsynch protocol was as follows: prostaglandin (PGF), 21-27 d; PGF, 35-41 d; GnRH, 49-55d; PGF, 56-62 d; GnRH, 58-63 d; insemination 59-64 d, postcalving. Postsynch protocol was applied to cows not seen in estrus 21 d following first insemination (POSTAI): GnRH , 32 d POSTAI; rectal examination for pregnancy at 39 d POSTAI; if not pregnant, PGF, 39 d POSTAI; GnRH, 41 d POSTAI; appointment inseminated, 42 d POSTAI. Results for number cows inseminated (Nins), pregnant (Npreg), days to first breeding (DFB), days open (DO), first service conception rate (FSTCR), and DO survival analysis (DO_KM) were as follows:

Year	Group	Nins	Npreg	DFB	sem	DO	sem	FSTCR,%	DO_KM	
1999	CON	501	332	79.6	2.3	154.6	6.1	25.5	199.9	6.2
1999	SYNCH	580	415	77.5	1.8	154.6	4.8	23.4	179.0b	4.9
2001	CON	517	483	79.2	2.3	167.0	4.7	26.0	199.4	6.2
2001	SYNCH	529	502	68.2a	1.8	129.7a	5.0	33.1	157.0a	5.4

Poster C5.11

Ingestive behaviour of free grazing bovines in range lands. Method of intake by Balent and Gibon - a proposal of evolution

J.C-R Santos and R.A G. Pinheiro. Divisão Producão Animal (DRAEDM)-Quinta do Pinhó, 4800-875, Portugal.*

Beyond ingestive behaviour we present a development in the method proposed by Balent and Gibon (1986) in order to evaluate the intake (QI) of free-grazing bovines in Peneda´s mountain. After previous (2001) work we also studied the following parameters related to rumination: time (in seconds) spent in each period of rumination (DPR), number of regurgitations (NR) by rumination period; number of chewings in each regurgitation (NMR) and the time (in seconds) of each regurgitation (TR). To study ingestive behaviour we made direct observation and used focal-animal sampling method proposed by Altmann (1973) in 24 hour-periods. Our proposal is based on correlations and regression lines, between QI and DPR in 24 hours (r=0.74 with an R^2 adj.=0.99 for a $P<0.05$), between DPR and NR (r=0.97 with an R^2 adj.=0.92 for a $P<0.001$) and only in daylight (r=0.52), and between DPR and NR (r=0.72 with an R^2 adj.=0.5 for a $P<0.001$) in each period of rumination. Although more work needs to be done on this subject, a positive correlation was found between intake (QI) and time spent in rumination (DPR). Due to a good correlation between DPR and NR it is concluded that intake of free-grazing bovines on Peneda's mountain can be evaluated by counting the animal's NR while ruminating only during the daylight period.

Poster C5.12

Effect of the inclusion of low levels of salts of sulphite on the aerobic stability and intake levels of whole crop wheat and grazing of dairy cattle

J.K. Margerison and R.R. Edwards. University of Plymouth at Seale Hayne, Netwton Abbot, Devon. UK. TQ12 3LT.*

Two experiments were completed to measure the effect of salts of sulphite on the stability of whole crop wheat (WSW) buffer feed to dairy cattle. Experiment 1, 40 cows at 60 days postpartum, were allocated in pairs, 20 received WSW with no additive (NoSS), 20 received WSW with added sulphite salts (SS). Diets were fed for 42 days, with a 28 day measurement period. Pre-treatment milk yield and composition were used as covariates. Experiment 2, 1.5 kg of WSW from each treatment (experiment 1) was used for laboratory erobic styability studies and plate yeast culture. WSW intake levels (kg DM/d) were significantly lower in SS 6.9, NoSS 5.9 (sem0.19), grazing time (min/d) SS - 263.5, NoSS 296.0 (sem 6.911), ruminating time (min /d), SS 546.6, NoSS 530.8, 3.353 was significantly greater with NoSS. Diet had no effect on milk yield (kg/d), SS 33.3, NoSS 32.9, (sem 0.52), milk fat (g/kg), SS 40.5, NoSS 42.1, 0.07 or protein (g/kg), SS 33.6, NoSS 33.6, (0.03) content. Mean live weight (kg) was significantly greater in SS cows, SS 666.81, NoSS 660.14 (0.823). Time to peak temperature (h), SS 128.64, NoSS 82.89 (1.547), maximum temperature (°C), SS 6.76, NoSS 10.90 (0.372) heat generated (°C), SS 39744.0, NoSS 54938.0 (1171.00) and yeast numbers (NoSS 4.951, NSS 4.156 (0.62) log cfu/ml) were greater with NoSS. In conclusion, silage quality, live weight gain and eraobic stability of WCW was increased by the addition of salts of sulphite.

Theatre CM6.1

Design of large scale dairy cattle units in relation to management and animal welfare

R.W. Palmer, University of Wisconsin, 1675 Observatory Drive, Madison, WI 53706, USA.*

Large scale dairies have become very popular because of the adoption of new housing styles and management procedures which allow producers to enhance labor efficiency, increase profits, and improve the quality of life of dairy owners and workers. For a large dairy to be labor efficient and conducive to animal health and welfare it must be designed to: 1) group animals with like needs; 2) allow easy movement of animals; 3) allow easy selection and restraint of animals for health and reproductive treatments; 4) provide for physical separation of disease infected animals; and 5) provide easy access for feed delivery and manure removal. Far-off dry, close-up dry, maternity, just fresh, milking and sick groups of cows should be housed separately. The number and size of each group type depends on total herd size and the management practices expected. Milking group sizes should be based on expected parlor throughput values which are influenced by milk production levels, milking procedures, milking frequency, etc. Animal health and welfare issues relate directly to profitability in that unhealthy cows lead to high culling rates, low production levels and increased treatment costs. Cows are most susceptible to health problems during the transition phase (-21d to +21d of calving). To minimize health related problems proper freestall design, alley surface design, and transition cow facilities must be incorporated into the dairies facility design.

Theatre CM6.2

Changes of management in Slovak, Czech and Hungarian large-scale dairy farms after transition to market economy

S. Mihina[1], V. Matlova[2] and F. Szabo[3], [1]Research Institute for Animal Production, Hlohovska 2, 94992 Nitra, Slovak Republic, [2]Research Institute for Animal Production Pratelstvi 815, 104 Prague, Czech Republic, [3]Georgikon Faculty of Agriculture, Deak F.u. 16, 8360 Keszthely, Hungary

In the Slovak Republic, the Czech Republic and Hungary, dairy cattle farms are mostly of larger capacity, although smaller family farms also emerged after 1989. In many cases the farms have more than 400 dairy cows kept at one location. The larger number of animals and the different approaches of managers and hired workers, compared with family members, affect the whole management of the farm. In this paper, the real situation in the management of reproduction, nutrition and feeding, quality of products, health care of animals, housing and technology on larger farms in specific Central European countries is presented. On family farms with lower capacity, animals are treated much more individually than on larger farms. On farms with larger capacity, although the individual approach is also needed, herds are divided into groups, and reproduction and feeding are managed using a "group approach". Transition to the market economy in certain countries opened new possibilities of modernising the farms. It can have a positive effect on quality of products and on animal welfare. The respective advantages of the more individual approach on smaller farms, and the greater space and investment possibilities on larger farms, are discussed.

Theatre CM6.3

Health management in large-scale dairy farms

J.P.T.M. Noordhuizen[*1], K.E. Müller[2], [1]Dept. of Farm Animal Health, Faculty of Veterinary Medicine, Utrecht University, P.O.Box 80151, 3508 TD Utrecht, The Netherlands; [2]Klinik für Klauentiere, Fachbereich Veterinärmedizin, Freie Universität Berlin, Germany*

Large-scale dairy farms are found throughout the world. In public opinion they often are said to hamper animal health and welfare due to their level of industrialisation and the great potential for transmission of disease agents in the highly-dense population, and their focus on increasing profits and reducing costs. Especially within Europe there are various directives centering around animal hygiene, animal welfare and health, and food safety. Not in the least because consumer protection in the broadest sense is playing a paramount role. In this presentation it will be shown how managerial and organisational science principles apply to these farms by operationalising goals, conduct monitoring on animals and farm conditions, execute performance evaluation and risk assessment, and how as a consequence the herd health management can be designed and executed. By continuous monitoring of cattle and farm data for rapidly obtaining performance signals, and by inspection of farm risk conditions potentially contributing to disease occurrence, applied at the level of separate units within the dairy operation, the whole production process may be controlled. The ultimate target is to have an early warning system to detect pending problems and adjust in time, and to safeguard the products from becoming aberrant. It is concluded that by integrating herd health and welfare issues in an overall quality control programme at farm level the management efficiency is substantially increased and animal health safeguarded.

Theatre CM6.4

The effect of management factors on somatic cell counts and specific mastitis causing pathogens in large-scale dairy units

R.-D. Fahr[1], A.-A.A. Fadl-el-Moula[1], G. Anacker[2] and H.H. Swalve[1], [1]Institute of Animal Breeding and Animal Husbandry, University of Halle, D-06099 Halle, Germany, [2]Thüringer Landesanstalt für Landwirtschaft, Jena, Germany.*

Aim of the present study was to examine the frequency of specific pathogens under differential management situations and the relationship of type of pathogen with somatic cell count in the milk. 65,542 milk samples of 10,741 cows were analyzed during the period of June 1998 to April 2000. Cows originated from 48 randomly selected large-scale dairy units in the state ofThuringia. Somatic cell counts stemmed from the official milk recording scheme and information on management factors were collected via a questionnaire. S. aureus and CNS were the most frequent pathogens (35.5% and 32.7%, respectively) found in the quarter samples. Hygienic factors were stronger associated with the frequency of contagious pathogens than with environmental pathogens. In all samples, somatic cell counts were lowest for samples without bacteriological findings. Samples with environmental pathogens had lower cell counts than those with contagious pathogens. Bacteriological examinations are of great help when interpreting somatic cell counts from milk recording schemes and should also be used when selecting for resistance to mastitis.

Theatre CM6.5

Animal health of herds converting to automatic milking

M.D. Rasmussen[1] and F. Skjøth[2], [1]Danish Institute of Agricultural Sciences, Foulum, DK-8830 Tjele, Denmark, [2]Danish Cattle, Skejby, DK-8200 Aarhus C, Denmark*

Treatments of diseases in 404 herds were recorded and analysed in respect to change of housing and milking system. 234 herds changed from stanchion barn to loose house with a milking parlour, 65 herds had loose housing but changed from parlour to automatic milking, and 105 herds changed from stanchion barn to automatic milking. Recordings of veterinary treatments, cow cell counts, and bulk milk quality were included in the analysis from 9 to 3 months before a shift and from 3 to 9 months after.
Bulk milk cell count remained unchanged no matter the housing or milking system. The frequency of acutely elevated cell counts decreased of herds changing to parlour milking but increased for herds milking automatically. The frequency of teat tramps was reduced about 50% by the change of housing system indicating that this frequency was highest for tied cows. Stanchion barns also had the highest frequency of manually birth help, which may explain why the frequency of retained placenta was lower after changing to loose housing. Automatic milking did not improve udder health as expected with the higher frequency of milking and a change in housing system did not improve udder health as seen for herds converting from stanchion barn housing to loose housing with parlour milking.

Theatre CM6.6

Genetic and nongenetic influences on fertility traits in large scale saxinian dairy cattle units

U. Bergfeld, St. Pache, K. Heidig and U. Müller, Saxonian Federal Institution of Agriculture, Am Park 3, 04886 Köllitsch, Germany.*

Fertility is knows as a trait which is mainly influenced by management factors. However several studies have shown that parts of the fertility complex are much more genetic determained.
In this study different traits of the calving interval are investigated using multivariate statistical methods. Data of the saxonian dairy cattle population from several years were used. Different conditions concerning herd size, herd performance, feeding and management conditions were included. The herd sizes ranged from fewer than 100 up to much more then 1000 cowes per herd. With a multivariat animal model with all relationship included genetic and nongenetic variances und covariances between the different conditions were estimated. The herds were classified depending of the different conditions and the performances under the different conditions were considered as different traits.

Theatre CM6.7

Association of type, efficiency of herdlifetime performance and longevity in selection of Holstein-Friesian cows

J. Püski[1], I. Györkös[2], E. Szücs[1], S. Bozó[2], T. A. Tuan[1] and J. Völgyi Csík[2], [1]Szent István University, Páter Károly street 1, 2103 Gödöllö, Hungary, [2]Research Institute for Animal Breeding and Nutrition, Gesztenyés street 1, 2053 Herceghalom, Hungary*

Conclusions of this study reveal that, lifetime production of wide cows with average stature, deeper trunk, more strength and larger body capacity exceeded that of narrow ones by 3,257 Kgs of milk. The efficiency of lifetime production of narrow cows seemed to be smaller than that of wide cows by 13-15%. In narrow cows, under identical environmental conditions, in wide ones this highly improved efficiency can be decreased considerably in case of high level of load, the explanation of which might be due to their depressed adaptation ability in comparison with their wider counterparts. For narrow and wide cows, this phenomenon results in significant decrease in stayability, the figures of which were 19.3% and 0.5%, i.e. 30.0% and 1,7%, respectively. As for longevity, the same figures of narrow and wide cows were 696 and 807days, respectively. In addition to total milk yield, due to the considerable contribution of wide cows in terms of efficiency of lifetime milk production, the size of cows has to be taken in selection, too. Cows with medium stature, average or above average rump width and trunk depth perform best in terms of long productive life, lifetime production and milk production efficiency on lifetime basis. The authors emphasise the superiority of medium sized cows from the viewpoint of efficiency.

Poster CM6.8

Influence of housing systems on fertility and longevity of Swiss Brown cows

J.C. Bielfeldt[1],K.-H. Tölle[1], R. Badertscher[2], J. Krieter[1],[1]Institute for Animal Breeding and Husbandry, Christian-Albrechts-University,24098 Kiel, Germany, [2]Swiss Federal Research Station for Agricultural Economics and Engineering, 8356 Tänikon, Switzerland*

During the last years dairy cattle housing systems changed from tie-stall barns to cubicle houses. Therefore the aim of this investigation was to analyse the influence of housing systems on bovine fertility and longevity.

212,656 records from Swiss Brown cows in eastern and central Switzerland that calved from January, 1988 to May, 2002 were analysed concerning days to first service, days open and conception rate. The intervals from calving to first service and to successful insemination were 69 and 86 days, resp., for loose-housed animals. Cows in tied systems had significant longer intervals (72 and 99 days, resp.). Conception rate was approximately 4% lower for cows in tie-stall barns (46%) compared with cubicle systems (50%).

For survival analysis records of 79,357 Swiss Brown cows that calved from January, 1987 to May, 2002 were used. Data contained 32.4% right-censored records. Besides the random effect herd-year-season, the Weibull model included effects of age at first calving, parity, lactation stage, relative sum of fat and protein yield within herd and housing system. The probability of animals being culled increased with high age at first calving (1.06) and in low producing cows (2.10). The relative risk of being culled was about 15% lower for cows in loose housing systems (0.87) than in tied systems (1.02).

Poster CM6.9

Evaluation of health udder status and economy of selected systems of prevention

L. Stádník and R. Tousová, Department of Cattle Breeding and Dairying, Czech University of Agriculture, Kamycká 129,165 21, Prague 6 - Suchdol, Czech Republic

The health of the lacteal gland is one of the secondary selection indices considered for cattle selection and breeding in the near future. Suitable prevention is a prerequisite for optimum economy and achieving high-quality production. Average production value of investigated herd was on the level of 9,353 kg of milk. Dairy cows with increased content of somatic cells in milk have been selected as experimental group. The analyses of somatic cells content in individual milk samples have been made. The aim of our investigations has been to evaluate the possibility of applying selected preparations in the system of prevention and sanitation of lacteal gland. Average milk efficiency of the whole herd during the inspection day in May was 30.9 liter of milk, and in the experimental group 38.1 kg of milk. During the first month of treatment the content of somatic cells in the experimental group decreased onto 34.68 per cent of original level. In the whole herd there was no decrease - just to the value of 78.05 per cent of original level. In the experimental group the content of somatic cells decreased onto 88.30 per cent during the whole investigated period. In the same period the average content of somatic cells in the whole herd increased to 111.6 per cent of original level.

Poster CM6.10

The intensity and causes of culling Black and White cows in commercial herds with various forms of ownership

I. Antkowiak, J. Pytlewski,Z. Dorynek. Chair of Cattle Breeding, Agricultural University 60-625 Poznan, ul.Wojska Polskiego 71A, Poland.

The investigations were conducted in the years 1997-2000 in two commercial farms with differing forms of ownership. The analysis concerned the intensity and causes of culling of Black and White cows with differing shares of Holstein-Friesian cattle genes in their genotypes. One farm belonged to the Breeding Centre Ltd. (Osrodek Hodowli Zarodowej Sp. z o.o) [I], whereas the other was privately owned [II]. The average annual stocking in the farms was 126 and 224 cows, respectively. The mean milk yield in the analyzed herds was similar, with approx. 6400 kg of milk with the fat content of approx. 4,10% and protein content of approx. 3,30%. In both farms the adopted housing system was indoor keeping. Cows were milked twice a day using milking pipeline machines. During the analyzed period in farm I 26,69% of cows were culled, whereas in farm II it was 22,52%. The most frequent reason for the removal of cows from the herds in both farms was their sterility (I - 44,03% and II - 55,94%). Another cause of culling were accidents: 25,37% and 28,22%, respectively. Other important reason for removal of animal in farm I were udder diseases (18,66%) and low milk yields (10,45%), whereas in farm II they were low yields (9,90%) and sale for further breeding (2,97%).

Poster CM6.11

Selected reproduction indexes of Black and White cows in the farm of the „Lubiana" Breeding Centre

J. Pytlewski, I. Antkowiak, Z. Dorynek. Chair of Cattle Breeding, Agricultural University 60-625 Poznan, ul.Wojska Polskiego 71A, Poland.

Selected breeding indexes of 438 primiparous cows of the Black and White breed with differing shares of Holstein-Friesian cattle genes in their genotype. The average milk yield of the cows was approx. 5900 kg of milk with the fat content of 4,19% and protein content of 3,18%. Breeding performance of cows was analyzed taking into consideration the age at calving, the calving interval, the interpregnancy period, the gestation length and number of sperm doses per successful conception. The obtained results were subjected to statistical analysis using the SASÒ software package. The average age at the first calving was 856 days. The lowest value of this index, i.e. 839 days was observed in the cows with share of the Holstein-Friesian cattle genes below 50%. While analyzing the use of sperm form the first successful conception, the worst result (2,31) was found in the cows with the highest share of Holstein-Friesian genes (over 75%). The average calving interval for all the genotypic groups was 405 days, whereas the lowest value of this period (371 days) was found in the cows the 50,01 -75% share of the Holstein-Friesian cattle genes. The longest interpregnancy period (146 days) was observed in the cows with genotype with over 75% of Holstein-Friesian cattle genes.

Poster CM6.12

The breeding of various performance types of cattle in identical technological conditions

A. Jezková, Czech University of Agriculture, Department of Cattle Breeding and Dairying, Prague, Kamycka, 165 21, Czech Republic

The work assessed the effect of rearing quality on milk production of a herd of Holstein (H) and Czech Pied (C) cattle. An evaluation was made of the impact of selected factors (breed, lactation sequence, age at first mating, live weight at the ages of 3, 6, 9, 12 and 15 months) on indices of milk production and reproduction (quantity of milk and contents of the milk components, age at first calving, length of calving interval, insemination index). We measured 8 bodily dimensions to characterize the growth of calves-heifers (height at withers, height at sacrum, direct body length, chest circumference, length of pelvis, front, middle and rear width of the pelvis). The results were evaluated statistically using a linear model in SAS software, with a correlation analysis for evaluating dependencies between the individual bodily measures.

The work included monitoring the behaviour of dairy Holstein and Czech Pied cows. In the course of ethological monitoring the dairy cows were found to behave calmly, without manifestations of aggressiveness while maintaining stereotypical behaviour. The chosen technology of housing and treating the dairy cows of both performance types (open cubicle-type stable) can be considered appropriate based on ethological observations.

Theatre SH3.1

Impact of horses on pastures and consequences for management

G. Fleurance[1], P. Duncan[2], D. Durant[2], G. Loucougaray[3], [1]Station Expérimentale des Haras Nationaux, 19370 Chamberet, France. [2]Centre d'Etudes Biologiques de Chizé, CNRS-UPR 1934, 79360 Beauvoir-sur-Niort, France. [3]UMR-CNRS 6553, Université Rennes 1, France.*

1. Impact on the vegetation and on wild animals

Pastures grazed by horses are characterised by strong spatial heterogeneity. This pattern contrasts sharply with cattle. Both species have an impact on colonisation of grasslands by shrubs and trees, but use different species. Horses kill a few species by bark stripping (e.g *Salix, Populus*) and trampling (*Vaccinium)*, while cattle eat a much wider range of dicotyledons. The quality of the resulting swards (N content) is often greater under horses as is plant species richness and diversity. Some vertebrates (and invertebrates) benefit from the spatial structure created by horse grazing, small mammals and waterbirds which prefer short swards and obtain higher rates of nutrient acquisition (e.g. wigeon, barnacle geese). Greylag geese prefer the taller, homogeneous swards (c. 12cm) produced by cattle grazing which allow them to feed faster.

2. Mechanisms involved in these contrasts between horses and ruminants

The foraging strategy of horses differs strongly from ruminants : horses maintain high rates of nutrient intake on pastures difficult for cattle (short and/or coarse). Cattle use plants with secondary metabolites which protect them from horses.

3. Consequences for the management of multiple use grazing systems

Horses and ruminants, singly or together, can be used to achieve a wide range of objectives, for conservation and production.

Theatre SH3.2

Conservation grazing in Scotland: a change in emphasis from stocking rate prescription towards management to achieve conservation targets?

A. Waterhouse and M.Pollock, SAC, Hill and Mountain Research Centre, Environment Research, Kirkton, Crianlarich, Perthshire, Scotland, FK20 8RU*

The majority of Scotland is grazed by livestock, or in remoter areas by managed red deer. Designated land covers 40% of the country. Many of these protected areas have habitats heavily influenced, if not created, by grazing. Appropriate grazing is thus important, with too little or too intense grazing being detrimental. Historically, cattle, horses, sheep and goats were all important in the uplands, but sheep are now dominant, though cattle are of considerable importance locally. Grazing by horses and goats is very limited. Considerable controversy exists over the best approach to establish appropriate management. Current practice in conservation grazing includes; (i)statutory controls to avoid 'over-grazing' under Less Favoured Areas Support Scheme; (ii) voluntary schemes e.g. Environmentally Sensitive Areas, Natural Care, Stewardship and Forestry Schemes; (iii) site specific management agreements to manage protected sites (e.g. Natura 2000); and (iv) voluntary approaches often managed by nature conservation NGO's. In the first two decades of large-scale conservation grazing, management options were restricted and usually prescribed by stocking rates. However, now a change in emphasis is occurring towards objectively measured criteria considering animal species, breed and seasonal timing of grazing to target conservation objectives. Better understanding of relationships between grazing, pastures and biodiversity is enabling this more objective approach though significant issues and problems remain.

Theatre SH3.3

Sustainable use of grassland with sheep in alpine regions

F. Ringdorfer, Federal Research Institute of Agriculture in Alpine Regions, Gumpenstein, Departement of Small Ruminants, A-8952 Irdning, Austria

The Alps are the greatest natural and cultural landscape in Europa. 13 million people live in an area of 191.287 km_, 8 countries are included. Sustainable development is one of the most important demand in future. Sustainable development means, that people who live in the Alps today can satisfy all their needs without diminishing the possibilities for the future generations to satisfy all their needs.
The steep pastures in the alpine regions can be used very well by sheep. In Austria, the Mountain Sheep is the most popular breed for alpine pasture. Particular qualities of this breed are its secure step and good mother instinct. The Mountain Sheep has an aseasonal oestrus cycle and, therefore, is very well suited for production systems with continuous lambing over the year. The alpine pasture period reaches from June to middle of September. During this time, animals can move freely in the Alps. Once a week or once in two weeks, the farmers control the sheep and bring some salt and minerals up to the mountain.
To keep the animals on the mountains has three positive effects. The first is a positive effect on animal health (claws, parasites), the second is low costs and the third is landscape conservation. On particularly steep areas, sheep grazing is very important. Thereby, the plants are kept short and the soil will be compressed without destroying the stand of grass. This protects from avalanches and landslides.

Theatre SH3.4

Use of small ruminants for landscape conservation in Swiss Alpine area

R. Lüchinger Wüest[1], M. Schneeberger[2], J. Troxler[3], [1]Extension and health service for small ruminants, P.O. Box 399, CH-3360 Herzogenbuchsee, [2]Animal Sciences, ETH, CH-8092 Zurich, [3]Swiss Federal Research Station for Plant Production, Changins, CH-1612 Nyon*

The Alpine area is a complex and fragile ecological system. Approx. half of the Swiss sheep population (420,000 total) are pastured during summer in alpine area, 1600-2700 m a.s.l. The mountain pasture represents an important part of Swiss sheep production systems. Sheep have a tendency to follow the melting snow and overgraze the young plants while lower parts of pastures remain undergrazed. Sustainable use of mountain pastures is essential to avoid negative effects, such as erosions and loss of botanical diversity. The main elements of sustainable use of mountain pastures are: 1) Demarcation of the pastured area, moderately steep, covered by close vegetation. 2) System of pasture and flock management. Generally, pastures should be changed weekly. Equal use of pasture can best be achieved by flocks permanently guided by shepherds and sheep dogs. This system is limited to large flocks for economical reasons. Similar results are obtained by dividing the pasture in paddocks. In the frequently applied system of free grazing, the stocking rate has to be reduced to avoid partial overgrazing. 3) Stocking rate, depends on elements 1) and 2) and the productiveness of pastures. From summer 2003 the subsidies for sheep on alpine pasture will be attributed according to the system of pasture.

Theatre SH3.5

The conservation and sustainable use of biodiversity in Vlasina lake region

M. Savic[1], S. Jovanovic[1], R .Trailovic[1] and N. Adzic[2], [1]Faculty of Veterinary Medicine, Belgrade, [2]Institute of Biotehnology, Podgorica, Serbia and Montenegro*

The region of lake Vlasina is very picturesque, high altitude area in South East Serbia. Concerning that several factors play an important role in degrading mountain biodiversity, the Municipal of Crna Trava, the regional centre designed program for protection of natural and genetic resources. Natural reserves like Vlasina Lake, surrounded by ancient forests and fields rich in medicinal herbs and endemic fauna are of special interest for preservation. The presence of mineral water springs with trademark licence, allows development of eco-tourism and organic agriculture in this part of Europe.

The identification and monitoring of animal genetic resources revealed a great number of rare wild birds, mammals, reptiles, fishes, and other animals in the region. The long tradition in extensive breeding of pasture animals, especially locally adapted livestock breeds allows implication of eco-friendly utilisation programmes for protection of economically non-important domestic animals and also for non-agricultural use of for example horses in landscape tourism, hunting, riding tours etc. Genetic characterisation of the well adapted Zackel sheep; robust Balkan goat and Yugoslav mountain pony has been performed in the scope of National project for conservation of autochthonous breeds. Pasture livestock co-existing with natural ambiance in Vlasina district, allow linking of safe animal production, recreation and environmental energy input into a system of sustainable development of this protected area.

Theatre SH3.6

Use of sheep for conservation of wasteland in the north of Poland

R. Niznikowski, Warsaw Agricultural University, ul. Ciszewskiego 8, PL 02-786 Warszawa, Poland.*

A change in Poland from controlled to market economy caused reduction of land used agriculturally. As a result, in Poland 10% of this land comprises of wasteland. This has made way for areas which can be used for sheep grazing in order to prevent growth of trees and bushes. Because in the north of Poland there are the largest areas of this kind, real dietary value of the close sward during vegetation period was estimated and their usefulness to sheep breeding and lamb production was checked. Chemical composition and energetic value of the close sward in June, July and August on an eight-year-old wasteland was analysed and usefulness of a few sheep breeds to utilisation of this kind was compared. The breeds used in the research were as follows: Black Mutton Sheep, Pomeranian Sheep, Leine and Polish Heath Sheep. Their reproduction traits underwent estimation (when ewes were kept on the pasture all the time during vegetation period). Their usefulness to fat lamb production with estimation in the above mentioned environmental conditions was also researched. The acquired data show a possibility of utilisation of Polish sheep in fat lamb production in conditions of extensive farming on wasteland.

Diet selection by goats: implications for landscape conservation in Central Italy

S. Verzichi[1], M.Trabalza-Marinucci[1], V. Abbadessa[2], M. E. Piciollo[2], O. Olivieri[1], [1]Dip. Tecnologie e Biotecnologie delle Produzioni Animali, University of Perugia, Via San Costanzo 4, 06126 Perugia, Italy, [2]ENEA CR-Casaccia, via Anguillarese 00060, Roma, Italy.*

It is recognised that ungulate herbivores can have a profound effect on the vegetation of marginal areas. This frequently results in conflicts between foresters, nature conservationists, and farmers. The aim of this study was to examine the effect of stocking rate on diet composition by Angora goats and the impact on the vegetation of a marginal hilly area in Central Italy. The area was subjected to goat grazing for 3 consecutive years at either 1.7, 3.3 or 4.5 heads/ha. Diet composition was determined using both the *n*-alkanes technique and the faecal plant cuticle technique. Plant communities were characterised using transect in the woodland and randomly placed quadrates in the grassland. Shrub/tree species were predominant in goats' diet except in springtime, when grass species were preferentially selected. *Hedera helix* was the dominant species in the diet across areas and seasons. The intake of several individual plant species was significantly affected by experimental factors. Sward biomass was negatively correlated to stocking rate and progressively increased along the trial. Results indicate that, at the experimental conditions of the trial, grazing by goats can significantly affect vegetation in marginal areas. Grazing pressure can be used as a tool to differentially modify plant communities development and increase biodiversity.

Poster SH3.8

A bio-park type mountain refuge for ruminants as an element of landscape protection - maintaining animal welfare without buildings

A. Dobicki[1], P. Nowakowski[1], A. Zachwieja[1] K. Chudoba[1], J. Twardon[2], R. Mordak[3] and J. Pacon[4], [1]Institute of Animal Breeding, [2]Department of Animal Reproduction, [3]Departmnent and Clinic of Internal Diseases, [4]Department of Parasitology and Invasive Diseases, Agricultural University of Wroclaw, Chelmonskiego str. 38 C, 51 630 Wroclaw, Poland.

The refuge for animals covered 3.2 ha (4 paddocks, wooden 2 m high posts, wire netting), was located on a southern slope (450 m over see level), had a set of gates, roofing for hay and straw and access to water (mountain stream). Observations were conducted over the years 1998-2002 and included sheep (4-12 head), goats (4-0), fallow dears (4-3), lamas (4-3) and crosses mouflon x sheep (2-1). The flock hierarchy gave priority in accordance with the animal's body weight: lamas, mouflon, sheep and goats. The fallow dear created a separate and independent group.
Three years without using any preparations against parasites resulted in a parasite infestation (30-300 eggs/oocysts according to the method by McMaster) - sheep and goats (40-100), fallow dear (30-70) and lamas (200-300). It was confirmed that offering for one day, four times a year, salt licks with an anti parasite preparation *Fenbenat* is justified (0.008% of an active factor). Such a procedure limited the parasite infestation: *Eimeria sp.* almost totally (in 2 sheep out of 10 up to 10 eggs were found), *Trichostrongylidae* - small infestation (in 4 sheep out of 10 up to 10-20 eggs and in 2 fallow dear out of 3, up to 20 eggs/oocysts).

Sustainable conservation of animal genetic resources in marginal rural areas: integrating molecular genetics, socio-economics and geostatistical approaches

The ECONOGENE Consortium, P. Ajmone-Marsan, M. Bruford, S. Dunner, G. Erhardt, G. Hewitt, J.A: Lenstra, G. Obexer-Ruff, P.Taberlet, A. Valentini, R. Caloz, A. Georgudis, G. Canali, J. Roosen, P. Crepaldi, I. Togan, A. Vlaic, R. Niznikowski, L. Fésüs, O. Ertugrul, M. Abo-Shehada, M.A.A. El Barody, A. Hoda, M. Trommetter, Istituto di Zootecnica, Università Cattolica del S. Cuore, 29100 Piacenza, Italy.*

The ECONOGENE project is funded by the European Union under the V Framework Programme.
ECONOGENE combines a molecular analysis of biodiversity, socio-economics and geostatistics to address the conservation of sheep and goat genetic resources and rural development in marginal agrosystems in Europe. To assist in situ conservation and address the relevant socio-economic factors, a co-ordinated approach is developed to define strategies of genetic management and rural development. Knowledge of sheep and goat genetic diversity will be greatly extended at the molecular level, examining many unstudied, local breeds, and identifying gene pools to map conservation priorities. A map of development perspectives will be produced, to identify areas where sustainable conservation of valuable populations could succeed. Maps of conservation and development priority will be overlayed and the value of biodiversity estimated, to justify economic intervention, and suggest appropriate guidelines and actions.

Theatre S4.1

Genetic study on pelt quality traits in the Gotland sheep breed

A. Näsholm, Swedish University of Agricultural Sciences, Department of Animal Breeding and Genetics, P.O. Box 7023, S-750 07 Uppsala.*

In the Swedish Sheep Recording Scheme lambs are inspected at around 4 months of age. For Gotland lambs six pelt quality characteristics are judged: colour of fleece, size of curl, distribution of the colour, curl distribution and firmness, quality of hair, and hair density. Since year 2001 a subjective overall score of the pelt is also made. To study the genetic relationship between the overall score and the other pelt quality traits, genetic parameters were estimated using multiple-trait animal models. Data included observations on about 47 000 lambs born during the period from 1991 to 2002. The overall score was recorded for close to 2 200 lambs. Genetic correlations between the overall score and scores for curl distribution and firmness and quality of hair, respectively, were strong (0.90 to 0.94), whereas genetic correlations with distribution of colour, hair density, and size of curl were moderate (0.39 to 0.50). The genetic correlation between overall score and colour of fleece was close to zero. Estimates of heritability for the overall score were moderate to high and varied between 0.32 and 0.51 in the different analyses, whereas they were 0.21 to 0.47 for the individual pelt characteristics. To improve pelt quality in lambs of the Gotland breed, the overall score should preferably be included as a trait in the genetic evaluation.

Theatre S4.2

Effect of the method of rearing on sexual activity and libido of Awassi ram lambs

A.N. Al-Yacoub and R.T. Kridli, Department of Animal Production, Faculty of Agriculture, Jordan University of Science and Technology, Irbid 22110, Jordan*

Thirteen Awassi ram lambs of the same age were raised in either an all-male group (n=7) or in a group mixed with females (n=6) from weaning to puberty to examine the effect of rearing method on sexual performance. Libido testing was performed at 9 and 14 months of age. Bouts of anogenital sniffing and the frequency of mount attempts were greater ($P<0.05$) in the all-male group. Mounting frequency was numerically greater in the all-male group. The frequency of raising the fat tail of females was similar ($P>0.05$) between the two treatments. At 14 months of age, all sexual performance parameters were only numerically higher for all-male group than the mixed group ($P>0.05$). Body weight (BW), and scrotal circumference differed ($P<0.01$) between treatments. Ram lambs in the all-male group were heavier ($P<0.01$) than those mixed with females throughout the trial. Scrotal circumference was greater ($P<0.01$) in the all-male group when compared with the mixed group. Sampling week affected BW and body condition score ($P<0.05$). Semen evaluation revealed no differences between the two treatments. Results of the current study indicate that rearing Awassi ram lambs in all-male groups may increase their aggressiveness during libido testing.

Theatre S4.3

Reproductive performances in primiparous Awassi, F_1 Romanov x Awassi and F_1 Charollais x Awassi ewes bred in Jordan

M. Momani Shaker[1], A. Y. Abdullah[2], R. T. Kridli[2], I. Sáda[1], R. Sovják[1], [1]Czech University of Agriculture Prague, Institute of Tropical and Subtropical Agriculture, Czech Republic, [2]Department of Animal Production, Faculty of Agriculture, Jordan University of Science and Technology, Irbid.*

The objective of this study was to evaluate the effect of genotypes on reproductive performances, including the effect of ewe age and year of rearing.
50 A (Awassi), 36 F_1 R50A (Romanov x Awassi) and 46 F_1 Ch50A (Charollais x Awassi) were compared. For the 3 genotypes, the percentage of conception (lambing ewe per ewe mating) was 58.0 %, 88.89 % and 67.39 % respectively, prolificacy (lambs born per ewe lambed) 113.79 %, 143.75 % and 103.23 %, fecundity (lambs born per ewe mating) 66.0 %, 127.78 % and 69.56 % respectively. Differences in reproductive indicators according to genotypes were significant ($P \leq 0.01$). The influence of age of ewes and year of rearing on reproduction proved to be highly significant ($P \leq 0.01$). In general, results obtained from this study revealed that crossbreeds F1 A x R and crossbreds F1 A x Ch excelled pure Awassi ewes.

Theatre S4.4

Comparison of transrectal ultrasonography and pregnancy protein (PAG) tests for diagnosis of early pregnancy in sheep

A. Karen[1], J.F. Beckers[2], J. Sulon[2], B. El-Amiri[2], K. Szabados[4], S. Ismail[1], J. Reczigel[4], O. Szenci[1]. [1]Clinic for Large Animals, Faculty of Veterinary Science, H-2225 Üllö-Dóra Major, Hungary. [2]Department of Physiology of Reproduction, Faculty of Veterinary Medicine, Sart Tilman, Belgium. [3]Awassi Corporation, Bakonszeg, Hungary. [4]Department of Biomathematics and Informatics, Faculty of Veterinary Science, Budapest, Hungary.

Two hundred sixty eight ewes synchronized for estrus were used in the present study. The ewes were fasted overnight and scanned in a standing position by transrectal ultrasonography (5 MHz) at days 24, 29 and 34 after AI. Recognition of the embryonic fluid was used as a positive sign for pregnancy. Simultaneously with transrectal ultrasonographic examination, blood samples were collected from each ewe. PAG concentrations were determined by RIA. The cut off value of the PAG-RIA test to detect pregnancy was ≥1 ng/ml. The sensitivity (100 %) of PAG test for detecting pregnant ewes was significantly ($P<0.05$) higher than that (81%) of transrectal ultrasonography at day 24 after AI. However, on days 29 and 34 of gestation, the accuracy of transrectal ultrasonography and PAG tests for detecting pregnant (96.8 % and 96.8% vs. 100% and 100%, respectively) and non-pregnant ewes (98.7 % and 98.5 % vs. 98.7 % and 99.5%, respectively) were not significantly different. In conclusion, PAG-RIA test is a highly accurate and reliable method to distinguish between pregnant and non-pregnant ewes from day 24 of gestation. Transrectal ultrasonography is an accurate alternative test for early pregnancy diagnosis in Awassi x Merino ewes from day 29 of gestation.

Theatre S4.5

Effects of some environmental factors on lactation curves of Sarda dairy goats

N.P.P. Macciotta[1], P. Fresi[2] I. Pernazza[2], A. Cappio-Borlino[1]. [1]Dipartimento di Scienze Zootecniche, Università di Sassari, Italia, [2]Associazione Nazionale della Pastorizia, Roma, Italia.*

The Sarda breed is an autochthonous goat population characterised by the existence of three subpopulations related to the geographical location of flocks. In order to estimate possible relationships between milk yield of animals and subpopulation they belong to, test day (TD) records of 14,928 lactation of Sarda goats were analysed with a mixed linear model that included test date, parity, number of kids born, altitude of location of flocks, flocks within altitude and lactation stage as fixed, and individual lactation as random effect. All factors considered in the model affected milk yield significantly. Lactation curves of goats of flocks located at different altitudes were markedly different, with plain and mountain having the highest and the lowest production respectively, thus suggesting a possible relationship among yield and type of subpopulation. Moreover, differences in management, in general environmental conditions and the effect of crosses with specialised breeds should not be neglected. First parity goats showed the lowest productive level whereas the goats at fifth kidding were the most productive. The number of kids affected milk yield in the first part of lactation, with goats with two kids having the highest yield. The average phenotypic correlation between TD within lactation was 0.34, lower than in dairy cattle and sheep, probably reflecting the main incidence of environmental factors in the extensive farming system of this autochthonous breed.

Theatre S4.6

Application of a management system aimed at continuous production in dairy ewes

A. Bonanno, A. Di Grigoli, M. Bongarrà, B. Formoso, G. Tornambè, M.L. Alicata. Dipartimento S.En.Fi.Mi.Zo., sezione Produzioni Animali, Università di Palermo, Viale delle Scienze, 90128 Palermo, Italy.

A continuous productive system (CPS) of ewes based on an uniform distribution of lambing (September, December, February, May) and aimed at continuous milk and cheese production, was compared with Sicilian traditional seasonal system (TSS), in which lambings occur in September mainly and less in February. CPS and TSS groups consisted of 60 Comisana ewes grazing on the same pastures. CPS ewes fed concentrate with two levels based on their milk yield. Milk and cheese yield and milk quality were evaluated during a year. The lambing rate between systems was analogous. Lambing season affected lactation length and milk production in both systems. The average milk yield per year was higher in CPS than in TSS (662 *vs* 571 g/d/ewe; $P \leq 0.05$). In winter, when forage availability at pasture was low, the concentrate supplementation provided CPS ewes on the basis of productive level, improved milk yield (782 *vs* 610 g/d/ewe; $P \leq 0.05$), reducing casein (4.7 *vs* 5.1%; $P \leq 0.05$) and cheese yield (16.5 *vs* 18.6 %; $P \leq 0.05$) in comparison with TSS ewes. Finally, the CPS gave 5% higher milk production than TSS, uniformly distributed during the year, without productive shortage. Therefore, the CPS permitted to achieve a net profit higher than TSS by 14.5% with milk sale and 21.8% with cheese sale.

Poster S4.7

Estimation of white clover and grass intake in grazing lambs

R. Sormunen-Cristian[1] and P. Nykänen-Kurki[2], [1]MTT Agrifood Research Finland, Animal Production Research, 31600 Jokioinen, Finland, [2]MTT Agrifood Research Finland, Ecological Production, 50600 Mikkeli, Finland*

Herbage intake by lambs was evaluated on three grass (mixture of *Phleum pratense* L., *Lolium perenne* L. and *Festuca pratensis* Huds.) pastures with annual nitrogen rates of 0 (G0), 120 (G120) and 250 (G250) kg ha^{-1} and on a white clover-grass pasture without nitrogen fertilization (CG0) by total collection, sward cutting method and using n-alkanes C_{32} and C_{33}.
Pasture white clover content averaged 12-32% in fresh herbage. Due to the sowing method, sward height for grazing was higher (20 cm) than recommended (5-8 cm) for dense sward under continuous sheep grazing. Accurate estimates of herbage intake in grazing lambs were not obtained by sward cutting method. Not more than 25% of lambs acclimatized well to harnesses and dung bags, and daily herbage dry matter (DM) intake measured by total faecal collection was relevant only on CG0 swards, 84 g $(kgW^{0.75})^{-1}$. By alkanes C_{32} and C_{33} estimated herbage intake averaged 106, 79 and 64 g DM $(kgW^{0.75})^{-1}$ in CG0, G0, G120 and G250 swards, respectively (CG0 *vs*. G, $p<0.05$). Some findings have shown the alkane method to be more appropriate in ryegrass monoculture than in mixed sward and a combination of markers C_{32} and C_{33} to predict herbage intake the most precisely. In this study, an overestimation of white clover intake was assumed by alkanes.

Poster S4.8

The influence of different levels of by-pass protein on the performance and wool characteristics of Sanjabi sheep

A. Farahpoor[1], Y. Rouzbehan[1], N. Taherpoor-Dori[2], [1]Animal Science Dept., Agriculture College, Tarbiat Modaress University, Tehran P.O. Box 14155-4838, Iran, [2]Animal Science Research Institute, P.O. Box 1483, Karaj.*

To assess the effect of fish meal (FM) on the growth performance and wool yield, twenty Sanjabi male lambs with an initial weight of 28 kg (sd 1.34) and age of 6 months were used. The animals which were individually penned were divided into four groups (n = 5). Each group was offered either 0 (a), 50 (b), 75 (c) or 100 (d) g FM/day. The basal diet which was based on barley, wheat straw, wheat bran, cottonseed meal and lucerne hay was formulated according to AFRC (1995). The dry matter intake (DMI) and weight gain were measured throughout the trial which lasted for 100 days. The wool of the animals which were sheared at the beginning and at the end of the trial was characterised. The data were statistically analysed using completely randomised design. Mean values for animals' performance for the diets a, b, c and d were as follows: LWG 201, 199, 237, 242 g/day (s.e.m. 11.5, P<0.01); DMI 1715, 1704, 1742, 1813 g/day (s.e.m. 2.4, P<0.01); feed conversion ratio 8.5, 8.6, 7.3, 7.5 (s.e.m. 0.03, P<0.05); fleece weight 684, 694, 817, 874 g (s.e.m. 46.7, P<0.01); fiber diameter 27, 26.8, 27.9, 30.9 micron (s.e.m. 0.9, P<0.01); fiber length 48.7, 42.4, 49.8, 48.8 mm (s.e.m. 1.7, P<0.05); wool yield 66.5, 66.2, 67.8, 73.4 percent. Economically, adding FM to the basal diet had no beneficial effect, although there was an improvement in the animals' performance and wool yield.

Poster S4.9

Efficiency of using dried groundnut vine in rations of growing Barki lambs under desert farming system

N.M. Eweedah, S. A. Mahmoud, G. E. El-Santiel and S. F. Killany. Department of Animal Production, Faculty of Agriculture, Kafr El-Sheikh, Egypt.*

Thirty Barki lambs, with an average live bodyweight 31.8±1.89 kg and aged 9-11 months, were divided into three similar groups in feeding trial to investigate the effect of replacing alfalfa hay by dried groundnut vine at levels (0,50 and 100%) on lambs performance. The animals in all groups were fed on cracked barley at level 2% of live bodyweight. Quantities of roughage were given to complete the nutritional requirements according to NRC (1985). Digestibility trials were carried out by using nine Barki rams to evaluate these rations. Rumen liquor and blood samples were collected at the end of the experimental period. Results indicated that no significant differences in the digestion coefficients and nutritive value between rations containing dried groundnut vine or alfalfa hay with barley. However, dried groundnut vine ration showed higher ether extract and lower crude fiber digestibility. Ruminal pH value was lower (5.49) for lambs fed alfalfa hay plus dried groundnut vine, which was coincided with significantly higher total volatile fatty acids (12.74 meq/100 ml). Total gain, average daily gain and feed conversion were not significantly different. However, the economic efficiency was the best for lambs consumed the dried groundnut vine which due to the low cost (40%) of the daily ration.

Poster S4.10

Evaluation of quantitative and qualitative characteristics of spontaneous and seeded pastures

P. Secchiari[1], A. Pistoia[1], L. Casarosa[2], P. Poli[1] and G. Ferruzzi[1], [1]DAGA Sezione Scienze Zootecniche, Università di Pisa; [2]CIRAA Centro Interdipartimentale "E.Avanzi", Università di Pisa.

The trial was carried out on two different farms located in the sublittoral area of Tuscany (Livorno, Italy). It was based on six experimental plots, two for each pasture: sown, uncultivated and becoming naturalized pastures. Fodder samples were cut, using the Corral method, in order to value the forage production. On the forage samples, botanical characterisation and chemical analysis to calculate the instant stocking and the mean season stocking rate were carried out. The rational management of the different pastures through cutting and simulated grazing trials was valued. The sown pastures gave a high production, but mostly in the Spring season, so they have to be cut in the growing period, and the regrowth can be grazed only for a short period, so they are best used as meadow-pastures. The uncultivated pastures are characterised by a low forage production, but they present a good regrowth which permits to graze till the Autumn season. As the becoming naturalized pastures have intermediate characters between the other two, they can be used in both ways according to the farm managing requirements. The sown pastures bear, in average, the highest season stocking rate (39 sheep/ha) followed by the becoming naturalized pastures (25 sheep/ha) and than by the uncultivated pastures (19 sheep/ha).

Poster S4.11

The nutritive effect of probiotic Pioner(r)PDFM on haematological values and some serum parameters in growing lambs

Marcela Speranda[1], B. Liker[2], Z. Antunovic[1]. [1]Agricultural Faculty, Trg Svetog Trojstva, Osijek, Croatia. [2]Agricultural Faculty, Sveto_imunska 25, Zagreb, Croatia.*

The nutritive effect of probiotic Pioner®PDFM on haematological value (RBC, haemoglobin , haematocrit, WBC) and on some other parameters in blood serum (calcium, phosphorus-inorganic, sodium, potassium, chloride, iron, UIBC, total protein, albumin, triacylglycerols, cholesterol, glucose, urea, creatinine, bilirubin, ALT, AST, GGT, AP CK and LDH) was investigated. Fattening results were also investigated. The trial lasted 35 days.
Forty-eight lambs, initial body weight of 20 kg, divided in two groups equal in number: one control (C) and one, experimental group (E) were included in trial and were fed hay, and fodder mix (16% CP). Added to the fodder mix (0.1%), the group E received probiotic Pioner®PDFM. Blood samples were collected et 19th. and 35th.day of trial.
Calcium ($p<0,01$) of E group was decreased, and potassium ($P<0,01$), phosphorus ($P<0.05$) chloride ($P<0.05$) and iron ($P<0.05$) increased. The values of glucose and urea were significantly lower ($P<0,01$) and bilirubin ($P<0.01$) and triacylglycerols ($P<0.05$) significantly higher in the E group. The activity of ALT, AST and CK were highly significantly lower ($P<0.01$) in the E group. Enterococcus faecium from Pioner®PDFM caused compensated metabolic acidosis.

Poster S4.12

Nutritional level, body weight and ovulation rate in the ewe

F. Wergifosse, J.L. Bister, C. Pirotte, R. Paquay, Department of Animal Physiology, The University of Namur, B-5000 Namur Belgium*

An experiment was conducted with 48 adult fertile Ile-de-France ewes allotted in 4 groups according to their nutritional program. This program consisted in two periods of 10 weeks of high (H) or low (L) level of nutrition; H level consisted in 2 kg hay and concentrate ad libitum, L level, in 0.8 kg hay par day. The ewes were weighed and scored for body condition weekly, the food consumption was calculated, blood was sampled for hormone measurement and ovulation rate (OR) was estimated according to the number of corpora lutea on the ovaries at the end of the experiment.

The weight at the beginning of the assay was similar in the different groups (between 60 and 65 kg) and the weight gain for the 2 periods was respectively for the HH group: +9.7 and +4.9 kg, HL: +10.3 and -7.3 kg, LL: -2.6 and -1.6 kg, LH: -3.5 and +16.2 kg. For these groups, the ovulation rate was respectively 2.1, 1.9, 0.8 and 1.9; the final weight 76.4, 66.1, 59.1 and 77.5. Without regards on the group of the ewes, a positive correlation is calculated between the ovulation rate and the body weight ($P<0,01$), and between OR and the weight gain during the second period ($P=0,08$). Plasma leptin levels are now being measured and will be correlated with the other parameters.

Poster S4.13

Effect of electron-charging of feed and water on the blood characteristics in fattening lamb

H. Tobioka[1], M. Morimoto[1], A. Nagao[1], R. Pradhan[1] and K. Niidome[2], kyushu Tokai University, Choyo-son, Aso-gun, Kumamoto, 869-1404, [2]JEM Co., 341-2- Kamiyoshida, Yamaga-shi, 861-0524, Japan.*

In order to establish the environmentally friendly system of animal production without using any chemical, electron-charging system of feed and water was applied to the fattening lambs and blood characteristics of metabolites and enzymes were measured.

Fifteen heads of lamb of 6 months, weighing 38 kg were allocated to 3 groups of reference (RE), electron-charged feed (EF) and electron-charged feed and water (EW) with 5 heads each. The feed were fed at the rate of 70 % formula feed and 30 % Bermuda hay on DM basis. Feed and water were charged by the system developed by JEM Co., Japan. The experiment was divided into 3 one-month terms. The blood samples were taken before feeding and 4 hr after feeding in each term. Serum urea and glucose of EF and EW groups tended to be higher than those of RE group and cholesterol before feeding tended to be lower in EW group. The GOT and γ-GPT of EF and EW groups were lower or tended to be lower compared to that of RE group. The SOD in red blood cell and plasma GSH-Px tended to be higher in the order of EW, EF and RE groups. In conclusion, electron-charging of feed and water seemed to have some influence on blood constituents as one of the overall effect in whole body.

Poster S4.14

Carcass composition of Awassi ram lambs in comparison to its crossbreds with Romanov and Charollais slaughtered at marketing age

A.Y. Abdullah[*1], M. Momani Shaker[2], R.T. Kridli[1], I. Sada[2], [1]Department of Animal Production, Faculty of Agriculture, Jordan University of Science and Technology, Irbid, Jordan [2]Insititute of Tropical and Subtropical Agriculure, Czech University of Agriculture, Prague, Czech Republic*

This study was designed to compare carcass composition of Awassi (A, n=6) with F1 Awassi X Charollais (AC, n=6) and F1 Awassi X Romanov (AR, n=6) ram lambs slaughtered at an average marketing age of 180 ± 15 days and final live weight of 36.18 ± 6.1 kg. Following slaughtering, the chilled carcass was divided into eight primal cuts. The leg cut of the right side of each carcass was physically dissected. Genotype affected fasting weight ($P<0.05$), cold and hot carcass weights ($P<0.001$), tail fat % ($P<0.05$), fore and hind quarter % ($P<0.001$), rack and loin cut % ($P<0.01$), fasting dressing % ($P<0.001$) calculated with tail fat weight. Awassi had higher dressing % and tail fat % compared with AC and AR ram lambs. Leg, loin, rack and shoulder cut percentages were higher in AC and AR compared with A ram lambs. Awassi carcasses had the lowest total dissected leg muscle and bone weight and the highest total dissected leg fat weight than the two genotypes. Results of this study demonstrate that AC and AR were superior to A ram lambs in all cuts and muscle weights and percentages and had lower fat weights and percentages which increases the value of meat produced from crossbreeds.

Poster S4.15

Relationships between carcass weight, carcass dimensions and tissues thickness on Churro Galego Bragançano and Suffolk lambs

A. Teixeira[1], V. Cadavez[1], M.S. Bueno[2] and R. Delfa[3]. [1]Escola Superior Agrária de Bragança, Área de Zootecnia, Apartado 172, 5301-855, Bragança, Portugal, [2]Instituto de Zootecnia, CP 60, CEP 13460-000, Nova Odessa, Sao Paulo, Brazil, [3]Unidad de Tecnologia en Producción Animal, Servicio de Investigación Agrária, Diputación General de Aragon, Apartado727, 50080, Zaragoza, Spain*

This study was carried out on 46 male lambs, 26 Churro Galego Bragançano and 20 Suffolk breed. Following slaughter, carcasses were weighed and cooled at 4 ºC for 24 h, and a set of eighteen carcass dimension and tissues measurements were recorded. Data were subjected to a common factor analysis procedure. The carcass width and perimeter showed high positive correlations with the hot carcass weight (0.736 to 0,911) and between them (0,546 to 0,802). Otherwise, the hot carcass weight showed low correlation (0.171) with leg length and average correlation (-0.387 to 0.563) with measures that characterise carcass length and perimeters. Subcutaneous fat thickness at different positions showed low correlations with hot carcass weight (<0.200), but high correlations between themselves (>0.666). Four common factors were identified as carcass weight (factor I), sternal tissue thickness (factor II), subcutaneous fat (factor III) and conformation (factor IV) and explained 81,9% of the variation of the eighteen original variables, leaving 18,1% of variability to the 18 unique factors. The information present in the 18 original variables can be condensed in four common factors.

Poster S4.16

Relationships between carcass weight, carcass dimensions and tissues thickness on Churro Galego Bragançano lambs

V. Cadavez[1], A. Teixeira[1], M.S.Bueno[3] and R. Delfa[2]. [1]Escola Superior Agrária de Bragança, Área de Zootecnia, Apartado 172, 5301-855 Bragança, Portugal, [2]Instituto de Zootecnia, CP 60, CEP 13460-000, Nova Odessa, Sao Paulo, Brazil, [3]Unidad de Tecnologia en Producción Animal, Servicio de Investigación Agrária, Diputación General de Aragon, Apartado727, 50080 Zaragoza, Spain*

This study was carried out on 126 lambs (86 male and 40 female) from Churra Galega Bragançana local breed. Lambs were slaughtered in the experimental slaughterhouse of the Escola Superior Agrária de Bragança, after 24-h fasting. Following slaughter, carcasses were weighed and cooled at 4 °C for 24 h and a set of eighteen carcass dimension and tissues measurements were recorded. Data were subjected to a common actor analysis procedure. All variables in the study presented high and positive correlations with the hot carcass weight, especially the carcass dimension measurements with correlations coefficients superior to 0.751 ($P<0.001$). The carcass dimension measurements showed high correlations among themselves (>0.888, $P <0.001$). There was a high positive correlation between the subcutaneous fat thickness and sternal tissues thickness measurements (>0.580, $P<0.001$). Three common factors were identified as carcass weight (factor I), subcutaneous fat (factor II) and sternal tissue thickness (factor III) and explained 83,5% of the variation on the eighteen original variables, leaving 16,5% of variability to the 18 unique factors. The information present in the 18 original variables can be condensed in three common factors.

Poster S4.17

The evaluation of the basic characteristics of lamb meat quality on the base of musculus triceps brachii analysis

J. Kuchtík and F. Horák, Mendel University of Agriculture and Forestry Brno, MSM 4321 00001, Department of Animal Breeding, Zemedelska 1, Brno 613 00, Czech republic.

The goal of the study was to evaluate the basic characteristics of lamb meat quality at five genotypes with different proportions of Oxford Down breed (OD), German long-wool breed (GL) and Merino (M). The evaluation was carried out on the base of *musculus triceps brachii* analysis. There were not differences among the groups in the contents of dry matter and of protein and in energy values in the origin matter in the muscle. The content of protein varied from 18.62 % (GL 75 OD 25) to 19.56 % (OD 75 GL 25). The highest energy value in the origin matter was found in (M x GL) x OD (549.47 kJ/ 100 g). Concerning the content of intramuscular fat (IF) and ash, the significant difference ($P \leq 0.05$) among the groups were found. The highest and the lowest contents of IF were found in (M x GL) x OD (3.56 %) and in OD 75 GL 25 (2.59 %). The content of ash was the highest in OD 75 GL 25 (1.05 %), while the lowest content was in (M x GL) x OD (0,97 %). It is possible to conclude that all observed characteristics were found as the best in crosses with the highest proportion of OD (OD 75 GL 25).

Poster S4.18

The growth rate and carcass quality of Lithuanian native coarsewooled sheep

B. Zapasnikiene, V. Juskiene, Lithuanian Institute of Animal Science, R. Zebenkos 12, LT-5125 Baisogala, Radviliskis distr., Lithuania.

A small herd of native coarsewooled sheep (approx. 40 heads) is conserved and studied at the Lithuanian Institute of Animal Science. In 2000-2002, the analysis of the growth rate of the sheep and the first test slaughterings indicated that the growth rate of the sheep was rather high (daily gain from 80 to 200 g), fat content of meat low, but the meat percentage was low, too. The weight of lambs at birth, 20 days, 2.4 (at weaning), 7 and 12 months of age were, respectively, 2.5-4.0, 5.0-8.0, 10.0-13.0, 15-25, 22-35 and 31-42 kg. However, the average preslaughter weight of 9-11 month-old male lambs was 39.9 kg, but their dressing percentage accounted for only 41.4%. The weight of internals was 10.7 kg, that of skin - 5.8 kg, head - 2.9 kg, limbs - 0.8 kg, blood - 1.6 kg and fat in the abdominal cavity - 0.5 kg. The chemical composition of M. *longissimus dorsi* was 22.4% dry matter, 20.6% protein and 1.2% fat. The pH - value of meat was 5.8, colour intensity 123.1 units, water binding capacity 60.1%, cooking losses 40.2% and fat melting temperature amounted to 48.6%.
Though our native coarsewooled sheep are not characterized by high meatiness and their dressing percentage is low, these animals have good prospects in the EU market due to the low fat content in meat.

Poster S4.19

Estimation of live body weight, conformation and compactness from body measurements of indigenous sheep and goats under marketing conditions in Faranah, Guinea

M. Mourad, Institute of Agricultural Research of Guinea, (IRAG), P.O. Box 1523 Conakry, Guinea

Estimation of body weight, conformation and compactness(body weight / body length) from chest girth and body length was studied for 301 lambs of Djalonkè sheep (DB) breed and 223 kids of the West African Dwarf goats (WADG) in the market and at marketing weights. Both sexes of DB had a better grade of conformation than those of WADG. The coefficient of determination (R^2) for the simple regression and the coefficients of variation (C.V.%) showed that chest girth of the animal is much better than body length in predicting body weight of the animal in both species and gender. The coefficients of determination increased and the coefficients of variation decreased when both chest girth and body length were used as independent variables in the regression equations. The body weight was highly correlated ($P<0.01$) with chest girth, body length and body compactness. Species affected significantly ($P< 0.001$) body conformation and body compactness, however, gender affected ($P< 0.001$) only the body conformation and did not significantly ($P> 0.05$) affect the body compactness. The interaction (Species x Gender) was significant ($P< 0.01$) for body conformation and not for body compactness.

Poster S4.20

Modelling learning performance of African dwarf goats

G. Nürnberg, G. Dietl, K. Siebert[1], J. Langbein[1], Research Institute for the Biology of Farm Animals, Division Genetics and Biometry, [1]Division Behavioural Physiology, Wilhelm-Stahl-Allee 2, D-18196 Dummerstorf, Germany.*

Animal cognition is currently attracting interest in the context of environmental enrichment. In this context, a wider and deeper knowledge of the learning abilities of animals is required. African dwarf goats were studied for visual discrimination learning using a computer based learning device integrated in the home pen of the animals. To get a reward (water) goats had to choose the correct stimulus by pressing a button in front of the screen. Visual stimuli (geometrical signs) were presented on a computer screen in a four-choice design, over test period of 12 to 14 days. Individual learning performance was measured as rate of correct choice due to all choices per testday. Starting with short mathematical considerations of a class of four-parametric growth functions (Tangenshyperbolicus-, Arcustangens-, Janoschek- and Bertalanffy-Richards function) the goodness of fit due to learning data was analysed for this four functions. The best fit was found for the Arcustangens- and Janoschek-function. Several types of learning curves, modeled by the same function, are presented. Data of individual learning curves of several groups of goats are analysed. Different mean learning curves of male and female goats are found and discussed. Furthermore a selection experiment on learning performance with dwarf goats is described.

Poster S4.21

Presence of CAEV infection in Hungarian goat industry as an effect of livestock import

S. Kukovics[1], A. Molnár[1], M. Ábrahám[1], Z. Dani[1], Sz. Kusza[2], and Fülöp[3], [1]Research Institute for Animal Breeding and Nutrition, Gesztenyés u. 1. 2053 Herceghalom, Hungary; [2]University of Debrecen, Centre of Agriculture, Böszörményi u. 138. 4015 Debrecen, Hungary; [3]Hungarian Goat Breeders' Association, Gesztenyés u. 1. 2053 Herceghalom, Hungary.*

The CAEV infection was discovered a couple of years ago in the Hungarian goat sector after the importation of livestock import from Holland (Saanen) and France (Alpine). In order to determine the level of infection 96 goat farms were selected out and 5,100 blood samples were taken (every single animal was sampled in the farms). The selection was made based on the size of the farm (1-10; 11-30, 31-50, 51-100, 101-150, 151-200 and above 200), breed in the herd (purebred and crossbred Saanen, Alpine, Boer, and Hungarian White, Hungarian Brown, Hungarian Multicolour), as well as the region of the farms. The samples were examined at the Central Veterinary Institute (Budapest) using ELISA and AGID tests.
SPSS for Windows and Microsoft Excel programmes were used for processing the data. According to the results, the breed had a strong effect on the presence of CAEV infection. The size of farms also effected the level of infection: the ratio of infected animal was increased with the number of animals on the farms. There were significant differences found among the regions (county) concerning the herds attached by CAEV infection.

Poster S4.22

The weaning stress response in lambs of different age

J. Sowinska, H. Brzostowski, Z. Tanski, J. Szarek. University of Warmia and Mazury, 10-718 Olsztyn, ul. Oczapowskiego 5, Poland*

Responses to weaning were studied in 50- and 100-days-old lambs of Ile-de-France Sheep. Blood samples were collected before weaning and 15 h after weaning. Levels of cortisol and glucose as well as haematocrite were determined in the collected blood samples. Weaning caused a significant increase in cortisol levels in both groups of lambs. More sensitive than 100-days-old lambs were 50-days-old lambs in which an increase in cortisol level from 30.21 to 55.33 nmol/l was found. On the contrary, in 100-days-old lambs the cortisol level increased from 21.43 to31.81 nmol/l. Weaning stress caused an increase in glucose content in 50-days-old lambs (from 3.68 to 3.99 mmol/l), while in 100-days-old lambs it remained on the nearing level (4.25 and 4.35 mmol/l, respectively). Neither age of lambs nor weaning stress influenced the haematocrit value.

Poster S4.23

The stress response to weaning and pre-slaughter transport of lambs

J. Sowinska, H. Brzostowski, Z. Tansk, K. Majewska. University of Warmia and Mazury, 10-718 Olsztyn, ul. Oczapowskiego 5, Poland*

The present study was carried out on 3 genetic groups of 50-days-old lambs: of Pomeranian Sheep breed (P), Ile-de-France (IF) and crossbreds F_1 of Pomeranian ewes with Ile-de-France rams (PIF) (10 in each genetic group - 30 lambs in total). Blood samples were collected three times: I - before weaning, II - 15 h after weaning and III - after pre-slaughter transport. The level of cortisol, glucose and haematocrit was determined in the blood samples.

We have not found significant differences in the level of cortisol and haematocrit between the genetic groups. The level of glucose in IF lambs (5.83 mmol/l) was significantly higher than the level in P lambs (4.66 mmol/l) and crossbreds PIF (4.96 mmol/l).

The term of blood sampling caused a significant differences of cortisol (34.07, 51.30 and 105.80 nmol/l, respectively) and glucose levels (5.67, 4.42 and 5.36 mmol/l, respectively).

Poster S4.24

Variability of values of plasmatic proteinase inhibitors in sheep with chronical form of mastitis

J. Buleca Jr.[1], I. Sutiaková[1], J. Szarek[2], J. Bíres[1], E. Pilipcinec[1], V. Sutiak[1], J. Trandzík[3], [1]University of Veterinary Medicine, Komenského 73, 041 81Kosice, Slovakia, [2]Agricultural University of Cracow, Al. Mickiewicza 21, 31 103 Cracow, Poland, [3]State Breeding Institute, Hlohovská 5, 95 141 Luzianky, Slovakia

In our work the values of plasmatic proteinase inhibitors in sheep of improved Valaska breed (n=7+7), with microbiologicaly confirmed chronical form of mastitis (Staphylococcus aureus, Streptococcus agalactiae, beta heamolytic streptococci) were analysed. Electrophoretical analyses on polyacrylamide gel were measured on horisontal electrophoresis (Pharmacia LKB). Plasmatic inhibitors in mammals are localised in plasma in high concentration and plays key role in regulation of several physiological processes. They are component of non-specific reaction of organism by proinflamatory cytokines, which are typical by some systemic reactions. Concentration and induction of new electrophoretic fractions can be affected, except other factors, also by pathological conditions of organism. In sheep with mastitis were registered reorganisation of the fractions with very intensive activity to acidic zone (pH 3,75-3,50). In addition in sick animals lower intensity of fractions with lower activity in the area of pH 5,85, from pH 6,55 to pH 6,85-7,35 respectively were registered. In healthy animals 12-13 protein fraction of trysine were noted. Occurrence of the fractions with highest activity was found in the zone of isoelectric points with pH 3,75-6,0. Presented partial results show the possibility of application of plasmatic proteinase inhibitors knowledge in diagnostic practice and in prevention of animal health disturbances.

Poster S4.25

Effect of anthelmintic treatments on milk production and on rennett coagulation properties in goats

L. Rinaldi[1], V. Veneziano[1], M. Pizzillo[2], V. Fedele[2], G. Cringoli[1], R. Rubino[2], [1]Dipartimento di Patologia e Sanità Animale, Facoltà di Medicina Veterinaria, Università degli Studi di Napoli "Federico II", Via Della Veterinaria 1, 80137 Napoli, Italy, [2]Istituto Sperimentale per la Zootecnia, Via Appia, 85054 Bella Scalo (PZ), Italy*

A field trial was conducted at the Istituto Sperimentale per la Zootecnia, on 75 goats with naturally occurring infections of gastrointestinal strongyles.
The gastrointestinal strongyle population consisted of *Teladorsagia circumcincta*, *Haemonchus contortus*, *Trichostrongylus colubriformis*, and *Oesophagostomum venulosum*.
Three treatments groups of 25 goats each were performed: eprinomectin pour-on group (E-group), albendazole drench group (Al-group), and control untreated group (C-group).
The efficacy of eprinomectin and albendazole was determined by faecal egg counts (FEC) performed on each study animal on the day of treatments (day 0) and on days 7, 14, 21, and 28.
Milk production (ml) and rennett coagulation properties were recorded for each study animal weekly from day 0 until day 63 (9 weeks).
With respect to FEC, eprinomectin was more effective than albendazole.
The milk production of E- and Al-groups was statistically significant higher than milk production of C-group goats. No significant differences were found between milk produtions of E- and Al-groups. With respect to the rennett coagulation properties, no differences were found between C-, E-, and Al-groups.

Poster S4.26

Level of inbreeding and its effects on some performance traits in teddy goats

M. Afzal, K. Javed and M. Shafiq. Livestock Production Research Institute, Bahadurnagar, Okara, Punjab, Pakistan.

1643 pedigree and performance records of Teddy goats kept at Livestock Production Research Institute, Bahadurnagar, Okara during 1976-1998 were used. The inbreeding coefficients were calculated using DFREML computer programme. For estimation of effect of inbreeding on performance traits, Harvey's LSMLMM software was used. Year and season of birth, birth type and sex as fixed effects and inbreeding coefficient as covariate were included in the model for all the traits, weaning age as covariate for weaning and yearling weight. Overall means for birth, weaning and yearling weight (kg) were 1.65±0.37, 10.48±2.34 and 19.60±3.57. Overall inbreeding coefficient was 0.030. About 29 percent of animals were inbred (average inbreeding coefficient 0.111). Inbreeding had no effect on birth, weaning and yearling weight. Least squares means for birth, weaning and yearling weight were 1.59 ± 0.01, 10.30 ± 0.91 and 19.88 ± 0.18 kg. Spring born kids were generally heavier than kids born in autumn for all traits. Male and single born kids had heavier weights compared to female and twin or triplet born kids. Year of birth was significant source of variation for all traits while season of birth and sex of kid had significant (P<0.01) effect on weaning and yearling weight. Birth type had a significant effect on birth weight only. Weaning age had a significant effect on weaning (P<0.01) and yearling (P<0.05) weights. There was an increase of 0.023±0.005 and 0.026±0.010 kg in weaning and yearling weight per day increase in weaning age.

Poster S4.27

Genetic correlations between reproduction and production traits of Polish dairy goats

E. Bagnicka[1], M.L. Lukaszewicz[1], Tormod Ådnøy[2], Ewa Wallin[3], [1]Polish Academy of Sciences Institute of Genetics and Animal Breeding, Jastrzebiec, 05-552 Wólka Kosowska, Poland, [2]Agricultural University of Norway, Department of Animal Science, N-1432 Ås, Norway, [3]Norwegian Association of Sheep and Goat Breeders, Postboks 2323 Solli, 0201 Oslo, Norway

The aim of study was to estimate the genetic correlations between reproduction and production traits in first parity.
Data on 5917 reproduction and 7927 production records served to analyse genetic correlations between number of kids born alive (NBA), total losses after first kidding (TL), fat (FY) and protein (PY) yields in first lactation. Data were analysed employing REML with multiple-trait animal model approach. The means of NBA and TL were 1.47 (sd=0.59) and 0.11 (sd=0.36), and of fat and protein yield were 18,2 (sd=7.0) and 15.0 (sd=5.4) in first parity, respectively. Genetic correlations between NBA and FY, and TL and FY were 0.118 (se=0.145) and -0.262 (se=0.164), respectively. The genetic correlation in first parity between NBA and PY was -0.019 (se=0.152), and between TL and PY -0.351 (se=0.171). Genetic correlations between yields and number of kids born alive tended to be negative.

Poster S4.28

Prospects of dairy goat breeding improvement in the North-West of Russia

T.I. Kuzmina[1], R. Laski[2] and L. Volkova[2], [1]Research Institute for Farm Animal Genetics and Breeding, St.Petersburg-Pushkin, 19625 Russia, [2]Heifer International,1015 Louisiana St.,Little Rock, AR, U.S.A. 72202, [3]The Goat Breeder's Society of Northwest Russia, St.Petersburg-Pargolovo, 194362, Russia.*

One of the mission of the Heifer International (International Charitable Organization) is to assist genetic improvement of dairy goats in order to increase milk production, and (2) marketing goat milk in order to increase incomes. In the agreement between Heifer International and the Goat Breeder's Society of North-West Russia, the Small Scale Dairy Goat Breeding Project was started in 1999. 100 highly productive Saanen goats were bought. During this period, number of animals increased from 296 to 992. Increasing the amount of goat milk was achieved by three approaches which were used singularly or in combination. They were: 1.Increase the number of animals in production. 2.Increase milk yield per animal. 3.Increase milk component yield per animal. 11 Saanen pure bred bucks were imported from U.S.A. Milk production (MP) increased by 136%, average milk yield per goat increased by 1020 kg (2002), in compare 1999 (750 kg). There are 3 groups of animals with different milk production: low MP (1,5 -1,7 kg - 460 animals), middle MP (3 - 3,2 kg - 378), high milk production (4-4,2 kg - 154 animals) in population. The further strategy of genetic improvement will based on the genetic evaluation procedures and the dissemination of the improved genetic material in the population.

Poster S4.29

Sex distortion and monozygosity rate in Valle del Belice sheep twins

J.B.C.H.M. van Kaam[1], R. Finocchiaro[1], B. Portolano[1], P. Giaccone[1], [1]Dipartimento S.En.Fi.Mi.Zo-Sezione Produzione Animale, Viale delle Scienze, 90128 Palermo, Italy.*

First parity Valle del Belice dairy ewes have 30% of twin lambing and higher parities 70%. Three sex combinations are possible among twins, both males, male and female, or both females. If some equal sex twins are monozygotic breeding value estimation is more complicated because the relationship matrix is singular. Statistics enables derivation of the percentage of monozygotic and dizygotic twins. The probability of a dizygotic twin is nearly twice the probability of a twin with different sex, whereas the probability of a monozygotic twin is 1 minus that. A data set consisting of 5276 single and 3040 twin births with sex of each offspring identified has been utilized. In single births 52.4% males were found, whereas in twin births this was 52.5%. Of the twin births 794 were both males, 1604 were male+female and 642 were both females. This means that the number of unequal sex twins is higher than would be expected if all twins would be dizygotic. Simulation showed a probability below 0.1% for this number of unequal sex twins. Conclusions from this analysis are (1) monozygotic twins are very rare, (2) the percentage of male births is higher than the percentage of female births, unlike results in literature and (3) the percentage of male+female twins is higher than expected, which is in agreement with literature.

Poster S4.30

Effect of gonadotrophin treatments on follicles size and oocytes quality in goats

G.M. Terzano, E.M. Senatore, G. Ficco, R. Stecco and A. Borghese ,Istituto Sperimentale per la Zootecnia (ISZ), Via Salaria 31, 00016 Monterotondo, Roma, Italy.

Forty-two Derivata di Siria goats were subjected to 2 ovarian stimulation protocols: group A (n=23) was synchronized by 45 mg FGA sponges (10d) plus 3 mg PGF2a (8^{th}d); starting 72 h before sponge removal, does were administered pFSH (250 IU) injected (i.m) 12h apart in a decreasing dosage over 4d. Sponges were removed on the morning of the last pFSH injection and the aspiration was performed 26h later. Group B (n=19) was treated similarly to those in (A) but was implanted for only 3d before starting the pFSH injections and the aspiration was performed 9d following sponges implant. The ovaries of donor females were evaluated laparoscopically for follicle number and diameter prior to the oocytes aspiration. Group B, in comparison with group A, showed a higher number of observed follicles (20.2 vs 16.4; P≤0.001); a lower percentage of small (≤3mm) follicles (8.8 vs 24.0; P≤0.05); a higher percentage of medium (<4-6 mm>) follicles (79.5 vs 62.1; P≤0.05). Treatments significantly affected neither the percentage of large (≥7mm) follicles (13.9 vs 11.8) nor the number of recovered oocytes (11.2 vs 12.5), (A vs B groups); nevertheless treatment B showed a higher percentage of viable oocytes (84.0 vs 36.7; P ≤0.001).

In conclusion we found the treatment B as a suitable stimulatory protocol for oocyte donor females, as it stimulates the growth of a higher percentage of medium follicles and the production of higher percentage of viable oocytes.

Poster S4.31

Effect of royal jelly on puberty of winter-born Awassi ewe lambs

M.M. Al-Molla and R.T. Kridli, Department of Animal Production, Faculty of Agriculture, Jordan University of Science and Technology, Irbid 22110, Jordan*

This study was conducted to evaluate the effect of using royal jelly (RJ) paste, a honeybee product, on puberty induction and metabolic hormones in prepubertal Awassi ewe lambs. Twenty seven Awassi ewe lambs were randomly assigned into three groups (n=9) to receive 0 (RJ 0), 200 (RJ 200), and 400 mg of RJ (RJ 400). Each animal in the RJ 200 and RJ 400 groups received 47 equal doses of RJ (orally) every other day for 3 months beginning on June 5th. Blood samples were drawn from each animal, via jugular venipuncture, every other day throughout the experiment. Five ewe lambs in each group were randomly selected to receive 50 µg GnRH (i.m.) on the last day of the RJ administration period. There were no differences among treatments in terms of body weight change. Body weight increased (P<0.05) as the experiment advanced. Royal jelly treatment did not influence puberty age, while GnRH had a slight tendency (P=0.14) to advance it. Mean age at the time of puberty among the three treatments was 273 ± 8.7 days (39 weeks). Thyroid hormones were not affected by RJ treatments. In conclusion, results of the current study demonstrate that RJ treatment neither advanced puberty age in Awassi ewe lambs nor did it influence animal growth. Awassi ewe lambs reached puberty at a body weight and age similar to those previously reported in the literature.

Poster S4.32

Physiological adaptation of sheep maintained in severe conditions of eastern Poland

C. Lipecka, K. Patkowski, Agricultural University, Faculty of Biology and Animal Breeding, Akademicka 13, 20-950 Lublin, Poland.

The aim of study was to evaluate the contents of some haematologic and biochemical blood indices of sheep maintained outdoor with a possibility to hide under island station roof (group P) and indoor (group A). The experiment was performed using 30 ewes at the age of 8 months that were randomly divided into groups A and P at the beginning (September 1, 2001). They were maintained under such conditions till the end of September 2002. Investigated ewes were mated at the first year of age. Blood for tests was taken three times: in the fifth month of pregnancy (March), in the second month of lactation (June) and before next tupping (September). Contents of Hb and Ht were determined in full heparinized blood; activities of ALAT, AspAT and LDH enzymes, as well as total protein, cholesterol and triglyceride contents in blood serum. It was found that the system of sheep maintenance significantly differentiated the level of hemoglobin in blood, activity of enzymes involved in metabolism (ALAT and LDH) and cholesterol content in blood serum, particularly at the final stage of pregnancy and lactation. During lactation, Hb, ALAT and LDH were respectively by 2.75mg%, 24% and 26% higher at ewes maintained whole year outdoor, than those living in inventory buildings. Higher cholesterol content in blood serum by 21.2 mg/dl was found in the latter ones. Taking into account the number of embryos and reared lambs, it was proved that mothers with double pregnancy and rearing two lambs were distinguished with significantly lower activities of tested enzymes, as well as higher content of cholesterol as compared to those with single pregnancy and rearing only one lamb and sterile mothers.

Poster S4.33

Use of does body measurements to predict does weight, litter size and kids birth weight in Zaribi X Baladi crossbred goats

A.E. Fekry, Biological Applications Department, Nuclear Research Center, Cairo 13759, Egypt.*

45 Zaribi X Baladi crossbred does (10 mono- and 35 multi-parous) were used to verify the relationships between body conformation and each of gestation length (GL, day), litter size (male, LSm and female, LSf), kids mortality (male, Mortm and female, Mortf), and kid birth (male, BWm and female, BWf) weight (kg). Body weight (Wt) was recorded monthly throughout the gestation period along with the following body measurements: back length (BL), height at withers (HW), height at hip (HH), heart girth (HG), abdominal girth (AG) and pelvic girth (PG). Stepwise regression analyses were performed between pregnancy traits (X) and body measurements (Ys).
In mono-parous does, LSm can be predicted using: PG & AG (1st, 4th and 5th months), Wt (2nd month), and HH (3rd month). While in multi-parous does: (1)GL can be predicted using: PG & AG (1st month), HW (2nd & 5th months), and BL & HH (4th month); (2)LSm can be predicted using: HH (1st, 4th & 5th months), HW (2nd month), and HG & PG (3rd month), Wt (2nd month), and HH (3rd month); (3)LSf can be predicted using: HH (1st, 3rd & 4th months), and HH & HW (5th month); (4)BWm can be predicted using: HH & BL (2nd month), and HH & HW (3rd month); and (5)BWf can be predicted using: Wt & HG (2nd month), and HH, HG & HW (3rd & 5th months), and BL & HH (4th month).

Poster S4.34

Characterisation of phospholipids ovine milk fat globule membrane (MFGM)

P. Secchiari[1], F. Paoletti[1], M. Mele[1], A. Serra[1], A. Buccioni[2], M. Antongiovanni[2]. [1]DAGA Università di Pisa; [2]Di.Sc.Zoo. Università di Firenze.

Aim of the work was to characterise the phospholipids (PL) fraction of ovine MFGM from two Italian sheep breeds (Massese and Sarda) reared in Pisa Province. Bulk milk samples were collected from 10 flocks (5 Massese and 5 Sarda) during the second month of lactation. The PL classes of the MFGM were separated by TLC and quantified by GC. Linoleic acid content was higher in milk fat of Sarda breed (1.76 vs 1.05g/100g Total Lipids -TL-), while a-Linolenic acid, Vaccenic acid and Rumenic acid were higher in milk fat of Massese (respectively 0.78 vs 0.62g/100g TL; 2.20 vs 1.22g/100g TL and 1.17 vs 0.74g/100g TL). On the contrary, PL classes distribution (as percent of total Fatty Acids -FA-) resulted similar from the two breeds: Phosphatidyl Ethanolammine (PE) 37.63% vs 36.65%; Shingomyelin (SM), 26.66% vs 27.90%; Phosphatidyl Choline (PC), 17.41% vs 17.14%; Phosphatidyl Inositol (PI) 10.91% vs 12.24%; Phosphatidyl Serine, 8.92% vs 7.50% in Massese and Sarda. The FA composition of SM and PC was quite constant. The PE, PI and PS FA composition, on the contrary, changed with the FA availability, because the nutritional role of these PL in the MFGM. The PE provides, in fact, the major part of PUFAs of PL which play an important nutritional role in growth and in brain development of new born.

Poster S4.35

Changes in wool production traits of the six top quality Merino flocks during the last two decades

S. Kukovics[1], J. Megyer-Nagy[2], A. Domanovszky[2], P. Székely[2], A. Jávor[3] [1]Research Institute for Animal Breeding and Nutrition, Gesztenyés u. 1. 2053 Herceghalom, Hungary; [2]National Institute of Agricultural Quality Control, Keleti K. u. 24. 1024 Budapest, Hungary; [3]University of Debrecen, Centre of Agriculture, Böszörményi u. 138. 4015 Debrecen, Hungary*

In order to investigate changes in wool production traits in the Hungarian Merino industry during the last two decades, an analysis was carried out. For this work, the top six nucleus flocks were selected from the national flock, which survived the affects of re-organisation of the industry and the production data of which have not disappeared during almost fifteen years of privatisation process.

Wool production data from almost fifty thousand Merino ewes were evaluated covering the period between 1982 and 2000. This period was divided into three year sections and the data were pooled (across the flock firstly and then across the whole studied population within the three years sections). Greasy wool weight, rendement (clean wool yield), staple length and fibre diameter were determined concerning these sections.

Significant differences were found among the studied flocks, but the overall examination showed declining tendency in average raw wool yield, and increasing rendement, staple length, and fibre diameter with time.. Strong time and farm effects were observed on these traits, which could be followed in the relationships among them.

Theatre S5.1

Use of major genes in small ruminants selection: the French examples of as1-cas in goats and PrP gene in sheep

I. Palhière[1], A. Piacère[2], J.M. Astruc[2], [1]INRA, SAGA, BP27, 31326 Castanet-Tolosan, France, [2]Institut de l'Elevage, INRA, SAGA, BP27, 31326 Castanet-Tolosan, France.*

For a few years, molecular genetics has been taking a growing importance in livestock selection (Marker Assisted Selection, major genes, parentage verification).
In small ruminants, few cases of utilisation of major genes, at a large scale, already exist. The paper presents two examples in the French situation: use of αs1-cas in goats and PrP gene in sheep. The αs1-cas gene explains a significant part of the variability of a quantitative selected production trait (protein content) within a polygenic background. The PrP gene, which is associated to scrapie resistance, corresponds to a non quantitative trait, to be taken into account as an additional trait in the selection goal, in the context of increasing interest in transmissible spongiform encephalopathies (TSE).
The different ways of utilisation of these major genes are presented in the framework of the context of production, as well as the questions that occurred in their utilisation in breeding schemes : indirect effects (loss of genetic variability, possible pleïotropic effect), strategy of selection, cost-effectiveness.
The strategies adopted are described (type and number of genotyped animals, use in the selection process) and the efficiency of the programs is discussed.

Theatre S5.2

Taking account of scrapie in the usual genetic improvement scheme of Causses du Lot sheep breed

G.Perret[1], H.Issaly[2], J. Bouix[3], I. Palhière[3]. [1]Institut de l'Elevage, BP 18, 31321 Castanet Tolosan, France, [2]UPRA Causses du Lot, BP 199, 46004 Cahors, France, [3] INRA-SAGA, BP 27, 31326 Castanet Tolosan, France.*

The Causses du Lot breed (108000 ewes) is a hardy breed in the south west of France, with frequent extensive management. The sheep breeding association (UPRA) started a breeding program in the 70's with the development of sheep recording on farm and the setting up of a ram centre. Then in the 80's , thanks to the use of AI, about 15 rams per year were progeny tested for prolificacy and suckling ability. In 1998, scrapie occurred in a breeding flock.
The original frequency of Prp's alleles was 15.1% ARR, 17.4% AHQ, 60.4% ARQ and 7.1%VRQ. Very quickly, all the tools and the genetic organisation were mobilized to increase the genetic resistance to scrapie and the safety of meat lambs. According to the national scrapie plan, the new breeding scheme aims at eliminating animals with VRQ, producing ARR/ARR rams and ewe lambs in the selected population first and distributing them to infected commercial flocks. In 2002, 4500 animals have been genotyped in the 30 breeding flocks. All the rams should be homozygous in 2004-2005 and the progeny for maternal ability is going to start again in 2003 with such rams. Some attention has been paid to the genetic level and variability of the previous traits. The success of this program is a priority because of a large diffusion of young females used in terminal crossbreeding for meat production.

Theatre S5.3

PrP genotyping in a flock of Assaf sheep: polymorphisms and relationship with milk yield

N. Marcotegui, A. Parada, L. Alfonso and A. Arana*. Dpto. Producción Agraria, Universidad Pública de Navarra. Campus de Arrosadía. 31006 Pamplona. Spain.*

Resistance/susceptibility to scrapie has been linked to polymorphism at codons 136, 154 and 171 of the prion protein (PrP) gene. The aim of this work is to study polymorphism at these codons in a flock of Assaf sheep in Spain and to analyse the existence of association between PrP variants and milk yield. The most frequent genotype ARQ/ARQ was present in 47% in females and 33% in males indicating that this population could be highly susceptible to the disease. Other frequent genotypes were ARQ/AHQ (15% in females, 20% in males) and ARQ/ARH (16% in females, 7% in males). Allele ARR related to high resistance only occurs at low frequency (<15%) and it has not been found in homozygosis. Allele VRQ related to high susceptibility was not found. There was no found association between PrP genotype and milk yield.

Theatre S5.4

Characterization of prion protein (PrP) gene polymorphisms of TSE-positive sheep flocks in Germany

G. Lühken[1], A. Buschmann[2], M. Groschup[2] and G. Erhardt[1], [1]Department of Animal Breeding and Genetics, Ludwigstrasse 21B, 35390 Giessen, Germany, [2]Federal Research Centre for Virus Diseases of Animals, Boddenblick 5a, 17493 Insel Riems, Germany.*

International findings suggest that the occurrence of scrapie / TSE in sheep flocks is associated with polymorphisms at codons 136, 154 and 171 of the prion protein (PrP) gene. The aim of this study was to validate this for the TSE-situation in the German sheep population.
TSE-diagnosis was confirmed by immunoblot and/or immunohistochemistry. After DNA-extraction from brain tissue of TSE-positive sheep and tongue tissue or leukocytes of TSE-negative or clinical healthy sheep, polymorphisms at codons 136 (A;V), 154 (H; R) and 171 (R; Q; H) were identified as haplotype by two restriction fragment length polymorphism (RFLP) analyses.
The genotype known to be most resistant to natural scrapie / TSE in sheep, ARR/ARR, has been found in any of TSE-positive sheep (n = 28), while TSE-positive sheep of the breeds Suffolk and Texel had the genotypes ARQ/ARQ and VRQ/ARQ respectively, which internationally are known to be associated with high susceptibility in these breeds. Within TSE-positive sheep of German Merinolandschaf-type, the AHQ-haplotype occurred, which until now never has been identified in German scrapie / TSE cases.
The results indicate that the sheep breed has to be considered by selection against TSE-susceptibility on the basis of PrP-alleles.

Theatre S5.5

Breeding goals and new perspectives in dairy sheep programs

A. Carta[1] and E. Ugarte[2]. [1]Instituto Zootecnico e Caseario per la Serdegna. I-07040 Olmedo, Itlay. [2]NEIKER, A.B. Basque Institute for Agricultural Research and Development. Arkaute. Apdo 46. 01080, Vitoria-Gasteiz. Spain.*

The current state and future perspectives for the dairy sheep breeding programs will be discussed in this paper. Traditionally, dairy sheep production has been based on native breeds, very well adapted to their local conditions and production systems. Therefore, most of the breeding programs currently going on are based on pure breed selection. These programs have been focused on milk production features (milk yield and composition traits). However, as a consequence of the increasing interest in traits related to the reduction of production costs and the increasing consumer's demand for safety and healthy food products, udder morphology traits, somatic cell counts and resistance to scrapie disease are being considered within the breeding programs.

In addition, the development of DNA molecular techniques, the appearance of microsatellites and genetic maps have opened the possibility to detect genomic regions involved in the genetic determinism of quantitative traits (QTL).

This approach, together with candidate gene studies, is currently explored in several research projects. Depending on the results, either the marker assisted or the gene assisted selection strategies could be implemented in dairy sheep breeding programs in the near future.

Theatre S5.6

Implementation of a genetic improvement program for Comisana dairy sheep population in Sicily: challenges, solutions and results

F. Pinelli[1], P.A. Oltenacu[2], M. Scimonelli[1], G. Iannolino[1], A. D'Amico[1], A. Carlucci[3], [1]Istituto Sperimentale Zootecnico per la Sicilia, Palermo, Italy, [2]Department of Animal Science, Cornell University, USA, [3]Associazione Provinciale Allevatori di Matera, Italy.*

A breeding program to improve milk production in Comisana breed was successfully implemented in Sicily since 1998. The program was designed to overcome the major limitations faced by dairy sheep improvement programs: poor animal identification, limited control of production, use of multiple rams in flocks and lack of a genetic structure in the flock population. The program started with a selection nucleus of 3000 ewes in 7 flocks where 40 young rams are progeny tested each year and the best 6 are selected. Records are collected and stored using a software package that consists of a data base management program, an electronic animal identification system and a field interface program that facilitates the collection of records on farm and their transfer to the data base. An autoregressive test day animal model is being used for the genetic evaluation of the animals. Based on 2003 genetic evaluation, the range in the breeding value for milk/day in the nucleus was 800 g and the average of best 4 progeny tested rams was +200 g. The multiplication and dissemination phase are ongoing. The next goal is to increase the testing, multiplication and dissemination capacity of the program by expanding the size of the nucleus.

Theatre S5.7

Development of a national breeding programme for milk sheep in Germany

B. Zumbach and K.J. Peters, Humboldt University Berlin, Department of Animal Breeding in the Tropics and Subtropics, Philippstr. 13, Haus 9, D-10115 Berlin, Germany.*

Milk production from dairy sheep is of increasing importance in Germany. Nevertheless the establishment of an efficient breeding programme still remains a problem mainly for structural and economical reasons. Not only the limited population size which is distributed among 15 breeding associations, each of them conducting their own programme, but also the small herds where breeding males are generally utilised only within farm pose serious constraints with regard to genetic evaluation. The new legislation of the EU commission in order to enhance TSE resistance in sheep has to be considered as a chance for the establishment of a national breeding programme. Prerequisites are the establishment of a unique animal identification system, a cost effective standardised recording system covering performance and functional data, pedigree data, systematic effects and PrP genotyping data. The programme system APIIS seems to be most appropriate as a universal common data basis for breeding purposes and others (e.g. EU requirements).

Breeding value estimation should be based on a BLUP test-day model. The introduction of AI with fresh semen for best rams carrying at least one ARR allele seems to be necessary to achieve satisfying genetic response and to increase the ARR allele frequency in the population. The most appropriate breeding scheme seems to be a young sire programme.

Theatre S5.8

Test-day model and genetic parameters in Slovenian dairy sheep

A. Komprej, G.Gorjanc, S. Malovrh, D. Kompan, M. Kovac, University of Ljubljana, Biotechnical Faculty, Zootehnical Department, Groblje 3, 1230 Domzale, Slovenia*

Validation of multiple-trait animal test-day model and the estimation of (co)variance components in Slovenian dairy sheep were performed. For the period 1994-2002, 41145 test-day records of 3317 ewes (2081 Bovec, 525 Improved Bovec and 717 Istrian Pramenka) were used. The model contained days in milk, parity and litter size as covariates. In joint analysis across breeds, the model contained also breed as a fixed effect. Random part of the model consisted of common flock environment within test month as flock-year-month, permanent environment as ewe within parity and additive genetic effect. Heritabilities for all breeds together were 0.25 for daily milk yield, 0.14 for fat (FC) and 0.12 for protein content (PC). New estimates of (co)variance components are proposed for regular genetic evaluations in Slovenian dairy sheep. In addition, there are indications for specific lactation curves within flock as well as animal suggesting random regression models for further research.

Theatre S5.9

Use of meat sheep sire lines in order to improve product quality in national sheep breeding systems

O. Vangen[1], T. Kvame[1,2] and F. Avdem[2], [1]Department of Animal Science, Agricultural University of Norway, P.O.Box 5025, N-1432 Aas-NLH, Norway, [2]Norwegain Meat Cooperation, P.O.Box 360 Økern, N-0513 Oslo, Norway.*

The Norwegian sheep breeding has been characterized by one large population of dual purpose sheep, including maternal, growth and carcass traits in the same breeding programme. In order to improve product quality, a meat sire line has been established based on crosses between Texel and Norwegian sheep. In the selection line (120 breeding ewes), preselection of male lambs is done on ultrasound. Computer tomography results (CT-results) on meat, fat and bone content in addition to special measures of meatiness and product quality has been the final selection criteria of young rams. The 8-10 selected rams are used in the herd the first year, and the best half of them is selected for AI the second year. Semen from these NOR-X rams is distributed through the national programme to produce crossbred lambs for improved meatiness and product quality (1/2 or 1/4 NOR-X lambs). The first carcass results on offspring from NOR-X rams was presented in 2002 and show improved slaughter weight, carcass percentage, carcass class and economic benefit both per kg meat and per carcass. The future optimization of this crossbreeding programme will include discussions on the size of the nucleus and genetic improvement of the nucleus with new imports of genes from meat sheep breeds versus use of rams with extreme EBVs for carcass traits (through AI) from the national breeding scheme for the dual purpose sheep.

Theatre S5.10

Computerized tomographic study of the body composition in different sheep genotypes

D. Mezöszentgyörgyi[1], R. Romvári[1], L. Fésüs[2], I. Komlósi[3] and I. Repa[1], [1]University of Kaposvár Institute of Diagnostic Imaging and Radiation Oncology, H-7400 Kaposvár, Guba S. u. 40, Hungary; [2]Association of Hungarian Sheep Breeders and Sheep Breeder Organisation, P.O. Box 365, H-1242, Budapest, Hungary; [3]University of Debrecen, Faculty of Agriculture Sciences, Department of Animal Breeding H-4315 Debrecen, Hungary

The whole body composition of different sheep genotypes (Charollais (C), Texel (T), C × (British Milk Sheep x Hungarian Merino (BH)), Texel × BH) were studied, by means of *in vivo* computerized tomography (CT). 50 to 60 scans were taken of each animal, from the first cervical *vertebra* to the *os tarsus* at a mean body weight of 30 kg. Regarding cross sectional fat area T × BH showed the highest, while T the lowest values, with significant differences between T - C and T - T × BH. In muscle area, the T showed the highest values, then C, T × BH, and C × BH. Significant differences were found between the T - C × BH, C - C × BH and T × BH - C × BH groups.
An index was developed for expressing the muscle/fat ratio (MF). The highest MF values were obtained for the two breeds selected for mutton production. Significant differences were found between T - C and T - T × BH. The MF index is suitable for the incorporation into breeding programmes.

Theatre S5.11

Meat and wool production of progeny of Dorper (D) and White Alpine (W) rams mated to crossbred ewes

M. Schneeberger[1], C. Hagger[1], H. Leuenberger[2], K. Tschümperlin[2] and G. Stranzinger[1].* *[1]Institute of Animal Sciences, ETH, CH-8092 Zurich, [2]Research Station Chamau, ETH, CH-6331 Hünenberg.*

51 crossbred ewes of Black Brown Mountain, Charollais and W sheep breeds were mated to 3 D and 3 W rams. 79 progeny were visually appraised for conformation and wool traits at the average age of 56 days. All D progeny and 50% of W progeny had pigmented wool, 39% of D progeny showed white spots. In tendency, wool of D was less dense and shorter than that of W progeny. D lambs were 0.3 kg lighter at birth, and grew only slightly less than W lambs. Considerable differences were observed between sires. 26 D and 18 W lambs presently slaughtered at a life weight of 41 kg, reached at the average age of 125 d and 120 d resp. Higher slaughter yield (45% and 42%), better carcass grade (5 E, 18 U and 3 R vs. 5 U, 12 R, 1 O) and 20 SFr higher selling price per lamb (0.1 SFr/kg slaughter wt) was obtained for D than for W progeny. Average fat class was 3.0 for D and 2.8 for W, no difference was observed for percentage of valuable cuts in the carcass. Further studies will include chemical analyses of meat samples, segregation of haplotypes, and their relationships with observed phenotypic characteristics.

Theatre S5.12

Effect of body weight changes on some productive and reproductive performances in Egyptian native sheep

R. Salama[1] and A.A. El-Shahat[2], [1]Animal Prod. Dept. Faculty of Agric Al-Azhar University, Nasr City and [2] Animal Prod. Dept. National Res. Centre, Dokki (12622). Cairo,*

The main objective of the present work was to evaluate the critical live body weights of the Egyptian local ewe lambs which might influence its productive and reproductive performances thereafter. Therefore, native animals were weaned at 8 weeks of age and were fed on concentrate mixture and hay ad. lib. To detect the sexual maturity in ewe lambs, the animals were mated at the first regular cycle, and ages and weights of ewes were recorded.

Correlations among average live body weights of ewe lambs from birth to maturity were calculated. The results showed that the average live body weight at twenty weeks of age was significantly correlated with birth weight, weaning weight, weights at puberty and at lambing.

Upon the basis of the present finding it can be suggested that live body weight at twenty weeks of age may be more important than other weights, and selection for heavier body weight at this age (20 weeks) would result in younger age at puberty and at first lambing and longer reproductive life thereafter. The results will be discussed on the basis of sheep production and animal breeding.

Poster S5.13

Proposal for breeding programs for TSE-resistance in sheep in Saxony-Anhalt

K.-H. Kaulfuss[2], B. Hoffmann[2], H.-J. Rösler[1], and L. Döring[1], [1]MRA of Saxony-Anhalt, Angerstraße 6, D-06118 Halle; [2]Institute of Animal Breeding with Veterinary Clinic, Martin-Luther-University Halle-Wittenberg, E.-Abderhalden-Str. 28, D-06108 Halle, Germany

Transmissible spongiform encephalopathies are degenerative diseases which affect the central nervous system of many mammals including scrapie in sheep. Genetic susceptibility to scrapie is associated with polymorphisms in three different codons of the ovine prion protein (PrP) gene (136, 154, 171). Breeding for disease resistance (PrP^{ARR}/PrP^{ARR}) is now the most powerful means of controlling scrapie in sheep. For this reason in 2002 a project for the development of breeding strategies for the pedigree breeding in sheep was started in Saxony-Anhalt; Germany. The project will be running over three years and included the breeds: German Mutton Merino, German Improved Land Merino, German Blackheaded Mutton, Suffolk and some local breeds. A total of nearly 10.000 genotypings (male and female animals) for scrapie resistance are planed (5.000 until august 2003). The project is subdivided into four steps: analysis of the PrP genotypes; analysis of correlated effects between the scrapie genotype and other important production traits; development of breeding strategies for scrapie resistance for the included breeds; transfer of the breeding progress into commercial breeding. Based on present results in German Mutton Merino, German Blackheaded Mutton and Suffolk, the resistant pedigree flocks can be achieved during the project period. Only in German Improved Land Merino, the necessary time is much longer. Until now, we could not find negative effects of the selection on scrapie resistance to other production traits.

Poster S5.14

Genetic parameters of claws of Merinolandschaf and Rhönschaf

S. Erlewein, M. Gauly and G. Erhardt. Department of Animal Breeding and Genetics, Justus Liebig University of Giessen, Ludwigstr. 21 B, D-35390 Giessen, Germany.*

Claw parameters of Merinolandschaf (n = 132) and Rhönschaf (n = 105) were measured at the left fore and hind leg at an age of 8 to10 and 16 to 20 weeks and heritabilities were estimated for claw hardness (1), dorsal border length (2), posterior wall length (3), diagonal length (4) and dorsal angle (5). In addition histological and chemical claw parameters (average no. of horn tubules per mm2, area of individual horn tubules, total area of horn tubules, water content, water absorption capacity) were analysed in randomly selected lambs (Merinolandschaf n = 89, Rhönschaf n = 68) between 12 to 32 weeks of age at slaughtering. Rhönschaf claws were in average significantly harder, shorter and lower, had a greater total area of horn tubules and a lower water content compared with Merinolandschaf claws. The estimated heritabilities of the parameters at the first measurements (8-10 weeks) showed, oin average, medium values (1: 0.10 - 0.33, 2: 0.26 - 0.43, 3: 0.07 - 0.54, 4: 0.11 - 0.32, 5: 0.29 - 0.39) while the values of the second measurement (16-24 weeks) were significantly lower (1: 0.01 - 0.18, 2: 0.04 - 0.26, 3: 0.01 - 0.34, 4: 0.10 - 0.30, 5: 0.20 - 0.56). Heritabilities for histological parameters ranged from 0.01 to 0.81, for water content from 0.07 to 0.29 and for water absorption capacity from 0.09 to 0.14, respectively.

Poster S5.15

The relationship between the outer aspect of the dam sheep fleece and the curling quality of black Karakul lambs

V. Tafta[1], *Elena Filoti*[1], *I. Raducuta*[1], [1]*University of Agronomical Sciences and Veterinary Medecine, Bucharest, Str. Marasti 59, Romania.*

The Black Karakul sheep, in general with gross fleece having a conic fleece thread (Tsurcana type), includes 10 % - 15 % individuals with semi-fine fleece all over the body or only over a part of the body, named *''pârve sheep"*. The particularity of these sheep is the loss of the thick and long threads in the first 4-5 months. This research has been performed on 229 Black Karakul sheep, 143 *''pârve sheep"* and 86 individuals with the Tsurcana type fleece, resulting in the 4 following Karakul variants: ''*pârve* male" x ''*pârve* female", ''*pârve* male" x Tsurcanous female, Tsurcanous male x ''*pârve* female" and Tsurcanous male x Tsurcanous female. The results of the experiment revealed a close connection between the parents' fleece features and the curling quality of the descendants. The red-black curling, with lustreless brightness, rough and friable fibers, is inferior to the Karakul sheep with Tsurcanous-type fleece, probably because of some specific genes, not yet studied. Taking into account that even the productive capacity of such phenotypes is also inferior, it is recommended that, for the time being, these individuals should not be taken into the reproductive processes.

Poster S5.16

Results from a two-year sequence of three lambings in Merinos de Palas sheep

V. Tafta[1], *N. Cutova*[1], [1]*University of Agronomical Sciences and Veterinary Medecine, Bucharest, Str. Marasti nr. 59,Romania.*

A two-year sequence of three lambings is one of the main methods employed to increase meat production in a shorter time period. The research was carried out at ICPCOC Palas on a lot of 70 sheep (Merinos de Palas, age 4-6 years) whose feding consisted mainly of fresh fodder. After the end of suckling period, ovulation oestrus occured naturally on groups, as a result of introducing three rams into the lot for two weeks. The research proves that the two-year sequence of three lambings is recommended especially for sheep of a longer reproduction period (6-8 months), under favourable feeding and maintenance conditions leading to out-of-season ovulation oestrus. The 70 Merinos de Palas sheep included in the experiment produced 214 lambs (3.6 lambs/sheep) with a final body weght of 35.27 kg/lamb after 150 days of fattening, compared with only 150 lambs resulted from a two-year sequence of one lambing per year. The body weight of the mother sheep remained relatively constant (53-55 kg) irrespective of the reproduction season, while the quantitative and qualitative wool production was not influenced by any of the above-mentioned parameters. Taking into account the advantages, the two-year sequence of three lambings is recommended in Merinos de Palas for a rapid increase in meat production, particularly in the units that provide adequate feeding and maintenance conditions.

Poster S5.17

The transmission of main structural components of the fleece at the crossbred individuals resulted from the crossing of Merinos and Tzigaia

V. Tafta[1], I.Raducuta[1], [1]University of Agronomical Sciences and Veterinary Medecine, Str. Marasti nr. 59, Bucharest, Romania

The experiment has the aim to study the transmission of the main structural components of the fleece (that is: thickness of the skin, fiber diameter, implantation depth and density of pilous folicles) of crossbred individuals resulting from the crossing of Merinos with Tzigaia. The experiment has been carried out on a lot of 58 sheep as follows: 10 Tzigaia females (with semifine fleece, 30-35 microns), 4 Romanian Merinos rams, 10 crossbred individuals type F_1, 9 crossbred individuals type F_2 (crossing Merinos with F_1), 11 crossbred individuals type F_1 x F_1, 6 crossbred individuals type F_2 x F_2 and 9 crossbred individuals type F_2 x F_1, aged 15 months. The main histological skin elements have been intermediarly transmitted to the crossbred individuals compared to the parental breeds. Nevertheless, the resulting values are rather closer to the Merino breed. The pilous folicle density of the crossbred individuals is almost double compared to the Tzigaia individuals (the ratio of the number of secondary to primary folicles is, for Tzigaia, 4.6, while for the F_2 individuals it is 9.9). This represents a positive result as regards both quality and quantity of wool production, especially of F_2 x F_2 crossbred individuals. However, in the case of F_2 x F_2 the absorption breeding must be stopped, especially in pre-mountain and mountain areas.

Poster S5.18

Some production traits of Karayaka and Bafra (Chios x Karayaka B_1) Sheep

N. Unal[1], H. Akçapinar[1], F. Atasoy[1], M. Erdogan[2], [1]Ankara University, Faculty of Veterinary Medicine, Department of Animal Science, 06110, Diskapi, Ankara, Turkey, [2]Afyon Kocatepe University, Faculty of Veterinary Medicine, Department of Animal Science, Afyon, Turkey*

The study was carried out to investigate the fertility of ewes, survival and growth of lambs in Karayaka and Bafra genotypes reared in Gokhoyuk State Farm in Black Sea Region.
Chios breed is raised in the western coastal regions of Turkey. It is poorly adapted in other parts of the country. It has a high milk yield and outstanding prolificacy. Karayaka is an indigenous breed of Black Sea Region. Productive performances of the breed are generally low.
Bafra was obtained in Karakoy State Farm by crossings between Chios and Karayaka to increase lamb crop.
The fertility for Karayaka and Bafra ewes was 92.3 and 93.7% for birth rates, and 1.08 and 1.78 for litter size, respectively. The survival rates of Karayaka and Bafra lambs at weaning (90 days) were 93.6 and 91.9%, respectively. The least squares means obtained for Karayaka and Bafra lambs were 3.1 and 3.7 kg for birth weight, 19.5 and 22.5 kg for weaning weight and 29.6 and 32.6 kg for 180 days weight ($P<0.001$), respectively.
The results showed that the litter size of ewes and growth of lambs in Bafra genotype were better than in the Karayaka, while the survival rate of Karayaka lambs was better than Bafra.

Poster S5.19

Estimation of live weight by multivariate ratio type estimation methods using body measurements, in Merino sheep

I.S. Gurcan[1] and H. Akcapinar[2], [1]Ankara University Faculty of Veterinary Medicine,Department of Biometrics,06110 Diskapi, Ankara, Turkey. [2]Ankara University Faculty of Veterinary Medicine, Department of Animal ScienceBreeding, 06110 Diskapi, Ankara.

A suitable fiber for textile industry is obtained from fiber type sheep families. The Merino sheep has played an important role to obtain the fiber type sheep.
The main purpose in raising Merino is to maximize the meat and the fiber yield. The German Merino sheep was created for this purpose.
Because of its highly adapted capability in different climatic regions, Merino is a preferred breed of sheep in Turkey. The German Merino sheep has been raised in Turkey since the 1930s. Also, it played an important role to obtain crossbred Merino variants in Turkey with local breeds of sheep.
The body measurements give important information about animal's morphological frame and development ability. The meat production is highly related with body size. In order to increase the meat production, the main target should be obtaining the animals which have big and wide frame.
Many statistical methods have been developed for the estimation of live weights of the animals.
In this study, the live weights of German Merino and Karacabey Merino sheep of the age groups 1.5 - 2.5 years and 3.5 - 5.5 years were estimated using body measurements by multivariate ratio type estimation methods. The comparisons were made among the estimates of the different methods.

Poster S5.20

Morphometric characteristics of milk fat globules from Massese ewes raised in northwestern Tuscany

M. Martini, C. Scolozzi, F. Cecchi, P. Verità. Dipartimento di Produzioni Animali, Università degli Studi di Pisa, Viale delle Piagge 2, 56124, Pisa, Italy.*

This study evaluates the morphometric characteristics of fat globules (number/ml, diameter) from the milk of Massese ewes raised in northwestern Tuscany. A pool of samples was taken from 13 different herds during the morning milking; the samples, refrigerated until use and placed in a Burker chamber, were observed under fluorescence microscope and by an image analyser system (Leica Ortomat Microsystem). The results were obtained from the measurement of 41,972 globules.
The mean number of fat globules/ml from all samples was 2.21×10^9, while the mean diameter was 5.18 μm, ranging from 0.4 to 16 μm.
For all herds, frequency distribution of measured milk fat globules according to size shows ten size classes of 1 mm class widths (from <1 to >9μm); class widths were further utilized to define small (from <1 to 2μm), medium (>2 to 5μm) and large globules (>5μm).
The distribution of percentage of measured fat globules indicates that in all herds considered, the percentage of measured milk fat globules increased up to the sixth class (5-6μm) and then decreased progressively until the last width class.

Poster S5.21

Influence of several variability factors on morphometric characteristics of milk fat globules from Massese ewes

M. Martini, F. Cecchi, C. Scolozzi, P. Verità. Dipartimento di Produzioni Animali, Università degli Studi di Pisa, Viale delle Piagge 2, 56124, Pisa, Italy.*

The study evaluated the influence of several variability factors, such as altimetric location (plain and hills up to 500m above sea level), province (Lucca, Massa Carrara and Pisa) and the individual farm (13 farms in total), on morphometric characteristics [number of globules/ml, average diameter, frequency distribution of globules according to size: small (from <1 to 2μm), medium (>2 to 5μm) and large globules (>5μm)] of fat globules in milk collected from ewes of the Massese breed. The analysis revealed that in subjects raised in the hills, the number of globules/ml was nearly double that of animals raised on the plain (3.07×10^9 vs 1.67×10^9; $P<0.01$), while the difference relative to diameter was less marked (5.12μm vs 5.22μm). The territory of origin appeared to have a highly significant influence ($P<0.01$): the higher number of globules/ml characterized the milk of sheep reared in the province of Lucca (2.43×10^9), while the lower number pertained to the milk of sheep reared in province of Pisa (1.60×10^9). However, the medium diameter presented an opposite trend. Massa Carrara presented a greater percentage of large globules and a smaller percentage of those of medium size ($P<0.05$). Finally, the individual farm, depending on a complex of genetic and environmental conditions, always presented a statistically significant effect.

Poster S5.22

Milk protein variants in goat breeding

A. Caroli[1] S. Chessa[2], E. Budelli[3], O. Jann[4], E. Prinzenberg[4] and G. Erhardt[4], [1]Department SBA, Strada Prov. per Casamassima km 3, 70010 Valenzano, Bari, Italy, [2]Department VSA, Milan, Italy, [3]CERSA - Segrate, Milano, Italy, [4]Department for Animal Breeding and Genetics, Justus-Liebig University, Giessen, Germany.

Milk protein polymorphisms are of economic interest due to their direct relationships with milk quality, milk production traits and human health.

Within Vigoni project (CRUI-DAAD), a research was carried out from 2001 to 2002, on the variability of goat milk proteins representing an interesting and extremely complex qualitative and quantitative genetic system and model.

A high variability was found at κ-casein (*CSN3)* locus, confirming the presence of the B allele, which is detectable at protein level by isolectrofocusing. Further polymorphisms were identified at DNA level by PCR-SSCP technique. Molecular data analysis indicates that the *CSN3* polymorphisms are not randomly distributed within the gene sequence, the caseinomacropeptide being much more conserved than para-κ-casein.

Moreover, IEF analysis allowed to detect a novel allele at α_{S2} locus (*CSN1S2*). The new variant, showing an isoelectric point between *CSN1S2**A and *CSN1S2*C*, was named *CSN1S2*G.*

The study was finally directed to the definition of goat casein haplotypes at the casein cluster, by an accurate screening of milk protein loci in different Italian and German breeds.

 Poster S5.23

Comparison between two different transcervical insemination techniques in Sarda ewes

S.P.G. Rassu[1], G. Enne[1-2], M.T. Zedda[3], A. Carluccio[4], G.M. Schiaffino[3], S. Pau[3]. [1]Dipartimento di Scienze Zootecniche, via De Nicola 07100 Sassari, Italy, [2]Istituto Spallanzani, Milano, Italy, [3]Clinica Ostetrica Veterineria, Sassari, Italy, [4]Clinica ostetrica veterinaria, Teramo, Italy.*

Two different transcervical insemination techniques were compared using 47 Sarda ewes. Within 24 h after lambing (November), the cervical folds were cut out by surgery on 22 ewes: 11 ewes had 2 cuts for every cervical folds (group CFC2) and the other 11 ewes had 4 cuts for every cervical folds (groups CFC4). During the breeding season (May), the 22 ewes treated surgically and other 25 ewes with normal cervix (group NCF) received a progestagen pessary for 14 d and 300 IU of PMSG i.m. at the time of pessary removal. After 56-58 h from pessary removal, all the ewes were subjected to transcervical artificial insemination with frozen semen (about $80x10^6$ spermatozoa/dose) using the Cassou pistolet for CFC2 and CFC4 groups, and "Guelph System" with a modified instrument for NCF group. Penetration rate in uterus and time required for insemination were: 100% and about 25±6 sec. for CFC groups; 32% and 205±61 sec. for NCF group. Fertility was similar between CFC2 and CFC4 (73%) and higher than in the NCF group (28%). However, fertility of penetreted NCF ewes was satisfying (63%).In conclusion, with the aid of a surgery to cut cervical folds the efficiency of transcervical insemination was greatly improved.

Poster S5.24

Influence of prolonged conservation in liquid nitrogen upon pregnancy rate obtained from freezing - thawing ram and buck semen

*Stela Zamfirescu[1], *Vicovan Gabriel[1], Gore Iancu[1], Pop Aurelia[2], Fatu Nicolae[2]. [1]University Ovidius Constanta, Bd. Mamaia, 124, Romania. [2]Research and Development Institut for Sheep and Goat, IC Bratianu, 248, Constanta, Romania.*

The sperm cell after freezing procedure remains viable for years at the temperature of liquid nitrogen. The cryopreservation of semen is now considered to be a commonplace technology in sheep and goat industry because it is applied to international movements of genotype. Moreover, owing to the occurrence of some heavy diseases, the freezing semen has a very serious social implication in the local and international exchange. The aim of our study was to compare the conception rate after intracervical and intrauterine insemination of freezing - thawing semen of ram and buck conserved more than 10 years in liquid nitrogen. The semen from Palas and Australian Merinos ram was preserved for 21 years, from Awassi 19 years, from Angora bucks 14 years and Saanen bucks 12 years. The conception rate after intracervical insemination ranged from 41.3 - 56.5% (n=83) for the frozen semen from Palas and Australian Merinos rams, and 34.8% for Awassi semen (n=95). The conception rate after intracervical insemination of local breed was 62.9% for Saanen and 18.2% for Angora semen. After intrauterine insemination of Merinos Palas ewes with freezing semen the conception rate was 62% (n=138). Regardless of the preservation time of semen conserved in liquid nitrogen the conception rate was acceptable, except the Angora semen. The conception rate depended on the motility and viability after thawing of the semen.

Poster S5.25

The superovulation response treatment with Stimufol of ewes and goats

Stela Zamfirescu[1], Gore Iancu[1], J.F. Bekers[2], [1]University Ovidius Constanta, Bd. Mamaia, 124, Romania. [2]University of Liege, Bd Colonster, 20, Liege, Belgium.

Within in the last two years, Stimufol was used for the superovulation of ewes and goats (J. F. Bekers, 1998). The superovulatory treatment with Stimufol was demonstrated in the ovulatory response in ewes of various age (n=28) and adult goats (n=12). The treatments were performed in October 2001 - March 2003 in the Research Institute for Sheep and Goat Palas. After the oestrus synchronization with Chronogest, Stimufol was injected in total doses of 150, 200 and 250 μg. Treatment with Stimufol was given in 6 decreasing doses, the last being given after 10 hours from the removal of the Chronogest sponges. The mean number of usable embryos from 18 treated adult ewes was 5.36 and from 12 goats were 6.01 embryos. The ewe's ages 8-10 month were refractory after superovulatory treatment. The superovulatory response was affected by the body weight of young females, and in adult female the ovulatory response was influenced by the number of doses and procedure of administration of Stimufol. The optimal ovulatory response (OR = 8) was obtained by 6 decreasing doses of Stimufol.

Poster S5.26

The kidding rate with local does synchronized with Chronogest and inseminated with semen preserved under different forms

Stela Zamfirescu[1], Nadolu Dorina[2], Sava Iris[2], Fatu Nicolae[2], [1]University Ovidius Constanta, Bd. Mamaia, 124, Romania. [2]Research and Development Institut for Sheep and Goat, IC Bratianu, 248, Constanta, Romania.

In October 2002, 223 does of local breed raised in 5 herds were intracervical and intrauterine inseminated with frozen semen, diluted semen (+12°C) and refrigerated semen (+4°C). The frozen semen came from France (the Saanen and Angora breeds) and from the own laboratory of the Research and Development Institute for Sheep and Goats Breading Palas, Constanta. The diluted and refrigerated semen came from bucks crosses of local breed and Saanen and was diluted and preserved at +12°C for 8 hours and at +4°C for 24-36 hours, respectively. Fertility (F%) calculated after kidding within the normal term varied depending on the origin of the frozen semen, motility of the thawed semen, type of insemination and herd. Thus, after the insemination with the frozen semen coming from France, the lambing rate was 62-69.11% (n=85) and 58.2% - 61.5% (n=35) after the insemination with the semen frozen in the own laboratory. The frozen semen which was inseminated in the uterus (n=28) has achieved a lambing rate of 72.65%. Sperm motility after thawing regardless of the semen origin ranged between 34.43% - 48.27%. The kidding rate with does after intracervical insemination with diluted semen (n=45) was 88.94% and 73.50% after insemination with refrigerated semen (n=30). The type of semen did not influence prolificacy which was 127-181%.

SHEEP AND GOAT PRODUCTION [S] Theatre NS6.1

Relationship between feeding system and goat milk and cheese quality

R. Rubino[1] and Y. Chilliard[2], [1]Istituto Sperimentale Zootecnia, 85054, Bella Scalo, Italia, [2]INRA-Theix, F-63122, France*

One of the most important factors influencing the quality of milk and cheese is the feeding system. Grazing and the free choice of some specific herbs influence the flavour, the nutritional and pharmacological composition of cheese. In different trials comparing an outdoor flock grazing natural pasture and an indoor flock eating hay from the same pasture, the cheese produced with milk from grazing animals showed a higher content of mono-terpenes, sesqui-terpenes, unsatured fatty acids (Fedele et al. 2000), CLA, and the anti-oxidants (Pizzoferrato et al. 2000) than cheeses from indoor goats. Goats receiving a diet rich in *Borago officinalis* produced a milk with higher content of β-sitosterol and 5,7,4-tri-flavonol while group receiving *Crataegus oxyacanta* produced a milk with higher content of rutin than control group (Rubino et al. 2002). Other studies were done to investigate the effects of alfalfa hay (H) or maize silage (MS), and interactions with high oleic sunflower (OSO) or linseed (LO) oil. LO addition increased mainly trans-vaccenic acid (TVA) and rumenic acid (RA) percentages. OSO increased mainly C18:0 and oleic acid. Some effects were higher with H diet (Chilliard et al. 2002). Milks (raw or pasteurised) obtained from the same goats were transformed in fresh or ripened, lactic or soft cheeses. Intensities of the sensorial descriptors were generally higher for H than for MS, and more affected for LO than OSO and for H/LO and MS/OSO than H/OSO and MS alone (Gaborit et al. 2002).

Theatre NS6.2

Digestibility and milk production of goats fed a no forage diet

L. Rapetti, L. Bava., G. Galassi., A. Tamburini and G.M. Crovetto, Istituto di Zootecnia Generale, Università degli Studi, via Celoria 2, 20133 Milano, Italy*

Six lactating Saanen goats were used, in a Latin Square design, to compare a no forage (NF) diet with more traditional diets with grass (G) or hay (H) contributing to 55% of total DM. Diets averaged 17% CP and 32% NDF on DM. Diet NF included 26.5% dried beet pulp, 25.8% cracked carrobs, 12% soybean meal, 11.3% whole cotton seeds, 9.8% ground maize grain, 9.6% maize grain, 2% maize gluten meal and min/vit supplements; 35% of its feed particles were >4 mm.
Grass quality was lower than expected, for conservation problems. With diets G, H and NF the DM intakes were 104, 116 and 106 g/LW$^{3/4}$, respectively. DM digestibility was similar for diets G and H (69.7 and 70.5%) and higher with diet NF (74.1%; $P<0.05$). A similar trend was registered for OM and energy digestibility.
Milk production results with diets G, H and NF, respectively: milk yield 3011, 3688, 3212 ($P<0.05$) g/d, milk fat 3.37, 3.24, 2.96% ($P<0.05$), milk protein 3.21, 3.35, 3.32%, milk urea N 18.8, 18.6, 12.7 mg/100 ml, ($P<0.001$). When fed NF diet the goats produced a milk with a higher content of short and medium and a lower content of long chain fatty acids.
Diet NF proved to be "safe" for rumen function, but a good forage was more effective in promoting milk yield and quality.

Theatre NS6.3

Influence of level of rumen undegredable protein on milk yield of dairy goats

C. Kijora, K.J. Peters and H. Rexroth, Institute of Animal Sciences, Humboldt-University Berlin, Philippstr. 13, Building 9; 10115 Berlin*

The practice of increasing the ratio of rumen undegradable protein (UDP) in diets of dairy cows to raise milk yield is disputed in dairy goats, like the controversial literatur shows. The objective of this experiment was to estimate the influence of UDP content in diets with different protein levels for dairy goats.

A total of 24 dairy goats (German Fawn) were fed in two trails diets with low protein content (V1; CP: 12%) or high protein content (V2; CP: 16%) and balanced average energy content of 11.3 MJME/kg DM. The soya bean meal in the diet was either protected (P) or unprotected (UP) resulting in different ratios of UDP. The feed intake, milk yield and content of nutrients and urea were estimated over a period of 150 days.

The UDP ratio in both experiments amounted to 30% in the UP group and 40% in the P group, respectively. A higher protein content in the diet (V2) increased the feed intake significantly at 120% independent of protein protection, although the feed supply was identical in both experiments. The milk yield in the order of experiments: V1 UP; V1 P; V2 UP and V2 P amounted to 1600, 2254, 2739 and 3268 kg FCM resp. The urea content in the milk indicated a shortage of protein in the first experiment and a surplus (during late lactation) in the second experiment.

Protein protection in diets for dairy goats is a possibility to increase the milk yield.

Theatre NS6.4

Effect of diet botanical composition of grazing goats on mono and sesqui-terpene content in milk

S. Claps, G.F. Cifuni, L. Sepe, V. Fedele, Istituto Sperimentale per la Zootecnia, Via Appia- Bella Scalo; I-85054 Muro Lucano*

The aim of this research was to assess the effect of plants ingested by grazing goats on mono and sequi-terpene content in milk. Forty-five Siriana goats, in their 3rd lactation, were divided into 3 groups fed as follows: G (grazing) for 8 hours/day; GRD (grazing plus 600 g/d of rapidly degradable concentrate); GNRD (grazing plus 600 g/d of less rapidly degradable concentrate). A native pasture of 6 ha was used for this experiment. The contribution of the different species to the diet was estimated on four sampling units of 2x2 m. For each species, after visual assessment, the ratio between the number of grazed plants and the number of available plants was calculated. Mono and sequi-terpene content was determined on three milk samples for each season.

The results showed that season and selected diet influenced milk characteristics. Mono-terpene content was higher in winter than in summer (on average, 1288.7 vs. 584 µ/l), while sesqui-terpene was higher in summer than in winter (on average, 9724.9 vs. 2258.0 µ/l). Principal component analyses showed that plants selected by goats during winter have not influenced mono and sesqui-terpene content in milk. On the contrary, during summer, sesqui-terpene content was positively influenced by the percentage in the diet of *Daucus carota*, *Cichorium intybus*, *Foeniculum* sp. and level of forbs intake. Grasses intake and *Centaurea* sp. influenced positively mono-terpene content.

Interactions between raygrass preservation and linseed oil supplementation on goat milk yield and composition, including *trans* and conjugated fatty acids

Y. Chilliard[1], J. Rouel[1], J.M. Chabosseau[2], P. Capitan[1], P. Gaborit[3] and A. Ferlay[1], [1]INRA-Theix,63122, France, [2]INRA-Lusignan, France,[3]ITPLC-Surgères, France*

Forty-eight multiparous mid-lactation goats were used indoor in a 2x2 factorial design, including 2 forages *ad libitum* : fresh raygrass + raygrass hay (.26 kg DM/d) (FR) or raygrass hay (RH), and 2 lipid intakes (0 g/d, control, C, or 130 g/d, i.e. 5-6% of diet DM, of linseed oil, LO) for 5 weeks. Diets LO, compared to C, increased (P<0.05) milk fat (+4.8 g/kg), protein (+1.5 g/kg) and lactose (+2.9 g/kg) content and milk fat (+21 g/d) and protein (+10 g/d) yield. Effects on milk fatty acid (FA) composition were large. Diets LO, compared to C, decreased 6:0 to 16:0, branched-chain (BC) and odd-numbered (ON) FA, 18:2n-6, 20:3, 20:4n-6 and 22:2n-6, and increased 4:0, 18:0, *trans*9-16:1 (+955%), *trans*6+7+8-18:1, *trans*9 to *trans*13-18:1 (+944% for *trans*11-18:1), *cis*11 to *cis*15-18:1, *cis*9,*trans*13-18:2, *cis*9,*trans*11-18:2 (+645%) and 18:3n-3 (+114%). Diets LO decreased the normalized delta-9 desaturation ratios for 14:0, 17:0, 18:0 and *trans*11-18:1. Numerous significant interactions were observed : the effects of LO on *trans*11,*cis*15-18:2 and the delta-9 desaturation ratios for 14:0, 16:0 and 17:0 were more important with RH, whereas the effects on the isomers of 18:1 (particularly trans10 and trans13) and *cis*9,*trans*13-18:2 were more important with FR. In conclusion, diets LO improved largely production performances, increased n-3 and *trans*-FA, particularly *trans*11-18:1 and *cis*9,*trans*11-18:2, and decreased delta-9 desaturation ratios, short and medium-chain, and BC+ON FA, and interacted with raygrass preservation.

Theatre NS6.6

Correlations between milk fat content and fatty acid composition in goats receiving different combinations of forages and lipid supplements

Y. Chilliard[1], J. Rouel[1], P. Capitan[1], J.M. Chabosseau[2], K. Raynal-Ljutovac[3] and A. Ferlay[1], [1]INRA-Theix,63122, France, [2]INRA-Lusignan, France, [3]ITPLC-Surgères, France*

Eighty-four multiparous mid-lactation goats received indoor one of 7 diets differing in either forages : fresh raygrass + raygrass hay (.26 kg/d) vs. raygrass hay vs. alfalfa hay, or lipid intakes (O g/d, control vs.130 g/d, i.e. 5-6% of diet DM, of either linseed oil or high-oleic sunflower oil) for 5 weeks. Milk yield and fat content (MFC) were 2.87- 3.54 kg/d and 28.7-35.7 g/kg, respectively, for the different diets. MFC was significantly (P<0.05) increased by lipid supplementation. Individual MFC values were 32.3 +/- 5.2 (mean +/- SD, n=84).

Correlations between MFC and fatty acid (FA) percentages were significant (P<0.05) and positive for 18:0 (0.34) and 20:0 (0.22). Significant negative correlations were observed for *cis*9-14:1 (-0.35), 10:1 (-0.25), *cis*9-16:1 (-0.25), 24:1 (-0.23), for normalized delta-9 desaturation ratios (r= -0.49, 36, 36, 27 respectively for 18:0, *trans*11-18:1, 14:0 and 17:0), for 16:0 (-0.29), 15:0 (-0.29), 14:0 (-0.28) and iso14:0 (-0.23), and for polyunsaturated n-6 FA (-0.32, 29, 26, 25 respectively for 22:4, 18:2, 20:3 and 20:4). These correlations were due to differences between diets rather than between goats.

In conclusion, this study suggests that the regulation of MFC differs between goat and bovine species (no significant correlation was observed with any *trans*-18:1 or 18:2 isomer). Our working hypothesis is that 18:0 arising from the digestion of lipid supplements triggered the associated increase in MFC.

 Theatre NS6.7

Feeding the dairy ewe

G. Caja[1], E. Molina[2], C. Flores[1], M. Ayadi[1], A. Salama[1], T.T. Treacher[3], H. Hassoun[4] and F. Bocquier[4]. Grup de Recerca en Remugants, Universitat Autònoma de Barcelona, Bellaterra, Spain; [2]Departament de Producció Animal, Universitat de Lleida, Lleida, Spain; [3]51 Western road, Oxford, UK; [4]UMR Élevage des ruminants en régions chaudes, INRA-ENSAM, Montpellier, France.*

World dairy sheep are basically localized around the Mediterranean Sea where they mainly produce cheese and fermented milk products. Production systems are characterized by using local breeds and poor or seasonal pastures. Moreover, milk composition and artisan practices give own characteristics to sheep dairy products. Modernization of dairy sheep focuses on machine milking jointly with improvement of management, genetics and feeding. As a result, traditional scenarios change to intensive systems in which feeding becomes a key point. The French INRA feeding system (UFL and PDI), with feed intake estimated as fill units (UEm), is the most used feeding system in practice. Although main knowledge on dairy sheep nutrition comes from suckling ewes and dairy cows, in which nutrient partitioning and efficiency for milk production can be different, recent research allowed to know differences in nutrient requirements, intake, milk composition, body reserves, as well as in the use of nutrients (fats, aminoacids, etc.). Nutrition of ewe-lambs and pregnant ewes has also been updated. Effects of nutrition on milk composition as a consequence of feeding strategies, concentrate level, energy balance and dietary fat and protein supplements are also discussed.

Theatre NS6.8

Effects of dietary non-fiber carbohydrates concentration on intake, in vivo digestibility and milk yield in Sarda ewes

A. Cannas[1], A.Cabiddu[2], G. Bomboi[3], S. Ligios[2] and G. Molle[2], [1]Dipartimento Scienze Zootecniche, Via De Nicola, 07100 Sassari, Italy, [2]Istituto Zootecnico e Caseario per la Sardegna, 07041 Olmedo, Italy, [3]Dipartimento Biologia Animale, Via Vienna, 07100 Sassari, Italy*

The effects of dietary non-fiber carbohydrates (NFC) were studied on 20 Sarda ewes (BW 42.5±3.9 kg) in mid-lactation (89±1 d). They were divided into 2 groups and fed 400 g/d of chopped alfalfa hay and pellets *ad libitum* in metabolic cages. The pellets differed in NFC concentration (36% of DM: group NFC36; 23% of DM: group NFC23), due to the substitution of cereal grains with soybean hulls. DM intake was very high throughout the experiment, with larger values (P<0.01) for NFC23 (2943 g/d) than for NFC36 (2593 g/d). DM digestibility was higher in NFC36 than in NFC23 (68.4% vs. 62.9%, P<0.001), while the contrary occurred for NDF digestibility (52.9% vs. 56.1%, P<0.05). NE intake did not significantly differ between groups. Dietary NFC concentration negatively affected milk yield (1926 ml/d vs. 2143 ml/d; P<0.01) and positively affected milk protein (4.81% vs. 4.68%; P<0.09). Milk fat did not differ between groups (5.19% vs. 5.06%; P>0.1). Milk urea was lower in NFC36- than in NFC23-group (57 mg/dl vs. 65 mg/dl; P<0.001). Body fat tended to increase more in the NFC36- than in NFC23-group (P>0.1). Overall, the high dietary NFC concentration had negative effects on milk yield in ewes in mid-lactation.

Efforts in utilising locally available agro-industrial by-products and crop surpluses in dairy sheep feeding

M. Volanis[1] and P.E Zoiopoulos[*2], [1]National Agricultural Research Foundation, Agrokipio, Chania 731.00,Greece, [2]University of Ioannina, Seferi 2, Agrinio, 301.00, Greece.*

For the last 5 years efforts were made in the Greek island of Crete to utilise locally produced whole orange fruit surpluses or fresh orange juice industry by-products for feeding the local dairy type Sfakian breed of sheep. Due to the high moisture content of these materials, ensiling was preferred as less costly method of conservation. For the first 2 years preliminary work was carried out to study quality characteristics of orange silage produced. The latter had an exceptionally pleasant odour. Silage pH value dropped, from approximately 4.2 before to around 3.5 at the end of ensiling period. The effects of diets containing either 80% ensiled chopped oranges or 90% ensiled orange pulp were tested in 3 lactation periods using dairy Sfakian ewes, compared to ewes fed control diet. Live weight changes, as well as milk yield and composition were measured. Both silage materials proved to be particularly palatable for ewes fed the experimental diets. Fat content of milk was significantly higher for ewes fed the ensiled chopped orange and orange pulp diets. Results showed that feeding of high amounts of orange surpluses or pulp to lactating dairy ewes is a very promising proposition. The implications of the findings of these studies on the local dairy sheep production and feta cheese making industry are discussed.

Theatre NS6.10

Feeding level before puberty affects milk production during first lactation in Lacaune and Manchega ewes

M. Ayadi, G. Caja, X. Such, and J. Ghirardi. Grup de Recerca en Remugants, Departament de Ciència Animal i dels Aliments, Universitat Autònoma de Barcelona, 08193 Bellaterra, Spain.

Fifty seven ewe-lambs of Manchega (n=35) and Lacaune (n=22) breeds were used to study the effects of growth before puberty on milk yield. Feeding treatments were: 'high' (H, concentrate and straw) and 'medium' (M, rationed concentrate and alfalfa pellets). M ewe-lambs were switched to H treatment after puberty. Milk yield during suckling was estimated by the oxytocin method. After weaning of the lambs (wk 5), the ewes were machine milked and the yield recorded weekly. Milk was sampled bi-weekly for composition. Growth during pre-puberty (wk 7-22) varied according to treatments (H vs. M): Lacaune (293 vs. 189 g/d) and Manchega (254 vs. 164 g/d). No differences in reproductive performances or ewes condition at first lambing were reported within breeds. Milk yield and lamb growth during suckling were not affected by treatments, but M Manchega ewes yielded more milk in the first 2 wk of lactation. During milking (wk 5 to 16) milk yield in Lacaune ewes did not differ between treatments (137 vs. 132 L; for H vs M) but the M group produced 41% more milk than the H group in Manchega ewes (46 vs 66 L). We conclude that a medium level of feeding after weaning and before puberty may affect positively the development of the mammary gland and improve the milk yield in the first lactation in dairy ewes.

Theatre NS6.11

A mechanistic model to predict nutrient requirements and feed biological values for sheep in each unique production situation

A. Cannas[1], D.G. Fox[2], L.O. Tedeschi[2], A.N. Pell[2], and P.J. Van Soest[2], [1]Dipartimento Scienze Zootecniche, via De Nicola, 07100 Sassari, Italy; [2]Department of Animal Science, Morrison Hall, Cornell University, Ithaca, NY 14852, USA*

The Cornell Net Carbohydrate and Protein System, a mechanistic model that predicts nutrient requirements and feed biological values for cattle in each unique production situation (CNCPS-C) was modified for use with sheep (CNCPS-S). Published equations were added to predict energy and protein requirements of sheep. The CNCPS-C equations used to predict the supply of nutrients were modified to include new solid and liquid ruminal passage rates for sheep and new estimates of metabolic fecal nitrogen. Equations were added to predict energy and protein reserves fluxes from BW and body condition score.
When evaluated with data from 7 published studies, the CNCPS-S predicted OM digestibility, which is used to predict feed ME values, with no mean bias (1.3; $P > 0.1$; n = 19) and a low root mean squared prediction error (RMSPE; 3.7 g / 100 g of DM). The ability of the CNCPS-S to predict energy balance was evaluated with gains and losses in shrunk BW (SBW) in 6 studies with adult sheep. Gains and losses in SBW were accurately predicted when diets had a positive ruminal N balance (mean bias of 9.7 g/d; $P>0.1$; RMSPE of 32.1 g/d; n = 18).

Theatre NS6.12

Pasture percentage in the diet and milk fat composition in dairy ewes

M. Avondo, I.R. Pagano and A. Criscione. University of Catania, DACPA sez. Scienze delle Produzioni Animali, Via Valdisavoia 5, 95123 Catania, Italy*

Fourty ewe bulk samples were collected from 40 sheep farms located in eastern Sicily. For each farm, information on the diet supplied was detected and dry matter intake at pasture was estimated applying an intake model previously developed for dairy sheep. Fatty acid composition of milk fat was affected by pasture percentage in the diet. We found that C16:1, C18:1*n*-9 and C18:2*n*-6 decreased, whereas CLA and C 18:3*n*3 increased as pasture percentage in the diet increased. However weak significance was found in regression analysis using pasture percentage or estimated herbage intake as independent variables. Analysis of variance subdividing pasture percentage in three classes (0%, 1-50%, >50) gave rise to significant differences ($P<0.05$) between classes. Results respectively for 0%, 1-50% and >50%, were: C16:1, 1.39, 1.02, 1.05 % of total fatty acids; C18:1*n*-9, 17.5, 18.3, 15.9 %; C18:2*n*-6, 2.5, 1.8, 1.6 %; CLA, 1.4, 1.2, 1.8%; C18:3*n*3, 0.9, 1.9, 1.9%.

Poster NS6.13

Effect of three levels of herbage allowance on voluntary intake and milk production of dairy ewes at pasture: preliminary results

P. Hassoun[1], P. Autran[2], C. Marie-Etancelin[2], F. Barillet[2] and F. Bocquier[1], [1]UMR_ERRC, INRA, 2, Place Viala, 34 060 Montpellier Cedex 1, France, [2]INRA SAGA, BP 27, 31 426 Castanet-Tolosan Cedex, France*

Three groups of 16 multiparous Lacaune dairy ewes in late lactating stage (175 d) were initially balanced on body weight (BW: 70 kg) and milk yield (MY: 0.9 l/d) basis. For 3 weeks, each group has been offered: Low: 1.4, Medium: 1.9 or High: 2.4 kg DM/ewe/day allowances of a cocksfoot pasture. Ewes grazed only 6 h/d with no other food but 0.1 kg of dehydrated alfalfa given in the milking parlour. Dry matter intake (DMI, kg/ewe/d) was estimated through ytterbium oxide and faecal nitrogen on four ewes per group.
Average daily grass DMI was identical for M (1.5 ± 0.3) and H (1.5 ± 0.2) allowances and declined with the lowest allowance (1.2 ± 0.30). Out of the natural decline of milk yield, there were no significant (P>0.05) differences between groups. Unexpectedly, both milk fat and protein contents decreased without (P>0.05) difference between groups. BW decreased, without significant differences between groups.
Even in late lactation, a limitation of herbage allowance had an impact on MY, BW changes and milk content. Surprisingly, at highest grass allowance, a 6h daily access to pasture may not allow to fulfil requirements as suggested by both BW and milk content evolutions.

Poster NS6.14

Effect of Soy Bean Meal substitution with cotton by-products on nutrient digestibility of sheep rations

D. Liamadis[1], Ef. Lales[1] and Ch. Milis[2]. [1]Aristotle University of Thessaloniki. [2]Ministry of Agriculture, Greece

An in vivo digestibility trial using a Latin Square 4x4 experimental design with castrated rams was conducted to evaluate effects of replacing protein from Soy Bean Meal (SBM) with Whole Cottonseed (WCS), Cottonseed Meal (CSM) and Cottonseed Cake (CSC), protein, respectively, on nutrient digestibility. Rams were fed four isonitrogenous rations differing in main protein source, which corresponded to maintenance requirements for energy. Statistical analysis was performed by the use of SPSS, and significance was declared at P<0.05. The SBM ration had higher Dry Matter (DM), Organic Matter (OM), Crude Protein (CP) and Nitrogen Free Extract (NFE) digestibility from all other rations (61.3, 65.3, 78.8 and 65.8%; 58.3, 62.3, 75.2 and 61.9%; 56.5, 60.1, 73.9 and 63.5%; 56.9, 59.8, 72.6 and 63.3% for the SBM, WCS, CSM and CSC ration, respectively). The WCS ration had higher Ether Extract (EE) digestibility from all other rations (43.1, 85.2, 43.5 and 53.5% for the SBM, WCS, CSM and CSC ration, respectively). The SBM and WCS rations had superior Crude Fiber (CF) digestibility from the other two rations (48.9, 49, 44.7 and 45.6% for the SBM, WCS, CSM and CSC ration, respectively). Replacement of SBM with WCS, CSM, CSC could have negative effects on DM, OM, CP and NFE digestibility whereas replacement of SBM from WCS has no negative effect on CF digestibility. Moreover, replacement of SBM with WCS is beneficial on digestibility of EE.

 Poster NS6.15

Responses in blood characteritics, milk constituents and growth of offspring to dietary protein in Rahmani ewes rations

Y.A. Maareck[1] and Y.M. Hafez[2], [1]Animal Production Department, National Research Center, Egypt, [2]Animal Production Department, Faculty of Agriculture, Cairo University, Egypt.*

Eighteen pregnant Rahmani ewes (40.7 ± 1.2 Kg) were used starting 4 weeks before lambing till weaning to investigate the effect of 3 different levels of dietary protein (100%, 80% and 120% of NRC, 1985) on blood charateristics, lactation performance and offspring growth.
Blood hematocrit of ewes was not significantly affected by dietary protein Hemoglobin increased with 120% dietary protein (CP). Plasma total protein and globulin increased while plasma albumin decreased due to decreasing CP by 20%. Changes in plasma urea showed an increase due to increasing CP. Decreasing protein content of the diet by 20% increased plasma creatinine. Activity of GOT and GPT decreased with the high level of CP.
Ewes daily milk production changed from -6.0% to +7.9% relative to the control for 80 and 120 % CP, respectively. Better milk constituents and milk gross energy accompanied the highest CP.
Final body weight of ewes fed the highest CP level was the highest (34.7 kg). Decreasing CP in ewes diets decreased lamb birth weight by 7.4% and lamb growth performance till weaning.
Ewes fed on NRC, 1985 allowences showed satisfactory performance, but those fed on 120% CP showed better performance which reflected on greater growth of lambs.

Poster NS6.16

Variations in the constituents of colostrum, transitional milk and blood of Rahmani ewes in relation to dietary protein and days relative to parturition

Y.M. Hafez[1] and Y.A. Maareck[2], [1]Animal Production Department, Faculty of Agriculture, Cairo University, Egypt, [2]Animal Production Department, National Research Center, Egypt.*

Eighteen pregnant Rahmani ewes (40.7 ± 1.2 Kg) used to study the effect of 3 levels of dietary protein (100%, 80% and 120% of NRC, 1985) starting from 28 days prepartum till the 10th day post-lambing on composition of colostrum, transitional milk and blood.
Ewes fed 120 % CP produced the best colostrum. Colostrum obtained immediately after lambing had the highest values of gross energy and concentrations of all constituents except lactose. Total solids, protein, fat, solids not fat and gross energy of colostrum decreased by days post-lambing while lactose showed a reversed trend.
Changes in blood hematocrit and hemoglobin of ewes due to CP levels were not significant. Plasma total protein and globulin concentrations increased while plasma albumin and A/G ratio decreased due to decreasing or increasing CP level by 20%. Plasma urea was not significantly affected by dietary CP. Plasma creatinine significantly decreased by feeding the low CP diet (80%). Activities of GOT and GPT showed no obvious trend due to dietary CP. Time of parturition was accompanied by the lowest values of tested blood measurements except the values of albumin, A/G ratio, urea, creatinine and GOT activity.

 Poster NS6.17

The effect of different ratios of effective rumen degradable nitrogen: sulphur (ERDN: S) on the microbial production in the Raini goats

Y. Rouzbehan[*1], F. Fatahnia[1] and K. Rizayazdi[2], [1]Animal Science Dept., Agriculture College, Tarbiat Modaress University, Tehran P.O. Box 14155-4838, Iran, [2]Animal Science Dept., Agriculture College, Mohaghegh Ardabili University, University Sreet, P.O. Box 179, Ardabil, Iran.*

Little information is available on the ERDN: S ratio for the determination of optimal ruminal microbial protein of goat. Therefore, this trial was carried out to assess the influence of five different ratios of ERDN: S (12:1, 7.6:1, 5.9:1, 4.9:1 or 4.9:1) on the amount of microbial protein produced in the rumen of Raini goat. Fifteen Raini male kids of 13.5 months age weighing 32 kg (sd 1.7 kg) were kept individually in metabolic cages for two weeks. During the second week, their urine samples were collected for the estimation of urinary purine derivatives (allantoin, uric acid, xanthine and hypoxanthine). The trial was conducted using a completely randomised design with five diets (n=3), which were isocaloric and isonitrogenous. The metabolisable energy and the metabolisable protein of the diets were 9.57 MJ/kg DM and 84.2 g/kg DM respectively. The results show that the highest concentration of purine derivatives was found in the urine of kids fed the diet containing the ERDN: S ratio of 6.7:1. Hence, this diet had the maximum microbial protein produced in the rumen. Using the regression analysis between the ratio of ERDN:S and ruminal microbial protein, the optimum ratio was 6.3:1.

Poster NS6.18

Effects of fresh raygrass, raygrass hay or alfalfa hay on goat milk yield and composition, including *trans* and conjugated fatty acids

J. Rouel[1], A. Ferlay[1], J.M. Chabosseau[2], P. Capitan[1],P. Gaborit[3] and Y. Chilliard[1], [1]INRA-Theix,63122, France, [2]INRA-Lusignan, France, [3]ITPLC-Surgères, France*

Thirty-six multiparous mid-lactation goats received indoor one of 3 diets based on either fresh raygrass + raygrass hay (.26 kg DM/d) (FR), raygrass hay (RH) or alfalfa hay (AH) *ad libitum*, and 1.3 kg/d of concentrates, for 5 weeks. The mean forage intake was 1.23, 1.33 and 1.74 kg DM/d for diets FR, RH and AH, respectively. Diet FR, compared to RH, tended ($P<0.10$) to decrease milk yield (-290 g/d), increased ($P<0.05$) milk protein (+1.2 g/kg) and decreased lactose (- 2.5 g/kg) content. Diet AH, compared to RH, increased milk yield (+380 g/d), and milk protein content (+1.9 g/kg) and yield (+16 g/d).
Effects on milk fatty acid (FA) composition were small but significant. Diet FR, compared to RH, decreased 11:0 to 14:0, *cis*9-14:1, *cis*9-16:1, 17:1, branched-chain (BC) and odd-numbered (ON) FA, and increased 22:2n-6 and the ratio *cis*9,*trans*11-18:2: *trans*11-18:1 (RA:TVA). Diet AH, compared to RH, decreased 14:0, *cis*9-14:1, *cis*9-16:1 and BC+ON FA, and increased 20:0, 21:0, 22:0, 24:0, 18:2n-6, 18:3n-3, 20:5n-3, and RA:TVA.
In conclusion, AH improved largely production performances, whereas indoor FR decreased them, compared to RH. Fresh grass *vs.* hay changed delta-9 desaturation ratios, and decreased medium-chain FA and BC+ON FA, whereas alfalfa *vs* raygrass hay changed delta-9 desaturation ratios, and increased polyunsaturated FA and long-chain saturated FA. Studies on sensorial quality of cheeses are in progress.

Poster NS6.19

Interactions between raygrass preservation and high-oleic sunflower oil supplementation on goat milk composition, including *trans* and conjugated fatty acids

A. Ferlay[1], J. Rouel[1], J.M. Chabosseau[2], P. Capitan[1], K.Raynal-Ljutovac[3] and Y. Chilliard[1], [1]INRA-Theix,63122, France, [2]INRA-Lusignan, France,[3]ITPLC-Surgères, France*

Forty-eight multiparous mid-lactation goats were used indoor in a 2x2 factorial design, including 2 forages *ad libitum* : fresh raygrass + raygrass hay (.26 kg DM/d) (FR) or raygrass hay (RH), and 2 lipid intakes (0 g/d, control, C, or 130 g/d, i.e. 5-6% of diet DM, of high-oleic sunflower oil, OSO) for 5 weeks. Diets OSO, compared to C, increased ($P<0.05$) milk fat (+3.0 g/kg), protein (+1.9 g/kg with RH diet) and lactose (+3.8 g/kg) content, and milk fat yield (+13 g/d). Diets OSO, compared to C, decreased 6:0 to 16:0, *cis*9-16:1, branched-chain (BC) and odd-numbered (ON) FA, 18:2n-6, 18:3n-3, 20:4n-6, and 20:5n-3 and increased 4:0, 18:0 (+148%), 20:0, 22:0, 24:0, *cis*9-18:1 (+79%), *trans*9-16:1, *trans*6+7+8-18:1 (+1543%, up to 1.15% of total FA), *trans*9 to *trans*13-18:1 (+666% for *trans*10-18:1, up to 1.15% of total FA, +170% for *trans*11-18:1), *cis*9,*trans*11-18:2 (+79%), and probably *trans*7,*cis*9-18:2 (up to 0.12% of total FA) . Diets OSO decreased the normalized delta-9 desaturation ratios for 14:0, 17:0, 18:0 and *trans*11-18:1. The main significant interactions were that OSO decreased more cis9-14:1, cis9-16:1 and 17:1 with RH, whereas it decreased more the *cis*9,*trans*11-18:2 : *trans*11-18:1 ratio with FR.
In conclusion, diets OSO improved production performances, increased stearic, oleic and some *trans*-18:1, and decreased delta-9 desaturation ratios, polyunsaturated FA, short-chain, medium-chain and BC+ON FA, with few interactions with raygrass preservation.

Poster NS6.20

Influence of feeding system and season on CLA content in goat milk

A. Di Trana[1], G.F Cifuni[2], A. Braghieri[1], V. Fedele[2], S. Claps[2], R. Rubino[2], [1]Università degli Studi della Basilicata, Dipartimento di Scienze delle Produzioni Animali, Via N. Sauro 85, 85100, Potenza, Italy, [2]Istituto Sperimentale per la Zootecnia, Viale Basento106, 85100 Potenza, Italy.*

Milk fat of ruminants is considered the richest natural source of conjugated linoleic acid (CLA), a group of isomers of linolenic acid. The predominant isomer (cis-9, trans-11 CLA) has powerful anticarcinogenic, antiatherogenic and antioxidative properties. The objective was to examine the effects of feeding system and season on milk fat content of CLA under southern Italy conditions. In spring, summer and winter seventy-two samples of raw goat milk from four feeding systems: G (grazing), GMB (grazing, maize, broadbeans), GBC (grazing, barley, chickpeas) and ZG (hay, mixed grains) were analysed. The highest level of CLA was detected during winter and it increased 144% in G, 103% in GMB and 39% in GBC compared to ZG. In spring, G and GMB showed higher increase in CLA than GBC and ZG. During summer, GMB and G exhibited an increase in CLA compared to other groups. Feeding system and season affect CLA content. High seasonal variability of CLA value in milk fat of goats fed at pasture was observed, this trend may be attributable to polyunsaturated fatty acid content in the fat of herbage in season progress; also, herbage at early growth stage play a main role on CLA increase compared to diets including late-growth herbage.

Poster NS6.21

The effect of omega-3 fatty acids supplemented to the diet of goats on milk composition

D. Kompan[1], A. Oresnik[1], J. Salobir[1], K. Salobir[1], M. Pogacnik[2], [1]University of Ljubljana, Biotechnical faculty, Groblje 3, 1230 Domzale, Slovenia, [2]University of Ljubljana, Veterinary faculty, Gerbiceva 60, 1000 Ljubljana, Slovenia.

Supplementation of octadecatrienoic (ALA), eicosapentaenoic (EPA), and docosahexaenoic (DHA) fatty acids (FA) to the diet of goats and its effect on milk composition, and fat content of goat milk. The experiment included 62 goats, from 28 to 105 days after kidding. After the adaptation period the animals were divided into four groups, the fourth was the control group. The other three groups were fed the FA supplemented diet (20 g/day) in the five successive days. Milk yield of each milking was recorded up to ten days before FA supplementation and in the next five days, and later, measurements of two milking were taken every fifth day. Samples of all recorded measurements, and each animal, were analysed for milk composition, somatic cell (SC) count, and the number of micro-organisms. It has been established that the supplementation of ALA over a short period of time decreased the somatic cell (SC) count. Statistically significant decrease lasted 29 days after the fifth supplementation of 20g/day ALA. In the group with added ALA (group ALA), the fat content percentage increased from 3.0 to 3.4 during FA supplementation. In the group with added EPA (group EPA), as well as in the group with added DHA (group DHA) the percentage decreased from 3.10 to 2.40.

Poster NS6.22

Metabolic profiles of goats on alpine grazing

A. Gaviraghi[1], L. Noè[1], A. D'Angelo[1], G.F. Greppi[2], [1]LEA Laboratory of Applied Epigenomic, Institute L. Spallanzani. Lodi, Italy, [2]Department of Veterinary Clinical Science, University of Milan

This research was aimed at determining the influence of alpine grazing on the metabolic profiles of goats. The trial was performed on a natural alpine pasture area from 1400 to 2100 m elevation (Val Fontana, Sondrio) in the Central Alps.

Metabolic profiles were tested in 32 goats - out of herd of 70 lactating goats - of the local breed Frontalasca. Blood samples were collected from the jugular vein both during alpine grazing and after stabling. Plasma samples were separated within 20' and kept refrigerated till stored at -20°C. Samples were analysed for albumin, β-OH-butyrate, cholesterol, creatinine, NEFA, glucose, calcium, inorganic phosphorus, triglycerides, total protein, urea, aspartate aminotransferase activity, alanine aminotransferase activity and gamma glutamyl transferase activity, alkaline phosphatase and creatinphosphokinase. Plasma globulins were calculated as the difference between total protein and albumin. The results show higher concentrations of both protein and urea in the middle period of grazing. Since in ruminants urea commonly reflects the protein content of pasture the results could therefore be related to a protein overload probably due to an excess of protein intake during grazing. In the same period an increase in both NEFA and β-OH-butyrate together with a decrease in blood glucose could reflect a low energy intake and therefore suggest using a supplementation with lower protein and higher fibre content.

 Poster NS6.23

Goat cheese production under semi arid rangeland seasonal grazing with protein or non protein urea supplementation

M.A. Galina and M. Guerrero, Facultad de Estudios Superiores Cuautitlan, UNAM, Cuautitlan, México 54000, Deprtamento de Ciencias Pecuarias FES.Cuautitlan UNAM Km 3.5 Carretera Teoloyucan-Cuautitlán Estado de México, México 54000.*

Pasture 110 goats (PG) and 20 in zero grazing (AG). Goats weighted 52.410 kg with 455 kg of milk/ 210 d for UG and 401 for AG. PG used balanced concentrate (BC) December to May, thereafter a multinutritional urea block (MB) 45% molasses and 10% urea and slow intake urea 5 % supplement (SIUS). BC was 60% corn; 16% barley and 20% wheat barn and 4% soybean. Animals pastured until November and 200 g of SIUS was added. BC goats were fed 55% alfalfa hay and 45% with 14% CP concentrate. UG average voluntary feed intake (VFI) was 1.880 kg DM/d with an annual total of 828 kg; of those 248 kg DM was provided by alfalfa hay 29.9 % of the total feed intake; 182 kg or 21.9 % of the diet was concentrate, (BC; MB; SIUS) and 398 kg or 48.0 % was from pasture (grasses, shrubs and tree leaves) or corn stubble. AG goats VFI was 1.650 kg DM/d 603 kg/year 331 kg alfalfa and 271 kg BC. It was possible to improve biosustainability from 33% before to 48% increasing milk from 401 (AG) to 455 (UG) kg/year and diminishing cost from 20 to 17 US cents per litter. Days of lactation, total solids of milk per day, nitrogen profile and supplementation had a significant ($P<0.01$) effect on cheese yield, from 6 to 9 kg. of milk in UG and 7 to 9.5 kg in BC.

Poster NS6.24

Kids growth on pasture with non protein urea supplementation

M.A.Galina and M. Guerrero, Facultad de Estudios Superiores Cuautitlan, UNAM, Cuautitlan, México 54000 Deprtamento de Ciencias Pecuarias FES.Cuautitlan UNAM Km 3.5 Carretera Teoloyucan-Cuautitlán Estado de México, México 54000.*

Voluntary dry matter intake (VDMI), organic matter intake (OMI), rumen digestion, passage rate, rumen NH_3 and VFA's, apparent digestibility, pH, fermentable carbohydrates, and weight gain of 50 young Alpines (15.5 ± 0.272 kg BW) and 4 rumen cannulated goats in pasture studied. Twenty five plus two cannulated goats were pastured with 200 g/head/day of a slow intake 5% urea supplement (SIUS) Second (n=25) plus two cannulated goats with 300 g/head of a balanced concentrate (BC) (2% salt, 1.5% commercial mineral salt, 60% corn, 32.5% wheat bran, 4% soybean oil meal). Stocking rates varied from 1.45 to 1.85 animal units (AU)/ha. VDMI and OMI were higher ($P<0.05$) in the SIUS goats. NH_3 and passage rate were augmented ($P<0.05$) by SIUS. Rumen pH rose when SIUS was offered while in BC fed goats decreased to 5.57. Growth averaged 105 g/d (±3) for CF and 87 g/d (±5) in BC ($P<0.05$). In SIUS goats, fermentable carbohydrate (FC) intake produced 31g BW gain/g FC, compared to the BC fed goats averaging 10 g BW gain/g FC ($P<0.05$). SIUS supplies critical nutrients to the rumen, improves DM intake, passage rate, ruminal pH, ammonia concentration, NDF degradabililty and better weight gain than those obtained by supplementing with BC while grazing on shrub rangeland. High fiber forages could be used efficiently (up to 70 to 80% DMI) when ruminal fermentation is improved with a continuous nitrogen supplementation.

Evaluation of the application of radiography and ultrasonography as diagnostic tools for reticulorumenal foreign bodies in goats

T.A. Abdou[*1], *I. Salah*[1], *W.M. Kelany*[1], *K.A. Farag*[2] *and A.H. Otman*[3], [1]*Dept.of Medicine Fact. of Vet. Med Cairo University* ,[2]*Dept of surgery and radiology, Fact. of Vet. Med Cairo University,* [3]*Dept of pathology, Fact. of Vet. Med Cairo University.*

95 goats were examined for the presence of ruminal foreign bodies by deep abdominal palpation. Fifteen of them were free (control group). The animals were subjected to thorough clinical examination, rumen liquor analysis, radiography and ultasonography which revealed that foreign bodies in the rumen caused severe unnoticed digestive disorders which resembled picture of subacute ruminal acidosis, only disclosed by rumen liquor analysis without any clinical sign except unnoticed growth retardation and sometimes illtherftiness. It was recorded that 55 of the examined goats were confirmed by X-ray and ultasonography that they contained foreign bodies in their reticulorumens, and the other were misdiagnosed or pregnant or having pregnancy disorders. The study could emphasize that ultrasonography and radiography are often complementary, and in many cases ultrasonography provides more useful information than radiography. Ultrasonography is entirely safe to the animal and the examiner. As, most of the female animals were suspected, by the owner, to be pregnant, therefore ultrasonographic examination was important for differential diagnosis without risk of radiation. The most limiting feature of ultrasonography in its application to the abdomen is the limitation of penetration and the economic value.

Theatre P1.1

Genetic and nongenetic factors influencing feed intake in growing pigs under conditions of a testing station

U. Bergfeld, C. Barbe and U. Müller, Saxonian Federal Institution of Agriculture, Am Park 3, 04886 Köllitsch, Germany.*

In a performance testing station for growing pigs feed intake is monitored using a computerized feed intake recording system of type ACEMA. The pigs are housed under group-conditions of 12-15 animals. In the station 450 testing places can be used. Growing pigs of different races (German Landrace, Large White and Pietrain) were tested.

Data from 1996 with alltogether 10.600.000 records from 6324 testing pigs could be analized. Daily feed intake was modelized using a regression animal model with all relationship included. Influences of race, sex and environmental factors in the testing station were investigated.

In a multi trait animal model the relationship of the daily feed intake between different testing periods and to other single measured performance traits of growing and slaughtered pigs were analized. Heritabilities and genetic correlations were estimated.

Theatre P1.2

RYR1 genotype and terminal sire line effects on feeding patterns in growing pigs

E. Fàbrega[1], J. Tibau[1], J. Soler[1], J. Fernández[2], J. Font[3], D. Carrión[4], A. Diestre[1], X. Manteca[2]. [1]Institut de Recerca i Tecnologia Agroalimentàries, 17121 Monells, Spain, [2]Unitat de Fisiologia Animal, 08193 Bellaterra, Spain, [3]Pinsos Baucells, 08551 Tona, Spain, [4]Pig Improvement Company, 08190 Sant Cugat del Vallès, Spain*

Differences in feeding behaviour between breeds or lines of growing pigs associated with their genetic background have not been widely studied. The aim of this study was to investigate the effects of RYR1 genotype and terminal sire line on feeding patterns and growth performance. A total of 130 castrates were monitored for 70 days in a *Pig Testing Centre*. The distribution of RYR1 genotype and terminal sire line was: 63 Large White x Pietrain (LWPi) sired pigs (32 NN and 31 Nn) and 67 Pietrain (Pi) sired pigs (34 NN and 33 Nn). Individual records of daily food intake, total eating time per day and number of visits to the feeder per day were taken using an IVOG®-station (Hokofarm, The Netherlands). Pigs were weighed and backfat thickness and loin-muscle depth were measured every 21 days throughout the test period. Under the present conditions, the feeding patterns evaluated (feed intake per day and rate of food intake) and average daily gain were found to be more affected by terminal sire line than RYR1 genotype, showing LWPi sired pigs a higher feed intake and body weight compared to Pi sired pigs. These results suggest that terminal sire line may affect feeding patterns more than RYR1 genotype.

Theatre P1.3

Modeling health status-environmental effects on swine growth

A.P. Schinckel, M.E. Spurlock, B.T. Richert, and T.E. Weber, Purdue University, Department of Animal Sciences, 915 W. State St., West Lafayette, IN 47907-2054 USA*

Pigs reared under commercial environments have substantially lower growth rates than those reared under research conditions. Commercial environments via the combined effects of pathogen exposure, social interactions, stocking density, and air quality; limit the expression of pig's genetic potential for growth rate, lean tissue deposition, and feed intake. The maximum achievable lean growth rates of modern pigs are reduced 20 to 40% under commercial conditions. Pigs from populations with above average percent carcass lean have been found to have a greater percentage reduction in live weight and carcass lean growth than pigs of average percent carcass lean. Genetic variation exists between genetic populations in their response to environmental, immune system activation, and health status stressors. Genetic population × environment interactions have been found for daily feed intake, lean growth, carcass lean percentage and death loss. The pig's response to stressors can reduce protein accretion and carcass muscle gain to a greater extent than lipid accretion. The pig's response to stressors down regulates growth and feed intake, likely at the gene expression level. The pig's genetic potential for protein accretion and feed intake are less important than the pig's response to encountered stressors when pigs are reared in commercial environments. For these reasons, farm × genetic population specific growth and feed intake parameters are required.

Theatre P1.4

Consequences of genetic selection for growth and body composition on the food intake of pigs

I. Kyriazakis[1], I.J. Wellock[1], G.C. Emmans[1] and P.W. Knap[2], [1]Animal Nutrition and Health Department, SAC, West Mains Road, Edinburgh EH9 3JG, UK, [2]PIC, PO Box 1630 24826 Schleswig, Germany*

Selection of growing pigs has been aimed mainly at increasing growth rate and reducing fatness at a market weight. These changes can be achieved through changes in either the material efficiencies of nutrient use, or maintenance, or food intake. There is little evidence that selection has changed material or energetic efficiencies. Although selection for growth rate may change maintenance requirements, this effect is relatively small compared to the changes in food intake. At a weight, improved genotypes will have higher rates of retention of protein and, in the absence of selection against fatness, also lipid. Higher retention rates will lead to higher requirements and intake. Selection against fatness, directly or indirectly through selection for efficiency, will lead to substantial reductions of food intake. These reductions will be only partly offset by the correlated effects (increase) on food intake seen due to selection for increased growth rate. For these food intake effects to be seen, genetic changes must be accompanied by changes in the environment, including the nutritional environment. Wrong conclusions about the effects of selection on food intake may be drawn if, for example, improved genotypes are kept in relatively hot environments or are given access to foods with limiting protein content.

Theatre P1.5

Predicting the consequences of genetic and social stress on intake and growth in growing pigs

I.J. Wellock, G.C. Emmans and I. Kyriazakis. Animal Health and Nutrition Department, Scottish Agricultural College, Edinburgh, EH9 3JG, U.K.*

The effects of the main social stressors, group size, space allowance, feeder space allowance and mixing on the intake and gain of growing pigs were described by conceptual equations derived on biological grounds. The values of their parameters were estimated from experimental data whilst avoiding the problems of using a strictly empirical approach. The equations were integrated into a general growth model in a logical way. The extended model allows the effects of interactions between social stressors and the other variables, such as the type of pig, feed composition and environment, that exist to be explored and, at least in principle, predicted. Genetic variation between breeds in their ability to cope with social stressors is represented by an extra genetic parameter in the model to describe the 'excitability' of the pig. The value of this adjusts both the intensity of stressor at which the animal becomes effectively stressed, and the extent to which stress reduces performance and increases energy expenditure (activity) at a given stressor intensity. The model is able to predict the feed intake of pigs differing in both genetic potential for growth and in excitability when raised under given dietary, physical and social environmental conditions. The social equations developed may be incorporated into other pig growth simulation models.

Theatre P1.6

Effect of energy density and energy source on the performance of lactating sows in hot environment

P.J.L. Ramaekers, Nutreco Swine Research Centre, P.O. Box 240, 5845 AE Boxmeer, The Netherlands.*

Sixty-six Hypor sows were used to examine the effect of the energy density and energy source in lactation diets on the performance in hot environment. During gestation all sows received the same diet. Sows were moved one week before farrowing to the farrowing room and allotted to one of three treatments, Treatment 1, control diet, 2290 kcal NE/kg, Treatment 2, High energy starch diet, 2450 kcal NE/kg, Treatment 3, High energy fat diet, 2450 kcal NE/kg. Sows received the Treatment diets and had free access to water the moment they entered the farrowing room. The first week after farrowing, minimum room temperature was maintained at 23 °C. After the first week, minimum room temperature was maintained during 7.00 -17.00 h, at 28 °C and during 17.00-7.00 h, at 23 °C. During lactation, sows had similar (P>0.1) feed intake of 4.7, 4.7 and 4.8 kg/d for Treatments 1, 2 and 3, respectively. Treatment 3 had a higher (P<0.05) energy intake than Treatment 1. The piglets in Treatments 1, 2, and 3 had similar (P>0.1) daily growth of 221, 236 and 229 g/d, respectively. Body weight, backfat thickness and condition score changes were similar among Treatments. It is conclude that energy density or energy source had no effect on feed intake and performance of lactating sows in hot environment.

Poster P1.7

Genetic geterogenity of pig breeds in heavy metals accumulation

S.A. Patrashkov, V.L. Petukhov, O.S. Korotkevich, E.Ya. Barinov, Novosibirsk State Agrarian University, 160 Dobrolubov Str., 630039, Novosibirsk, Russia*

The aim of our investigation is to determine the breed genopool stipulated part of the geterogenity in heavy metals (HM) accumulation in 2-month old pigs.
5 pig breeds from West Siberia region of Russian Federation were studied to determine Zn, Cu, Pb and Cd concentration in the bristle. The local Sibirskaya Severnaya and Kemerovskaya breeds of pigs, adapted to extreme Siberian conditions were the special interest.
The influence of breeds genopool on HM accumulation in hair was established.
The highest level of Zn was detected in Landras hair - 1.7 times higher, than in Sibirskaya Severnaya bristle. At the same time Cd content in Landras hair was 3 times lower than in Sibirskaya Severnaya and Big White pigs.
The parts of genofond influence on Cu concentration were significantly higher (36%), than Zn, Pb and Cd (6, 7 and 9%).
The distribution of breeds according to integral HM accumulation can be presenting in the following way: Big White > Landras > Dyurok > Sibirskaya Severnaya > Kemerovskaya.

Poster P1.8

Estimation of genetic parameters in Estonian pig breeds in animal recording

M. Kruus, Estonian Animal Recording Centre, 48a Kreutzwaldi Str., 50094 Tartu, Estonia

Genetic Parameters for backfat (BF), muscle depth (MD) and daily gain (DG) were estimated from pigs in farm-test in Estonia. Test data were recorded since 1998, Pietrain test data since 2000. For Landrace (L) 15 000 tested progenies, 20 000 Yorkshire (Y) tested progenies in 40 herds and 500 Pietrain (P) tested progenies in 2 herds were available. Backfat and muscle depth were measured with ultrasonic equipment PIGLOG 105. Daily gain was precorrected to 90 kg. At least two generations of pedigree information was taken into consideration to ensure the relationship between tested pigs. The three populations were estimated separately. The method used for genetic parameters estimation was REML. The same multitrait animal model (3 traits) was used for estimation of covariance components and for the genetic parameters estimation. The model contains sex as fix effect; litter group, herd*year*season and animal as random effects; and a regression of test weight is fitted for backfat and muscle depth.
Landrace and Yorkshire heritabilities were similar. Landrace shows stronger genetic correlations between traits than Yorkshire. Pietrain heritabilities differ from Landrace and Yorkshire breeds.

Theatre P2.1

Improvement of piglet survival by optimisation of piglet individual birth weight and reduction of its variation

R. Roehe, Institut für Tierzucht und Tierhaltung, Universität Kiel, Hermann-Rodewald-Str. 6, D-24118 Kiel, Germany.*

Piglet individual birth weight was highly associated with preweaning mortality with odds ratios increasing from 1.4-16.1 when birth weight decreased from 1.8-1.0 kg. Genetic parameters of individual birth weight were 0.08 and 0.22 for direct and maternal effects, which were nonsignificantly genetically correlated with -0.22. Thus, birth weight can be efficiently improved. Optimisation of piglet birth weight should be based on weight at which lowest stillbirth and preweaning mortality occurred, and was in the present population 1.6 kg. Reduction in variance of piglet birth weight is expected to decrease when selecting on optimal piglet birth weight by using e.g. nonlinear profit function. Selection for litter weight is less efficient because of biased parameter estimation by not taking into account covariances among full-sibs and unconsideration of variation of piglet birth weight within litter. Selection directly for survival of piglets is expected to be inefficient due to low heritability, low information content of the binary trait, and difficulties to disentangle direct and maternal effects. Further improvement of piglet survival can be obtained by selection on individual weaning weight and its variation; optimal feed intake, backfat thickness, weight loss of sows. Correct modelling uses the direct-maternal effect model for piglet survival or birth weight, whereas litter derivatives such as percentage of survival and mean birth weight will result in biased results.

Theatre P2.2

Sireline selection to improve pre-weaning survival of piglets: birth weight or vitality

E.F. Knol[1] and R. Bergsma[1], IPG, Institute for Pig Genetics, P.O. Box 43.6640 AA Beuningen, The Netherlands.*

There is debate on the best route to improve preweaning survival (PWS) of piglets, one approach is increasing birth weigh (BW), another is direct selection for PWS. Genotypes of sow, foster sow, service sire and piglet could be relevant. We chose to analyse the influence of the sire to study the best selection strategy for a sireline. Two datasets were available. Dataset 1 contained almost 80,000 observations on individual purebred piglets of a sireline and dataset 2 more than 5,000 observations on crossbred commercial piglets on an experimental farm with the rotational use of 4 sirelines. PWS was defined as a binary trait of the piglet.

Sire variances in dataset 1 were low, but significant for BW and PWS. Inclusion of BW in the survival model resulted in an increased sire variance estimate for PWS. The genetic correlation between BW and PWS was 0.09 (ns). Analysis of dataset 2 revealed a significantly lower PWS of Pietrain (Hal-) offspring, a difference that remained after correction for BW. The fenotypic relation between BW and PWS was different for Pietrain offspring than for the other sirelines.

Extrapolation of the results indicated that direct selection for increased PWS, especially with correction for BW, will outperform selection for increased BW by a factor 5 or more. Results are discussed between and within sire lines.

Theatre P2.3

Genetic parameters for litter traits derived from individual birth weight recordings

H. Täubert[1], H. Eding, H. Henne[2] and H. Simianer[1], [1]Institute of Animal Breeding and Genetics, University of Göttingen, Germany, [2]Züchtungszentrale Deutsches Hybridschwein GmbH, Lüneburg, Germany*

Individual piglet weights were recorded from 13'019 piglets of line 01 (LR) and 13'794 piglets of line 03 (LW) over two years. In total 1416 litters of line 01 and 1486 litters of line 03 were analysed. Genetic parameters for individual birth weights were estimated with random effects of animal, sow and litter. Litter size, mean and standard deviation of birth weight were analysed as traits of the sow. Results for individual birth weight were $h^2 = .098$ in line 01 and $h^2 = .147$ in line 03. Heritabilities for litter size, mean and standard deviation of birth weight were .119, .354 and .104 in line 01 and .114, .276 and .130 in line 03 resp. Genetic correlations in line 01 and line 03 between litter size and mean birth weight was -.254 and -.661, between litter size and standard deviation of birth weight .563 and .280. Selection only on litter size reduces the average birth weight and increases the variation of birth weights within a litter. with respect on number of piglets weaned, an optimum litter size and birth weight has to be found, to avoid too many dead piglets in large litters.

Theatre P2.4

Selection for sow fertility accounting for animal welfare aspects: possibilities to improve litter size without increasing piglet mortality in the pre-weaning phase

H. Simianer[1], H. Täubert[1], H. Eding[1], and H. Henne[2], [1]Institute of Animal Breeding and Genetics, Albrecht Thaer-Weg 3, 37075 Goettingen, Germany, [2]Zuechtungszentrale Deutsches Hybridschwein, Stadtkoppel 6, 21337 Lueneburg, Germany.*

Selecting for litter size leads to unbalanced litters with an increase of piglet mortality in the pre-weaning phase. Assuming the typical information structure in a commercial breeding herd, different selection strategies to improve sow fertility without impairing piglet welfare were compared. Selection based exclusively on the number of live born piglets leads to an increase of litter size by 0.4 piglets, while pre-weaning losses are also increased by 0.1 piglets. Adding information on average birth weight for the animals in the breeding nucleus reduces the genetic gain in litter size, but leads to an even higher reduction of piglet losses, so that the genetic progress in the number of weaned piglets is increased by 8.7%. Adding information on the standard deviation of birth weights leads to a further slight increase in the number of weaned piglets (+1.4%), but requires expensive recording of individual birth weights. It is recommended to select based on litter size and mean birth weight and to use a restriction on piglet losses. Compared to unrestricted selection on litter size only, the expected economic gain per sow and litter is increased by 17%, while piglet mortality in the pre-weaning phase is reduced.

Theatre P2.5

Genetic studies of weight changes, milk production and piglet production of sows based on data from nutritional experiments

O. Vangen[1,2], V. Danielsen[1] and I.M. Mao[1], [1]Danish Institute of Agricultural Sciences, Research Centre Foulum, DK-8830 Tjele, Denmark, [2]on leave from Department of Animal Science, Agricultural University of Norway, P.O.Box 5025, N-1432 Aas-NLH, Norway.*

Milk production and weight loss of lactating sows is regarded as important factors affecting sow productivity. However, these type of traits are costly to record and there are seldom large datasets from recording systems to do genetic analyses of such traits.
The present paper deals with a cross- disiplinary approach of utilising data from nutritional experiments, where weight changes, milk production, milk composition and efficiency of piglet production of sows have been recorded, to calculate genetic parameters to be used for further evaluation of such traits in breeding programmes for increased fertility and longevity. By genetic links between two nutritional experiments, with records on 282 observations on 212 sows of criss-cross Landrace and Yorkshire origin, from 74 sires of the two breeds, a DMU-AI REML programme, based on a full relationship matrix, was used to calculate heritabilities for weight changes during lactation, milk production, milk composition and efficiency of producing weaner pigs. Correcting for fixed effects like breed of sire, batch, parity and feed treatment, heritabilities for weight changes were found to be 0.32-0.36, milk production 0.24-0.32 and efficiency of weaner piglet production of 0.23-0.47.
The results were promising for breeding sows for more efficient piglet production.

Theatre P2.6

Relationships between reproduction and production traits in Norwegian landrace; estimation of variance components

B. Holm[1,2], M. Bakken[2] and G. Klemetsdal[2]. [1]Norsvin, P.O. Box 504, NO-2304 Hamar, Norway, [2]Department of Animal Science, Agricultural University of Norway, P.O. Box 5025, NO-1432 Aas, Norway.*

The objective of this study was to investigate if selection for production traits has affected the sows' reproductive performance. Reproductive traits investigated were; age at first service (AFS), return-rate primiparous sows (RR_p), gestation length, piglets born alive first litter (NBA_1), weaning to service interval after first litter (WTS_1), return-rate after first litter (RR_1), piglets born alive second litter (NBA_2), weaning to service interval after second litter (WTS_2). Number of records ranged from 13792 to 56932. The main production traits in the breeding goal were; age at 100 kg live weight (A100), back fat (BF), lean meat content (LMC), bacon side quality (BSQ), feed conversion ratio (FCR). Number of records ranged from 12992 to 190454. Parameters were estimated with a multivariate animal model using AI-REML procedures. 220000 animals were included in the pedigree file. Data were analysed in batches, first all the reproductive traits, then each reproductive trait with A100 and BF, then each reproductive trait with LMC, BSQ and FCR. The average heritablilities for the reproductive traits were: AFS; 0.38, RR_p; 0.016, gestation length; 0.35, NBA_1; 0.11, WTS_1; 0.06, RR_1; 0.015, NBA_2; 0.12 and WTS_2; 0.03. Genetic correlations between NBA_1/NBA_2 and production traits were unfavourable; A100 (r_g=0.60 and r_g=0.42 respectively), LMC (r_g=-0.12 and r_g=-0.24) and FCR (r_g=0.23 and r_g=0.20). BF was uncorrelated to all reproductive traits.

Theatre P2.7

Bayesian genetic analysis of differently transformed weaning-to-oestus interval in pigs

S. Malovrh[*1], M. Kovac[1] and R. Roehe[2]. [1]Animal Science Department, Biotechnical Faculty, University of Ljubljana, Domzale, Slovenia, [2]Institute of Animal Breeding and Husbandry, Christian-Albrechts-University of Kiel, Kiel, Germany*

Genetic parameters for weaning-to-oestrus interval (WOI) were estimated on 11,026 sows from pig selection farm Ptuj (Slovenia). Univariate analyses of observations of WOI across parities and two-trait analyses of records of primiparous (PP) and multiparous (MP) sows were performed applying Bayesian approach. WOI was analysed on original scale, transformed using a natural log transformation (lnWOI) and considered as a mixture of normal and exponential distributions (trWOI). Statistical model included genotype, season of service as year-month interaction, and parity as fixed effects, and previous lactation length and number of piglets weaned as covariates. Direct additive genetic effect and permanent environment were considered as random effects. (Co)variance components were estimated by Bayesian analyses. Gibbs chains of length between 130,000 and 180,000 were run. Univariate analysis for sows across parities resulted in heritability estimates of 0.06, 0.07, and 0.07 for WOI, lnWOI and trWOI, respectively. Permanent environment (PE) accounted for 26% of phenotypic variation for WOI and 19% for both lnWOI and trWOI. In bivariate analysis, heritability was 0.19 in PP and 0.06 in MP. Genetic correlation for WOI between PP and MP was 0.80. The PE proportion was 0.10 in MP sows. Based on genetic parameters, selection on improved rebreeding performance in pigs is expected to be most efficient considering WOI in primiparous and multiparous sows as different traits. Transformation of WOI increased the genetic parameters only slightly.

Theatre P2.8

Lactation feed efficiency

R. Bergsma and E.F. Knol. IPG, Institute for Pig Genetics, P.O. Box 43, 6640 AA Beuningen, The Netherlands.*

Lactation is a critical phase in the life of both sows and piglets. Piglets should survive easy and grow quickly. Sows should facilitate this through milk production and simultaneously prepare themselves for the subsequent litter. Feed intake of sows during lactation is often not high enough to realise the necessary milk output, resulting in a loss of body reserves.
From a genetic point of view it is not only necessary to quantify the genetic variation in lactation traits, but also be able to understand the biological background of the traits under selection. Therefore we implemented an intensive information collection protocol on our experimental farm to record input and output variables of sows during lactation.
First results are promising. Output increases proportionally with input to a certain level. Above this level extra input has a minor effect on the output. There are significant differences in efficiency (output/(input-maintenance)) between sows. The 50% most efficient sows produce as much output as the rest, but with a 15% lower intake. Nevertheless high energy intake is favourable for piglet growth, pre-weaning survival, and litter size in the subsequent cycle. Clear phenotypic differences in intake and efficiency exist. Selection for increased feed intake and efficiency should be investigated.

Genetic correlations between litter size and weights, piglet weight variability and piglet survival from birth to weaning in Large White pigs

M. Huby[1], L. Canario[1], T. Tribout[1], J.C. Caritez[2], Y. Billon[2], J. Gogué[3], J.P. Bidanel[1], INRA, [1]Station de Génétique Quantitative et Appliquée, 78352 Jouy-en-Josas Cedex, France, [2]INRA, Domaine expérimental du Magneraud, Saint-Pierre d'Amilly, 17700 Surgères, France, [3]INRA, Unité expérimentale porcine, domaine de Galle 18520 Avord, France*

Genetic parameters of litter size, litter weight, mean and heterogeneity (within-litter standard deviation) of individual piglet weights at birth, 3 weeks of age and at weaning, of proportion of stillbirths and of survival rate from birth to weaning were estimated in a Large White population using restricted maximum likelihood methodology applied to a multiple trait animal model. A total of 4055 litters produced by 1552 sows was analysed. All traits had low to moderate, but significant, heritability values. Proportion of stillbirths and birth to weaning survival rate had a low genetic correlation. A genetic antagonism was obtained between birth to weaning survival rate on one hand, litter size and weight at birth on the other hand. Similarly, piglet weight heterogeneity at birth was genetically associated a higher litter heterogeneity at 3 weeks of age and at weaning, with a higher proportion of stillbirths and a lower survival from birth to weaning. Mean piglet weights had moderate favourable genetic correlations with birth to weaning survival rate, but unfavourable genetic relationships with the proportion of stillbirths.

Poster P2.10

Genetic strategies to improve sow fertility of Norwegian Landrace

B. Holm, D. Olsen and H. Tajet, The Norwegian Pig Breeders' Association (Norsvin), P.O. Box 504, NO-2304 Hamar, Norway

The Norwegian Pig Breeders' Association, Norsvin, is in charge of the pure breeding as well as the national recording scheme, the herdbook and all AI-services in Norway. The Norwegian Landrace population consist of approximately 2100 and 2300 sows in 57 nucleus- and 110 multiplying herds respectively. The use of artificial insemination (AI) is 100% in both categories of herds. In 2001 compulsory recordings of several new fertility traits were introduced; intensity of pro-oestrus symptoms and ability to show standing reflex (none, weak, moderate, strong), dystocia and its reason (inertia, featal oversize, deviations of the uterus, inadequate dilations, etc), and duration of parturition (two hours' intervals). The farmers record the data and report them electronically to Norsvin on a weekly basis through the national recording scheme (In-Gris). This provides a unique opportunity to detect potential unfavourable genetic responses of the current breeding goal, re-optimise this if necessary, including economically important fertility traits.
In 2001 the nucleus and the multiplying herds in addition began to record individual weights of piglets at three weeks of age. These data are also sent to Norsvin through the national recording scheme. Approximately 100 000 piglets are weighted annually. Since the weights are recorded on an individual basis, a multivariate genetic evaluation of mother abilities and early growth of the piglets can be performed.

Poster P2.11

Genetic relationships between litter traits, piglet growth and sow feed consumption and body reserves mobilization in Duroc pigs

J. Tibau[1], J.P. Bidanel[2], J. Reixach[3], N. Trilla[1], J. Soler[1], [1]Institut de Recerca i Tecnologia Agroalimentàries, 17121 Monells, Spain [1]INRA - Station Genetique Quantitative et Appliquee 78352 Jouy-en-Josas, France [3]Selecció Batallé, Riudarenes 17421 Spain*

Data from 717 Duroc gilts purebred litters where used to estimate genetic parameters for number pigs born alive (NBA), piglets weaned (NPW), average weight at birth (AWB) and weaning (AWW), as well as sow feed consumption during the last week of lactation (SFC) changes in sow backfat (IGD) and loin (IGL) depth during lactation REML methodology was applied to a multivariate animal model including herd x year x season and mating type as fixed effects, additive genetic effect of each animal as a random effect and sow body weight as a covariate. Additional analyses were performed including sow body condition traits as covariates. Heritability estimates were 0.05; 0.01; 0.14; 0.19; 0.09; 0.10 and 0.19 for NBA, NPW, AWB, AWW, IGD, IGL and SFC, respectively. NBA had negative genetic correlations with AWB and AWW. IGD and IGL were positively correlated. SFC had a moderate positive genetic correlation with IGL, but a strongly negative one with IGD. Moderate to strong positive genetic correlations were obtained between AWW and IGD, IPL and SFC. These results illustrate and quantify the major role of sow feed consumption and ability to mobilize its body reserves on preweaning piglet growth.

Poster P2.12

Relationships between piglet survival and breeding values for dry-cured ham production

L. Degano, B. Contiero, G. Tonin, L. Gallo, and P. Carnier. Department of Animal Science, University of Padova, Italy

Logistic regression and survival analysis were used for investigating the relationship between piglet survival at birth (SB) or from birth to weaning (SBW), and breeding value class of the piglet (n=11089; Large White Gorzagri C21 boar line) for live weight at 270 d (LW270), for raw ham traits (round shape, fat thickness and marbling), and for backfat. Effects of sex, parity of the nurse sow or dam, year, season, cross-fostering, size of born or nursed litter (NL), and piglet total merit selection index (TMI) were also considered. SB was not affected by sex, size of the born litter, and by breeding values of the piglet, but year and season of birth and parity of the sow were significant risk factors. Cross-fostering (Hazard ratio = 0.39, Odds ratio = 0.81, P<0.01) increased SBW whereas a size of NL greater than 12 decreased SBV (Hazard ratio = 6.76, Odds ratio = 7.96, P<0.01). For all breeding values, at least one class exhibited different risk from the reference class, but relations between top breeding value classes and piglet survival were favourable. For piglet TMI, which includes also piglet survival, significant differences between the reference class and the worst (Hazard ratio = 1.36, Odds ratio = 1.40, P<0.01) or the best TMI class (Hazard ratio = 0.59, Odds ratio = 0.58, P<0.01) were detected.

Poster P2.13

Serum β-lactoglobulin content during pregnancy as an early indicator of reproductive efficiency in gilts

A. Sabbioni[1], M. Lavarini[1], M. Baratta[2], V. Beretti[1], C. Sussi[1], A. Summer[1] and P. Superchi[1], [1]Dipartimento di Produzioni Animali, Biotecnologie Veterinarie, Qualità e Sicurezza degli Alimenti, Università di Parma, Via del Taglio 8, 43100 Parma, Italy, [2]Dipartimento di Morfofisiologia Veterinaria, Università di Torino, Via L. da Vinci 44, 10095 Grugliasco (TO), Italy.*

The relationship between β-lactoglobulin (β-LG) serum concentration in sows during the last 8 weeks of pregnancy and subsequent piglets performance was investigated on 10 Dunel gilts. Two classes of gilts were identified with low (<150 ng/ml) and with high average β-LG content (>150 ng/ml). For both low and high content groups, power equations were calculated to describe trends in serum β-LG content, respectively [$y_1=141.07*x^{-0.3167}$ ($R^2=0.9433$) and $y_2=623.4*x^{-0.3494}$ ($R^2=0.6433$) , where x is no. of weeks from parity]. Differences in β-LG content between the two groups were highly significant at all weeks ($P<0.01$ from week 8 to 6; $P<0.001$ from week 6 to farrowing). No significant differences ($P>0.10$) between groups were shown for number of total born, born alive, stillborn or mummified and piglet survival rates until d 21 after farrowing; the group with high β-LG content during pregnancy showed higher litter weight at d 5 ($P<0.05$) and 21 ($P<0.10$) and higher milk production from farrowing to d 5 ($P<0.10$). The results indicate that serum β-LG content could be used as an early indicator of reproductive efficiency, and that gilts could be selected for high contents so to improve herd productivity.

Theatre P4.1

Associations of chemical body composition with body tissue content of growing pigs in a three generation full-sib design

M. Mohrmann[1], R. Roehe[1], S. Landgraf[1], P.W. Knap[2], U. Baulain[3], H. Looft[2], E. Kalm[1], [1]Institute of Animal Breeding and Husbandry, University of Kiel, 24098 Kiel, Germany, [2]PIC Deutschland, Ratsteich 31, 24837 Schleswig, Germany, [3]Federal Agricultural Research Center (FAL), Institute for Animal Science Mariensee, 31535 Neustadt, Germany.*

Body composition of 454 pigs from three generation full-sib design to identify QTL was measured by three methods, in vivo using isotope dilution technique (IDT) or Magnetic Resonance Imaging (MRI), and by serial slaughter with chemical analysis of the entire body (CAEB) from 15 to 140 kg body weight (BW). Correlations between chemical body composition using IDT and CAEB were high at 0.92, 0.90, 0.85 for empty body water, lipid, protein, respectively. IDT based on lean-fat tissue fraction only showed BW-dependent correlations with MRI up to 0.67 or 0.71 for protein to lean and lipid to fat tissue content. Prediction equations were established to relate lean and fat tissue content to protein and lipid content or vice versa. Allometric functions relating these body components to live weight showed high coefficients of determination. Based on body composition, protein, lipid, lean and fat tissue deposition rates ranged from 95-154 g, 146-328 g, 373-420 g and 129-254 g with highest values between 90-120 kg. Between-animal variation in protein (lean) and lipid (fat tissue) deposition rate was large which can be exploited in order to identify QTL of these traits.

Theatre P4.2

Future scenarios for sustainable pig production, which way ahead?

S. Stern[1], S .Gunnarsson[2], I. Öborn[3], U. Sonesson[4] , [1]Department of Animal Breeding and Genetics, [2]Department of Animal Health and Environment, [3]Department of Soil Sciences, Swedish University of Agricultural Sciences, Funbo-Lövsta, SE-75597 Uppsala,[4]SIK P.O. Box 5401, SE-42902, Göteborg, Sweden*

The Swedish research program Food 21 aims at making Swedish food production more sustainable and thus to present solutions for future production systems. Sustainability is a multidimensional issue. Hence to study this, a step-wise method for scenario construction was used to create three future scenarios of pig production. The purpose was to provide a platform for discussions between researchers from different disciplines and stakeholders from the food chain. In these groups the scenarios will be discussed and modified to result in more detailed descriptions and solutions for the short (using today's knowledge and technology) and long term (desired directions, approximately 20 years ahead). The three scenarios were deliberately chosen to be extreme with different goal visions. The first scenario has the focus on animal welfare, natural behaviour of the animals and a good working environment for the farmer/caretaker. The second scenario focuses on low impact on the external environment and an efficient use of natural resources, including energy. The third scenario focuses on high efficiency, quality and safety of the product. Finally, the three scenarios will be evaluated from an environmental aspect using Life Cycle Assessment. The economic effects will be calculated and possible social impacts of the different scenarios will be evaluated.

Theatre P4.3

Influence of husbandry methods on animal welfare and meat quality traits in pigs

B. Lebret[1], S. Couvreur[1], J.Y. Dourmad[1], M.C. Meunier-Salaün[1], P. Mormède[2] and M. Bonneau[1*], [1]INRA UMRVP, 35590 Saint-Gilles, France, [2]INRA-INSERM Neurogénétique et Stress, 33077 Bordeaux, France.*

A total of 120 pigs (castrated males and females) were used to evaluate the influence of an alternative husbandry method for growing-finishing pigs on animal welfare, growth performance, carcass and meat quality traits. Sawdust-shave bedding with free access to an outdoor area (2.4 m^2/pig) (**O**) was compared with a conventional system (totally slatted floor, 0.65 m^2/pig) considered as control (**C**). The experiment was repeated three times in spring, summer and winter, each replicate involving 2 groups of 10 pigs in each system.

During rearing, O pigs spent twice more time on exploration activities (specially towards the bedding) and showed twice lower urinary cortisol level than C pigs, suggesting that the O system would improve animal welfare. Growth rate was higher for O than C pigs (+10%) due to their higher feed intake, resulting in a higher body weight at slaughter for the formers (+ 7 kg). O pigs exhibited higher mean back fat depth (+ 3 mm) and lower lean meat content (- 2.5 points) than C pigs. The O system did not influence pH1, but led to lower pHu, higher drip losses but also higher intramuscular fat content. Sensory analyses and consumer tests remain to be performed to evaluate the influence of husbandry methods on eating quality and product acceptability.

Theatre P4.4

Effect of managemental factors on piglet mortality with focus on herds with loose-housed sows

G.M. Tajet[1], I.A. Haukvik[2], I.L. Andersen[3] and S. Kongsrud[1]. [1]Norsvin, P.O.Box 504, N-2304 Hamar, Norway, [2]Gilde Fellesslakteriet BA, P.O.Box 2009, N-3103 Toensberg, Norway, [3]Department of Agricultural Engineering, P.O.Box 5065, N-1432 Aas, Norway.*

The aim of this study was to identify and quantify the effect of farrowing environment and managemental routines on postnatal piglet mortality. In the project 113 herds were visited and the stockperson was interviewed. Information on piglet loss and number of live born per litter in 2001 was provided from the national pig recording system (In-Gris). Average piglet loss in these herds was 14.1 +/- 4.9 %, and average number of live born was 12.0 +/- 0.8. Of these herds 39 had loose-housed sows between farrowing and weaning. Average piglet loss and number of live born per litter in the loose-housed herds were 15.2 +/- 4.4 % and 11.9 +/- 0.7, respectively.
Generalised linear models were used to analyse the data. Factors affecting postnatal piglet loss in herds with loose-housed sows were: Number of walls in the farrowing pen with rails ($P<0.05$), liquid or dry feed ($P<0.01$), access to roughage ($P<0.01$), additional heat to cold piglets ($P<0.01$), filing the teeth of the piglet ($P<0.10$) and automatic *ad libitum* feeders ($p<0,10$). Number of live born per litter, length and width of the farrowing pen and total space available to the sow had no significant influence on piglet loss in this study.

Theatre P4.5

Effect of design of farrowing pen and housing on behaviour of sows and piglets

L. Botto, S. Mihina, P. Kisac and V. Brestensky, Research Institute of Animal Production, Hlohovska 2, 949 92 Nitra, Slovakia.*

Evaluation of behaviour of sows and piglets in three different types of farrowing pens was carried out. Two of them were as individual type, non-bedded pens with crate (C-pen) and straw-bedded pens with free movement of sows (F-pen). The third type was a straw-bedded group pen for six sows with feeding in the EFS (G-pen). Sows were observed before farrowing and in the first and second week after farrowing during 24 hours, when as well the piglets were observed.
The longest period of lying of sows was in the G-pen (1356 minutes). Sows lay longer time in the C-pens compared with the F-pens. The longest period of lying of sows was noticed in the first week after farrowing in all three types of pens. Sows were more active before farrowing. Sows had greater possibility of exploration and of manifestations of maternal behaviour in the F-pens than in the C-pens.
In the individual pens piglets lay shorter in the F-pens, but at the udder they lay longer. Total sucking was longer in the G-pen (413 minutes), but the sucking of own dam dominated. Sucking of alien sows was more marked in the older piglets ($p<0.05$). Piglets were more often occupied by sucking in the individual pens; total time of one sucking was longer in the G-pen.

Theatre P4.6

Breeding for environmental-friendly pigs, an opportunity?

E. Kanis, Department of Animal Sciences, Wageningen University and Research Centre, P.O. Box 338, 6700 AH Wageningen, The Netherlands.*

Pig production can have negative and positive effects on the environment. Negative effects are related to: 1) regional over-production of manure, 2) the use of fossil energy, and 3) others, like residues of medicines and feed additives that accumulate in the environment. The use of pigs for converting various kinds of waste into high quality pork has a positive effect.

The amount and composition of manure produced per kg of pork depends on the amount and digestion of the feed eaten, as well as on sow reproduction and longevity. Feed efficiency of growing pigs and litter size of sows are common breeding goal traits but digestion of specific nutrients, feed efficiency and longevity of sows are usually not. Fossil energy is used for production and transport of feed and for light and climate control in pig houses. Breeding of pigs that perform well with locally produced and less processed feed, in housing systems with little climatic control, contributes to a lower use of energy. Breeding for healthy and robust pigs will reduce the use of medicines and feed additives. Also the capabilities of pigs to grow on various kinds of organic waste and by-products from other food chains can probably be improved by breeding.

It is concluded that breeding for environmental-friendly pigs is already successfully applied in most common pig breeding programs. Further environmental profit requires other production systems with respect to feeding and housing, and breeding of pigs that fit well in those systems.

Theatre P4.7

The effect of environment enrichment with straw or hay on the productive traits of fattening pigs

D. Jordan, I Stuhec and K. Hrastar, University of Ljubljana, Biotechnical Faculty, Zootechnical Department, Domzale, Slovenia*

In intensive housing systems pigs are kept in slatted floor pens, where their only possible occupation is short time feeding on concentrate feed mixture. Therefore the addition of straw or hay to the nutrition enriches their living environment. This kind of enrichment and its influence on growth rate and carcass composition of fattening pigs was studied in two repetitions. Each repetition included 96 fattening pigs (three pens of 16 females and three pens of 16 male castrates) from 60 kg to slaughter with average weight 96 kg. Environment enrichment represented daily addition of 100g/animal of hay or straw laid in a rack. Such treatment had no significant influence on growth rate and lean meat percentage. The average daily gains were 765 g in control group, 759 g in straw and 773 g in hay group. The corresponding average lean meat percentage rates were 53.68 %, 53.46 % and 53.75 %. Fattening pigs preferred hay to straw as they liked chewing and eating hay more than straw.

Theatre P4.8

The energy intake limiting effects of alfalfa in gestation diets of sows

M.J. Van Oeckel[1], N. Warnants[1], M. De Paepe[1], S. Robert[2], F. Tuyttens[1] and D. De Brabander[1]. [1]Agricultural Research Centre, Department Animal Nutrition and Husbandry, Scheldeweg 68, B-9090 Melle, Belgium, [2]Dairy and Swine Research and Development Centre, P.O. Box, 2000 Route 108 East, Lennoxville, QC JIM 1Z3, Canada.*

The effect of alfalfa on the ad libitum feed intake of pregnant hybrid sows was studied in three trials. A control diet, a diet with 25% alfalfa and one with 47% alfalfa with, respectively, 5, 10 and 15% crude fibre were tested in a Latin square design. In the first trial (12 sows), the three diets were isoenergetic (8,6 MJ/kg feed), in the second (12 sows) and third trial (14 sows), the energy content decreased with increasing alfalfa content, from 8.6, 7.9 to 6.7 MJ/kg feed. The adaptation and feed intake registration period were, respectively, 10 and 5 days in the first two trials and 14 and 7 days in the third trial. The average energy intake over the three trials for the control, medium and high alfalfa treatment was, respectively, 2.1 (s.d. 0.6), 1.7 (s.d. 0.5) and 1.3 (s.d. 0.6) times the daily energy requirement, according to CVB (2002). With the high alfalfa diet a close to optimal average energy intake was realised, however, the variation between the sows was considerably high: 37% and 8% of the sows ate more than 150%, and less than 50% of the energy requirement, respectively.

Theatre P4.9

Effects of supplemental phytase and formic acid on the performance of weaning piglets and on the excretion of P, Ca and N

J. Balios[1] and V. Stravogianni[2], [1]School of Agriculture, Dept. of Animal Science, Aristotle University of Thessaloniki,Greece, [2]Lab of Animal Feed Inspection, Ministry of Agriculture, Greece*

A feeding trial was conducted to study the effects of phytase and formic acid on the performance of weaning piglets and on the faecal excretion of P, Ca and N. Ninety six crossebred piglets (Landrace X Large White) of an average body weight of 8,5 Kg were randomly allotted into four treatments in a completely randomized feeding trial. The four diets used were A (control), B (0,01%Phytase), C (0,8% Formic acid) and D (Phytase +Formic acid). The body weight of the piglets (individually) and feed consumption was recorded every week. Faeces was collected every day.

There was a strong synergy between phytase and formic acid. As a result of this synergy, both growth rate and feed efficiency were significantly improved. Growth rate was improved by 27 and 22% respectively for the first two weeks and feed efficiency by 9 and 12% for the same periods. For the whole period (0-28 days) growth rate was improved by 10% and feed efficiency by 8.5%. Phosphorus, Calcium and Nitrogen excretion was reduced by 30, 35 and 10% respectively for the first week of the trial. By the end of the fourth week the reduction in the excretion was in the order of 5, 2 and 2,5% for P, Ca and N respectively.

Poster P4.10

Reproductive performance of Bísaro sows in outdoor system along the year

J. Santos e Silva[1], Patrícia Gomes[2] and J.S. Pires da Costa[3], [1]DRAEDM, DPA, Quinta do Pinhó, S. Torcato, 4800, 875 S. Torcato, Portugal, [2]Escola Superior Agrária de Coimbra, Bemcanta, 3040 Coimbra, [3]INIAP, Estacao Zootécnica Nacional, Fonte Boa, Vale de Santarém.

32 Bísaro sows were used for evaluating the reproductive performances in outdoor breeding system and its adaptation to this system. This study was carried out in northern Portugal for 5 years (1997-2001). Prolificacy traits show an average of 8, 7 live born piglet per sows, a high mortality rate at weaning (20,5%) and a low farrowing rate (1,8 farrowing/year, as a result of a large weaning-to-oestrus interval 49 days).

A piglet mortality rate of 14, 2% occurred within the third day of life and was significantly higher ($P<0, 05$) in seasons with high levels of temperatures and rainfall (Autumn 12, 4 ^{0}C; 601 mm and Spring 14, 8 ^{0}C; 340 mm).

The period of farrowing was concentrated at the end of spring (32%) as a result of the high levels of oestrus in winter (42%). Possible this is associated with a high infertility rate observed in some sows in summer time (33% of cases) and the (early) autumn (43%).

In our opinion the inefficient in reproductive management, a natural synchronization of oestrus in winter and the bioclimatic seasonal factors (temperature, precipitation and photoperiod) seem to have a large influence on reproductive parameter in our experimental sows.

These factors need to be investigated in the Bísaros sows which showed a similar effect already demonstrated in Iberian and wild pigs.

Poster P4.11

Relationships between GPI and PGD locus genotypes and selected meat quality traits of Polish Large White pigs

B. Orzechowska and M. Tyra, National Research Institute of Animal Production, 32 083 Balice, Poland

This study attempted to determine the effect of GPI and PGD gene alleles on meat quality traits in 163 PLW gilts station tested in 2000-2002. The following meat quality traits were analysed: pH measured 45 minutes postmortem, pH measured 24 hours postmortem, meat colour in L* a* b*, water holding capacity, and electric conductivity 45 min. and 24 h postmortem.

The aim of the experiment was to analyse the effect of different GPI and PGD locus alleles on meat quality traits. The results of statistical analysis are inconclusive as to which allele of these loci could markedly affect the meat quality traits. For the GPI locus, significantly higher pH values of meat in animals with the $GPI^{B/B}$ genotype were observed. Animals with the $PGD^{B/B}$ genotype showed a similar tendency, but the differences were not significant. A significant effect on electric conductivity was exerted by the GPI^B allele. In the case of other traits, no significant differences between the genotypes were observed.

The present findings indicate the advisability of undertaking breeding work aimed to increase the frequency of GPI^B and PGD^B alleles in the population of PLW pigs. This might favourably affect the indicators of pH and electric conductivity of meat. However, this task may prove difficult to carry out considering the low (about 4%) frequency of animals with the $GPI^{B/B}PGD^{B/B}$ genotype.

Poster P4.12

Relationships between GPI and PGD locus genotypes and some fattening and slaughter traits of Polish Large White pigs

B. Orzechowska, M. Tyra, M. Kamyczek, National Research Institute of Animal Production, 32 083 Balice, Poland

This study attempted to determine the effect of GPI and PGD gene alleles on selected fattening and slaughter traits.

163 PLW gilts were investigated in the years 2000-2002. Rearing, feeding, slaughter and dissection were according to methods used by pig testing stations. Prior to slaughter, blood was drawn from each animal to genotype the animals for GPI and PGD genes. The results of these analyses were used for further statistical calculations aimed at determining the effect of genotypes of particular genes on selected fattening and carcass traits.

The results of statistical analysis for fattening traits showed that GPI and PGD locus alleles had no effect on these traits. Significant correlations were observed for slaughter traits. A favourable and significant effect of the PGD^{B} allele on loin eye area was found. $PGD^{B/B}$ genotype animals were characterized by considerably heavier loin than $PGD^{A/A}$ and $PGD^{A/B}$ animals. Among the meatiness traits, the weight of meat of primal cuts and meat percentage in carcass showed a considerable but non-significant influence of the GPI^{B} allele.

To improve the meatiness of pigs, it would be necessary to use information on the PGD gene locus, whose PGD^{B} allele showed a positive effect on this group of traits in most of the cases.

Poster P4.13

Reproductive usefulness of young boars reared in standardized litters of hyperprolific sows of the Polish Synthetic Line 990

R. Czarnecki, M. Kawecka, A. Pietruszka, M. Rózycki, M. Kamyczek, B. Delikator, Department of Pig Breeding, Agricultural University of Szczecin, Dr. Judyma 10 str., 71-460 Szczecin, Poland

The standardization to 8 piglets (63 litters) or 12 piglets in litter (69 litters) was performed on the first day after birth. In the both groups the sows were born the similar total and alive number of piglets in litter, respectively: 14.00, 12.98 and 13.75, 12.94. The evaluation of sperm value of the analysed boars was performed at about 7 months of age on a base third ejaculates (67 boars from "smaller" litters and 56 boars from "larger" litters). Weight of boars during weaning at 28 days, reared in "smaller" litters shaped 7.73kg and reared in "larger" litters 6.92kg. Volume of both testes at 180 days (cm^3) shaped, respectively: 262.82 and 256.14; concentration of spermatozoa in cm^3 x 10^6 235.16 and 233.84; total number of spermatozoa x 10^9 28.56 and 25.54; percentage of spermatozoa with major defects 9.72 and 12.33; percentage of spermatozoa with normal acrosome 86.00 and 80.31; AspAT enzyme activity 120.91 and 113.61. The boars reared in "smaller" litters were havier during weaning, had higher volume of testes and better sperm.

The study was financed by Committee for Scientific Research (grant No 6 P06E 035 20)

Poster P4.14

Relationship between body weight of young boars at age of 21, 28 or 64 days and their future reproductive usefulness

J. Owsianny, B. Matysiak, R. Czarnecki, B. Delikator. Department of Pig Breeding, University of Agriculture, ul.Dr.Judyma 10, 71-460 Szczecin, Poland.

The main objective of the research has been to determine relationship between body weight of young boars during their first two months of life and their future reproductive value characterized with quantitative and qualitative characteristics of sperm from first three ejaculates. 110 young boars of synthetic line 990 have been examined. They have been weighed at the age of 21 days, during weaning at the age of 28 days and at the age of 64 days at the beginning of the survival estimation test. Quantitative and qualitative tests of sperm have been carried out three times. The first sperm sampling has been carried out at the age of 180 days and the other two with 7-days' intervals. There were analysed the following traits: ejaculate volume, concentration of spermatozoa, total number of spermatozoa, spematozoa with major and minor defects.
A statistically significant relationship ($P \leq 0.01$) between concentration and the total number of spermatozoa on the one hand and body weight of young boars at the age of 28 days on the other hand has been found. The correlation coefficients between mentioned traits shaped, respectively: -0.22** and -0.21**.
*The study was financed by the Committee for Scientific Research (grant No.6 P06E 035 20).

Poster P4.15

The influence of nutritive regime on the meat performance and meat quality of pigs

S. Sevcíková, M. Koucky, V. Kudrna and P.Lang, Research Institute of Animal Production, Prague, Uhríneves, Czech Republic

The objective of the present study was to investigate the effect of high-crude fibre-diet on the carcass and chosen characteristics of meat quality and comparison with commercial diet. The diet with high-crude fibre content was feed to the pigs of final hybrid combination (Norway Landrace x Landrace) x (Large White x Pietrain) in the final period of fattening from 65 kg of live weight to average slaughtered weight - 111 kg (K = control group) and 109 kg (P = experimental group).
The slaughter values of P group were nonsignificantly better in comparison with the control group. The SEUROP classification of meatiness, using the two-point method, showed the evaluation 55% of lean meat in the P group, being included in class E, as compared with the K group (class U, 53% lean meat). The meat:fat ratio in the P group (1:0.25) was better than in control group (1:0.28). The experimental group with higher-crude fibre diet had decreased content of intramuscular fat (13.8 $g.kg^{-1}$) and cholesterol (0.56 $g.kg^{-1}$), higher ($P \leq 0.5$) content of crude protein (219.7 $g.kg^{-1}$), and lower ($P \leq 0.5$) content of hydroxyproline (0.44 $g.kg^{-1}$) in comparison with K group (14.3 $g.kg^{-1}$; 0.63 $g.kg^{-1}$; 214.6 $g.kg^{-1}$; 0.51 $g.kg^{-1}$, respectively).
This study was supported by the Ministry of Agriculture of the Czech Republic (project No. M02-99-04).

Poster P4.16

Seasoning effect on the chemical and acidic composition of the "*S. Angelo*" salame processing with pork meat belonging to the Nero Siciliano pigs

B. Chiofalo, L. Liotta, L. Venticinque, D. Piccolo, L. Chiofalo, Dept. MO.BI.FI.P.A., Faculty of Veterinary Medicine, Polo Annunziata, 98168 Messina, Italy.

The effect of seasoning on the chemical and acidic composition of "*S. Angelo*" salame (Messina, Italy) processing from the Nero Siciliano pig was studied. The chemical and the fatty acid composition, the oxidative stability (TBARS) were determined on the fresh mix (day 0) and after 7, 21 and 39 days' manufacturing. Data were subjected to statistical analysis (GLM - SAS). Seasoning effect showed a reduction ($P<0.001$) in water percentage (day 0: 62.67%; day 39: 37.13%) and an increase ($P<0.01$; $P<0.001$) of protein (day 0: 19.74%; day 39: 21.92%), NPN (day 0: 10.03%; day 39: 10.57% of total nitrogen), fat (day 0: 15.05%; day 39: 18.58%) and ash (day 0: 3.73%; day 39: 6.22%) percentages and of TBARS (day 0: 0.20; day 39: 0.38, measured at 532 nm). Seasoning also influenced fatty acid composition which showed the greatest differences ($P<0.001$) at day 21 for SFA and MUFA classes, for UFA/SFA ratio and for Atherogenic and Thombogenic indices. PUFA showed no significant difference during seasoning. These findings may represent a starting point for better knowledge of the quality characteristics of this typical product ("*S. Angelo*") and show that the meat of Nero pig is qualified to salami processing deserving a larger market with the support of a quality label.

Poster P4.17

Nero Siciliano pig for the production of the "*S. Angelo*" salame: sensorial characteristics

L. Liotta, B. Chiofalo, A. Zumbo, V. Chiofalo., Dept. MO.BI.FI.P.A., Sect. Animal Production, Faculty of Veterinary Medicine, Polo Annunziata, 98168 Messina, Italy.

The research was carried out on "*S. Angelo*" salami (Messina, Italy) processed with pork meat of the Nero Siciliano pigs living in extensive conditions. The mix, 70% of muscle and 30% of fat, was divided into two different lots: A with 3.4% and B with 3.2% NaCl content. The salami were dried and seasoned in a natural environment. Sensory analysis was performed by a tasting panel on salami after 45 days' seasoning and by a jury of 11 tasters. Data were subjected to statistical analysis considering the variables: salt percentage and taster, using GLM procedure of SAS. Taster judgement was not influenced by the salt percentage, though the overall judgement was "very satisfactory" for the A lot and "good" for the B lot. Sensorial profile of "S. Angelo" salame is: meat/fat ratio: ideal; fat colour: satisfactory; flavour: aromatic; tenderness: ideal; juiciness: slightly juicy; crust of slice: absent; meat colour: ideal; saltiness: to the right degree; different tonalities of the meat: absent; grain and structure of slice: ideal.

Poster P4.18

Intensity of formation of lean tissue in pigs and correlation with backfat thickness

R. Klimas, Siauliai University, P. Visinskio 25, LT-5400 Siauliai, Lithuania.

Fat deposition in pigs is an indicator of their leanness. The lower is the backfat thickness, the higher is the lean meat content (r=-0.6-0.9). At the control fattening performance test station, pigs (n=49) of some breeds were used in a study to determine the formation intensity of subcutaneous fat and lean tissue using the ultrasonic apparatus *Piglog 105*. Backfat thickness was measured for pigs of 30 to 80 kg weight, and from 80 to 100 kg weight determination of the lean meat percentage was added. At the start of control fattening, backfat thickness of Norwegian Landrace and Swedish Yorkshire pigs was, respectively, by 4.5 and 4.0 mm lower than that of purebred Lithuanian Whites. Lean tissue deposition was more intensive for the pigs of the imported breeds. During the period of control fattening (from 30 to 100kg), fat deposition in Norwegian Landrace pigs increased by 4.73 mm, Swedish Yorkshire by 6.57 mm, meat-type Lithuanian White by 7.29 mm and purebred Lithuanian White by 7.83 mm. The average lean meat percentage of 100 kg pigs was, respectively, 56.16, 52.48, 49.07 and 48.0%. Thus, under the same feeding and housing conditions, the intensity of subcutaneous fat (backfat) and muscle deposition was different at different weight periods for pigs of various breeds. Furthermore, higher weight of pigs led to higher backfat thickness and relatively lower content of lean meat.

Poster P4.19

Body water in sows during pregnancy and lactation

M. Neil, Department of Animal Nutrition and Management, Swedish University of Agricultural Sciences, Funbo-Lövsta, S-755 97 Uppsala, Sweden.

If sows are to give many and large litters of prospering piglets they must maintain their body reserves over time and should be fed accordingly. Hence effects of feeding should be measured not only as litter size and liveweights of piglet and sows, but also as composition of the liveweight. In a feeding experiment sows were fed standard (St) or low (L) protein diets during pregnancy, and standard (St) or high (H) diets during lactation in a 2*2 factorial design. The study comprised 13 blocks of 4 litter sisters during parity 1 to 3. In 3 of the blocks, water dilution space was measured using D_2O as marker, in early, mid and late pregnancy, and 1 and 3 weeks after farrowing during parity 1 and 3.

The water dilution space (kg) showed the same pattern as sow liveweight, it increased from early to late pregnancy and decreased after farrowing, being larger during parity 3 than parity 1. The proportion of water in the body, i.e. water dilution space as percent of liveweight, was not constant over time, it increased during pregnancy to a maximum in late pregnancy, and decreased after farrowing. There was no difference between parities. StH sows - highest dietary protein level - had larger proportion of body water than LSt sows - lowest protein -, with StSt and LH sows intermediate.

Poster P4.20

Analysis of muscle fibre thickness in relation to the gender and live weight of pigs during fattening

T. Cervenka, J. Cítek, T. Neuzil, R. Stupka and M. Sprysl, Czech University of Agriculture Prague, Faculty of Agronomy, Department of Pig and Poultry Science, Czech Republic

Pork is comprised of cross-striped muscle tissue whose functional and morphological construction unit is a muscle fiber. The goal of the work was to document the effect of the gender and live weight of pigs on muscle fiber thickness. Eight hybrid pigs (4 male pigs/female pigs with a live weight of 25 kg and 105 kg) of the VEPIG firm product were subject to two completed VJH experiments. Muscle fiber thickness was measured by means of section preparations of the following m. semimembranosus, adjuctor, serratus ventralis, cleidocephalicus and MLLT. Regardless of the gender, the average detected thickness of MLLT muscle fiber was 34.52 μm (25 kg) and 54.48 μm (105 kg). The biggest fiber diameter ($P<0.05$) was detected in the group of female pigs (34.48 μm; 34.48 μm) with a live weight of 25 kg compared to male pigs (36.62 μm; 34.48 μm). During the second series of experiments the biggest muscle fiber thickness was demonstrated by the monitored male pigs (66.54 μm; 58.4 μm) compared to female pigs (59.38 μm; 57,5 μm).

Poster P4.21

The physicochemical properties of the two-breed hybrid fattener meat

A. Litwinczuk, M. Florek, P. Skalecki and Barlowska J, Department of Evaluation and Use of Animal Raw Materials, Agricultural University of Lublin, Akademicka 13, 20-950 Lublin, Poland

The studies comprised 38 heads of fatteners divided into following genetic groups: I - wbp♂ x Pulawy♀ (n=15), II - pietrain♂ x wbp♀ (n=8) i III - pietrain♂ x pbz♀ (n= 15). In the samples of the longest dorsal muscle and of the semimembranosus muscle were determined the physical properties (ph, electrical conductivity, trichromatic values in the L*a*b* colour space, the percentage of loose water, as well as drip loss and cooking loss) and chemical composition of meat. On the basis of the obtained results we found out that genetic groups significantly influenced the discriminants of physicochemical quality of pork, although it is difficult to conclude that there is an explicit influence of a certain genotype on all the meat quality parameters. Generally, the best quality features (and especially water absorption) were found in group I (wbp♂ x Pulawy♀) hybrid meat. It probably resulted from the beneficial influence of Polish local Pulawy breed.

Poster P4.22

Comparison of lean meat content estimation methods of living and slaughtered pigs

M. Baltay, V. Pfaff and Z. Csörnyei, National Institute for Agricultural Quality Control, Keleti K. u. 24., 1024 Budapest, Hungary

Some years ago account method of Self Performance Test of pigs was based on the measurement of weight gain and estimation of valuable meat parts. The basis of estimating valuable meat parts was the measurement of fat depth. For more exact prediction of breeding value and the integration of estimation methods we entered the determination of lean meat content of living pigs. The measurement is done on the same measuring points on living pigs like in EUROP classification method of carcasses in the slaughterhouse. Objective of our examination was to find the correlation between parameters of EUROP Self Performance Test measured by ultra-sonic equipment and the data measured by FAT-O-MEATER in the slaughterhouse. Altogether we have evaluated data of 180 animals from 7 genotype, which had been tested on the Animal Performance Testing Station of National Institute for Agricultural Quality Control in 2003. We have estimated all of the living animals' lean meat content by ultrasonic equipment SONOMARK 100S previous day of slaughtering and after the slaughtering we have measured the lean meat % of their carcasses by FAT-O-MEATER machine on the same measurement points. The results of our trial showed that both of the measuring methods are acceptable and their correlation assures the exact estimation of lean meat content of living animals at the end of the Self Performance Test period.

Poster P4.23

Effect of iso-malto-oligosaccharide on gut flora and animal performance of piglets

M.J. Van Oeckel[1], N. Warnants[1], M. De Paepe[1], K. Cauwerts[2], L. Devriese[2] and F. Haesebrouck[2].*
[1]Agricultural Research Centre, Department Animal Nutrition and Husbandry, Scheldeweg 68, B-9090 Melle, Belgium, [2]Faculty of Veterinary Science, Salisburylaan 133, 9820 Merelbeke, Belgium.

As an alternative for in-feed antibiotics, non-digestible oligosaccharides were tested for their capacity to enhance beneficial bacterial species in the gastrointestinal tract of piglets. Three weeks prior to parturition until four weeks after parturition 21 pregnant hybrid sows were supplied with a top-dressing of 45 g iso-malto-oligosaccharides (IMO) two times a day. From two up to ten weeks of age their piglets received a diet supplemented with 3% of IMO. The piglets of sixteen control sows received a diet with 3% maltodextrine instead of IMO. Only sows with litters of 8 to 12 piglets were withhold in the trial. The piglets were weaned at 4 weeks of age and further raised in groups of 6 littermates. At 4, 6, 8 and 10 weeks of age, four piglets of both groups were euthanised and sampled for the contents of duodenum, jejunum, ileum, caecum and colon. The treatments were compared for significant performance differences with the LSD-test. Counts of *E. coli*, *C. perfringens*, *E. faecium*, *E. faecalis, E. hirae* and *S. gallolyticus* were analysed with the Rank Sum test at each sampling time. No significant effect of IMO was observed on the intestinal tract microflora, daily feed intake, daily gain and feed conversion ratio.

Poster P4.24

Efficiency of crossbreeding on production of lean pork meat

A. Klimiene, Siauliai University, P. Visinskio 25, LT-5400 Siauliai, Lithuania.

Higher demand for lean pork and introduction of the EUROP requirements for slaughtered animals, require to use rationally all the available pig breeds in the breeding system. In Lithuania, the genetic potential of pigs and current breeding system create favourable conditions for commercial crossbreeding. Comparative evaluation of the leanness of crossbred pigs has been carried out and the most effective combinations of crossbreeding determined. According to the *Piglog 105* data, the crossbred pigs (n=2301) produced by crossing Lithuanian White pigs with boars of the imported breeds had by 0.8-4.1% higher lean meat content (P<0.05-0.001) compared with that of purebred Lithuanian Whites. German Landrace and Swedish Yorkshire had the lowest influence on the lean meat percentage of crossbreds, respectively, 51.6 and 51.7%, while Norwegian Landrace (54.9%), Duroc (54.4%) and Pietrain (54.3%) breeds had the highest influence. The average lean meat percentage or crossbreds (n=566) produced by crossing the pigs of imported breeds varied from 51.9 to 59.0%, depending on the combination of breeds. Norwegian Landrace x Norwegian Yorkshire, Norwegian Landrace x Hampshire and Hampshire x Pietrain crossbreds were distinguished by the highest lean meat content, respectively, 59.0, 58.7 and 58.5 %. Crossbreds produced by crossing imported breeds are suitable for three- or four-way commercial hybridization. The analysis of the lean meat percentage of crossbred pigs indicated that rational use of various breeds in crossbreeding combinations usually produces carcasses of desirable leanness.

Poster P4.25

Effect of boar semen extenders on insemination dose quality

A. Jezková, Czech University of Agriculture, Department of Cattle Breeding and Dairying, Prague, Kamycka, 165 21, Czech Republic

The aim of this study was to compare the influence of Kare, Androhep, BTS, MR-A extenders, and new diluent (our name D-XY) on spermatozoa motility. The spermatozoa survival tests (thermo-resistance test) and insemination dose thermal endurance tests were made.
Laboratory tests revealed higher survival rate of Androhep diluted spermermatozoa decisively in comparison with spermatozoa from the same collection diluted by other diluents.
Spermatozoa survival test and test of thermal endurance in insemination doses proved the differences between Kare and Androhep dilutents (4 boars) with various degrees of significance but always in favour of Androhep diluent. Similar results were found in comparing Androhep, BTS, and D-XY diluents (11 boars). Spermatozoa motility in Androhep dilutent was also arguably supreme during a long-time thermal endurance test. The difference in spermatozoa motility in these diluents is increasing with the duration of storage interval.
Individual differences exist between different boars not only in survival rate and endurance, but also in a response to particular diluter. In spite of the fact that dilution ratio higher than 1:10 are commonplace in some stations, according to the results of laboratory tests of spermatozoa motility with dilution 1:16, higher dilution ratio than 1:10 may be used only in selected boars.

Poster P4.26

Relationship between semen value and slaughter value of young boars at different levels of their meatiness

M. Kawecka, R. Czarnecki, M. Rózycki, A. Pietruszka, E. Jacyno, J. Owsianny, B. Delikator, Department of Pig Breeding, Agricultural University of Szczecin, Dr. Judyma 10 str., 71-460 Szczecin, Poland

Many authors think that better meatiness value of the boars can decrease their reproductive ability. The aim of the study was comparison the relationship between meatiness of young boars and their semen traits within the limits of two groups: group I (161 boars) with average meat content in body 54.5% (from 51.2 to 56.0); group II (261 boars) with average meat content in body 59.0% (from 56.1% to 64.7%). The evaluation of sperm value of the analyzed boars was performed at about 7 months of age on a base third ejaculates. Correlation coefficients between meatiness and traits of semen of the boars in analyzed groups was obtained: volume ejaculate after filtration in group I - r=0.095 in group II - r=-0.061 and respectively: percentage of motile spermatozoa 0.116 and -0.138*; concentration of spermatozoa 0.007 and -0.154*; total number of spermatozoa in ejaculate 0.137 and -0.182**. Results of the study suggest that antagonism between slaughter value and reproductive usefulness of the boars can appear in relation to male population which characterized higher level of meatiness.

Poster P4.27

Evaluation of progeny performance from purebred and crossbred terminal boars

I. Bahelka, P. Flak, L. Hetényi and E.N. Blanco Roa, Research Institute of Animal Production, Hlohovská 2, 949 92 Nitra, Slovak Republic*

Data were obtained from progeny (160 and/or 182 respectively) sired by 5 purebred (Slovakian Meaty breed - SM) and 6 crossbred (SM x Pietrain - PN, Duroc x PN, PN x York-
shire) terminal boars. Boars were tested in field conditions and following traits were evaluated: average daily gain (ADG) from birth to the 100 kg live weight, backfat thickness (BF) and lean meat content (LMC) at 100 kg live weight.

Progeny traits were ADG from 30 to 100 kg live weight, days to the slaughter, feed conversion ratio (FC), BF, percentage of valuable meaty cuts (VMC) and eye muscle area (EMA). Regression coefficients of progeny traits on each sire trait and heritability estimates were calculated.

Purebred sires had significant effect (P<0.05) on BF and highly significant (P<0.01) on ADG and days to the slaughter of progeny. The days, BF and VMC of progeny were influenced (min. P<0.05) by crossbred boars.

Similar regression coefficients of progeny traits on sire BF and LMC in purebred and/or crossbred boars were obtained. However, regressions of progeny traits on sire ADG were different between the two types.

The heritability estimates for ADG, BF and LMC were 0.55 and/or 0.98, 0.66/0.75 and 0.67/0.88 for purebred and crossbred boars respectively.

Poster P4.28

Does low level laser cause a stress reaction in piglets' organism?

A.I. Serzhantova, Novosibirsk State Agrarian University, 160 Dobrolubov Str., Novosibirsk, 630039, Russia

Though low intensive laser therapy has been commonly applied, it is still unknown whether laser irradiation causes a considerable stress reaction. That point is especially important in pig breeding as pigs are known to be very stress-susceptible.
The 2-week old piglets (Early Meat breed) of experimental group were irradiated thrice with 24-hour intervals. Piglets' behaviour was measured according to the 6-grade scale from 1 (very quiet) to 6 (screaming and breaking away) with 4 mediate states. On the beginning of the experiment the reaction of the experimental animals was more intense than one of the control piglets (2.7 and 2.0 points, respectively, $P<0.05$). However, this difference disappeared on the 2nd day . On the third day the piglets of both groups behaved much more quietly in response to the procedure carried out (1.83 points on the average) compared to the first day (2.35 points on the average). The hematological analyses had shown the significant increase of erythrocyte rate in experimental animals' blood compared to control group (6.2 and $5.5*10^9$/L, $P<0.05$), that could be the sign of hemogenesis stimulation caused by the laser irradiation.
Thus, we can conclude that LLL itself produces very little stress reaction, if any, and on the contrary, it may precipitate the process of animals' adaptation to the stress factor, namely, the procedure conducted.

Poster P4.29

Meat content and quality in final pig hybrids fattened under conditions of the Czech Republic

J. Pulkrábek, J. Pavlík and L. Valis, Research Institute of Animal Production, Prátelství 815, 104 01 Praha 10 -Uhrnees, Czech Republic.

Totally 60 gilts and 60 barrows were included into the analysis. The average slaughter weight was 106,9 ± 1,18 kg. Values of lean meat content determined by the FOM device and pH_1 of meat were recorded. The average values of lean meat percentage and pH_1 were 57,10 ± 0,376 % and 6,18 ± 0,031, respectively. The results of meat content show a high level of carcass conformation in pigs involved in the experiment. However, the observed pH_1 values are somewhat surprising when the relationship between pH_1 and lean meat content in individual animals is investigated. The calculated correlation coefficient ($r = 0,03 \pm 0,092$) indicates that there is almost no relation between these two traits. Some previous studies, however, documented that higher meat content in carcass is often accompanied by deteriorated values of meat quality traits. Only when the carcasses were classified into two groups with pH_1 higher than 5,80 and lower than 5,80, a slight tendency towards reduced pH_1 in carcasses with a higher lean meat content was observed. Totally 85 % and 15 % of carcasses with average lean contents of 57,04 ± 0,403 and 57,47 ± 0,995 % were included into the group with $pH_1>5,80$ and $pH_1<5,80$, respectively. In case that the observed relationship is confirmed in further analyses of currently produced pig carcasses, this result will be significant for future development of selection programmes.

Poster P4.30

The growth of young boars and gilts until two months of age reared in litters standardized to 8 or 12 piglets

R. Czarnecki, M. Rózycki, M. Kamyczek, A. Pietruszka, J. Owsianny, B. Delikator Department of Pig Breeding, Agricultural University of Szczecin, Dr. Judyma 10 str., 71-460 Szczecin, Poland

The aim of the study was comparison the growth of young boars and gilts obtained from hyperprolific sows of Polish Line 990, reared in “smaller” and “larger” litters. The standardization was performed on the first day after birth. In both of groups the sows were born the similar total and alive number of piglets in litter, respectively: 14.00, 12.98 and 13.75, 12.94. Weight of boars reared in “smaller” litters at 21; 28 and 63 days shaped, respectively: 5.75; 7.73 and 19.39kg and reared in “larger” litters, respectively: 5.12; 6.92 and 16.83kg. Weight of gilts from “smaller” litters shaped, respectively: 5.58; 7.56 and 18.80kg and reared in “larger” litters 5.16; 6.97 and 17.01kg. In “smaller” litters the young boars and gilts were growing faster. In more favourable rearing conditions (“smaller” litters) the boars grew faster in comparison with gilts. However, the boars could not utilize of that potential to faster growing in worse rearing conditions (“larger” litters).

The study was financed by Committee for Scientific Research (grant No 6 P06E 035 20)

Poster P4.31

Outdoor rearing of gilts

Alexy Márta[1], J. Gundel[2], G. Nagy[1], [1]University of Debrecen, Centre of Agricultural Science, P.O. Box 36, 4032 Debrecen, Hungary, [2]Research Institute for Animal Breeding and Nutrition, 2053 Herceghalom, Hungary*

The applied technology is an alternative approach to pig keeping-systems. An outdoor pig production breeding sows are kept at pasture either year-round or in a certain period of the year. Nowadays the number of breeding sows are kept outdoor is increasing.
Within the scope of the study we are performing an experiment to examine how this system can be adapted to Hungarian circumstances. 28 gilts were kept on pasture all day and 28 gilts are kept in traditional indoor system. We performed weight measures monthly and gathered data about supplementary concentrate feed mass. Ethological observations and examination of grassland are included in the experimental data.
By gilts the average daily gain was higher in conventional system excepting winter months when this value was higher by outdoor gilts (313g vs 309g). The feed-consumption was 14,7 % higher by outdoor gilts. The age of outdoor gilts by artificial insemination was 20 days less than in conventional system. Pasturing sows became fertil 5,6 % more than control sows. Numbers and weights of live born piglets were better in outdoor group (9,6; 11,7), as in indoor-system (8,4; 7,8).

Poster P4.32

Effect of caprylic acid and Akomed R on shedding of oocysts of *Cryptosporidium parvum* in piglets

V. Skrivanová[*1], *M. Marounek*[1,2]; [1]*Research Institute of Animal Production, Prague 10;* [2]*Institute of Animal Physiology and Genetics, Prague 10, Czech Republic*

Medium-chain fatty acids (MCFA) exert a strong activity against rumen protozoa. Their effect on parasitic protozoa is not known. Thus, 120 piglets, just after weaning were divided into 3 groups and housed in pens. Piglets were fed a standard dry commercial feed without additives (Ist group, control) or supplemented with caprylic acid at 5g/kg (IInd group), or supplemented with Akomed R (oil containing triglycerides of caprylic and capric acid by Karlshamns, Sweden) at 5g/kg. In weekly intervals faeces of 10 piglets per group were examined microscopically for the presence of *Eimeria* and *Cryptosporidium* oocysts. Numbers of oocysts were scored on a 4-point scale. Two control piglets were infected with *C. parvum* in the 2nd week of the trial and another 3 control piglets in the 3rd week (++++). Oocyst shedding in treated groups was one week delayed. Three piglets were infected in the IInd group (+++), and one piglet only in the IIIrd group (+). Oocyst shedding ceased in the 4th week. It can be concluded that MCFA bound in triglycerides are more efficient toward cryptosporidia than free acid, probably due to their *in situ* release in the intestine. (This study was supported by the Ministry of Agriculture of the Czech Republic: project No. MZE-MO2-99-04).

Theatre PhP5.1

Lipid oxidation and meat quality

J. Buckley, J. Kerry and P. Morrissey, Department of Food and Nutritional Sciences, University College, Cork. Ireland.

Oxidation of lipids is a major cause of the deterioration in the quality of muscle foods and can directly affect many quality characteristics such as colour, flavour, texture, nutritive value and safety of the food. Lipid oxidation *in vivo* and in muscle foods is believed to be initiated in the highly unsaturated phospholipid fraction in sub-cellular membranes. Oxidative damage to lipids occurs in living animals because of an imbalance between the production of reactive oxygen species and the animal's antioxidant defence mechanisms. This may be brought about by a high intake of polyunsaturated fatty acids, or by a deficiency of nutrients involved in the antioxidant defence systems. Damage to lipids is accentuated in the immediate post slaughter period and, in particular, during handling, processing and storage. Dietary functions contribute to the antioxidant defence systems and protect biological membranes against lipid oxidation. A variety of nutrients and non-nutrients, including Vitamin E, ascorbic acid and tea catechins are available. This talk focuses on the chemistry of lipid oxidation in muscle foods and on the mechanisms of antioxidants. In addition the effect of lipid oxidation and antioxidant on colour, cholesterol oxidation and water-holding capacity will be discussed.

Theatre PhP5.2

Dietary prooxidants and antioxidants: From pig diets to human consumers with emphasis on antioxidative and oxidative status of pork

Charlotte Lauridsen and Martin Tang Sørensen, Danish Institute of Agricultural Sciences, Foulum Research Centre, DK-8830 Tjele

The effects of dietary copper (0, 35, and 175 mg Cu/kg feed) and vitamin E (0, 100, and 200 mg dl-a-tocopheryl acetate/kg feed) in diets containing 6% rapeseed oil were investigated with regard to the antioxidative and oxidative status of live pigs and the carcass. Several responses were used such as blood, liver and muscle concentrations of antioxidants, prooxidants, and lipids, and susceptibility to lipid oxidation. Meat quality was assessed under different storage conditions. Meat and meat products were served for healthy human subjects, and blood samples obtained before and at the end of a dietary period of 4 weeks were analysed for concentration of vitamin E, triglycerides, and cholesterol.

Major conclusions were that accumulation of vitamin E in muscle membranes plays an important role in the prevention of lipid oxidation in the muscle and in pork products. Supplemental copper accumulated in liver, but did not affect the oxidative stability of muscle or any of the pork products. Addition of 6% rapeseed oil changed the lipid profile of pork and increased the susceptibility to lipid oxidation. Consumption of pork products from pigs fed diets with addition of rapeseed oil reduced blood cholesterol concentrations in human subjects, and intake of pig fat with a high content of unsaturated fatty acids increased the requirement of vitamin E.

Theatre PhP5.3

Comparative effect of dietary fatty acid composition and vitamin E supplementation on meat quality characteristics in light and heavy pigs

C.J. López-Bote, A.I. Rey and J. Ruiz. Departamento de Producción Animal, Universidad Complutense, Ciudad Universitaria, 28040 Madrid, Spain.

Two parallel experiments were carried out with modern pig hybrids (Large White x Great York) slaughtered at 95 kg live weight an with Iberian pigs (an autochthonous breed from the Iberian peninsula) slaughtered at 160 kg. Each experiment was organised in a 3 x 2 factorial arrangement with mixed diets formulated to contain three dietary fat blends and a basal (20 mg kg^{-1} diet) or supplemented (220 mg kg-1) level of α-tocopheryl acetate. A significant effect of dietary vitamin E and fatty acid composition was observed for muscle α-tocopherol concentration and susceptibility of muscle and microsome extracts to lipid oxidation. The effect of dietary treatment on colour stability along storage (as assessed by the evolution of 'a' value, or redness) was dependent on the pig genotype: while no effect was observed in improved pig genotypes slaughtered at 95 kg live weight, a significant effect of dietary vitamin E was observed in Iberian pigs (160 kg).

Theatre PhP5.4

Dietary fat and its impact on quality traits of pork tissues

S. Gebert, M.R.L. Scheeder, C. Wenk, Swiss Federal Institute of Technology Zurich, Institute of Animal Sciences, Nutrition Biology, ETH Zentrum, Universitätstrasse 2, CH-8092 Zurich, Switzerland*

In monogastric animals ingested fats can be readily incorporated into body tissue. Therefore adipose tissue composition, its physicochemical properties and the nutritive value of meat and meat products from pigs are directly influenced by the dietary fatty acid composition. But it depends also on the genetic disposition of the animals. Nowadays the modern pigs have very lean carcasses and thus the proportion of polyunsaturated fatty acids (PUFA) is high. In several studies an increased susceptibility to oxidation and an impaired consistency of pork tissues have been reported. To overcome this undesired trend, the Swiss slaughter plants established an at-line method to measure the amount of double bounds in backfat, the so called fat score, fifteen years ago. It still plays part of the payment system for pork carcasses in Switzerland. As a consequence feeding guidelines were developed, recommending a maximum of 0.8 g PUFA/ MJ DE. Recent studies also showed that a high content of monounsaturated fatty acids (MUFA) in the diet could be even more detrimental than dietary PUFA. Therefore MUFA are now considered in Swiss feeding recommendations as well. Furthermore, today a grown interest exists in conjugated linoleic acids (CLA) as feed additive for pigs, as it was reported to reduce fat deposition. However, its potential for improving pork and lard quality by reducing endogenous fatty acid desaturation might be even more important, giving room for an increased proportion of valuable PUFA in pork products.

Poster PhP5.5

The effect of α-tocopherol acetate supplement in fatteners' feed mixtures fattened with corn oil on the fatty acids profile and cholesterol content in meat

M. Pieszka, T.Barowicz, National Research Institute of Animal Production, 32-083 Balice, Poland*

The feed experiment was carried out on 24 cross-breed fatteners [(Polish Large x Polish Landrace) x pietrain] randomly divided into two groups (12 animals in each, 6 gilts and 6 barrows). The fattening for both groups was based on the complete mixture fattened with 3% of corn oil. The addition of α-tocopherol acetate in amount of 200 mg/kg of mixture was used for the experiment group. The addition of α-tocopherol acetate to the diet caused the significant decrease of MUFA level in *longissimus dorsi* and *semimembranoeus muscles* ($P<0.05$) and also the increase the PUFA level in the *semimembranoeus muscles* and the *longissimus dorsi* respectively from 20.34% and 14.84% to 22.98% and 16.48%. The differences were not significant. The addition of α-tocopherol acetate to the diet for experimental animals caused the increase of unsaturated fatty acids from *n-6* family, mainly the linoleic (C18:2) and arachidonic (C20:4) acids. The significant decrease of the oleic acid (C18:1) in the *semimembranoeus muscle* of fatteners from the experimental group from 39.4% to 35.2% ($P<0.01$) was stated. The significant decrease of the total cholesterol level in the *semimembranoeus muscle* from 68.4 to 52.8 (mg/100g) and the tendency to reducing its content in the *longissimus dorsi muscle* were observed in this study. It was noted that the addition of the α-tocopherol acetate in amount of 200 mg/kg of mixture increased significantly the α-tocopherol level ($P<0.01$) in *longissimus dorsi* and *semimebranoeus muscles* respectively from 1.58 and 1.56 to 3.37 and 3.33 (μg/g of fresh meat).

Poster PhP5.6

Fatty acid composition and carcass characteristics of Iberian pigs fed in either free-range or in confinement with acorns and grass or a formulated diet

C. López-Carrasco[1], J.M. Contreras[1], A. Daza[2], A.I. Rey[3] and C.J. López-Bote[3], [1]Centro de Investigaciones Agropecuarias "Dehesón del Encinar", 45560 Oropesa, Toledo, Spain, [2]Dpto. de Producción Animal, Universidad Politécnica de Madrid, Ciudad Universitaria, 28040 Madrid, Spain, [3]Dpto. de Producción Animal. Universidad Complutense de Madrid, Ciudad Universitaria, 28040 Madrid, Spain.*

One group of Iberian pigs was fed in a free-range production system. The other 3 groups were fed in confinement with acorns, acorns and grass, and a formulated diet.At slaughter hams and longissimus dorsi and psoas major muscles were collected and weighted. At cutting, pigs fed the formulated diet had the heaviest meat yield and those fed in free-range the lightest. Measurement of the longissimus dorsi muscle perimeters and backfat by an ultrasound system showed that pigs fed in free-range had significantly highest values for the backfat measurement, however not significant differences were found for the longissimus dorsi muscle.
The subcutaneous fat from the pigs fed in free-range had higher C18:1n-9, C18:3n-3 and lower C18:2n-6 proportions than those from the pigs fed the formulated diet (inner and outer layers). Pigs fed acorns and grass in confinement had a C18:3 higher proportion than those fed with acorns or the formulated diet which was more marked for the inner fat. Neutral and polar muscle fatty acids showed a similar trend to that observed for subcutaneous fat.

Poster PhP5.7

Influence of dietary conjugated linoleic acid (CLA) on serum leptin concentrations and physiological variables of lipid metabolism in finishing pigs

T. Barowicz, M. Pieszka, M.P. Pietras, National Research Institute of Animal Production, 32-083 Balice, Poland*

The effects of conjugated linoleic acid (CLA) on serum leptin and lipid blood profile in fatteners was investigated. Twenty four Polish Landrace fatteners, 12 males, 12 females of mean 70 kg LW were assigned into two groups in which complete pelleted feeds were supplemented with 2% sunflower oil (control group), or 2% of CLA (experimental group). The CLA preparation contained 61%CLA isomers (Edenor UKD 6010, Henkel). Blood was collected at slaughter at 108 kg LW. Total cholesterol, triglycerides, HDL and glucose were determined in serum by enzymatic spectrophotometric assays. Serum leptin concentrations were determined with a commercially available radioimmunoassay procedure (Multi-Species Leptin RIA Kit, Linco Research, MO). CLA supplement caused the significant increase ($P< 0.05$) of total cholesterol and HDL level in serum with a trend to increased serum leptin ($P= 0.07$). The effect of fatteners sex on leptin level and studied fat lipid variables in blood serum was not stated. These data suggest that dietary addition of CLA in finishing pigs altered lipid metabolism to produce higher concentrations of serum total cholesterol, HDL and leptin.

Influence of dietary fat source on sows' reproductive traits and piglets' rearing

T. Barowicz, M. Pieszka, M.P. Pietras, National Research Institute of Animal Production, 32-083 Balice, Polan*

The study was carried out on 20 Polish Landrace sows being on average in 3,7 - 3,8 pregnancy, divided into two groups with the same number of sows. Animals were kept in the same zoohigienic conditions and fed with isoenergetic and isoprotein diets. Diets differed in composition; control animals from 70 days of pregnancy were fed with fodder fattened with calcium salts of fatty acids of utilization fat; experimental animals got fodder with different level of *n-3* PUFA (calcium salts of line seed fatty acids). Piglets were weaned in 42 days of their life. The significant influence of calcium salts of line seed oil addition on number of piglets born alive and reared piglets was stated in this study. Body weights of weaned piglets were 8,44 and 11,22 kg (P<0.01). Similarly, milk yield to 21 day of lactation for control sows was lower than for experimental sows, respectively 202,2 and 266,1 kg (P<0.01). Barren period was also shorter from 7,4 to 4,7 days (P<0.01). Lower loss of sows body weight was observed during lactation, in control group it was 29 kg, in experimental group - 26 kg. It is believed that calcium salts of line seed oil fatty acids, rich in *n-3* PUFA used in diets for sows as an addition of 6% from 70 to 90 day of pregnancy and 9% from 91 day of pregnancy to 42 of lactation, have an positive effect on sows' reproductive traits and piglets weaning traits.

Theatre H1.1

Research issues on horse welfare

E. Søndergaard[*1], J.W. Christensen[1], M. van Dierendonck[2], J. Ladewig[3], M. Minero[4] and E. Canali[4], [1]Danish Institute of Agricultural Sciences, P.O. Box 50, 8830 Tjele, Denmark, [2]Tolnegenweg 39, 3776 PT Stroe, The Netherlands, [3]Royal Veterinary and Agricultural University, Grønnegårdsvej 8, 1870 Frederiksberg C, Denmark, [4]Istituti Zootecnica, via Celoria 10, 20133 Milan, Italy*

The importance of horses as leisure, sports and companion animals is increasing and as a consequence many horses are kept and managed by people with no previous knowledge about their physical or behavioural requirements. Keeping horses within a stabled environment, and using them for riding and driving purposes require consideration about how these environments and activities affect the welfare of horses. Additionally, horse welfare is affected by handling and training techniques. However, until recently, very little research has been directed towards investigating the welfare of the domestic horse. Horse research would benefit from increased worldwide cooperation and agreement on the importance of the different issues, since a joint effort will give the biggest impact on horse welfare. With the aim of reaching consensus on recommendations for future horse research scientists within the field of animal behaviour and welfare research will meet in a workshop in conjunction with the 37th Congress of the International Society of Applied Ethology in June 2003. The workshop will actively involve all participants in identifying important welfare issues by means of a so-called MetaPlan method. The results from the workshop will be presented.

Theatre H1.2

Current topics in equine behavior: Where the United States stands

Jennifer Weeks, Centenary College, 651 Fox Farm Road, Asbury NJ 08802, USA

An assessment of recently published or presented work from American authors reveals several areas of interest in equine behavior and welfare. Much of this research appears to be influenced by public awareness of welfare problems as well as the popularity of "natural horsemanship" methods. Recently, huge advances were made in the assessment of welfare of horses being transported to slaughter by Friend et. al. (2001). However, the majority of research on the emotional well being of horses is being conducted outside of The United States. The second main area of interest involves alternative training methods such as imprinting and clicker training. Many horse owners are ascribing to these training methods without any empirical conformation of their efficacy on equine learning. Several groups are currently working to evaluate these training methods. Texas A & M University has been assessing imprint training in foals. Contrary to the purported benefits of imprint training, the researchers (Williams et.al, 2002) found that imprint trained foals did not perform significantly better than non-imprint trained foals on several tasks. The University of Georgia has begun to assess the efficacy of clicker training on basic tasks such as trailer loading and novel object approach in weanling foals. These studies are preliminary, but they suggest clicker training is no more efficacious than normal handling for the tested tasks. Further work is needed in all areas to better our understanding of equine learning capabilities and emotional well being.

 Theatre H1.3

Interplay between environmental and genetic factors in the behaviour of horses

M. Hausberger and M.A. Richard-Yris, Université Rennes 1, UMR 6552 Ethologie, Evolution, Ecologie, Campus de Beaulieu, F - 35042 Rennes Cedex, France

Behavioural genetics of horses are in their infancy. The importance of taking behaviour into account during selection appeared only recently. In addition, this is a difficult question to address for this species as the living conditions of these animals are very varied. We have no data on genetic determination, only indirect indications based on comparisons among races or lines. Greater similitudes among animals with the same father and/or of the race were observed in foals, as well as in adults, in freely expressed activities (play, distance from mothers) and in reactions to experimental situations. Stereotyped activities appear to be related, in addition to environmental conditions, to family and to race. The relative weights of environmental and genetic factors on the determinism of behavioural characteristics appear to differ in relation to the character considered. The differences observed between families or races could also be linked to epigenetic factors (maternal effect for example). Taking behaviour into account when selecting horses appears advisable and possible, on condition that the character considered is well defined, its measurement is standardized and the impact of epigenetic factors is evaluated.

Theatre H1.4

Effects of handling during neonatal period or at weaning on manageability and reactivity of foals

L. Lansade[1], M.F. Bouissou[1] and X. Boivin[2]. [1]Laboratoire du Comportement Animal, UMR 6073 INRA-CNRS-Université de Tours, F-37380, Nouzilly, France.[2]URH-ACS, INRA-Theix, F-63122, Saint-Genès-Champanelle, France*

The short and long term effects of handling, during two periods of foal development, was studied. In the first experiment, 13 Welsh foals were handled from birth for 14 days, 13 were non-handled controls. Two days, 3, 6 and 12 months after the end of handling, they were submitted to various behavioural tests aimed at measuring their manageability and various aspects of their reactivity. The results show that neonatal handling has only short term effect on manageability and fear reactions. Furthermore, there was no generalization to unknown frightening stimuli. These effects are similar to habituation and cannot be interpreted in terms of "imprinting".

In experiment 2, 16 Anglo-Arab foals were handled for 12 days either immediately following weaning (W0) or 21 days after (W21), 8 were non-handled controls. During handling sessions, W0 were easier to handle than W21. During tests conducted two days and three, seven or ten months after the end of the handling period, W0 did not differ from W21 but both were easier and less reactive than controls. The period following weaning can therefore be qualified as an "optimal period" for handling. Furthermore, contrary to the first experiment, the effects persist at least ten months. Taken together, these results would lead to minimize the success of neonatal handling in favour of handling at weaning.

Theatre H1.5

Contribution to the improvement in horse Behaviour and Well being using Parelli Natural Horsemanship method

A. Booth, J.P. Vergnier and W. Kieffer, Haras de la Cense 78730 Rochefort en Yvelines, France.

To understand what is good for a horse, one must think like a horse. In other words one must lose the notion of oneself as predator and to take on the identity of the preyed upon.
The most important thing for a horse is survival -security- then comes the search for comfort and finally the search for a playmate. In essence these characteristics define the spirit of the herd.
Consideration of a horse's well being is more than just about tending to a horse's physical requirements, it is about understanding a horse's emotional and mental well being as well.
It is out of this philosophy that the 7 games of the Parelli Natural Horsemanship method were created. Haras de la Cense presents the 7 games in order to inspire the mental, physical and emotional stimuli necessary to the horse's well being as well as to promote a greater understanding of horse behaviour.

Theatre H1.6

Introduction of a behavioural test for Franches-Montagnes horses

D. Burger[1], L. Jallon[2], J.-C. Ionita[1], I. Imboden[1], M. Doherr[3] and P.-A. Poncet[1], [1]Swiss National Studfarm, 1580 Avenches, Switzerland, [2]Swiss Franches-Montagnes Breeding Association, 1580 Avenches, Switzerland, [3]Department for Clinical Veterinary Medicine, University of Bern, 3001 Bern, Switzerland*

Along with conformation, paces and performance of horses, their character and behaviour are of greatest importance. To better provide for the needs of the clients of the Franches-Montagnes breed - mostly amateur pleasure riders and drivers - routine official behaviour testing for these horses was introduced in 2001. The tests are carried out in conjunction with the breed association's field tests for three-year-old Franches-Montagnes and the annual 40-day station test for young approved stallions. The testing procedure involves three randomly allocated tests, one of each of four tests designed on the standing horse, three on the ridden horse and four on the driven horse. The horses' reactions are assessed and graded by previously instructed experts. Some of the tests closely resemble already existing, well-documented methods, that have been adapted to field conditions.
Test procedures, their sensitivity and repeatability as well as the first results obtained from tests on 1555 three-year-old and 52 graded Franches-Montagnes stallions, 20 Trotters, 20 Thoroughbreds, 20 Warmblood and 20 Arab horses are being described and analyzed. First experiences gathered on the introduction of a behavioural test on the occasion of a breeding selection program and the effects and consequences for the breeders and customers are being illustrated and discussed.

Theatre H1.7

24-hours ambulatory electrocardiography in athletic horse

F. Porciello[1], F. Birettoni[1], F. Rueca[1]. Dip. Patologia, Diagnostica e Clinica Veterinaria, Sez. Med. Int., Centro di Studio del Cavallo Sportivo, Università di Perugia, Italia.*

Several kinds of ECG abnormalities as well as some cardiac dysrhythmias, has been considered causes of poor performances in the athletic horses for a long time.
Some of these arrhythmias, as first and second degree AV blocks, are recognized to be associated with high vagal tone in the resting horse, and not with cardiac disease.
Atrial fibrillation, ventricular tachycardia and some bradyarrhythmias, can occur during horse's exercise, causing poor performances, syncope or sudden death. The standard ECG examination is universally used to assess cardiac rhythm but it shows several limitations mainly due to its brief time of recording. Holter examination improves ECG sensibility to cardiac arrhythmias.We communicate our method for Holter examination in the horse that we use to enhance our knowledge about cardiac rhythm either at rest or during physical activity, and to rule out cardiac dysrhythmias as cause of poor athletic performances. The exam lasts 24 hours and allows records of the heart rhythm in many different condition, from the physiological bradycardia of the resting hours to the high heart rate expected during the exercise. We also present the analysis of the recordings obtained from four horses referred to our examination with an history of poor athletic performances, or because an arrhythmia was found out during physical examination, and again because of a sudden collapse.

Theatre H1.8

The effects on behaviour of the presence or absence of a familiar horse during feeding

S.E. Redgate[1] N.K. Waran[1], H.P.B.Davidson[2] C. Morgan[3], [1]IERM, and [3]Animal Biology Division, University of Edinburgh SAC, West Mains Road, EH9 3JG UK, [2]Equine Studies Group, c/o WCPN, Leicestershire LE14 4RT UK,*

Increasing visual contact between stables improves awareness of conspecifics, which has been linked to a decrease in abnormal behaviour. There has, however, been limited investigation into the relationship between neighbouring stabled horses especially during potentially stressful periods such as meal times.
Seven adult riding horses of mixed breed were used; six acted as observers and one as a demonstrator. Three treatments were applied: (1) (stable): observer eating alone; (2) (arena): observer eating, demonstrator not eating; (3) (arena): observer and demonstrator eating. Horses were fed a standardised plain concentrate feed; behaviour was recorded using instantaneous sampling every 5 seconds for the 5-minute test period.
Individual differences existed in the amount of vigilant behaviour recorded; three horses showed more vigilant behaviour in the presence of another horse than when stabled alone. Conversely, the second three horses showed more vigilant behaviour in the stable. As vigilant behaviour increased time taken to consume the feed decreased. These trends suggest that sub groups may exist in the population.
The results have implications for stable design. For certain horses during competitive activities such as feeding, the close presence of another horse may be either beneficial or stressful. As this is only a preliminary investigation further research is advocated.

Theatre H2.1

Analysis of gene expression in endurance horses using cDNA-AFLP

A.Verini-Supplizi, K..Cappelli, M. Silvestrelli. Sport Horse Research Centre, University of Perugia, Via San Costanzo 4, 06126 Perugia, Italy.*

In endurance horses strenuous exercise would be associated with modifications of gene expression. The nature of change - up or down regulation - is dependent upon intensity and duration of the exercise, as well as prior exercise training. In athletic horses, exercise-induced suppression of the pulmonary and systemic immune responses has been reported. In the present study cDNA-AFLP technique was applied to two Arab horses to visualise variation of transcriptional profiles during a 160 Km European Endurance Riding Championships. Blood samples were collected just before the ride and 0, 24 and 48 hours after the competition. Peripheral blood mononuclear cells (PBMCs) were isolated. Standard procedures for RNA extraction and cDNA synthesis were employed and AFLP procedure was realised using 43 primer combinations. 51 gene fragments, differentially expressed were cloned and sequenced. BLASTN evidenced homology with genes known to be important in normal cell growth and metabolism. Two of these gene fragments, which resulted news for horse, were full-lenght cloned using RACE-PCR and included in GenBank database (Equus caballus interleukin 8 (IL8) mRNA, AY184956; Equus caballus retinoblastoma binding protein 6 mRNA, AY184957).

Theatre H2.2

Estimation of genetic parameters of Osteochondrosis in Hanoverian Warmblood foals

M. Schober, E. Bruns. Institute of Animal Breeding and Genetics, 37075 Göttingen, Germany*

Osteochondrosis (OC) is defined as a disturbance of enchondral ossification and is characterised by loose flaps of cartilage that may be present within the joint space which can cause a continous lameness in horses. OC is recognised as having a multifactorial aetiology; main causes are supposed to be found in rearing-conditions, nutrition, hormonal aberrations and genetic predisposition. As a part of an interdisciplinary research project, the aim of the present investigation was to estimate genetic parameters concerning the occurence of OC, based on a sample of 624 Warmblood foals reared on 80 german breeding farms. After radiographic examination at an age of at least 5 months, 32% of the tested foals revealed positive findings in fetlock and hock.The genetic analysis was carried out using REML techniques. The applied animal-model included influences of fixed parameters such as sex, time of birth, nutritional grade, body weight and locomotion. Heritabilities have been estimated for OC in fetlock (h^2 =.10 -.13 ±.09) and hock (h^2 =.06-.07 ± .04). Furthermore, phenotypic correlations between OC and performance traits, e.g. dressage, jumping and rideability, have been estimated based on both recent breeding values of stallions- and mares performance tests and competitions in 2002. Most of these correlations tend to be zero and are therefore regarded as statistically insignificant. The evaluation results revealed no indication for any relation between performance traits and the occurence of OC.

Theatre H2.3

Heritabilities of locomotor and physiological traits related to endurance and three day events exercise

E. Barrey, INRA Sation de génétique quantitative et appliquée, 78350 Jouy-en-Josas, France.

With the development of equine science, more functional traits has been studied to be used for early evaluation of horses. The chalenge is to predict the level of performance that a young horse can reached by measuring some of its physiological characteristics during a specific test. For a breeding purpose, the heritabilities of the traits should be determined to know if the measurements of these traits are useful for early genetic selection. The purpose of this paper was to give a review of heritabilities available of these locomotor and physiological traits realted to long exercise ability. During long exercise activity several systems are functionally linked to produce economical and efficient gaits. The energetic aspect of the locomotion is determined by the muscular fiber types, the level of fitness and the locomotion characteristics. The heritabilities of some variables related to long exercise ability were :
Percentage of slow and fast twich fibers in gluteus medius = 0.13 to 0.28; Cardiac capacity velocity at 200 beats/min=0.46; Anaerobic threshold velocity at 4 mmol of blood lactate=0.10; Trot variables=0.12 to 0.44; Canter variables=0.32 to 0.50 ; Jumping variables=0.23 to 0.52
The heritabilities of these traits were low to high and indicated that some of them could be used for early selection. However, the phenotypic and genetic correlation with the performance in endurance and three-day-event should be further investigated.

Theatre H2.4

Physiological responses to physical exercise in training trotters

A. Barone[1], S. Diverio[1], C. Federici[1], N. Falocci[2] and C. Pelliccia[1],* 1Dpt. Scienze Biopatologiche Veterinarie, Faculty of Veterinary Medicine, Perugia University, Via S. Costanzo 4, 06126 Perugia, Italy, 2Dpt. Scienze Statistiche, Faculty of Economy, Perugia University, Via Pascoli, 06100 Perugia, Italy

The experiment was carried out on November-December 2001, on a group of 8 trotters (6 males and 2 females), all housed and feed in similar condition. The animals were equally divided in two groups, according to their training state: Group NT (Not Trained) and Group T (Trained). Once a week, over a period of 6 weeks, all animals were subjected to a "standard" training (ST) (15 minutes): after a warm-up of 3 laps horses went at steady trot for 2 laps. Blood samples were taken by venipuncture at the jugular vein before training (T0), at the end of training (T1), and at 60 minutes (T2), 120 minutes (T3), and 24 hours (T4) after the end of the ST. At the same time heart rate (HR) and respiratory rate (RR) were recorded. Blood samples were assayed for packed cell volume (PCV), cortisol, muscular and hepatic enzymes, blood urea nitrogen (BUN) and glucose. Data were analysed by GLM for group, weeks and sampling time.
There were no significant differences for all parameters between Groups. Immediately after training (T1) significant increases of HR ($P<0,001$), RR ($P<0,001$), PCV ($P<0,001$) and cortisol ($P<0,001$), glucose ($P<0,05$), LDH ($P<0,01$), CK ($P<0,01$) concentrations were registered.

Theatre H2.5

Adrenocortical and thyroid responses to training in trotters

S. Diverio, A. Barone, C. Federici, and C. Pelliccia,* Dpt. Scienze Biopatologiche Veterinarie, Faculty of Veterinary Medicine, Perugia University, Via S. Costanzo 4, 06126 Perugia, Italy

Aim of the study was to assess the effect of the physical exercise on the adrenal cortex and thyroid responses in trotters. At this purpose, an experiment was carried out on November-December 2001, on a group of 8 trotters (6 males and 2 females), all housed and feed in similar condition. The animals were equally divided in two groups, according to their training state: Group NT (Not Trained) and Group T (Trained). Once a week, over a period of 6 weeks, all animals were subjected to a "standard" training (ST) (15 minutes): after a warm-up of 3 laps horses went at steady trot for 2 laps. Blood samples were taken by venipuncture at the jugular vein before training (T0), at the end of training (T1), and at 60 minutes (T2), 120 minutes (T3), and 24 hours (T4) after the end of the ST. Plasma were assayed for cortisol, triiodothyronine and thyroxine by radioimmunoassays. Data were analysed by GLM for group, week and sampling time.
No significant differences in plasmatic cortisol, triiodothyronine and thyroxine concentrations were found between the Groups. Adrenocortical and thyroid responses significantly raised ($P<0,001$) immediatly (T1), but cortisol levels maintained elevated up to T2, whereas thyroid hormones up to T3. All parameters returned to pre-training values (T0) within a 24 hours period (T4).

Theatre H2.6

Glycolipidic profile assessment in endurance riding horses

F. Rueca[1], M.B. Conti[1], M.C. Marchesi[1], F. Porciello[1], C. Pieramati[2]. [1]Dip. Patologia, Diagnostica e Clinica Veterinaria, [2]Centro Studio Cavallo Sportivo, Università di Perugia, Italia.*

While it is accepted that aerobic training increases capacity for fat oxidation during the exercise, there are few studies evaluating glycolipidic modifications during the training in endurance riding horses. In order to assess usefulness of serum biochemistry in determining the relative contribution of fat to energy production, 6 Arabian horses (speed class, 160 km) were studied all over the training. Horses performed a standardised exercise test on a high-speed treadmill, which consisted of 3 trials, one month apart each other. In each trial blood samples were collected prior to (T0), immediately after (T1), 2 hour after (T2) and 24 hour after (T3) the exercise in order to determine serum levels of glucose, cholesterol, triglicerids and lactate. According to the records achieved in the subsequent race season, horses were then divided into 2 groups: group A (successfully endurance raced-performers) and group B (unsuccessfully raced-performers). Lactate and cholesterol levels showed statistical differences ($p < 0.05$) as group A had lower levels than the other group. These results could be related to a more effective training schedule, as the lowest lactate levels had confirmed the enhanced metabolism of fatty acid when energy demands increase. However it could be also related to the lowest cholesterol concentration, as the serum levels of cholesterol decrease when β-oxidation of Acetyl Coenzyme A increases.

Theatre H2.7

Oxygen consumption measured in Arabians tested in a field endurance exercise test

E. Barrey[1], N. Metayer[1], A.G. Goachet[2], V. Julliand[2], J. Slawinski[3] and V. Billat[3], [1]INRA Station de génétique quantitative et appliquée, 78350 Jouy-en-Josas, [2]ENESAD, Dijon, [3]LIGE, Université d'Evry Val d'Essonne, France.

The running economy in endurance horses should be a major factor of the performance. The aim of this study was to measure the oxygen consumption in endurance horses running in the field at speed recorded in endurance races in order to estimate the running economy around the specific endurance competition speed (i.e. 20 $km.h^{-1}$). Five Arabians trained for endurance racing were tested ridden at increasing speed in the field. Their speed was measured and controlled by the rider by a GPS logger (Garmin 12). Each horse was equipped with a respiratory mask that measured the ventilation variables by two turbines and collected O_2 and CO_2 expired. A portable analyzer measured the respiratory variables breath- -by-breath ($K4b^2$, Cosmed) and recorded the heart rate (Polar 610). The quality of the measurements was carefully checked for the mask, the ventilation and gas variables. The mean VO2 (s.d.) results were:

- at the trot 13 and 15.5 km/h : 28 (3.6) and 36 (5.4) ml/min/kg
- at the canter 18.7, 25,2 km/h: 42 (8.6) and 50 (3.3) ml/min/kg
- at the gallop 33.5, 36, 39.6 and 43.2: 60 (4.9), 63 (4.2), 71 (5.6) and 85 (4.6) ml/min/kg

The rate of respiratory ratio increased from 0.89 (0.1) at slow trot to 1.21 (0.1) at the fastest gallop. These respiratory results were in accordance with the previous results obtained in treadmill exercise. This portable respiratory analyzer allows to measure in the field the energy expenditure during moderate exercise.

Theatre H2.8

Effect of locomotion on the development of Osteochondrosis (OC) in Hanoverian warmblood foals

A. Wilke and E. Bruns, Institut of Animal Breeding and Genetics, Georg-August-University Göttingen, Albrecht-Thaer-Weg 3, 37083 Göttingen, Germany*

Osteochondrosis (OC) is a cartilage disease which is characterised by flaps or loose bodies. It is part of the "Developmental Orthopaedic Diseases" which describe a complex of skeletal problems associated with growth and development in the foal. The frequency of OC is up to a quarter in different Warmblood breeds. Affected foals have a higher risk for locomotion problems later on. The present study is based on a sample of 624 Warmblood foals reared under regular farm conditions which were monthly visited for half a year. The radiographic findings show 32 % of the foals being OC-positive. The time of birth affects the frequency of OC significantly. Early born foals are more frequently affected (+ 10 %) than late born foals. Because feeding management shows no significant effect, the main seasonal factor seems to be related to locomotion (free exercise) of the foals. Foals with very little locomotion (less than four hours per day) within their first months of life show highest incidences of OC. Therefore, current foal management under regular farm conditions has to be reviewed.

Theatre H2.9

Relationships between locomotor test and racing performances in Standardbreds

C. Leleu[1], C. Cotrel[1] and E. Barrey[2], [1] Pégase Mayenne, Département de médecine du Sport, Centre Hospitalier, 53 000 Laval, France, [2] INRA, Station de génétique quantitative et appliquée, 78 352 Jouy en Josas, France*

Few information are available about gait characteristics and level of performance in harness race horses. The aim of that cross-sectionnal experiment was to study the relationships between some locomotor variables measured during a standardized exercise test and the level of performance of Standardbred racehorses. A total of 104 horses from 3 to 7 year-old performed a 4 step-locomotor test on the track with an accelerometric device : Equimétrix TM. The population was divided into 2 groups on the basis of their official performance index based on earnings (ITR) : an elite performers group (n=52) and a medium performers group (n=52). The locomotor variables (stride, stance, braking and propulsion durations, stride length, symmetry, regularity, dorso-ventral, longitudinal and lateral activities) were calculated at 4 different speeds. The results were compared between the 2 performance-groups by an analysis of variance. Elite performers presented significantly higher stride frequency, longer stance and propulsion durations at submaximal speed ($p<0.05$). There was no significant difference between the 2 groups for braking duration, symmetry, regularity, dorso-ventral, longitudinal and lateral activities. In conclusion, some locomotor characteristics of Standardbred racehorses were significantly related to the racing performance and could be useful to identify gait efficiency in harness racehorses.

Theatre H2.10

Study of locomotion and conformation in the endurance horse

N. Métayer[1], S. Biau[2], J-L. Cochet[2] and E. Barrey[1], [1]INRA SGQA, 78350 Jouy-en-Josas, France, [2]ENE, 49411 Saumur Cedex, France.*

To identify specific locomotor and conformation attributes of endurance horses, accelerometric and photometric measurements were made (Equimetrix system, INRA) on 35 adult horses. The test group consisted of 27 endurance horses (16 national level and 11 pre-national level) and 8 horses without any experience in this discipline.

An accelerometric device fixed to the girth of the saddle against the sternum measured the dorsoventral and longitudinal acceleration of the running horse. The tests were made on a track at two different speeds: trot at 13 km/h and gallop at 18 km/h. To evaluate their conformation, digital photographs of lengths and angles were taken of points marked on the main articulations. The statistical study (variance analysis: GLM and discriminant analysis) made possible the characterization of gaits and conformation of the endurance horse. Correlation between conformation and gaits was also analyzed.

The endurance horse was a small, thin type with a short, hollow back. He had an inclined pelvis, open haunch and closed hock.

The endurance horse, which had a quicker cadence at the trot than a non qualified horse ($p<0.05$), had a shuffling gait. The horse which specialized in endurance had quicker galloping strides and shorter amplitude than a non qualified horse ($p<0.05$). It also had better longitudinal propulsion at the gallop ($p<0.01$).

Primary standards characterizing the locomotion of endurance horses were established.

Theatre H2.11

Influence of long distance ride conditions on the results

S. Pietrzak and P. Bereznowska, Agricultural University, Faculty of Biology and Animal Breeding, Akademicka 13 Str., 20-950 Lublin, Poland.

The primary problem concerned with preparing the horse to start in rides is long lasting exertion, which has to be shared, taking into consideration the speed and time of passing the succesive parts of the distance.
The results achieved during the events are final position as well as speed and marks pointed in veterinary cards. They depend to certain degree on the conditions defined by the riding rules (length of the distance, minimal speed) and also from additional conditions like the formation of area, quality of the ground and the weather.
The research involved 367 horses, which took part in national and international competitions from 2000 to 2002 (16 and 3 events, respectively).
The detailed analyse of 59 trekking routes (total length 4042 km) was carried out. Besides, the soil consistency measured with the striking probe and profile of routes with topography maps, were analysed. Considerable variability of ground quality was stated (from 3.47-17.11). The interdependence between ground quality indices and round speed was negative and statistically significant (r= -0.51). Significant influence of route configuration on horse physiological parameters was also defined.

Theatre H2.12

Repeatability of the horse's jumping parameters with and without the rider

D. Lewczuk, K. Sloniewski, Z. Reklewski, Institute of Genetics and Animal Breeding Jastrzebiec, 05-552 Wólka Kossowska, Poland*

The total number of 4323 jumps of 143 young stallions were filmed and measured using video image analysis. Horses were filmed during their usual work in the 8th, 9th and 10th month of training at the stallion's performance test station. The investigations were hold on the doublebarre fence (100, 110 and 120cm) with the same wide of 80cm. The repeatability of the jump's parameters were calculated as ratio of animal effect variance to the sum of all random variances received from the model included statistically significant fixed effects and regressions on the frame of horses. All analyses were done using SAS procedure MIXED. The jump's parameters were analysed as different traits for free jumping and jumping under the rider. The style of jump was characterised by measurements of taking off and landing distances, measurements of lifting horse's body over the obstacle and measurements of legs' lifting above the obstacle. The repeatability of distances of the jump's length were 0,40 - 0,58. Similiar repeatabilities were estimated for the bascule's measurements (from 0,37 to 0,56). The lowest repeatabilities (about 0,2) were received for the heights of legs' lifting above the fence. Traits measured under the rider were more repeatable then for three jumping. For most parameters the repeatability of the measurements were higher for fence of 120cm then for the lowest one.

Theatre H2.13

Horse and rider interactions during jumping

G. Giovagnoli[1]; M. Reitano[2]; M. Silvestrelli[3]. [1]Federazione Italiana Sport Equestri, Dipartimento Veterinario, Viale Tiziano, 74, 00196 Roma , Italy. [2]Raggruppamento addestrativo RSTA, Centro Militare di Equitazione, Montelibretti, 00010 Roma, Italy. [3]Centro di Studio del Cavallo Sportivo - Università di Perugia, Perugia, 06100 Italy.*

There are not information on horse and rider muscular interactions during jumping, although such of information can be crucial to be acquainted with their reciprocal influence during that specific athletic movement. EMG signals and video-synchronized images from a single horse and rider were collected by exploring biceps brachii and flexor carpi radialis from rider's left side muscles and from masseter, splenius and sternomandibularis horse's left side muscles. The highest jump was120 centimetres and was repeated four times.

Results show that the splenius activity is comparable to those reported in literature in not mounted horses. Sternomandibularis activity shows a single burst lasting all ending take-off phase. Masseter and sternomandibularis muscles are synchronous with the rider's biceps brachii in the take-off phase. The flexor carpi radialis of the riders is recruited immediately before and after biceps brachii. From first to fourth jump the rider's muscles activities seems to decrease progressively in intensity; whereas horse's muscles still recruited at the same intensity.

This sternomandibularis activation lets to suppose a complex function from both biomechanic and neurological points of view. The rider's muscles activity seems to be involved to control the speed and thus, indirectly, the balance between horizontal and vertical vectors.

Poster H2.14

Parametrès génétiques du rendement des allures des étalons demi-sang

M. Kapron, I. Janczarek, B. Kapron, E. Czerniak, Chaire d'Elevage et d'Utilisation des Chevaux, Académie d'Agriculture, ul. Akademicka 13, 20950 Lublin, Pologne.*

180 étalons demi-sang ont été soumis aux triples contrôles du rendement des allures: au pas, au trot et au galop (trois tours dans chaque allure) - entraînnés dans « le test de 100 jours ». On mésuraient la longueur des allures en se servant de la bande (avec de l'exactitude jusqu'à 0,01 m) - individuelement pour chaque démarche des différents étalons.

On a détérminé le haut niveau de l'héritabilité de la longueur des allures (pas - h^2 = 0,657; trot = 0,631; galop = 0,455) et de l'index d`allures (longueur d`allure: hauteur au garrot x 100; pas = 0,653; trot = 0,619; galop = 0,498). En outre on a détérminé encore plus haut niveau de la répétabilité des indicateurs motoriques: longueur d`allure (pas - $r^2$ = 0,863; trot = 0,818; galop = 0,728); l'index d`allure (pas = 0,861; trot = 0,812; galop = 0,719). Les corrélations génétiques entre les indicateurs de mouvement se renfermaient entre les limites: de 0,522 jusqu'à 0,977; et les phénotipiques: de 0,263 jusqu'à 0,966.

Poster H2.15

Effect of confinement in a stationary vehicle on haematological and functional values of horses

F. Cusumano, P. Medica, E. Fazio, V. Aronica, A. Ferlazzo. Department of Morphology, Biochemistry, Physiology and Animal Production, Unit of Physiology, Polo Universitario Annunziata, 98168 Messina, Italy.

Aim of the study was to provide informations concerning of the haematological and functional values of horses before and after confinement in a stationary vehicle.The study was carried on 12 healthy stallions, aged between 5 and 19 years, of different race, submitted to confinement for 3 hours.Blood samples were collected from jugular vein before (09.00 a.m.) and after the 1st, 2nd and 3rd hour of confinement and after 24 hours.To determine the effect of confinement an analysis of variance (ANOVA) for repeated measures was applied. To compare post-confinement to basal values the paired t-test was applied. Per cent differences (Δ%) were calculated. Significative increases of RBC (+17.09%; $p<0.02$), HGB (+15.09%; $p<0.05$) and HCT (+16.04%; $p<0.05$) after the 1st and after 3rd hour of confinement respectively (+13.0%; $p<0.05$), (+13.4%; $p<0.05$) and (+13.9%; $p<0.05$) as compared to basal values were detected. No significative differences were found regarding PLT, WBC, MCH and MCV values as compared to basal. Haematological values generally were superimposed to basal values after 24 hour. ANOVA for repeated measured showed a significant effect of confinement on rectal temperature ($F=28$; $P<0.001$) and heart rate ($F=6.71$; $P<0.05$). Data obtained showed that haematological and functional variables can be used as measures of welfare during confinement of horses. It is concluded that confinement is inevitably associated with a stress response.

Poster H2.16

Neuroendocrine adaptations to confinement in a stationary vehicle and to road transport stress of horses

F. Cusumano, E. Fazio, P. Medica, L. Grasso[1], A. Ferlazzo. Department of Morphology, Biochemistry, Physiology and Animal Production, Unit of Physiology, Polo Universitario Annunziata, 98168 Messina, Italy, [1]Laboratorio Centralizzato Policlinico Universitario, Messina, Italy.

The aim of this study was to evaluate the circulating β-endorphin, ACTH and cortisol response during confinement and after road transport of horses. The study was carried out on 12 healthy stallions submitted to confinement for 3 hours and then, two weeks later transported by truck on roads of short (<50 km), middle (50-150 km) and long (>150 km) distance. Blood samples were taken before (09.00 a.m.) and after the 1st 2nd and 3rd of confinement and after 24 hours and after transport. Circulating β-endorphin and cortisol levels showed higher concentrations after transport than after confinement. Statistical analysis showed a significant increase of β-endorphin after short ($p<0.05$) and long ($p<0.02$) distance as compared to post confinement after the 1st and 3rd hour. Cortisol level increased significantly after middle ($p<0.05$) distance as compared to 2nd hour of confinement. ANOVA for repeated measures showed a significantly effect of confinement on plasma β-endorphin ($F=8.35$; $p<0.01$) and of transport on serum cortisol ($F= 33.92$; $p<0.01$) concentrations. On the contrary, serum ACTH concentrations generally decreased after transport of different lengths as compared to the 1st , 2nd and 3rd hour of confinement. The results obtained confirm that transport stress influences the opioid system and adrenocortical function in horses and showed that confinement and transport induce a univocal response of β-endorphin and cortisol probably induced by permissive effects of β-endorphin on the adrenocortical secretions.

Poster H2.17

Plasma β-endorphin and cortisol variations in training trotters

S. Diverio[1], A. Barone[1], C. Federici[1], N. Falocci[2] and C. Pelliccia[1] , [1].Dpt. Scienze Biopatologiche Veterinarie, Faculty of Veterinary Medicine, Perugia University, Via S. Costanzo 4, 06126 Perugia, Italy, [2]Dpt. Scienze Statistiche, Faculty of Economy, Perugia University, Via Pascoli, 06100 Perugia, Italy*

Aim of the study was to assess the effect of the physical exercise on the adrenal cortex and endogenous oppioid responses in trotters. The experiment was carried out on November-December 2001, on a group of 4 trotters (2 males and 2 females), after the beginning of their annual training period. Once a week, over a period of 6 weeks, the 4 animals were subjected to a "standard" training (ST) (15 minutes): after a warm-up of 3 laps horses went at steady trot for 2 laps. Blood samples were taken by venipuncture at the jugular vein before training (T0), at the end of training (T1), and at 60 minutes (T2), 120 minutes (T3), and 24 hours (T4) after the end of the ST.

Plasma were assayed for cortisol and β-endorphin by radioimmunoassays. Data were analysed by GLM for group, week and sampling time.

There were no significant differences in cortisol and β-endorphin plasma concentrations between Groups. Plasmatic cortisol and β-endorphin concentrations significantly increased ($P<0,001$) immediatly after the standard training (T1), but only plasmatic cortisol levels remained elevated up to T2. After 24 hours the end of training (T4), both parameters presented values similar to those recorded as pre-training (T0).

Poster H2.18

Adrenal testosterone, progesterone and cortisol responses to physical excercise in training trotters

A. Barone, S. Diverio, C. Federici, and C. Pelliccia, Dpt. Scienze Biopatologiche Veterinarie, Faculty of Veterinary Medicine, Perugia University, Via S. Costanzo 4, 06126 Perugia, Italy*

Aim of the study was to assess the effect of training on the adrenal secretion of sexual hormones in trotters.

The experiment was carried out on November-Dicember 2001, on a group of 8 trotters (4 males and 4 females), all housed and feed in similar condition. Once a week, over a period of 6 weeks, all animals were subjected to a "standard" training (ST) (15 minutes): after a warm-up of 3 laps horses went at steady trot for 2 laps. Blood samples were taken by venipuncture at the jugular vein before training (T0), at the end of training (T1), and at 60 minutes (T2), 120 minutes (T3), and 24 hours (T4) after the end of the ST.

Plasma were assayed for cortisol, testosterone (only on females) and progesterone (only on males) by radioimmunoassays.

Significant increases of cortisol ($P<0,001$) and testosterone ($P<0,05$) immediatly after standard training (T1) were recorded. A similar trend was also observed for plasmatic progesterone levels, but differences among sampling times were not significant.

All plasma parameter levels returned to pre-training values (T0) after 24 hours the end of the standard training (T4).

Poster H2.19

Judges preferences in jumping style evaluation

D. Lewczuk, Institute of Genetics and Animal Breeding Jastrzebiec, 05-552 Wólka Kossowska, Poland*

The study was conducted on the group of 21 young stallions during 100 days performance test at the training station. Three qualified independent judges were asked to give notes for jumping style simulatelously while free jumping were filmed. Sixty-nine jumps were analysed by video image analyses. The style of jump was described by: measurements of taking off and landing distances, measurements of positions of the head, withers, croup during the bascule and height of leg's lifting over the obstacle. The partial correlations between measurements and judges' notes were calculated using SAS procedure GLM. The correlations were adjusted for height of the fence and successive number of the jump. The correlations between investigated parameters and notes of judges were 0,2 - 0,43. The measurements of body position and lifting over the obstacle were significantly correlated with the average note of judges. The correlations between individual notes of every judge and jumps parameters were also calculated. In some causes correlations for individual notes differed between jugdes. Two of judges payed more attention for the work of hind legs and length measurements of the jump. Third judge looked much more carefully for the work of the head during the bascule of the horse. All of them take a lot attention to the position of the withers and croup during the bascule of the horse.

Poster H2.20

Analysis of untrained colt's jumping parameters - preliminary study

D. Lewczuk, Z. Reklewski, Institute of Genetics and Animal Breeding Jastrzebiec, 05-552 Wólka Kossowska, Poland*

Free jumping of ten one-year-old colts was filmed twice with the interval of three months. During every trial horses jumped 2-3 times trough two different heights of the doublebarre (50 and 70cm) and 60cm wide. A hundred jumps were measured using video image analysis. The jumping style was described as measurements of taking off and landing distance, measurements of positions of the head, withers and croup above the obstacle (bascule) and measurements of legs' lifting over the obstacle. The data was analysed using SAS procedures. The three-month break was statistically significant for measurements of bascule positions, landing distance and front legs' lifting above the fence. In the second trial horses carried their body and front legs higher then in first one. The lifting of the hind legs was not influenced by the trial. In the second trial longer jumps were observed, in case of landing about 30cm father. The measurements made on successive number of the jump were different only for leg's lifting. With every successive jump lifting of the legs were lower. The height of the fence influenced only the landing distance. Horses landed about 30cm closer on the second height of the fence. Investigations are carried on.

Poster H2.21

Dorsal muscular activities during the horse jumping

G. Giovagnoli[1]; M. Reitano[2]; M. Silvestrelli[3]. [1]Federazione Italiana Sport Equestri, Dipartimento Veterinario, Viale Tiziano, 74, 00196 Roma , Italy. [2]Raggruppamento addestrativo RSTA, Centro Militare di Equitazione, Montelibretti, 00010 Roma, Italy. [3]Centro di Studio del Cavallo Sportivo - Università di Perugia, Perugia, 06100 Italy.*

Scarce information exists on muscles activities during jumping, although such information should be a prerequisite for pertinent training programmes. EMG muscles activities (synchronised with video-tape images) of Splenius, Longissimus Thoracis and Middle Gluteus from both sides (right and left) were recorded from six adult warmblood horses during jumping in circle on sand by lungeing rein. The highest jump was120 centimetres.
Results allow to recognise a general trend of the EMG patterns: 1) the muscles activity seems to be generally synchronous between right and left sides; 2) the Splenius muscles work before the others in take-off and landing phases; 3) the Longissimus thoracis recruitment, during the take-off, starts immediately after the Splenius recruitment and it is substantially synchronous with Middle Gluteus, even if it prolongs its action until landing when the horse flexes its hind leg to prepare next gallop step; 4) the Middle gluteus recruitment does not begin immediately after hind limbs touch ground during take-off phase, but seems to start approximately only when hock's perpendicular line overtakes the buttock's perpendicular line.
These results show a clear pattern in the muscular sequence of recruitment to optimise and coordinate the dorsal muscular chain during jumping.

Poster H2.22

Movement analysis as a basis for selection of traditional Gidran horse breed

S. Jónás[1], S. Mihók[2], Z. Gyürki[1], K. Altmár[1], I. Bodó[2] [1]Pannon Riding Academy H-7018 Kaposvár, Maróczpuszta, [2]Debreceni Egyetem H-4032 Debrecen Böszörményi út 138*

The Gidran is one of traditional horse breeds of Hungary. The breed, - although it is an endangered rare one - permanently produced succesful horses at international competitions. Its genetic value is, however, the isolation, the differentiation from international common gene basis of high performance sport horses.
The breeding goal of Gidran breeders is the selection for performance and simultaneously to maintain the original breed character and pedigree.
For accomplishing this aim and criteria the pretraining of foals and movement analysis by video technics were amalgamated in a system.
The recent research started 7 years ago in Maróczpuszta stud, testing 1.5, 2.5, and 3.5 year old Gidran fillies. The basic gaits, the willingness and ability for jumping and character were analysed by SELECTOR 1. video and PC program.There are 3 trials a year, 21 days each and later the tested foals are involved in show jumping and eventing.
The earliest day for effective estimation of quality and talent of fillies, the possible development of manifestation of inherited traits by permanent training, the advantage of pretraining in later results in sports and the applicability of the system for an effective preselection were analysed in order to to develop the sporting ability not neglecting the traditional breed character of Gidrans at the same time.

Poster H2.23

Influence of elettrolyte integration with diet on trotter horses' fitness

A. Falaschini[1], G. Marangoni[1] and M.F. Trombetta[2], [1]DIMORFIPA, Via Tolara di Sopra, 50, 40064 Ozzano Emilia, Bologna, Italy, [2] DIBIAGA, Via Brecce Bianche, 60131 Ancona, Italy.

Thermoregulation in athlete horses principally relies on perspiration. The resultant loss of large amounts of salts and water may create an imbalance and affect the subject's well-being, and performances.

To evaluate the effect of dietary supplementation of salts (Na^+, K^+, Cl^-) and Vitamins (C, E) four trotter horses were monitored during tests simulating a race. *Test 1* (day 1): subjects received the control diet; *Test 2* (day 6): subjects received the same complete feed supplemented with a commercial electrolyte beginning on day 5; *Test 3* (day 16): subjects had been receiving the supplement for 12 days.On test days, subjects were weighed at rest, immediately after the race, and at 24 h. Blood was collected at rest, 1 min, 20 min and 24 h after each test to determine pH, Hmt, Hb, GPx, PT, AST, LDH, PAO, electrolytes and lactic acid. Systematic administration of the dietary supplement allowed better recovery of weight loss in the first 24 h. The trend of blood parameters indicated a better overall condition of the horses and less oxidative stress in the subjects who had been receiving the supplement longer (12d *vs* 1d). The greater amount of available electrolytes and the stronger protection from stress provided by systematic dietary supplementation reflected favourably on the subjects' physical condition.

Theatre H4.1

Potential utilisation of Yugoslav Mountain Pony in Eco tourism in Natural reserves of Serbia and Montenegro

*R .Trailovic, *M. Savic, S. Jovanovic, Faculty of Veterinary Medicine, Belgrade, Bulevar JA 18, Serbia and Montenegro*

Yugoslav mountain pony is autochthonous horse breed developed on high mountain slopes in Serbia and Montenegro. This sturdy animal is exceptionally adapted to terrain, which is reflected in leg conformation.

Some animals within separate location have been rejected by humans and submitted to natural selection by predators. There is no contemporary interest in breeding of these horses, but their adaptability and resistance gave interest to evaluation of some isolated populations. Some preliminary test of biochemical polymorphism revealed extensive variability of this horse.

Having in mind that this horse was evolutively adopted to harsh climate and poor nutrition it can be used for transport of tourists in natural reserves like Kopaonik, Golija, etc. The only interest in organized breeding is through utilization of Yugoslav mountain pony in hunting tourism and eco-tourism and effects on landscape conservation in natural reserves. The grazing ponies on high mountain pasture are picturesque and give aesthetic grace to pastoral atmosphere of natural reserves in Serbia and Montenegro.

Theatre H4.2

Characterisation of the Irish Draught Horse population in Ireland

H. O'Toole[1], L.I. Aldridge[1], P.O. Brophy[2], D.L. Kelleher[2], K. Quinn[2], [1]Irish Horse Board, Block B, Maynooth Business Campus, Maynooth, Co Kildare, Ireland, [2]Dept of Animal Science and Production, Faculty of Agriculture, University College Dublin, Belfield, Dublin, Ireland.*

The Irish Draught Horse has historically been an intrinsic component in the production of farm horses and hunters in Ireland and in more recent times in the production of the modern Irish Sport Horse. Despite this important role, population numbers have been in decline in recent years and the breed is currently categorised as endangered. The objective of this project was to evaluate how falling population numbers and past breeding practices have affected the genetic composition and diversity of a reference population of 1,317 Irish Draught Horses born between 1997 and 2000 inclusive. A data set containing 16,310 records was analysed using *Pedig* (Boichard 2001). Population numbers continued to decline e.g. 804 Irish Draught mares produced foals in 1997 and 727 in 2000. Mean inbreeding coefficient was found to be low (0.86%). Overall, 17 ancestors contributed 50% of the genes to the reference population, indicating an unbalanced contribution from ancestors. The results show that the Irish Draught Horse population is at risk of losing more of its genetic diversity and should therefore be managed as a rare genetic resource.

Theatre H4.3

On breeding value of horses in Estonia

H. Peterson, Institute of Animal Science, Estonian Agricultural University, Fr.R. Kreutzwaldi 1, 51014 Tartu, Estonia

There are three local horse breeds and Trakehner, Hannover and other breeds in Estonia, but the objective of the study has been mostly the determination of breeding value of Estonian Native Horses and Tori Horse (expressed by indexes).
The study is based on the results of the 88 tests by Toric and 99 tests of the Estonian Native Horse, carried out by the Estonian Horse Breeders Society in 1995-2002. Most important qualities were investigated: general index of stallions, indexes of type, body, feet, pace, trot and free jumping. The best general indexes had the Estonian Native Horses, as the excellent state of feet of this breed guarantees their good pace and free jump qualities. The 6 years' average general index was 100.81, which dropped to 96.75 in 2002, as the Estonian Native Estimation Commission was too principal last year.
As regards Toric, the best indexes got stallions Premium and Hermelin (both born in Germany in 1989.) Four years' average was 98.59 by Toric, but last year it was 96.75. Number of tests with various sport horses has been rather small and their general indexes have been rather low.

Theatre H4.4

National genetic evaluation for horses in Germany

J. Jaitner and F. Reinhardt, United Data Systems for Animal Production (VIT), Heideweg 1, D-27283 Verden, Germany.*

On behalf of the German Equestrian Federation (FN) a new evaluation system was developed and introduced in 2001. The annual evaluation applies a BLUP multitrait repeatability animal model, combining data of horses being active in sport as well as information from own performance tests being conducted by breeding associations. 15 traits, describing performances of national sport and breeding events, are used simultaneously to estimate the genetic disposition of horses for jumping and dressage. With regard to sport events, all starts in competitions from 1995 onwards are considered, distinguishing show jumping and dressage competitions and in addition jumping and dressage competitions of young horses. The traits are the achieved rank, which is transformed, and the score (1-10), respectively. With regard to breeding events, the scores (1-10) for walk, trot, canter, rideability and free jumping, in addition for stallions also parcours jumping, being recorded during mare and stallion performance tests, are taken into account from 1986 onwards. For all horses having own performance at least two generations of ancestors are considered, if available. All breeding values are standardised to a genetic standard deviation of 20 points, all stallions being born from 1987-1991 and having passed a stallion's own performance test or having least 5 offspring, have on an average a breeding value of 100 points. Publication of breeding values depends on accuracy and number of offspring. The evaluation 2002 covered in total about 390,000 horses, out of which about 250,000 horses had altogether about 6.5 Mio. observations.

Theatre H4.5

Genetic evaluation of competition results of Dutch harness horses

E.P.C. Koenen[1], R.M.G. Roelofs[1] and J.M.F.M. van Tartwijk[2], [1]NRS, P.O. Box 454, 6800 AL Arnhem, The Netherlands, [2]Royal Dutch Warmblood Studbook, P.O. Box 382, 3700 AJ Zeist, The Netherlands.*

The breeding population of the Dutch harness horse includes 35 stallions and 1450 mares that are mainly selected for performance in driving competitions. The aim of this study was to analyse the suitability of competition data including earnings (high ranked horses only) and ranks (all started horses) for a genetic evaluation. The data included 26,160 earnings of 1529 horses (period 1983-1996) and 21,584 ranks of 1214 horses (period 1997-2002). These data were recorded at 3119 competitions. To improve normality, a logarithmic transformation (earnings) and a Blom-score transformation (ranks) were applied. Genetic parameters of transformed observations were estimated using a bivariate animal model including the fixed effects of competition, age*sex and the random permanent environment and genetic animal effect. The pedigree file included 8928 horses. Performance results improved by age. Stallions performed better than geldings and mares, especially at higher ages. Repeatability estimates were 0.30 for earnings and 0.54 for ranks. Heritability estimates were 0.10 for earnings and 0.23 for ranks. High correlations between earnings and ranks were found for the permanent environment effect ($r = 0.54$) and the genetic effect ($r = 1.00$). It was recommended to base a genetic evaluation for competition performance of harness horses on ranks, as these data have a higher heritability and are available at a higher frequency.

Theatre H4.6

Some factors affecting numerical productivity in French type horse breeding

B. Langlois and C. Blouin, Station de Génétique quantitative et appliquée, INRA-CRJ, 78352 Jouy-en-Josas cedex, France

195485 declarations of matings from 1989 to 1999 and 108583 consecutive declarations of birth were analysed by logistic regressions in order to determine the effects of year, breed, age of parents and status of the mare on the numerical productivity (Number of foals declared per mated mare per year). For the years 1994 to 1999, the Type of mating and month of first mating were also available. The effect of inbreeding and, for warm blooded horses, the effect of the level of performances or the effect of the level of breeding value estimation were also analysed.
The main results are the following :
- Numerical productivity is progressing in France more for draft breeds than for saddle breeds and trotters. Thoroughbreds are progressing less and just reach the level of significance.
- However Cold-blooded horse appeared less productive than warm blooded horse for which thoroughbreds were at the lower level. It cannot be concluded if this figure reveals biological differences in fertility or if it is only the result of differences in managing the official declarations.
- For Warm blooded horses, the absence of negative relationships between the trends of selection and numerical productivity results clearly appeared. A high performance level for the mare was positively associated with higher productivity results in sport and trotting and showed no significant influence for galloping. Relationships with breeding value estimation illustrated the same trends.

Theatre H4.7

Orthopaedic disease: effect of diet and stallion

S. Nannarone, C. Cavallucci, G. Macolino, M. Pepe, M. Bonanzinga. Sport Horse Research Center, University of Perugia, Via San Costanzo 4, 06126 Perugia, Italy.*

The aim of the research was to study the relationship among the ortophaedic disease (MOS) of Maremmano yearlings with their metabolic condition and stallion.
Foals fed with different copper integration of concentrate were divided in two groups (C and T). These foals were born by mares fed with same concentrates. At weaning and twelve months old, blood samples from the jugular vein have been collected for the determination of the metabolic profile.
Metabolic parameters (Ca, P, Mg, Fe, Cu, Zn, and Ceruloplasmin) were significantly influenced by integration and stallion ($p > 0,001$). .The stallion were licensed by the 100 day Station test
The six month old foals were examined for clinical status (physitis, angular and flexural limb deformities, wobbler syndrome) and at twelve month old they underwent radiographic evaluation (hock joint and stifle joint) for diagnosis of osteochondrosis.

Theatre H4.8

Variation of mare milk nitrogen fractions: distribution of the main whey-proteins in relation to lactation stage

A. Summer[*1], A. Tirelli[2], P. Formaggioni[1], F. Martuzzi[1], P. Mariani[1]. [1]Dip. PABVQSA, Università degli Studi, via del Taglio 8, I-43100 Parma, Italy. [2]DISTAM, Università degli Studi, via Celoria 2, 20133 Milano, Italy*

The aim was to study nitrogen fraction variations and whey-proteins distribution in relation to lactation stage in milk of Haflinger nursing mares, 7÷15 years old (4÷12 parities), 400÷540 kg live weight, fed mixed hay *ad libitum*. Samples were collected by hand-milking at d 4, 20, 40, 60, 80, 120, 150 and 180 *post-partum*. Nitrogen fractions were determined by Kjeldahl on 80 samples from 10 mares, as HPLC separation of whey-proteins regarded 40 samples from 5 mares. Data were analysed by ANOVA. Data were grouped in three lactation periods (4÷40 early, E; 60÷120 mid, M; 150÷180 late, L; days). Milk produced in the last two periods contained significantly less nitrogen compared to milk produced in early lactation. In particular (mg/100g): true protein N (330.2E *vs* 243.0M and 233.6L); casein N (189.5E *vs* 135.8M and 129.5L); non protein N (33.4E *vs* 29.3M and 29.2L). True whey-protein N decreased throughout lactation (140.7E *vs* 107.2M and 104.3L; mg/100g) and in the same way also its components (mg/100g): β-lactoglobulin+α-lactalbumin (107.3E *vs* 80.5M and 79.0L) and serum albumin+immunoglobulins (37.7E *vs* 25.6M and 25.1L). Whey-proteins percentage distribution on total whey-proteins was: β-lactoglobulin 45.20E, 46.29M, 47.04L; α-lactalbumin 29.22E, 29.49M, 28.47L; serum albumin 8.04E, 7.81M, 7.83L; immunoglobulins 17.54E, 16.41M, 16.66L.

Theatre H4.9

Diet selection by horses on paddocks with four different sward heights

A. Naujeck[1], J. Hill[1] and M.J. Gibb[2], [1]Faculty of Applied Science and Technology, Writtle College, UK, [2]Institute of Grassland and Environmental Research, North Wyke, Devon, UK*

Seven heterogeneous paddocks of perennial ryegrass pasture were created by mowing sixteen 4x4 m square patches. Patches were cut to four different sward heights (3.6, 5.3, 8.3 and 15.5 cm), replicated 4 times. Sward height and biomass were determined. For one hour, one horse (7 horses in total) was allowed to graze within a paddock. The number of visits, residence time and behaviour on a patch were recorded. After one week of re-growth, the same paddocks were used again. The experiment was repeated, but without mowing the pasture and with six horses, only.

In the first period of the study, patches differed in sward height and biomass, whereas in the second period, the re-growth of the sward reduced differences in grass height between patches. There was no significant difference in the number of visits per patch for most horses in either period. While foraging, residence time was longer on tall swards (taller than 8 cm) than on short ones. As tall swards allowed a greater short-term intake rate than short patches, it is suggested that the horses were maximizing their intake rate per unit time grazing. In order to maintain the highest possible energy intake, an animal has to sample the environment continuously, which may explain the movements of the horses between the patches.

Poster H4.10

The effect of Foot and Mouth Disease on eventing participation within the UK during 2001

T.C. Whitaker, R. Harris, P. Wallace C.L. Whitaker and J. Hill. Writtle College, Chelmsford, Essex CM1 3RR*

The discovery of an outbreak of foot and mouth disease in February 2001 had a devastating impact on UK agriculture; ancillary activities relying on the use of agricultural land were dramatically affected. British Eventing completely suspended its calendar of events between March and June 2001 in total 47% of all events were cancelled.

A survey was conducted amongst event competitors to quantify the effect of foot and mouth had upon their participation in the sport. A total of 76% of competitors stated they had performed at fewer events during 2001. Increased balloting (returning of entries based on over subscription to events) was reported by 41%. A failure to qualify for the next level of competition through limited opportunities to compete affected 35% of respondents. Of the 22% of competitors that reported they had some form of sponsorship deal, 20% had lost sponsorship as a direct result of foot and mouth.

In total 46% of respondents reported that they had suffered an extra cost burden. Furthermore 26% competitors who had event horses stated they had had to reduce the working hours of their staff as a direct result of the disease, 26% had made permanent redundancies whilst a further 9% had made temporary redundancies. In 85% of cases those competitors that bought and sold event horses stated their business had been negatively affected by the disease outbreak.

Poster H4.11

UK horse breeding society attitudes towards the use of *in-vitro* fertilisation

T.C. Whitaker, J. Alderman and J. Hill. Writtle College, Chelmsford, Essex CM1 3RR*

The recent successful use of *In-Vitro* Fertilisation (IVF) technologies within horse breeding has raised various ethical and procedural issues within horse breeding societies. A survey of the leading breed societies within the UK was conducted. Over 50% of societies completed the survey with a large number of the non-completers being from smaller breeding societies.

A total of 27% of societies had considered the use of IVF and already had policies in place for registration of any animals produced by this means. However, 33% would not allow IVF foals to be registered, whilst 40% of societies had not yet considered the situation. The use of IVF was seen as a positive development by 44% of societies, 28% expressed no opinion whilst a further 28% felt it might be detrimental. The largest concern over the use of IVF was the cost of the procedures involved in gaining IVF conceptions 91% of societies expressed this concern. It was felt by 66% of societies that cost might prevent IVF becoming commercially viable. Other areas where concerns were raised were over the issue of cloning where 66% of societies expressed concern. This raises issues of the perception of IVF amongst breeding societies and their understanding of what IVF exactly is. Further areas of concern reported by societies were genetic modification and reduction in gene pools 58% and sexing of foals 50%.

Poster H4.12

The effect of gender on performance of progeny of elite eventing stallions within the UK

T.C. Whitaker, S. Brook and J.Hill, Writtle College, Chelmsford, Essex CM1 3RR*

Data was collated from progeny groups of the top ten ranked stallions for eventing (by progeny winnings), for performance in the year 2000. A total of 339 horses performances were recorded. Of the progeny population 6% were stallions, 54% geldings, 40% mares. Performance was recorded via points gained in competition, these were then totalled to give a lifetime score for all horses; 1-20 novice level, 21-60 intermediate level, 61+ advanced level. A total of 31% of the population had failed to attain any winnings, 33% were competing at novice level, 17% at intermediate level and 19% at advanced level. Analysis of the level of competition in relation to gender showed, geldings to be fairly evenly distributed, with a large percentage of mares failing to win or in novice grade, stallions formed the largest group in advanced grade.
The data set was found to be abnormally distributed non-parametric statistical tests were applied. Kruskall-Wallis test showed a significant difference in median performances (mares, stallions, geldings) $K = 20.544$, $P = 0.001$. Mann Whitney U test showed a significant difference between the median performance of mares and stallions $Z = 2.1608$, $P<0.005$ and between mares and geldings $Z = -4.412$, $P<0.01$, no significant difference was found between stallions and geldings. The results from this study confirm that within the progeny group on average males perform at a superior level to females.

Poster H4.13

Investigations on standardizing evaluation of external conformation traits by cold-blooded horses in Croatia

A. Ivankovic, P. Caput, B. Mioc and M. Cacic, Department of Animal Production, Faculty of Agriculture, Svetosimunska 25, 10000 Zagreb, Croatia*

Cold-blooded horses in Croatia belong to the group of autochthonous endangered breeds whose preservation is financially supported by authorized state institutions. The cold-blooded group of horses in Croatia has been differentiated in three breeds: Croatia cold-blooded horse, Murinsulaner horse and Posavina horse. The population consolidation started fifteen years ago since breeds were badly structured and intercrossed. The aim of the research is to establish conformation features of the mentioned three cold-blooded breeds of horses in order to determine the actual condition, noticing progress in relation to previous researches, i.e. further direction of breeding. Apart from measuring 11 body measures of a horse, the method of linear evaluation of conformation features (39 features) and the evaluation of walk (at the hand) according to digital video camera, has been used. The research confirmed the significant difference in expressiveness of body measures of Posavina horse in relation to populations of the Croatian cold-blooded and Murinsulaner horse. Smaller number of linear evaluations of conformation features has been significantly different on a breed level. The significant population difference in the leg movement action was determined by movement analysis, but not also in a walk length. The established ideas will be implemented in the breeding programmes for further breed consolidation and profiling.

Poster H4.14

Involvement of homocysteine and related metabolites in horse lymphocyte proliferation

E. Chiaradia, L. Avellini, M. Silvestrelli, L. Terracina and A. Gaiti - Sport Horse Research Center, Department of Technology and Biotechnology of Animal Production, University of Perugia, Via S. Costanzo 4, 06126 Perugia, Italy.*

The pathogenesis of some diseases related to physical exercise in horses may be related to depressed immunological function. We previously reported, that: plasma levels of homocysteine (Hcy), a non-proteic sulfur-containing aminoacid, increase in horse after treadmill submaximal exercise; Hcy at concentrations similar to those measured in the plasma horse after exercise is able to inhibits mitogen activated proliferation of horse lymphocytes. In the above study, we tried to ascertain whether the involvement of homocysteine in proliferative horse lymphocyte pathways is due to an effect of either the thiol on cellular redox status or is related to the transmetylation reactions. To try to distinguish between the two above hypothesised effects, we tested the effects of homocysteine on the proliferative capacity of horse lymphocytes in the presence of different substances: buthionine sulfoximine a selective inhibitor of g-glutamyl-cysteine synthetase involved in GSH biosynthesis; N-acetylcysteine a pro-glutathione drug and exogenous thiol antioxidant, S-adenosyl-L-homocysteine a selective inhibitor of S-adenosyl-L-methionine-dependent transmetylation reactions. Lymphocytes were obtained from seven Anglo-Arab horses (3-7 years of age). Our results indicate that it may exclude the involvement of Hcy on transmetylation reactions, while it is possible to hypothesise that Hcy modulates the redox sensitive pathways involved in cell proliferation.

Poster H4.15

Development of body measurements of heavy horses in Czech republic during the 20th century

M. Hajkova, Z. Matousova -Malbohanova, J. Navrátil, Czech University of Agriculture Prague, Faculty of Agronomy, Department of Cattle Breeding and Dairying, 16 21 Prague 6, Suchdol, Czech Republic

The population of heavy horses in Bohemia and Moravia has been forming under specific climatic conditions during the last 120 years. This population has its origin in original Belgic and Noric stallions imported between 1880 - 1930, in less measure in Valon stalions imported between 1880 - 1900 and in few original Belgic mares. Today the population of heavy horses in the Czech Pepublic is devided into three breeds: Czech-Moravian Belgic, Noric and Silasian Noric. Czechmoravian Belgic and Silasian Noric are included in the genetic resource of the Czech Republic.

The development of four main body measurements (height at withers -measured with stick and tape, chest circumference, cannon circumference) of heavy stallions in the Czech Republic during the 20th century was evaluated. Also, the comparison of body measurements between Belgic and Noric stallions was done. Source data were raised from archives of the State stud farms in Pisek and Tlumacov and from the Central register for horse breeding in Slatinany.

Poster H4.16

Analysis of the Hucul Horse in the Czech Republic

Z. Matousova-Malbohanova and M.Hajkova, Czech University of Agriculture, Faculty of Agronomy, Department of Cattle Breeding and Dairying, 165 21 Prague 6, Suchdol, Czech Republic

Conservation of domestic livestock genetic resourses is a current consequential issue in the Czech Republic.
One of the breeds embraced in the genetic resource of the Czech Republic is the Hucul horse, classified as the genetic resource of the Czech Republic in 1993. This breed was also declared a FAO - protected genetic resource since 1979. On that account it is necessary to preserve this breed, to select and keep high quality studhorses, and to monitor pedigree composition of the stud. The objective of this study was to analyze population of hucul horses in the Czech Republic. Pedigree analysis, analysis of coat colours, and the study of average age of studhorses was done. The pedigree analysis comprises the level of inbreeding, proportional representation of main blood lines, and the proportional representation of blood of other breeds. For the evaluation of a level of inbreeding the Wright's inbreeding coefficient to the fifth and sixth ancestors' generation was counted.
The gained data were statistically processed for the whole population, and separatly processed for the population of horses classified as the genetic resource of the Czech Republic.

Poster H4.17

Linear assesment of conformation traits in Thoroughbred mares of Napajedla stud

I. Majzlík, V. Jakubec and M. Hájková, Department of Genetics and Animal Breeding, Faculty of Agronomy, Czech University of Agriculture, 165 21Prague, Czech republic

Linear assesment of conformation traits was used in 96 thoroughbred mares. The linear type traits were divided in 3 general traits, 6 traits describing forehand, 4 traits describing body, 3 traits describing hindquarters, 5 traits describing the formation of limbs. All traits were analysed by least squares analysis using GLM procedure with respect to age and origin of mares (CZ,US IRE, GB,FR) , correlations between traits were estimated.
Significant diferences between traits according to the age were found in „type", „back", „lenght of loins". Traits evaluated according to the origin shoved shoved significant diferences mainly in traits „lenght of whithers", „foreleg hoof", „hindleg pastern". Significant correlations were found in: type - nobility (r=0.62), type - length of neck (r=0.61), frame - length of back (r=0.62), frame - lenght of loins (r=0.65). Linear assesment of conformation traits seems to be very useful for breeding value estimation and selection in Thoroughbreds with their use in warmblood breeds.

Poster H4.18

Microbiological evaluations and morphologic features of endometrium in 15 barren mares

M. Sforna[1], F. Passamonti[1], M. Rubei[3], M. Coletti[2], L. Mechelli[1], [1]Dipartimento di Scienze Biopatologiche; [2]Dipartimento di Tecnologie e Biotecnologie delle Produzioni Animali, Facoltà di Medicina Veterinaria, Università degli Studi di Perugia, Via S. Costanzo 4, 06126 Perugia, Italy; [3]Libero Professionista.

A group of 15 mares with an anamnesis of subfertility and early foetal death were examined in order to obtain data regarding their reproductive status with particular attention on endometrial changes. The procedures used were: endometrial, cervical and clitoridal swabs for bacteriology; endometrial swab for cytology; endometrial biopsy for histology and scanning electron microscopy; serum collection for EHV1, EHV4, Equine Arteritis Virus and Taylorella *equigenitalis* tests. Citologic examination did not show any inflammatory process throught the uterus neither the presence of bacteria. Evaluation of biopsies showed a variable degree of endometrial periglandular fibrosis (EPF) and inflammation in most of the examined mares using the modified Kenney classification system. Furthermore these results were confirmed by scanning electron microscopy observations. Bacterial culture from clitoridal and/or cervical swabs were positive for *Streptococcus* spp., *Staphylococcus* spp., *Actinobacillus equuli, Pseudomonas aeruginosa, Klebsiella pneumoniae; Escherichia coli* that are usually associated with non-specific metritis of the mare ("dirty mare" syndrome). Two mares were positive for Streptococcus *equi* var. *zooepidemicus*, isolated from the endometrium. The results of the current study indicate that morphological and microbiological evaluations could be useful in pathogenesis investigations and in clinical management of barren mares.

Poster H4.19

Grow and evolution intensity of Shagya-arab foals

J. Navratil[1], M. Pobudova[2], [1]Pure Bred Shagya-arab Society International CZ, Slatinany, [2]Czech University of Agriculture in Prague, Faculty of Agronomy, Cattle and Horses Breeding Department, Kamycká 129, 165 21 Prague 6, Czech Republic

Shagya-arab represents onwards building up breeding of Arabs originated from former austrian-hungarian stud farms Bábolna and Radovec (Radautz) on the base of purebred breeding. At present the breeding is developed on the basis of 13 families in the Czech Republic, number of young and breeding mares was 216 at the end of year 2002 (worldwide number is approximately 1550). Step by step type analysis of our population is realised and we have one objective - follow up last notifications at EAAP conferences and to present farther issues.

Through the evaluation of basic body measurements regarding foal segment limited by natal day to adult age so called grow-zones of Shagya-arab mares and stallions were created as a background for future specification and amending of breeding standard.

Poster H4.20

Breeding analysis of the largest stud-farm of the Czech Warmblood in the Czech Republic

M. Pobudova, J. Navratil, Czech University of Agriculture in Prague, Faculty of Agronomy, Cattle and Horses Breeding Department, Kam_cká 129, 165 21 Prague 6, Czech Republic

Czech warmblood is the most common breed in the Czech Republic. It is based on blood of Austro-Hungarian cock-tailed breeds Furioso, Przedswit, Gidran and Nonius. Actual breeding standard determinate height at withers by staff for the mares from 161 to 167 cm, stallion's from 162 to 170 cm; mare's circumference of cannon in interval 19,5 to 22 cm and stallion's 21 to 22,5 cm.

To the prime stud-farms (and all at once the biggest) behoove „Selection horse breeding Meník Josef Kubi_ta" which produces eminent sport horses.

In 1993 - 2002 deailed analysis of breed herd was realised. Monitoring involved 27 original families, new families, number of breeding mares in each year, number of foals and stallions, their genetic lines and breed attachement. Basic body measurements (height at withers by type, by staff, circumference of cannon, thorax depth) used in Czech Republic were monitored and compared with current standard of the Czech warmblood. At present is developed monitoring also in other well-known keepings of Czech warmblood.

Poster H4.21

Effect of beta carotene integration on trotter mare in peripartum

M.F. Trombetta[1] and A. Falaschini[2], [1]DIBIAGA, Via Brecce Bianche, 60131 Ancona, Italy, [2]DIMORFIPA, Via Tolara di Sopra, 50, 40064 Ozzano Emilia, Bologna, Italy.

The resumption of the mare's breeding activity takes place in the winter, when preserved feeds are depleted of β-carotene. The influence of this provitamin on reproduction has been demonstrated in other species. We studied the effect of dietary supplementation with synthetic β-carotene in the peripartum. Subjects were 60 Italian trotter mares divided at calving into a Control and a Treatment group. Beginning on the day of parturition, the feed was supplemented with 1g/d β-carotene (ROVIMIX ® containing 10%b-carotene, supplied by Istituto delle Vitamine S.p.A., Milan, Italy) for 15 days. Blood was collected at partum and at 5, 10 and 15 days and analysed for β-carotene, Vitamins A and E, progesterone and 17-β-estradiol. Even though there were no significant effects on the resumption of the mares' reproductive activity, results evidenced interesting changes in the parameters studied that can be attributed to β-carotene supplementation.

Poster H4.22

Qualification status and EBV in french Trotters

T. Vrijenhoek[1,2] and B. Langlois[1], [1] Station de Génétique quantitative et appliquée, INRA-CRJ, 78352 Jouy-en-Josas cedex, France,[2] Animal Breeding and Genetics group, Wageningen University, The Netherlands

The objective of this study was to review the current selection model for French trotters. Data were obtained form the French central registration system for horses - and contained records of performance at the age of 2 through 6 of 183,955 trotters born between 1975 and 1994, and 46,629 of their mothers born after 1966. Genetic parameters were obtained for six traits that could be included in a revised model. Because of the absence of selection of mares in this breed maternal-offspring regression analysis was used to estimate heritabilities and genetic correlations. Parameters were estimated per age, per trait and over the whole career. Heritabilities were generally moderate except for number of starts, which were low (0.07-0.13) and earnings at the age of 6 (0.13). Regarding estimates per age, genetic correlations between binary traits and performance traits were generally high (0.52-0.99 for earnings and [-1.00]-[-0.53] for best time). Binary traits were all genetically similar in relation to performance traits. Regarding estimates per trait, genetic as well as phenotypic correlations decreased with increasing age difference. Heritabilities for career traits were generally higher than those for age traits. It was concluded that a model based on career traits could very well be used for the selection of French trotters, for both scientific and practical reasons. This model would then contain three traits: qualification status and standardized earnings as index traits and number of starts as covariable.

Poster H4.23

Lysozyme in Thoroughbreed and Haflinger mare's milk

M. Orlandi, G. Civardi, M.C. Curadi, Dept. of Animal Production, University of Pisa, Viale delle Piagge, 2 - 56123 Pisa, Italy

Mare milk protein composition could be interesting because is more similar to human than cow's, where lysozyme is present as traces; for its particular proteins characteristics mare milk could be used in pediatric dietetics in cow's milk allergic children nutrition as a substitute. Colostrum and milk samples from 5 Thoroughbreed and 5 Haflinger multiparous mares were collected from delivery until 105 days of lactation. Total nitrogen (NT), non-casein nitrogen (NCN), non-protein nitrogen (NPN) contents were determined by Kjeldhal method; protein fractions were analyzed by using CE-SDS and a Biofocus 3000 system (Bio-Rad). Lysozyme amounts were 4.20 g/L in Thoroughbreed colostrum samples and significantly decreased (1.86 g/L) at 12 days. Respectively 1.68 g/L and 1.49 g/L were founded at 30 and 60 days. In Haflinger samples lysozyme amounts significantly changed from 1.36 g/L in the first month of lactation until 1.13 g/L at 105 days. Whey-proteins/caseins ratio reached highest values in Thorougbreed colostrum samples as 5.5/1; at 30 and 60 days the same ratio in Haflinger samples were higher than in Thoroughbreed's (0.91/1 and 0.93/1 vs 0.81/1 and 0.79/1) corresponding with higher whey-proteins amounts (0.88% and 0.84% vs 0.86% and 0.75%).

Poster H4.24

Bibliometric study about equine research

F. Clément[1], M. Zitt[2], D. Lhostis[2], E. Bassecoulard-Zitt[2]. [1]Haras nationaux, F-61310 Le Pin-au-Haras. [2]INRA, BP 71627, F-44316 Nantes.

In order to map the international landscape of equine research, a bibliometric study has been performed on the relevant literature published between 1998 and 2000. Data have been extracted both from the CAB database and the ISI Current Contents. After unification of the two datasets, 6775 notices related to horses have been issued from scientific journals (64%), transfer publications (31%) or conference proceedings (6%). The topics of research interest have been identified by an automatic clustering of the key-words. Pathology, locomotion-training, reproduction, nutrition, genetics, social sciences, behaviour, feral-donkey species and doping represent 53.9%, 17.5%, 11.8%, 5.6%, 4.7%, 3.2%, 1.4%, 1.0% and 0.8 % of notices respectively. A publication has been assigned to the countries of contributing institutions. EU and USA are the main area of research with 35.9 and 31.7% of notices. The others notices are issued from Asia (8.7%), Europe outside EU (8.1%), South America (5.9%), Oceania (3.8%), Canada (2.9%), South Mediterranean countries (1.9%), Africa (1.3%). Besides USA (31.7%), the main producing countries are the United Kingdom (9.5%), Germany (7.2%), France (5.1%), Japan (4.0%), Brazil (3.9%), Canada (2.9%), Italy (2.7%), Australia (2.7%), Poland (2.6%), Netherlands (2.3%). Research profiles : pathology seems more studied in USA (58.1% of the notices inside USA) compared to in EU (50.3 %) and inside EU, in traditional "horse races" countries (United Kingdom, Ireland) (57.2%) compared to countries mainly involved in sport horses (North Europe) (47.6%).

Poster H4.25

Essai d'établissement de l'index prèsvital de la valeur de boucherie des chevaux de differents types

M. Kapron, H. Kapron, I. Janczarek, E. Czerniak, Chaire d'Elevage et d'Utilisation des Chevaux, Académie d'Agriculture, ul. Akademicka 13, 20950 Lublin, Pologne.*

On a examiné 154 cheveaux d'abattoire de differents type (demi-sang, métis et de sang froide), qui ont été soumis aux mensurations prèsvitales de: hauteur au garrot, tour de poitrine, tour du corps et des autres parties du corps qui permettaient l`estimation de degré de la musculature et de la dégénérescence graisseuse de chaque cheval (largeur aux bras, longueur de l`epaule, longueur et largeur de la croupe).

On a détérminé un niveau très varié des valeurs des coefficient des corrélations simples et multiples entre les dimentions analysées et le rendement de boucherie « chaud » et « froid » - suivant le type d'origine des chevaux - ce qui a provoqué la nécessité d'une élaboration des differents formules de «*l`index prèsvital de la valeur de boucherie des chevaux* ». Les corrélations multiples entre les dimentions analysées et le rendement de boucherie « chaud » étaient: chevaux demi-sang (0,391), métis (0,357), sang-froid (0,583), et pour le rendement de boucherie « froid » étaient: demi-sang (0,361), métis (0,300), sang-froid (0,716).

Poster H4.26

Parametrès génétiques des indicateurs d'avancement à l`entraînement des étalons demi-sang

M. Kapron, I. Janczarek, B. Kapron, E. Czerniak, Chaire d'Elevage et d'Utilisation des Chevaux, Académie d'Agriculture, ul. Akademicka 13, 20950 Lublin, Pologne.*

Les « indicateurs d'avancement à l'entraînement » des 180 étalons demi-sang (entraînnés dans « le test de 100 jours ») ont été estimés pendant les triples contrôles du rendement des allures: au pas, au trot et au galop (trois tours dans chaque allure).

On a constaté que l'héritabilité de l'indicateur « distance-pouls » au pas était 0,571, au trot 0,433 et au galop 0,515, pourtant dans le cas de l'indicateur « réaction à l`effort -1 »: au pas (0,838), au trot (0,385), au galop (0,366); pour l'indicateur « réaction à l`effort -2 » on a constaté: au pas (0,255), au trot (0,108), au galop (0,205). On a détérminé la répétabilité de l'indicateur « distance-pouls » au pas (0,662), au trot (0563), au galop (0758), et pour le cas de l'indicateur « réaction à l`effort -1 », c'étaient relativement dans les allures particulières: 0,923; 0,497; 0,412, et en ce qui concerne l'indicateur « réaction à l`effort -2 »: 0,491; 0,334 et 0,344. Les corrélations génétiques entre les traits se renfermaient dans les limites: de - 0,785 jusqu'à 0,867, quand les phénotipiques: de - 0,726 jusqu'à 0,589.

Poster H4.27

Parametrès génétiques du pouls des étalons demi-sang

M. Kapron, I. Janczarek, B. Kapron, E. Czerniak, Chaire d'Elevage et d'Utilisation des Chevaux, Académie d'Agriculture, ul. Akademicka 13, 20950 Lublin, Pologne.*

Dans les recherches on évaluait le changement du pouls des 180 étalons demi-sang pendant les triples contrôles du rendement des allures: au pas, au trot et au galop (trois tours dans chaque allure) - entraînnés dans « le test de 100 jours ». Les mensurations du pouls ont été faites en se servant d'un télémetrique appareil éléctronique « Accurex Plus ».

On a détérminé le bas niveau de l'héritabilité du pouls: au repos (h^2 = 0,131) et au pas (0,120), au trot (0,014) et au galop (0,205). On a remarqué plus haut niveau des valeurs de répétabilité: le pouls au repos (r^2 = 0,185), au pas (0,200), au trot (0,385) et au galop (0,356). Les corrélations génétiques entre les traits en question se renfermaient entre les limites (rG: de 0,092 jusqu'à 0,749), et les corrélations phénotipiques (rp: de 0,060 jusqu'à 0,533). Les paramètres génétiques du changement du pouls des étalos demi-sang démontrent également sur le fait, que les variations de l'indicateur mentionné sont surtout conditionnés par les facteurs d'environnement.

Poster H4.28

Parametres génétiques des traits biometriques des etalons demi-sang, entrainnés dans le test de 100 jours

M. Kapron, I. Janczarek, E. Czerniak, B. Kapron, Chaire d'Elevage et d'Utilisation des Chevaux, Académie d'Agriculture, ul. Akademicka 13, 20950 Lublin, Pologne.*

180 étalons demi-sang ont été soumis aux mensurations biométriques: hauteur au garrot, au dos, à la croupe et à la base de queue, tour et profondeur de poitrine, longuer et largeur de la tête, longuer: de la patte de devant, de l`épaule, du bras, de l`avant-bras, du canon de devant et de derrière, tour du canon de devant, longuer et largeur de la croupe, et aussi les distances: noeud de la hanche - jointure de la hanche, jointure de la hanche - jarret, jointure de la hanche - jointure du genou et jointure de la hanche - pointe de fesse.
Le niveau d'héritabilité de la majorité des traits biometriques (sauf la longueur de la patte de devant - l'héritabilité basse et la longueur d'épaule - l'héritabilité très haute) se façonne sur le haut niveau (hauteur de croupe, longueur et largeur de la tête, longueur et largeur de la croupe, tour du canon de devant, longueur du canon de devant et du derrière, ainsi que les distances: jointure de la hanche - jarret, jointure de la hanche - jointure du genou et jointure de la hanche - pointe de fesse) ou sur le niveau moyen: hauteur au garrot, dos, à la base de queue, longuer du bras, tour de poitrine, longueur de l`avant-bras, distance noeud de la hanche - jointure de la hanche.

Theatre HN5.1

***In vivo* methodology to measure the degradation profile and effects of processed feeds in different segments of the equine digestive tract**

J.J. Hyslop, ADAS Redesdale, Rochester, Otterburn, Newcastle upon Tyne, NE19 1SB, UK

In recent years both the *in situ* (IST) and mobile bag techniques (MBT) have been adapted for use *in vivo* in the pre-caecal, caecal and total tract of equines. Using disappearance of feed material from these porous bag techniques, degradation profiles can be fitted to MBT and IST data using existing feed degradation mathematical models. By combining the fitted model parameters with estimates of digesta passage through each digestive tract segment, the extent of feed degradation (ED) within each of these segments can be quantified and compared for a wide range of feeds or single feeds subjected to various degrees of processing. Data was combined from a series of experiments where ground samples of unmolassed sugar beet pulp (USBP), hay cubes (HC), soya hulls (SH) and a 2:1 mixture of oat hulls:naked oats (OHNO) were incubated *in vivo* using these porous bag techniques. Partitioned dry matter ED values (g/kg) for USBP, HC, SH and OHNO were 160, 312, 246 and 344 (s.e. 40.7) in the pre-caecal segment, 411, 124, 66 and 37 (s.e. 85.8) in the caecum and 90, 40, 177 and 11 (s.e. 36.4) in the colonic segments of mature ponies. Use of these techniques *in vivo* allows the quantitative partition of feed degradation amongst the major segments of the equine digestive tract.

 Theatre HN5.2

Starch digestion in horses: the impact of feed processing

V. Julliand[1], A. de Fombelle[2], M. Varloud[2]. [1]Enesad, Dijon, France, [2]Evialis, Saint-Nolff, France*

Neither the partition of digestion between the foregut and the hindgut nor the factors of variation for diverse starches of the feeds or rations are well documented in spite of their importance in term of nutrition and health for the athletic horse. At similar intake, feed processing is one of major factors, with the botanical origin, controlling the extent of prececal starch digestion.
Physical and biochemical changes occurring during the process influence both the mean retention time and the enzymatic activity in the foregut. Apparent digestibility of cereal starch varies from 20 to 90 % in the foregut depending on the process used. Physical processes have a lower effect than thermal and hydrothermal ones. Physical processes increase significantly the prececal digestibility of corn starch but have a moderate impact with other cereals. Starch digestibility is increased by thermal and hydrothermal processes whatever the botanical origin.
Feed processing was shown to affect the fermentescibility of starch in ruminant. In horses, a similar impact is expected not only in the hindgut but also in the stomach where numerous starch utilising bacteria have been observed. Further investigation is needed to identify the feed processing which allows the highest prececal digestibility and decreases the hindgut fermentescibility of starch.

Theatre HN5.3

Protein digestion and protein metabolism in the equine - selected aspects of feed source and preparation, amino acids and metabolic processes

M. Coenen, School of Veterinary Medicine Hannover, Institute of Animal Nutrition, Bischofsholer Damm 15, 30173 Hannover, Germany.

The differences in praecaecal and total tract digestibility, the impact of amino acids in energy metabolism and the endocrine system as well as the suggested link between amino acids and central fatigue indicate to have closer look in protein.
The crude protein (CP) digestibility (total intestinal tract) is a rather uniform figure for different feeds, but contain hidden differences; e.g. in roughage the highest lignin content is not related to the lowest, but the highest protein digestibility.
The limited value of total tract digestibility for protein is well documented in growing horses and confirmed by data about praecaecal amino acid and protein digestibility . Considering the effect of feed treatment on CP digestibility it seems logical to expect comparable effects (e.g. heat treatment) on CP digestion as for starch, but exact experimental data are missed.
The AA absorption in the small intestine can be of some importance for metabolic processes involving amino acid homeostasis or hormone secretion.
The described results present an impression on some details in protein digestion and metabolism in the equine, but more research is needed to improve the knowledge in amino acid absorption and metabolism as well as nitrogen trapping in the hindgut.

Theatre HN5.4

Equine feed industry in Italy

G. Predieri, ACME S.r.l., Via Portella della Ginestra 9, 42025 Cavriago, Reggio Emilia, Italy.

The manufacture of quality feeds suitable to sport horse breeding, requires deep knowledge such of nutritional profile, such of technological productive profile.

Taking into account of market consistency of industrial equine feeds, stable or breeding dimensions and correlated relationship between feed qualities and health status of sport horses, it is easy to know how the manufacture facilities must have limited sizes and technological advances to offer quality industrial feeds.

The coexistence of evolved technologies into small size equipment is seldom verifiable in the national and international industrial outline.

The above requirements make difficult or unproposable the transformation of the existing firms to manufacture horse feeds.

In particular this firms have been imagined and built to support big manufacture of feed to productive livestock.

The availability of technologies for thermo mechanical treatment of feed, the protection of gastro sensitive substances will help, in the next future, to resolve big problems concerning the critical phases of sport horses life, opening real possibility to manufacture industrial dietetic feeds which help to prevent and to manage the principal feed disorders.

Theatre HN5.5

Effects of high concentrate versus high fibre diets on equine digestive parameters in relation to performance, animal behaviour and welfare

A.D. Ellis[1] and E.K. Visser[1], [1]Research Institute for Animal Husbandry, P.O.Box 2176, 8203 Lelystad, The Netherlands

In practice working horses are often fed higher levels of processed concentrate than necessary. One of the reasons given is that excess gutfill will restrict performance in the top sport. For the horse this leads to a restricted time spent eating. Excess concentrates with low fibre intake reduce saliva production and increase acidity in the stomach. Furthermore, granulation of concentrates may change inter-compartmental retention times. An overspill of starches into the hindgut leads to an increase in lactic acid producing bacteria, creating an unhealthy, acidic environment. Recently a link has been made between stereotypic behaviour, gastric ulcers and high concentrate feeding.

The effects of type of concentrates on performance have been measured at maximum exercise levels. Little direct comparison between high and low concentrate feeding techniques at lower exercise levels has been carried out. Behavioural changes in animals on different diets have never been measured before in conjunction with increasing exercise levels, digestive parameters and health. An experiment was set up to highlight the differences in nutrient digestibility, passage rates, faecal pH and exercise performance of 36 horses at 3 exercise levels. The horses were fed iso-energetically, with one group (n=18) fed a high concentrate diet (0.70 grain-pellets) and the second group (n=18) fed a high fibre diet (0.80 haylage).

Theatre HN5.6

Feeding value of various processed oat grains

S. Sarkijarvi and M. Saastamoinen, MTT Agrifood Research Finland, Animal Production Research, Equines, FIN-32100 Ypaja, Finland*

Diets based on dried hay and variously processed oats (70:30 on dry matter basis) were fed in a digestibility trial. Processing methods were: 1) untreated oats, 2) hulled oats, 3) autoclave processed oats, 4) autoclave processed hulled oats, 5) dantoaster processed oats, 6) dantoaster processed hulled oats. Treatments were assigned in a 6 x 6 balanced Latin square design. A preliminary feeding of 23 days was followed by 5 day collection in each period. Faecal samples were taken twice a day during the collection period. Chromium was used as a marker for the estimation of apparent digestibility.

The apparent dry matter (DM) and organic matter (OM) digestibilities were significantly ($p<0.001$) better for diets containing hulled oats. The heat treatments didn't improve DM or OM digestibilities and there was no difference between the heat treatments. Hulling of oats improved significantly the digestibility of non-protein nitrogen ($p<0.001$), crude protein ($p<0.05$) and neutral detergent fibre ($p<0.05$). There was a tendency of heat treatment to improve crude fibre digestibility, but the difference was not statistically significant. Dantoaster heat treatment resulted better crude fat digestibilities compared to autoclave treatment ($p<0.05$). The feeding values were 0.96, 0.90 and 0.80 feed units in DM for hulled, hulled + heat treated and untreated or heat treated oats, respectively.

Hulling of oats seems to be the most effective way to improve the nutritive value of oats.

Theatre HN5.7

Effect of feedtechnological prosessing of grains on rate of passage in horses

I. Rosenfeld and D. Austbø, Department of Animal Science, Agricultural University of Norway, P.O.Box 5025, N-1430 Aas, Norway

Four different feedstuffs (barley, oats, maize and wheat) were each physically processed in four different ways (ground, pelleted, extruded and micronized). Four caecally cannulated geldings (Norwegian coldblooded trotters) were given daily rations of 7 kg hay and 3 kg concentrates (one of the 16 different concentrates each week). Following a 5 days adaption period, chromium mordanted hay and ytterbium labeled concentrates (ca.200 g each) were included in the morning meal (hay 2 kg, concentrates 1 kg). Fecal samples were collected 5-52 hours after feeding, dried and analyzed for chromium and ytterbium for modeling of digesta transit in the horse. The experiment was repeated for all diets, so that each horse was fed each of the 16 concentrates in a random matter. As the experiment is still running, results will be presented at the EAAP-meeting.

Theatre HN5.8

Effect of caecal cannulation on passage parameters in horses

D. Austbø and H. Volden, Department of Animal Science, Agricultural University of Norway, P.O.Box 5025, N-1432 Aas, Norway*

The effects of caecal cannulation on passage parameters were investigated using 4 geldings of Norwegian Coldblooded Trotter, body weight 460-530 kg. Horses were exercised 45 minutes daily (2-3 hours after the morning feed) in walk and trot in a rotary exerciser. The daily ration consisted of 7 kg grass hay and 3 kg pelleted concentrates offered in three meals per day (07.00, 14.00, 19.00h). The morning meal consisted of 1 kg of concentrates and 2 kg hay. After minimum 5 days of adaptation, the horses were fed ca 200 g of chromium mordanted hay and 200 g of ytterbium labelled concentrates immediately prior to the morning meal. Faeces were collected by rectal sampling from 4 hours until ca 50 hours after feeding the markers. The other meals were fed as normal. The experiment was conducted before the cannulation surgery, 3 and 6 months post surgery. The cannulas had a diameter of 40 mm and were made from silicone.
The results show no effect of cannulation on passage parameters. The mean total retention time was 27.1, 27,5 and 25,2 hours for pre-surgery, 3 and 6 months post surgery, respectively (NS). No differences in passage parameters between concentrates and hay could be detected. However, a significant difference due to date of experiment was found and could be explained by the change of hay quality.

Poster HN5.9

Effect of a new concentrate, rich in fibre, on horse rations digestibility

N. Miraglia[1], D. Bergero[2], M. Polidori[1], P.G. Peiretti[3] and G. Ladetto[2]. [1]Università del Molise,SAVA Department, Via De Sanctis, 86100 Campobasso, Italy, [2]Università di Torino,DIPAEE Department, Via L. Da Vinci 44, 10095 Grugliasco (TO), Italy, [3]ISPA-CNR, Via L. Da Vinci 44, 10095 Grugliasco (TO), Italy.*

Commercial mixed feeds for light horse feeding are more and more used and, in recent times, a particular role is played by mixed feeds characterized by high fibre percentages together with probiotic supplements. Consequently, more data about these new feeds are required. The apparent digestibility of a commercial mixed feed containing 18.3% of crude fibre (CF) as fed and lactulose 1% was determined by means of 3 in vivo digestibility trials each performed on 4 saddle horses weighting about 560 kg over a 6 days period with a previous 14 days adaptation period. The diets were based on a first cut meadow hay - whose digestibility was estimated in the first trial - and the mixed feed at a feeding level close to maintenance. The forage:concentrate ratio(FCR) was 100:0, 75:25 and 50:50. Digestibility of dry matter, organic matter, gross energy, crude protein, NDF, ADF and CF were measured by ingesta/excreta procedure. Data was processed by ANOVA; significant differences were found between the digestibility of the 100:0 and the 50:50 FCR ration for dry matter, organic matter, gross energy and crude protein. The gross energy digestibility was found different also between the 100:0 and the 75:25 FCR rations.

Poster HN5.10

Effect of physical treatments on the resistant starch content and in vitro organic matter digestibility of different cereals in horses

L. Bailoni, R. Mantovani and G. Pagnin, Department of Animal Science, AGRIPOLIS, Viale dell'Università, 16, 35020 Legnaro (PD), Italy*

Samples of corn, barley, and oat, whole (W) or subjected to flaking (F), rolling (R) or extrusion (E), wheat bran and cereal mix were collected from different feed companies. Feed samples were analysed for their proximate composition and fibrous fractions by Van Soest procedure. The total starch content was determined directly by liquid chromatography and as sum of resistant starch and non resistant (solubilised) starch by enzymatic procedure. In vitro organic matter digestibility (OMD) by pepsin-cellulase technique was also estimated. The mean value of resistant starch was about 2.1% of the total starch. The relationship between chromatographic and enzymatic methods for total starch determination was investigated. The OMD values ranged from 64.2 (black oat) to 98.7% (flaked barley). The effects of the physical treatments on the OMD was variable among the different cereals, i.e. the R treatment gave the highest OMD increase in oat (+ 8.9% between R and W) while the E treatment improved the OMD in barley samples (+8.8% between E and W). Only small differences in OMD were detected for corn when subjected to F and E treatments. Using the step-wise multiple regression method for all the chemical parameters, OMD of the cereals could be predicted by ADF and CP contents (R^2=0.988; r.s.d.=± 1.2%).

Poster HN5.11

New INRA-AFZ tables for predicting nutritive value of concentrates in equine

W. Martin-Rosset, INRA, Department of Animal Husbandry and Nutrition, Center for research of Clermont/Theix 63122 Saint Genes Champanelle ,France.

These tables (N=81 feeds) are an evolution of the previous tables (N=33 feeds) published by INRA in 1984 then revised in 1990.They are using the same nutritionnal concepts :UFC for energy and MADC for protein.

In a first step UFC values of 59 raw materials of these tables , where OMD were stated from in vivo measurements drawn from the litterature, were calculated according to the reference method (e.g.analytical method)designed by INRA. In a second step the UFC valus of these 59 feeds were predicted from their chemical composition and OMD or ED content using a set of INRA equations. Comparing the UFC values calculated with both methods, it arised that the discrespancies were very low and non linked to chemical composition . As a result UFC values of 81 feeds were calculated using this set of equations .

The MADC values of these 81 feeds , where Digestible Crude Protein were stated from in vivo measurements drawn from the literature,or/and predicted from CP content using INRA equations, were calculated using the reference method designed by INRA.

. The chemical composition of the feeds was mainly drawn from routine analysis conducted in laboratories specialised in animal nutrition. These analytical data were scrutinised by AFZ to check and improve their consistency.

Poster HN5.12

Feed intake in young riding horses fed a Total Mixed Ration

E. Søndergaard, Danish Institute of Agricultural Sciences, P.O.Box 50, 8830 Tjele, Denmark

Dry matter intake vary according to animal and feed factors and is for horses estimated to be within the range of 1.0 and up till 3.5% of body weight. For young riding horses a dry matter intake of 1.8% to 2.2% is expected at the age of 7 to 12 months, decreasing to a level of 1.6 to 1.8 at the age of 13 to 24 months (Meyer, H. 1996. Pferdefütterung. Blackwell.).
In this experiment 2x20 horses housed either singly (n=2x8) or in groups of three (n=2x12) were fed a Total Mixed Ration from weaning at 4.7 months until 24.5 months of age except for a 4 months pasture period. The Total Mixed Ration consisted of chopped grass silage, hay and barley straw mixed with a concentrate feed and molasses. Feed intake was recorded on a daily basis for each pen. Every 4 weeks the horses were weighed and measured. Feed intake was calculated for six periods throughout the experiment: I:4.7 to 6 months, II:6 to 9 months, III:9 to 12.5 months, IV:16.5 to 18 months, V:18 to 21 months, VI:21 to 24.5 months of age. Total feed intake in kg/day was estimated at 6.5, 7.4, 8.9, 13.2, 13.8 and 16.1 for the six periods. Dry matter intake in relation to body weight will be calculated for each period and related to the housing of the horses.

Theatre H6.1

Genetic evaluation for racing speed in Italian trotters

C. Pieramati[1], M. Silvestrelli[1], L. Buttazzoni[2], A. Verini Supplizi[1], [1]Sport Horse Research Center, University of Perugia, Via San Costanzo 4, 06126 Perugia, Italy, [2]Associazione Nazionale Allevatori Suini, via Lazzaro Spallanzani,4/6, 00161 Roma, Italy.*

Italian data on harness racing, spanning from 1992 to 2002, were analyzed; 1,316,316 starters in 133,358 races were included in the data set; 283,721 racing times of 23,219 horses 2- to 5- year-old ranked in the first three places of each race were used for genetic evaluations according to a repeated record BLUP Animal Model together with 122,069 horses included in the pedigree file. Fixed effects included in the model were sex (male, female, and gelding), age, race length (1,600-1,725 m and 2,000-2,200 m), starting type (auto or tapes), driver (2,011 levels), and fixture (15,655 levels). Racing times higher than 90s/Km, drivers with less than three observations with two different horses, and fixtures with less than 5 racing times were excluded from the analysis.
Males resulted to be 0.33 s/Km faster than females; 5-year old resulted 2.67s/Km faster than 2-year-old; 2,000-2,200 m races were 1.08 s/Km slower than 1,600-1,725 m races, and auto-start was faster than tapes by 0.70 s/Km. Differences between drivers accounted for a maximum of 6.37s/Km, whilst those between fixtures for 10.79 s/Km.
Heritability and repeatability estimates from the entire data set were .18 and .45 respectively, but they were .24 and .47 when a subset with only racing data since 1999 was used.

Theatre H6.2

A Presentation of the Italian Warmblood Stud Books: the Italian Saddle Horse ("Sella Italiano") and the Maremmano Horse

M. Silvestrelli[1], C. Pieramati[1], L. Buttazzoni[2], M. Reitano[3], [1]Sport Horse Research Center, University of Perugia, Via San Costanzo 4, 06126 Perugia, Italy, [2]Associazione Nazionale Allevatori Suini, via Lazzaro Spallanzani,4/6, 00161 Roma, Italy, [3]Italian Equestrian Military Center, via Montelibrettese, 00010 Montelibretti, Roma, Italy.*

Breeding goal of Italian Saddle Horse is to produce high quality sport horse particularly suitable for jumping: to this goal also immigration from foreign populations and indigenous stock (Maremmano) is used.
Warmblood foals are described and checked by an authorized veterinarian within 90 days from birth in order to discover congenital defects. Stallions selection is performed in three steps: 2 year old males are evaluated for gaits by measuring length and speed of their free trot and 3 year old males are evaluated for free jumping: these two steps are carried out in a unique location nationwide, but separately for Italian Saddle Horse and Maremmano Horse. The third step is a 100-day station test, where the best 30 Italian Saddle Horse and the best 12 Maremmano males, according to results from steps 1 and 2, are evaluated together for character, power and jumping. No more than 15 stallions in total for the two breeds can be approved each year, according to their performance test index and health (horses suffering from osteochondrosis dissecans or roaring are rejected). The Maremmano breed completes its selection program with a 30 day station test to choose the elite brood mares and it uses MT-BLUP indexes for morphological traits.

Theatre H6.3

The genetic selection of the Italian Haflinger Horse

A.B. Samorè, Associazione Nazionale Allevatori Cavallo di Razza Haflinger (ANACRHA), Via Lavagnini 4, 50129 Firenze, Italy.*

In 1990, the Italian Breeders Association of the Haflinger Horse revised its technical norms, reorganized its methods of type classification and specified selection criteria. Selection aimed for a taller, more distinct and better saddle horse. Breeding value estimations for height at withers have been estimated every year since 1990 and a selection program was adopted at the same time. A new type classification, based on linear scale, was also introduced. In 1996 a total merit index was defined. This index included height at withers, breed type, general harmony and gait. The total merit index was estimated and published every year and it was used to rank stallions and mares for the national selection scheme. Selection for height at withers was so successful that, in 2002, it was decided to re-define the selection index excluding height at withers from selection criteria and increasing the relative emphasis assigned to gait. Genetic and environmental covariances were re-estimated: general harmony resulted to have the highest heritability (0.35), followed by breed type (0.27) and gait (0.26). The new index will be officially introduced with the breeding value estimation of October 2003.

Theatre H6.4

A genetic global index for Bardigiano Horse selection

M. Fioretti[1], A.L. Catalano[2], A. Rosati[3], F. Martuzzi[2], [1]Associazione Italiana Allevatori, Via Nomentana 134, 00162 Roma, Italy, [2]Dip. Produzioni Animali, Università degli Studi, via del Taglio 8, 43100 Parma, Italy, [3]EAAP, Via Nomentana 134, 00162 Roma, Italy.*

The present selection goal of the Bardigiano Horse, an ancient horse breed used for draft in the mountain areas in Parma and Piacenza Provinces (Northern Italy), is producing horses for saddle service. A genetic index for "height at withers" is used to obtain taller horses; a global genetic index (IGG) has been created to consider more traits, each of them important for the Bardigiano horse typicalness, using data from the linear morphological evaluation form. To obtain IGG, 18 different traits were genetically evaluated by BLUP -AM. The following effects were included in the model: additive genetic, evaluation herd group by evaluation year, month of birth, age at evaluation, in months, and sex of the animal. Heritability, genetic and environmental correlation for the morphological linear evaluation form traits and withers height were estimated. To consider the different variability of analysed traits, the genetic index of each trait was standardized. Finally, each standardized index was corrected for a given weight in IGG composition and the corrected indexes were added to obtain IGG. Genetic trend, calculated from year 1985 to year 2000 for males and females, was positive.

Theatre H6.5

The Italian heavy draft horse breed

R. Mantovani[1] and G. Pigozzi[2], [1]Dept. of Animal Science, Agripolis, 35020 Legnaro (PD), Italy, [2]Italian Heavy Draft Horse Breeders Association, Via Belgio, 10, 37135 Verona, Italy*

The origin of the Italian Heavy Draft Horse (IHDH) is related to the need of developing a strain of heavy horse in Italy to use in rapid draft for both military and agricultural purposes. This idea was first supported by military programs based on crosses that used mainly Norfolk-Breton stallions on local heavy mares widespread in the north-east of Italy. In 1927 started an official mating registration program, but only in 1960 the herd book was established. During the 70s', the IHDH population was subjected to a quick decline in numbers due to the mechanization of agriculture, but the conversion into the meat production attitude has contributed to the recent increase in the population size. At present, the actual no. of registered animals is about 6400 (3100 mares and 400 stallions) in 950 registered herds widespread in almost all the country. Selection is for dual purpose, i.e. meat and rapid draft, using a linear type trait evaluation (14 traits) on newborn foals (about 6 month of age), and genetic indexes are calculated using an animal model. During the last decade of selection the genetic trend for main selected traits, i.e. muscularity and blood, has increased rapidly (+2.6% and +1.4% of phenotypic mean/year, respectively) and, despite the reduced population size, the annual increase in inbreeding coefficient was low (+0.03%/year).

Theatre H6.6

The Italian Lipizzan State Stud

A. Carretta[1] and L. Buttazzoni [2], [1]Istituto Sperimentale per la Zootecnia (ISZ), Via Salaria 31, 00016 Monterotondo, Roma, Italy, [2]Associazione Nazionale Allevatori Suini (ANAS), Via L.Spallanzani 4, 00161 Roma, Italy.*

At the end of WWI, Italy received from Austria 109 lipizzan horses and one of the two original record books from the Imperial Stud of Lipizza. Since then, Italy has maintained the herd and in recent years an extensive check on pedigrees was carried out. As a result, the Italian Lipizzan State Stud, named ASCAL, is currently made up by 38 mares tracing back, as mother line, to 10 out of the 15 recognized founder females and by 12 stallions tracing back, as sire line, to the 6 recognized founder sires. Pedigrees can be traced back up to 23 generations, and pedigrees of all horses in the stud are fully known back to the original imperial stud of Lipizza before WWI. The oldest recorded female is Golomba, born in 1738, while the most recent is Katl, a mare born in 1900. The current Italian Lipizzan State Stud is the result of nucleus mating, completely closed for 103 years. Inbreeding coefficient of horses currently bred ranges from 0,09 to 0,266. Females have been exchanged after WWII with the Austrian State Stud only if their pedigree fully traced back to Lipizza Imperial Stud. All nucleus horses recorded in the last century turned grey at an age ranging from 3 to 6 years. Currently, horses are kept on range conditions, natural mating is used, and they are mainly trained and used for sport driving.

Poster H6.7

The genetic structure of Murgese horse

[1]Dept. PROGESA, Via Amendola 165/A, 70100 Bari, Italy, [2] Dept. SBA, Strada Prov. per Casamassima km 3, 70010 Valenzano, Bari, Italy, [3] LGS, Via Bergamo 292, 26100 Cremona, Italy, [4]IRIP, Via Caggese 1, 71100 Foggia, Italy.

The Murgese horse has a rustic nature, necessary for survival in the arid and rocky hills of Apulia from which it takes its name: Le Murge, where the climate is cold in the winter and dry in the summer. One of the outstanding features of Murgese, as well as of all Apulian native livestock breeds, is the evolution of tolerance to endemic tick borne diseases (TBD). The first herdbook was produced in 1926 with only 47 founder mares and all the existing Murgese horses can be traced back to this date. Lately, in 1957, they numbered 265 and presently there are about 1200 registered brood-mares and 400 colts per year on the average. This work aims to monitor the genetic structure of the present-day population. The herd book genealogic data were analyzed. Coancestry and inbreeding coefficients were estimated. The inbreeding coefficient trend was evaluated and compared with the genetic information (FIS coefficient) from a data-set containing 563 typing records of 12 microsatellites. The overall FIS coefficient estimation was 0.025, in agreement with the inbreeding mean value related to the typing period. The obtained information was used to discuss future strategies of breed management.

ANIMAL NUTRITION [N] Poster N4.60

Plant enzyme mediated lipolysis of *Lolium perenne* and *Trifolium pratense* in an *in vitro* simulated rumen environment

M.R.F. Lee, E.M. Martinez, N.D. Scollan and M.K.Theodorou, Institute of Grassland and Environmental Research, Aberystwyth, U.K.*

We have questioned the assertion that in ruminants grazing fresh pastures, the first stages of lipolysis are mediated by plant lipases. Additionally, we have evaluated differences in lipolytic activity between *Lolium perenne* and *Trifolium pratense*, as the latter has been shown to reduce biohydrogenation in the rumen. *Lolium perenne* (cv. AberElan) and *Trifolium pratense* (cv. Milvus) from experimental plots, were harvested (3cm above ground level), bruised by minimal crushing, cut into 5mm segments and incubated in 25ml antibiotic-containing (5.0mg chloramphenicol/ml in 50% v/v ethanol) anaerobic buffer at 39°C for up to 24 h. At different times (0, 1, 2, 3, 4, 5, 6 and 24 h) the incubation bottles were destructively harvested, the lipid extracted and fractionated by thin layer chromatography. Lipolysis was calculated by expressing the percentage decrease in fatty acid content of membrane lipid. The data showed a curvilinear response for both *Lolium perenne* and *Trifolium pratense* suggesting a declining rate of lipolysis with time. Additionally, at 30%, *Trifolium pratense* had a significantly lower ($P<0.05$) overall lipolytic activity, in comparison to *Lolium perenne* at 25%. Increases in the amount of triacylglycerol, diglycerides and free fatty acids were observed with decreasing membrane lipid over time. These results support the view that plant lipases may play a role in lipolysis in the early stages of digestion of forages in the rumen.

ANIMAL MANAGEMENT & HEALTH [M] Poster M1.44

Biological and economic assessment of fattening Egyptian native bullocks

S.M. AlSheikh, A.A. Younis and M.M. Mokhtar, Desert Research Center, Mataria, Cairo 11753, Egypt

Data of 53 bullocks in summer and 201 bullocks in winter were collected from a commercial feedlot farm located in a newly reclaimed area, some 86 km from Cairo on the Cairo-Alexandria desert road during the agricultural year 1997-1998. The goal of the study was to evaluate the biological and economic performance of fattening enterprises of Egyptian native cattle in both winter and summer seasons. The average daily gain was 1.17 kg and 1.11 kg in summer and winter, respectively. The corresponding values of feed conversion (kg dry matter intake per kg body weight) were 9 kg and 10 kg. The values of return per animal were LE 392 and LE 316 in summer and winter seasons, respectively (1 US dollar = 5.50 LE). Feeding cost accounted for 86 % and 87% of total variable cost in summer and winter seasons, respectively. The return per LE per year value was 12%. It could be concluded that, the standard management practiced to obtain the high biological performance is not enough to improve the value of return per LE per year. Other criteria could be taken into consideration such as purchasing animal at the low price season and reducing the cost of feeding throughout using local feed ingredients.

Theatre PhG4.11

Combining genomics and biochemistry of muscle to predict beef quality

J.F. Hocquette, I. Cassar-Malek, A. Listrat, B. Picard, INRA, Herbivore Research Unit, Theix, 63122 Saint-Genès Champanelle, France

Genetic and environmental factors profoundly alter muscle characteristics, and hence beef quality. The advent of high-throughput sequence analysis, DNA chip technology and protein analysis has revolutionized our approach of muscle physiology. For instance, a global gene expression profiling at mRNA or protein level will provide a better understanding of the gene regulation that underlies myogenesis and its control by nutrition. The most powerful scientific strategies are certainly based on the combination of genomics with classical biochemical and physiological studies by using bioinformatic tools to understand the control of a wide variety of phenotypes of genetic, environmental or nutritional origin. One of the main challenges will be to solve the problems posed by the analysis and interpretation to large amount of data that will become available from structural (QTL, SNP) and functional (mRNA or protein levels) genomics. Major applications could be (i) the identification of new predictors of beef quality traits (for instance, tenderness and flavour), (ii) the monitoring of beef quality through the production systems (nutrition level, growth path, grass-feeding), and (iii) the improvement of animal selection (markers and gene assisted selection) by including quality traits.

Theatre PhG4.12

Identification of a quantitative trait nucleotide affecting body composition in the pig

M. Braunschweig, Department of Animal Breeding and Genetics, Swedish University of Agricultural Sciences, Box 597, BMC, S-751 24 Uppsala, Sweden

A paternally expressed quantitative trait locus (QTL) for muscle mass, fat deposition, and the size of the heart was mapped to the insulin-like growth factor II (*IGF2*) locus at the distal end of pig chromosome 2p in intercrosses between the European Wild Boar and Large White domestic pigs and between Piétrain and Large White pigs (Jeon et al., 1999; Nezer et al., 1999). The identification of causative mutations for QTLs is a challenge because of the task to achieve sufficient high resolution to positional clone the underlying genes. Here we show that this QTL is caused by a single nucleotide substitution in intron 3 of the *IGF2* gene. The mutation occurs in an evolutionary conserved CpG island that is hypomethylated in skeletal muscle. The mutation abrogates *in vitro* interaction with a nuclear factor, most likely a repressor. Pigs carrying the mutation have a three-fold increase in *IGF2* mRNA expression in postnatal muscle. The study provides the first example where the causal relationship between a single base pair substitution in a non-coding region and a QTL effect has been established. It provides a proof-of-concept for the importance of regulatory mutations for phenotypic diversity.

Theatre PhG4.13

Gene expression analysis as a tool for the investigation of the physiological and genetic background of metabolic and growth traits in cattle

Ch. Kühn[1], T. Goldammer[1], R. Brunner[1], U. Dorroch[1], J. Wegner[2] and M. Schwerin[1], [1]Res. Unit Molecular Biology, Research Institute for the Biology of Farm Animals, Wilhelm-Stahl-Allee 2, 18196 Dummerstorf, Germany; [2]Res. Unit Muscle Biology and Growth, Research Institute for the Biology of Farm Animals, Wilhelm-Stahl-Allee 2, D-18196 Dummerstorf, Germany*

Gene expression analysis can provide information on the genetic determination of metabolic and growth traits and also on the regulation of physiological pathways underlying these traits. In our study a comprehensive gene expression profiling was performed by mRNA differential display in twelve tissues of individuals from the Charolais and the German Holstein breed. The breeds representing divergent metabolic types of cattle differed substantially regarding tissue development and nutrient partitioning and served as founder breeds for an F_2-resource population. The mRNA differential display analysis revealed differentially expressed genes/ESTs and enabled, supported by results of Real-time-PCR, identification of physiological pathways putatively involved in trait differentiation. About 30% of the identified ESTs did not show significant matches to any entry in public genome databases, which might suggest a speciesspecific gene equipment. Physical mapping and mutation analysis enabled assessment of the differentially expressed genes/ESTs regarding positional and functional candidate gene character for metabolic and growth traits. Furthermore, these genes/ESTs identified by a comprehensive approach are also included into parallel expression studies of targeted genes of known functional relevance to complement physiological studies of tissue development and nutrient partitioning.

Theatre PhG4.14

Functiona genomics of mammary gland growth and development

T.S. Sonstegard[1], E.E. Connor[1], and A.V. Capuco[1], [1]USDA, ARS Bovine Functional Genomics Laboratory, BARC-East, Beltsville, MD, U.S.A.*

A series of complex physiological processes underlie bovine mammary gland development from embryogenesis through puberty, pregnancy, lactation, and involution. The involvement of hormones such as estrogen and progesterone in these processes has been demonstrated. However, the mechanisms that ultimately modulate gene expression patterns for mammary cell proliferation, differentiation or secretory activity are not well understood. For example, it was demonstrated that estrogen and progesterone receptor transcript expression is significantly down regulated during mid-gestation in pregnant heifers but not pregnant lactating cows. To better understand effects of hormone response on downstream regulation of gene expression, studies were initiated to survey the mammary gland transcriptome. First, over 25,000 expressed sequence tags were characterized from a normalized cDNA library encompassing all the major physiological processes of the mammary gland. These sequence data and corresponding cDNA clones have been made freely available for all researchers. After testing several different platforms for transcript profiling, a nylon-based microarray containing reporters corresponding to more than 5,000 transcripts expressed in the mammary gland was developed. This resource is being used to evaluate effects on the mammary transcriptome of treatments that influence mammary development and lactation persistency. Significant differences in expression are being validated by quantitative real-time RT-PCR and immunohistochemistry or *in situ* hybridization.

Theatre Ph6.10

Development of muscle fibers and collagen in non-ruminant mammals

F. Gondret[1], L. Lefaucheur[1], S. Combes[2] and B. Lebret[1], [1]INRA, UMR Veau et Porc, 35590 Saint-Gilles, [2]INRA Station de Recherches Cunicoles, 31326 Castanet Tolosan cedex, France*

Muscle characteristics may be an important source of variation in eating quality and overall acceptability of the meat. Especially, constituent muscle fibers and their interaction with connective tissue may influence meat tenderness, juiciness and flavour. This review will focus on the age-related development of muscle fibers and intra-muscular collagen content in non-ruminant mammals, such as pigs and rabbits. New insigths into muscle fiber-type classification, including type IIX fibers, will be presented. Total fiber number is fixed before birth in pigs and during the first postnatal month in rabbits. Postnatal period is characterized by the hypertrophy of muscle fibers, and changes in the relative proportions of fiber types, collagen content, and collagen heat solubility, both in a muscle-specific manner. Biochemical composition of fibers is also influenced by age, especially myocellular lipid content. Both pre- and post-natal events are able modify total fiber number, cross-sectional size and myofiber types. Because of the increasing use of alternative breeding systems (such as large scale pens versus confined pen), the influence of spontaneous physical activity on muscle fibers and intra-muscular collagen will be discussed in both species.

Theatre Ph6.11

Molecular genetic background of variation in muscle development: Candidate gene approach and microarraying

Marinus F.W. te Pas, Wageningen UR, ID Lelystad, P.O. Box 65, 1200 AB Lelystad, The Netherlands

Mammalian myogenesis (muscle fibre development) is an exclusively prenatal process. Postnatal muscle development only encompass length and thickness growth of pre-existing muscle fibres. Mammalian myogenesis is a genetically regulated pathway controlled by many genes. Multi-gene regulated processes can be studied using genome scanning techniques and or candidate gene techniques. Candidate genes can be determined using available physiological information of the genes (experiments of the past), or by new functional genomics techniques (experiments of the future). This presentation will present 3 types of experiments: (1) Candidate genes using available physiologic information about the MRF gene family - a gene family of 4 structurally related transcription factors known to directly regulate proliferation of myoblasts (muscle cell progenitors) and differentiation of myoblasts to multi-nucleated muscle fibres, (2) Chromatin immunoprecipitation (ChIP) experiments aiming to find the target genes differentially activated by the MRF genes, and (3) Microarraying to search for the genes that differentially regulate the MRF genes. Experiments in (1) can be characterised as "experiments of the past" while (2) and (3) describe more "experiments of the future". In (1) we will show that genetic variation in gene loci of the MRF gene myogenin is associated with meat mass traits. In (2) we describe how this method enriches genomic DNA fragments for MRF recognisable promoter sites. In (3) we show how microarray data can be used to recognise genes differentially regulated associated with meat quality traits.

Significance of muscle fibre characterisitics in the relation of birth weight with carcass quality in pigs

C. Rehfeldt, G. Kuhn, I. Fiedler and K. Ender, Research Institute for the Biology of Farm Animals, Wilhelm-Stahl-Allee 2, D-18196 Dummerstorf, Germany*

We investigated relationships between birth weight, carcass quality and skeletal muscle fibre. At birth, three piglets (lighest; middle-weight; heaviest) were selected from 16 litters. The lightest exhibited the smallest percentages of meat, total protein, total fat, the lowest *Semitendinosus* muscle (ST) weight and total fibre number, whereas percentages of internal organs, skin, bone, and total water were highest. The remaining piglets grown at *ad libitum* feeding exhibited differences in daily gains that paralleled those in birth weights. At day 182 of age 58 pigs were randomly selected for slaughter assigned to birth weight classes (25% low; 50% middle; 25% heavy). Low had lower live weights ($P<0.05$), smaller meat percentages ($P=0.09$) and loin areas ($P=0.08$), whereas percentage of internal adipose tissue tended to be higher ($P=0.11$). Low exhibited lower relative heart weights ($P=0.02$) and a higher drip loss ($P=0.08$) in *Longissimus* muscle (LD). They exhibited the lowest muscle fibre numbers, the largest fibre size, the highest myonuclear number per fibre, and the highest percentages of abnormal giant fibres in ST and LD muscles ($P<0.05$). The deficiency in muscle fibres in low birth weight piglets cannot be equalized by accelerated fibre hypertrophy. In these pigs, extremely large fibres may be one of the reasons for poor carcass quality at slaughter.

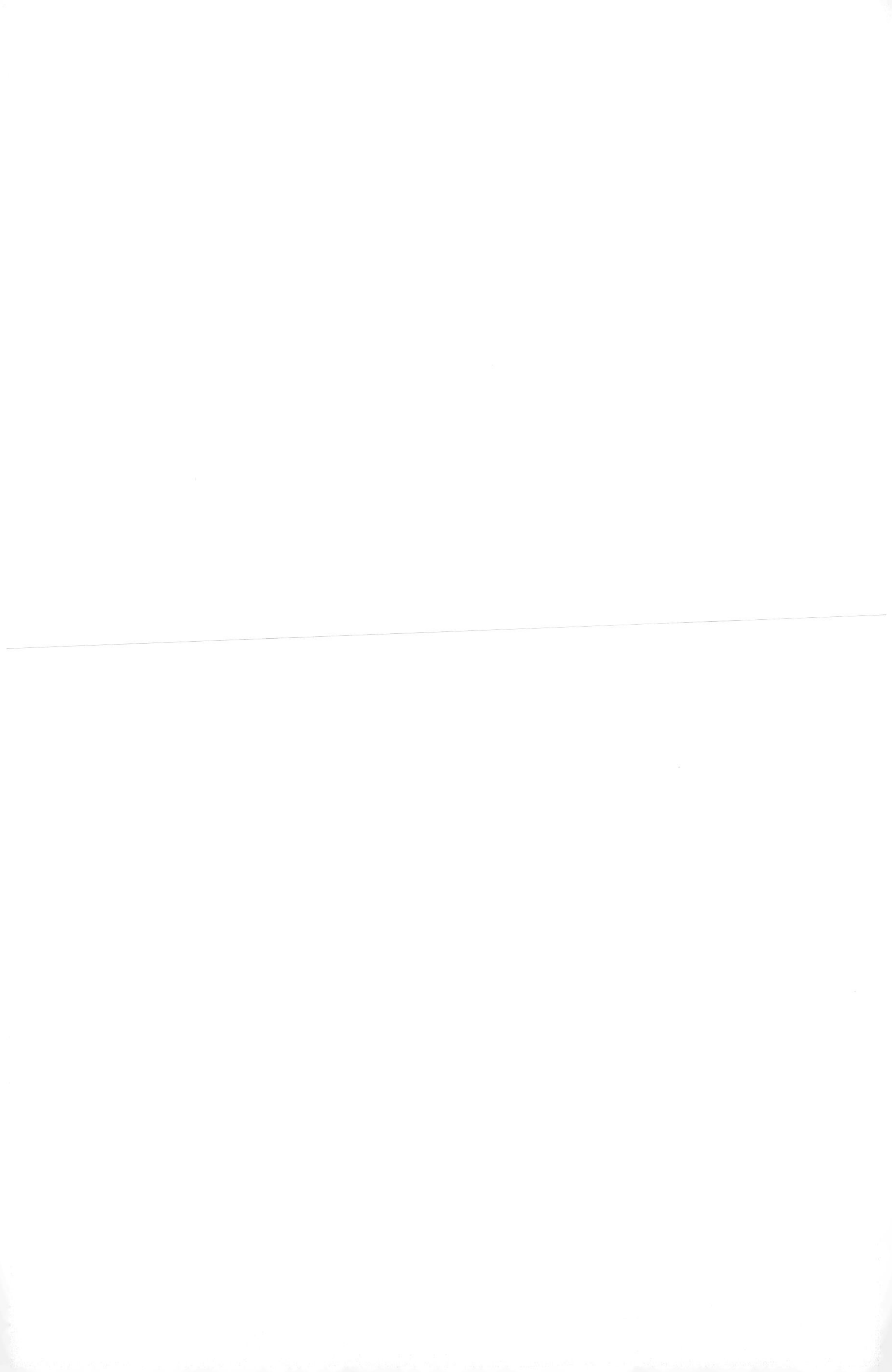

AUTHORS INDEX

F

I

J

	Page

L

S